MERRILL'S ATLAS OF

RADIOGRAPHIC POSITIONS and RADIOLOGIC PROCEDURES

Lumbar

accessory process	
inferior articular process	inferior apophyseal process
mammillary process	
superior articular process	superior apophyseal process

Sacrum and Coccyx

base	body
coccygeal horn	coccygeal cornu
lumbosacral junction	sacrovertebral junction
median sacral crest	medial sacral crest
pelvic sacral foramina	anterior sacral foramina
sacral horn	sacral cornu
superior articular process	articular process
vertebral canal	spinal canal

Chapter 9 Bony Thorax

body of sternum	gladiolus
jugular notch	manubrial notch
xiphoid process	ensiform cartilage

Chapter 10 Thoracic Viscera

cardiac impression	cardiac fossa
costodiaphragmatic recess	costophrenic, or phrenicostal sinus
hilum	hilus
impression	fossa
inferior lobe	lower lobe
jugular notch	manubrial notch
main bronchus	primary bronchus
pulmonary pleura	visceral
superior lobe	upper lobe
superior thoracic aperture	thoracic inlet

Chapter 11 Long Bone Measurement

limb	extremity

Chapter 12 Contrast Arthrography

limb	extremity

Chapter 13 Foreign Body Localization and Trauma Radiography Guidelines

limb	extremity

Chapter 14 Mouth and Salivary Glands

Mouth

frenulum of tongue	frenulum linguae
soft palate	velum
sublingual fold	plica sublingualis

Salivary Glands

parotid duct	Stensen's duct
sublingual caruncle	
sublingual ducts	ducts of Rivinus, or Bartholin's duct
submandibular duct	submaxillary, or Wharton's duct
submandibular gland	submaxillary gland

Chapter 15 Anterior Part of Neck

auditory tubes	eustachian tubes
choanae	
cricothyroid ligament	cricothyroid interval
inferior constrictor muscle	cricopharyngeus muscle
laryngeal inlet	laryngeal orifice
laryngeal pharynx	hypopharynx
lymphoid	lymphadenoid
piriformis recess	piriformis sinus
rima vestibuli	vestibular slit
valleculae epiglottica	epiglottic valleculae
vestibula folds	false vocal cords

Chapter 16 Digestive System
Abdomen, Liver, Spleen, Biliary Tract

Liver

hilum	hilus
porta	porta hepatis
visceral surface of liver	posterior surface of liver

Pancreas and Spleen

accessory pancreatic duct	duct of Santorini
pancreatic duct	duct of Wirsung
pancreatic islets	islets of Langerhans

Biliary Tract

gall bladder	gallbladder
hepatopancreatic ampulla	ampulla of Vater
sphincter of the hepatopancreatic ampulla	sphincter of Oddi

Chapter 17 Digestive System
Alimentary Tract

Stomach

angular notch	incisura angularis
cardia	
cardiac notch	cardiac incisura
esophagogastric junction	esophageal orifice
gastric folds	rugae
pyloric antrum	pyloric vestibule
pyloric canal	
pyloric orifice	

Small Intestine

first portion	superior portion
second portion	descending portion
third portion	horizontal portion
fourth portion	ascending portion
common hepatic duct	hepatic duct
duodenojejunal flexure	angle of Treitz

Large Intestine

left colic flexure	splenic flexure
right colic flexure	hepatic flexure

Chapter 18 Urinary System

glomerular capsule	capsule of Bowman
hilum	hilus
major calyces	infundibula
renal papilla	apex
spongy portion [of male urethra]	cavernous portion
straight tubule	descending and ascending limbs of the loop of Henle
suprarenal glands	adrenal glands
uriniferous tubules	

Chapter 19 Reproductive System

Male Reproductive System

ductus deferens	vas deferens
spongy portion [of male urethra]	cavernous portion

Female Reproductive System

cervix	neck
intestinal surface	posterior surface [of uterus]
isthmus	superior cervix, internal os
lateral angles	cornua
ovarian vesicular follicles	ovisac
perineal body	
uterine ostium	external os, or external orifice of cervix
uterine tube	fallopian tube [oviduct deleted]
vesical surface	anterior surface of uterus

Continued on inside back cover.

VOLUME TWO

MERRILL'S ATLAS OF

RADIOGRAPHIC POSITIONS and RADIOLOGIC PROCEDURES

Philip W. Ballinger, M.S., R.T.(R)

Director and Assistant Professor, Radiologic Technology Division
School of Allied Medical Professions
The Ohio State University
Columbus, Ohio

EIGHTH EDITION

with **2863** illustrations, including **9** in full color

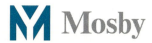 Mosby

St. Louis Baltimore Boston Carlsbad Chicago Naples New York Philadelphia Portland
London Madrid Mexico City Singapore Sydney Tokyo Toronto Wiesbaden

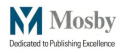

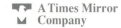

A Times Mirror
Company

Editor: Jeanne Rowland
Developmental Editor: Linda Wendling
Project Manager: Gayle May Morris
Production Editors: Deborah Vogel, Karen Allman
Manufacturing Manager: Theresa Fuchs
Design Manager: Susan Lane

EIGHTH EDITION

Printed in the United States of America
Composition by The Clarinda Company
Printing/binding by R.R. Donnelley

Mosby-Year Book, Inc.
11830 Westline Industrial Drive
St. Louis, Missouri 63146

International Standard Book Number 0-8016-7937-0

95 96 97 98 99 / 9 8 7 6 5 4 3 2 1

CONTRIBUTORS

Michael S. Bruckner, B.S., R.T.(R)(CV)
Angiographic Technologist
Radiology Department
The Ohio State University Hospitals
Columbus, Ohio

Terri Ann Bruckner, M.A., R.T.(R)
Radiographic Educational Consultant
Columbus, Ohio

Nina K. Kowalczyk, M.S., R.T.(R)
Associate Director
Radiology Department
The Ohio State University Hospitals
Columbus, Ohio

Rome V. Wadlington, R.T.(R)(M)
Supervisor, Mammography
    Department
The Ohio State University Hospitals
Columbus, Ohio

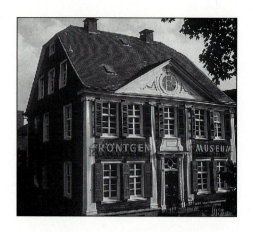

The Roentgen Museum
in Lennep, Germany.

PREFACE

With the 1995 centennial of the discovery of x-radiation, radiography students and practitioners throughout the world are reflecting on our history, celebrating our profession's contributions, and speculating about our future in the changing health care environment. *Merrill's Atlas of Radiographic Positions and Radiologic Procedures* has quite a history of its own. It has been recognized as a classic text in the field for almost half a century. In the eighth edition we believe we have successfully built on the pioneering work begun forty-six years ago by Vinita Merrill in the first edition of the atlas. Readers familiar with the atlas will find many improvements. For those using the atlas for the first time, our hope is that you will find it a highly reliable, comprehensive resource that will serve you well for many years to come.

The planning process for the new edition included soliciting input from *Merrill's Atlas* users and from many educators, who were teaching anatomy and positioning. In response to their insightful suggestions, we have made some significant improvements.

Standardization of terminology

The use of the important radiography terms, projection and position, has been standardized throughout the atlas. In particular, the comments of Eugene D. Frank, Radiography Program Director at Mayo Clinic/Foundation, provided the catalyst for these terminology changes. After many hours of discussion with Gene, who served as a special consultant on the revision, as well as Curt Serbus, who contributed greatly to our efforts, we worked out terminology we believe will be easier for students, radiographers and physicians to understand and use. The terminology continues to be in agreement with the American Registry of Radiologic Tech-

nologists and the Canadian Association of Medical Radiation Technologists. Chapter 3 provides a complete explanation of the modified terminology, and headers throughout the text reflect the improvements.

Essential projections

As a result of surveying all radiography programs in the United States and Canada, we identified 176 essential competency projections. These projections are the ones most frequently performed and are deemed necessary for competency of entry-level practitioners.

We have designated these with a special icon to alert students and instructors that these positioning skills are essential knowledge for the beginning radiographer. Instructors may, of course, modify the list of essential competency projections as appropriate to their specific geographic locations.

Bulleted positioning descriptions

Descriptions of positioning of patient and body part have been reformatted in bulleted lists for ease of reading and understanding.

Second color

Readers will notice that headings are set in color for emphasis. The second color has been incorporated in anatomic illustrations and is also used for demonstration of central ray angle and cassette positioning.

New and modified illustrations

The new edition has hundreds of new illustrations. Of particular note are the new photographs for cranium positioning. Also important is the inclusion of degree angulation information on most illustrations involving angulation of the x-ray

tube to assist the reader in quickly identifying the degree of central ray angulation or the degree of body rotation.

Historical photographs

In recognition of the 1995 centennial of the discovery of x-radiation, we have included historical photographs on the opening page of each chapter. Many are from the first edition of the atlas published in 1949, some were taken during a visit to the Röntgen Museum and birthplace of Dr. Röntgen in Lennep, Germany, and a few are from other credited sources. These photographs provide a historical perspective on the evolution of radiography and help us appreciate its significance.

Ancillaries

For the first time, the atlas has a comprehensive set of ancillaries. In addition to the third edition of *Pocket Guide to Radiography,* also available are an anatomy and positioning instructional program in slide/audiotape or CD-ROM format, student workbooks, instructor's manuals, and a 1000-question test bank on floppy disk and in bound form.

Anatomic terminology

With each new edition, anatomic terminology is updated to reflect the latest information from the International Congress of Anatomists. As in previous editions, this information is printed on the inside covers of the atlas for easy reference.

We hope you find this new edition the very best ever. Your comments and suggestions are always welcome. We are constantly striving to improve the atlas and are dependent on your input to help us in that process.

Philip W. Ballinger

ACKNOWLEDGMENTS

Dedicated to the memory of

Darrell Day Cardwell

Although he was not a radiographer, Darrell was a friend and neighbor who also assisted in producing this atlas

Sincere appreciation to the following individuals for having reviewed three or more chapters for the new edition:

Lana Andrews-Havron, B.S.R.T., R.T.(R)(T)
Baylor University Medical Center, Dallas, Texas

Michael Fugate, M.Ed., R.T.(R)
Santa Fe Community College, Gainesville, Florida

Linda Cox, M.S., R.T.(R)
Indiana University, Indianapolis, Indiana

Diane M. Kawamura, Ph.D., R.T.(R), RDMS
Weber State University, Ogden, Utah

Debra S. McMahan, B.S., PA-C, R.T.(R)
Daniel Freeman Memorial Hospital, Inglewood, California

Betty L. Palmer, A.A.S., R.T.(R)
Portland Community College, Portland, Oregon

Helen Marie Peters, ACR
Northern Alberta Institute of Technology, Edmonton, Alberta, Canada

Janet K. Scherer, DCR, RT(R), ACR,
McMaster University Medical Centre, Hamilton, Ontario, Canada

Curt Serbus, M.Ed., R.T.(R)
University of Southern Indiana, Evansville, Indiana

Donald C. Shoaf, M.Ed., R.T.(R)
Forsyth Technical Community College, Winston-Salem, North Carolina

O. Scott Staley, M.S., R.T.(R)
Boise State University, Boise, Idaho

James Temme M.P.A., R.T.(R)
University of Nebraska Medical Center, Omaha, Nebraska

I am grateful to the following professionals for their constructive comments on selected chapters:

Allan C. Beebe, M.D.

Scott A. Berg, B.S., R.T.(R)

Donald R. Bernier, CNMT

Janice M. Blanchard, R.T.(R)

Steven J. Bollin Sr., B.S., R.T.(R)

Dianna Childs, R.T.(R)

Joan Clark, M.S., R.T.(R)

Kathryn S. Durand, A.S., R.T.(R)

Kevin D. Evans, B.S., R.T.(R), RDMS

Sharyn Gibson, M.H.S., RT(R)

Ruth M. Hackworth, B.S., R.T.(R)(T)

Steven G. Hayes, B.S.R.T., R.T.(R)

Keith R. Johnson, R.T.(R)(CV)

John Raphael Kenney, R.T.(R)

Michael E. Madden, Ph.D., R.T.(R)

Elaine M. Markon, M.S., R.T.(N), CNMT

Darrell E. McKay, Ph.D., R.T.(R), FASRT

Rita M. Oswald, B.S., R.T.(R)(CV)

Robert Reid, M.S., R.T.(N)

Ken Roszel, M.S., R.T.(R)

Cheryl K. Sanders, M.P.A., R.T.(R)(T), FAERS

Nancy S. Sawyer, B.S., CNMT, R.T.(N)

Rees Stuteville, M.Ed., R.T.(R)

Tom F. Torres, B.S., R.T.(R)

Beverly J. Tupper, B.S., R.T.(R)(CV)

Melinda S. Vasila, B.S., R.T.(R)(N)

Special thanks go to **Eugene D. Frank, M.A., R.T.(R), FASRT,** who provided invaluable help standardizing the projection and position terminology and for reviewing galleys and pages for this edition. Thanks, Gene, for devoting generous amounts of time, effort and talent during the production process and for helping to bring consistency to the atlas.

To the professional staff of the medical illustrators, medical photographers and staff of the Biomedical Communications Division in the School of Allied Medical Professions at The Ohio State University. Thanks to you the quality of the illustrations in the atlas remains high. To **Harry Condry** and **Janet Nelms** who kept track of my many orders, thank you. Thanks also to medical illustrators **Dave Schumick** and **Robert Hummel** for their competent work. To **Theron Ellinger,** thank you for printing the illustrations to demonstrate the anatomy and positioning, and to **Jenny Torbett,** senior medical photographer, thanks for your photography of numerous atlas illustrations.

To **Eileen Buckholz,** I admire your ability to manage the Radiologic Technology Division at The Ohio State University. Your skills in keeping track of student schedules, clinical and academic records, faculty, due dates and my schedule continue to amaze me. You were always there when something was needed and you always pleasantly responded to my many requests like "Eileen I can't find my copy of . . ." You would retrieve the missing item and keep all of us on schedule in your own special, caring and gentle way. A sincere thank you is not enough, but thank you again.

For more than a decade I have had the pleasure of working with **Don Ladig** of the Mosby–Year Book family. Thanks, Don. Your support and encouragement have been a constant positive driving force. During the last few years I have had the rewarding experience of working with **Jeanne Rowland,** Editor at Mosby–Year

Book. Jeanne, I enjoy your honest and straight-forward manner of communicating, have found you to be readily available, and always striving to improve the atlas. Thank you, Jeanne, I have enjoyed working with you. Thanks to **Linda Wendling** for superb copyediting. You have really learned to talk like a radiographer in the last eighteen months. To **Debbie Vogel,** Project Manager, we have all appreciated your patience and calm demeanor in dealing with looming deadlines and revisions that just kept coming.

To **Terri Bruckner, M.A., R.T.(R),** where do I begin to say thank you. To keep current with the advancing profession of radiology, literally thousands of recent journal articles have been reviewed. Terri, while competently serving as my production assistant, you did an outstanding job in searching, screening, organizing and compiling the updated bibliographies for all three volumes. During the revision process, your ability to write, compile and critically evaluate new material was truly appreciated. During the production stages, your eye for consistency and detail was evident. It has indeed been a pleasure working with you, Terri.

The love and support provided by my family permitted my total involvement in this revision project. To my in-laws, **L. Neil and Ruth Hathaway,** thank you for accepting my absence too many times. I

plan to improve upon the time available to spend with you as I accept early retirement from The Ohio State University. To my parents, **Dwight W. and Mildred Ballinger,** this work would not have been possible had you not supported me after I initially made the decision to enter radiology. You were always there whenever I needed something, and your love and affection truly made the project easier.

To my son and daughter, **Eric and Monica Ballinger,** now that you are in college I hope you find professions that you will enjoy as much as I do radiology. There were many times I was not available to spend time with you because "I was working on the book." I hope you understand that in spite of my sometimes absence, I do love you.

To my wife of twenty-five years, **Nancy Ballinger,** thanks for always being there when I wasn't. And thanks for saying yes when I called "Hey Nanc, got a minute?" For all the times you dropped what you were doing to proofread, check, and double check a revised manuscript, thank you. For over half of our married life you have juggled the family schedule to accommodate my involvement with the atlas. Thank you, Nancy, for your tolerance, support and love. I do love you and appreciate your active involvement in my publishing efforts.

P.W.B.

CONTENTS

VOLUME ONE

VOLUME TWO

VOLUME THREE

MERRILL'S ATLAS OF

RADIOGRAPHIC POSITIONS and RADIOLOGIC PROCEDURES

Chapter 14

MOUTH AND SALIVARY GLANDS

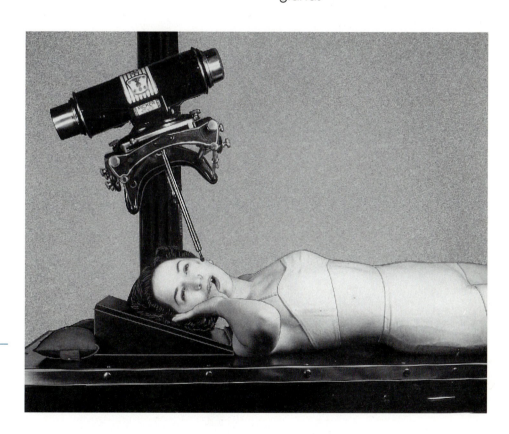

Patient positioned on a radiographic table for a radiograph of the upper bicuspids using head support.

Mouth

The *mouth* (Fig. 14-1) is the first division of the digestive system. It encloses the dental arches and receives the saliva secreted by the salivary glands. The cavity of the mouth is divided into (1) the *oral vestibule*, the space between the teeth and the cheeks; and (2) the *oral cavity*, or *mouth proper*, the space within the dental arches. The roof of the oral cavity is formed by the hard and soft palates. The floor is formed principally by the tongue, and it communicates with the pharynx posteriorly by an aperture termed the *faucial isthmus*.

The vault of the *hard palate* is formed by the horizontal plates of the maxillae and palatine bones. The anterior and lateral boundaries are formed by the inner wall of the maxillary alveolar processes, which extend superiorly and medially to blend with the horizontal processes. The height of the hard palate varies considerably, and it determines the angulation of the inner surface of the alveolar process. The angle is less when the palate is high and greater when it is low.

The *soft palate* (velum) begins behind the last molar and is suspended from the posterior border of the hard palate. Highly sensitive to touch, the soft palate is a movable musculomembranous structure which functions chiefly as a partial septum between the mouth and the pharynx. At the center of the inferior border, the soft palate is prolonged into a small, pendulous process called the *uvula*. On each side of the uvula, two arched folds extend laterally and inferiorly. The anterior pair of arches, which form the *faucial isthmus*, project forward to the sides of the base of the tongue. The posterior pair of arches project posteriorly to blend with the posterolateral walls of the pharynx. The triangular space between the anterior and the posterior arches is occupied by the palatine tonsil.

The *tongue* (Figs. 14-1 and 14-2) is situated in the floor of the oral cavity, with its base directed posteriorly and its apex directed anteriorly. The tongue is freely movable, composed of numerous muscles and covered with a mucous membrane that varies in character in the different regions of the organ. The extrinsic muscles of the tongue form the greater part of the oral floor. The mucous membrane covering the undersurface of the tongue is reflected laterally over the remainder of the floor to the gums. This part of the floor lies under the free anterior and lateral portions of the tongue and is called the *sublingual space*. Posterior movement of the free anterior part of the tongue is restricted by a median vertical band, or fold, of mucous membrane called the *frenulum of the tongue* (frenulum linguae), which extends between the undersurface of the tongue and the sublingual space. On each side of the frenulum, extending around the outer limits of the sublingual space and over the underlying salivary glands, the mucous membrane is elevated into a crestlike ridge called the *sublingual fold* (plica sublingualis). In the relaxed state the two folds (plicae) are quite prominent and are in contact with the gums.

The *teeth* serve the function of *mastication*, the process of chewing and grinding food into small pieces. During mastication, the teeth cut, grind, and tear the food, which is then mixed with saliva, swallowed, and later digested. The salivary glands produce approximately 1 liter of saliva each day. The saliva softens the food, keeps the mouth moist, and contributes digestive enzymes.

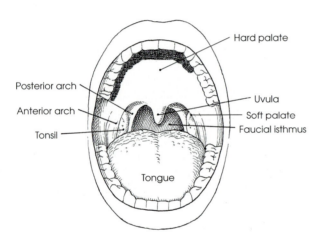

Fig. 14-1. Anterior aspect of oral cavity.

Hard palate

Posterior arch

Anterior arch

Tonsil

Uvula

Soft palate

Faucial isthmus

Tongue

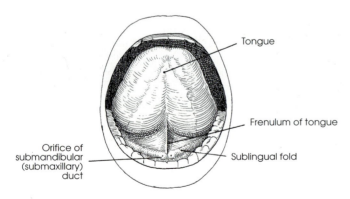

Fig. 14-2. Anterior view of undersurface of tongue and floor of mouth.

Tongue

Frenulum of tongue

Orifice of submandibular (submaxillary) duct

Sublingual fold

Salivary Glands

The three pairs of salivary glands are the *parotid*, the *submandibular* (submaxillary), and the *sublingual* (Fig. 14-3). The glands are composed of numerous lobes, each of which is made up of small lobules, the whole being held together by connective tissue and a fine network of blood vessels and ducts. The ductules of the lobules coalesce into larger tributaries, which in turn unite and form the large efferent duct, which conveys the saliva from the gland to the mouth.

The *parotid gland* is the largest of the salivary glands and consists of a flattened superficial portion and a wedge-shaped deep portion (Fig. 14-4). The superficial part lies immediately anterior to the external ear and extends inferiorly to the mandibular ramus and posteriorly to the mastoid process. The deep, or retromandibular, portion extends medially toward the pharynx. The *parotid duct* (Stensen's duct) runs anteriorly and medially to open into the oral vestibule opposite the second upper molar.

The *submandibular* (submaxillary) *gland* is a fairly large, irregularly shaped gland that extends posteriorly from a point below the first molar almost to the angle of the mandible (Fig. 14-5). Although the upper part of the gland rests against the inner surface of the mandibular body, its greater portion projects below the mandible. The *submandibular duct* (submaxillary or Wharton's duct) extends anteriorly and superiorly to open into the mouth on a small papilla at the side of the frenulum of the tongue, the *sublingual caruncle*.

The *sublingual gland*, composed of a group of smaller glands, is narrow and elongated in form (Fig. 14-5). This gland is located in the floor of the mouth beneath the sublingual fold (plica sublingualis). It is in contact with the mandible laterally, and it extends posteriorly from the side of the frenulum of the tongue (frenulum linguae) to the submandibular (submaxillary) gland. There are numerous small *sublingual ducts* (ducts of Rivinus), some of which open into the floor of the mouth along the crest of the sublingual fold and others of which open into the submandibular (submaxillary) duct. The main sublingual duct (Bartholin's duct) opens beside the orifice of the submandibular duct (submaxillary or Wharton's duct).

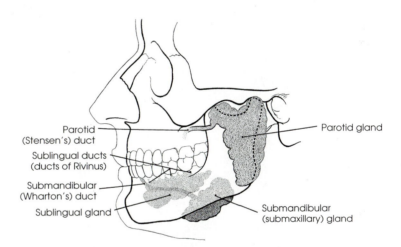

Parotid (Stensen's) duct

Sublingual ducts (ducts of Rivinus)

Submandibular (Wharton's) duct

Sublingual gland

Parotid gland

Submandibular (submaxillary) gland

Fig. 14-3. Salivary glands from left lateral aspect.

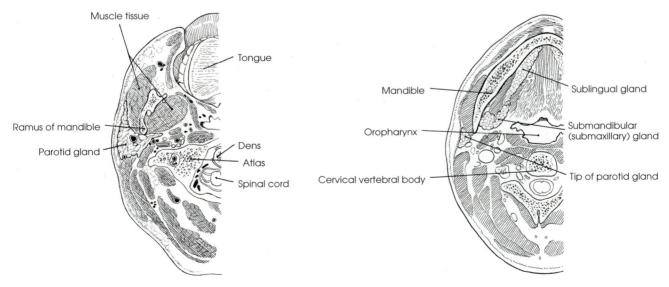

Muscle tissue

Tongue

Ramus of mandible

Parotid gland

Dens

Atlas

Spinal cord

Mandible

Sublingual gland

Oropharynx

Submandibular (submaxillary) gland

Cervical vertebral body

Tip of parotid gland

Fig. 14-4. Transverse section of face showing relation of parotid gland to mandibular ramus. (Auricle not shown on illustration.)

Fig. 14-5. Transverse section of face showing relation of submandibular (submaxillary) and sublingual glands to surrounding structures. (Auricle not shown.)

Sialography

Sialography is the term applied to radiologic examinations of the salivary glands and ducts with the use of a contrast medium, usually one of the water-soluble iodinated media. The frequency of performing sialograms has decreased during the past few years because of improvements in computed tomography (CT) and magnetic resonance imaging (MRI) techniques. When the clinician is evaluating a patient with a suspected salivary stone or lesion, CT or MRI is often the modality of choice. However, when a definitive diagnosis is needed involving one of the salivary ducts, sialography remains a viable diagnostic tool.

In performing a sialogram, the following steps are observed:

- Inject the radiopaque medium into the main duct; from there it flows into the intraglandular ductules. This makes it possible to demonstrate the surrounding glandular parenchyma as well as the duct system (Fig. 14-6). The procedure is used to demonstrate such conditions as inflammatory lesions and tumors, to determine the extent of salivary fistulae, and to localize diverticulae, strictures, and calculi. Because the glands are paired, and the pairs are in such close proximity, only one gland at a time can be examined by the sialographic method (Fig. 14-7).

- Obtain preliminary radiographs to detect any condition demonstrable without the use of a contrast medium and to establish the optimum exposure technique.

- Two or three minutes before the sialographic procedure, give the patient a secretory stimulant to open the duct for ready identification of its orifice and for easier passage of a cannula or catheter. Having the patient suck a wedge of fresh lemon serves this purpose and is repeated on completion of the examination to stimulate rapid evacuation of the contrast medium.

- Take a radiograph about 10 minutes after the procedure to verify clearance of the contrast medium, if needed.

Most physicians inject the contrast medium by manual pressure, that is, with a syringe attached to the cannula or catheter. Other physicians advocate that the medium be delivered by hydrostatic pressure only. The latter method requires the use of a water-soluble iodinated medium, with the contrast solution container (usually a syringe barrel with the plunger removed) attached to a drip stand and set at a distance of 28 inches (70 cm) above the level of the patient's mouth. Some examiners carry out the filling procedure under fluoroscopic guidance and obtain spot radiographs. The reader is referred to the articles listed in the bibliography for a detailed description of each of the numerous methods of performing sialography.

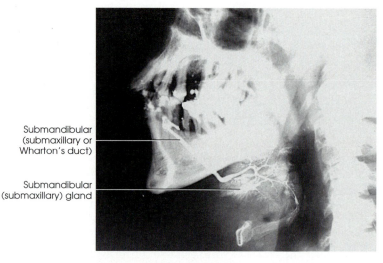

Submandibular (submaxillary or Wharton's duct)

Submandibular (submaxillary) gland

Fig. 14-6. Sialogram showing opacified submandibular gland.

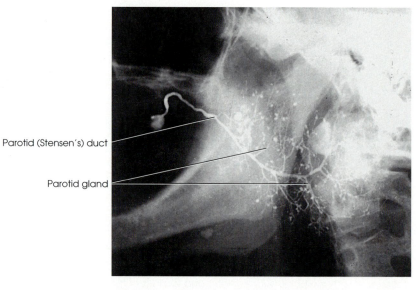

Parotid (Stensen's) duct

Parotid gland

Fig. 14-7. Sialogram showing parotid gland on patient without teeth.

Parotid Gland
TANGENTIAL PROJECTION

Film: 8 × 10 in (18 × 24 cm) lengthwise.

Position of patient

- Place the patient in either a recumbent or a seated position.
- Since the parotid gland lies midway between the anterior and posterior surfaces of the skull, take the tangential projection of the glandular region from either the posterior or the anterior direction.

Position of part

Supine body position
- With the patient supine, rotate the head slightly toward the side being examined so that the parotid area is perpendicular to the plane of the film.
- Center the film to the parotid area.
- With the patient's head resting on the occiput, adjust it so that the mandibular ramus is parallel with the longitudinal axis of the film (Fig. 14-8).

Prone body position
- With the patient prone, rotate the head so that the parotid area being examined is perpendicular to the plane of the film.
- Center the film to the parotid region.
- With the patient's head resting on the chin, adjust its flexion so that the mandibular ramus is parallel with the longitudinal axis of the film (Fig. 14-9).
- When the parotid (Stensen's) duct does not have to be demonstrated, rest the head on the forehead and nose.
- *Shield gonads.*
- *Respiration:* Improved radiographic quality can be obtained, particularly for the demonstration of calculi, by having the patient fill the mouth with air and then puff the cheeks out as much as possible. When this cannot be done, ask the patient to suspend respiration for the exposure.

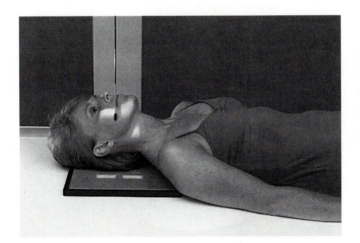

Fig. 14-8. Tangential partoid gland, patient supine.

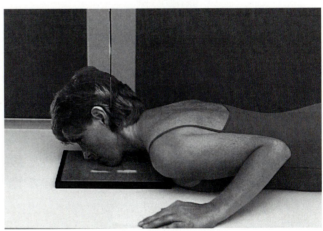

Fig. 14-9. Tangential parotid gland, patient prone.

Central ray

- With the central ray perpendicular to the plane of the film, direct it along the lateral surface of the mandibular ramus.

Structures shown

A tangential projection demonstrates the region of the parotid gland and duct. These structures are clearly outlined when an opaque medium is used (Figs. 14-10 to 14-14).

The following should be clearly demonstrated:

- Soft tissue density.
- Most of the parotid gland lateral to, and clear of, the mandibular ramus.
- Mastoid overlapping only the upper portion of the parotid gland.

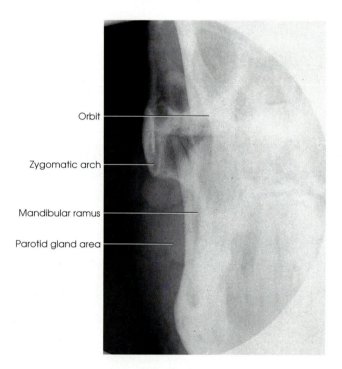

Orbit

Zygomatic arch

Mandibular ramus

Parotid gland area

Fig. 14-10. Tangential parotid gland. Examination of right cheek area to rule out tumor. Soft tissue fullness. No calcification.

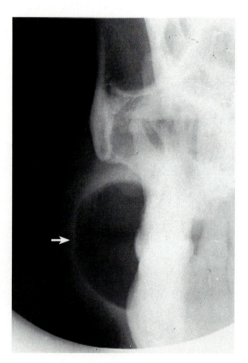

Fig. 14-11. Same patient as in Fig. 14-10. Right cheek *(arrow)* distended with air in mouth. No abnormal finding in region of parotid gland.

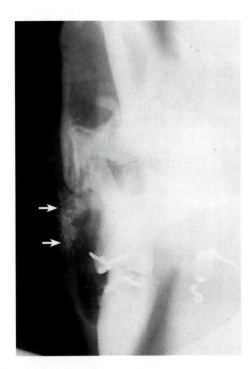

Fig. 14-12. Tangential parotid gland. Right cheek distended with air. Considerable calcification seen in region of parotid gland (arrows).

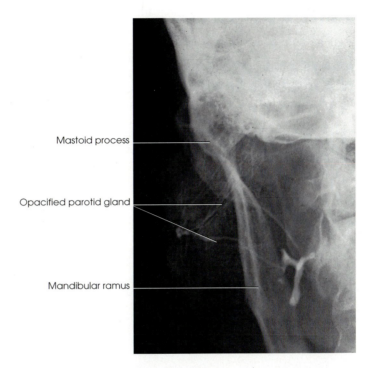

Mastoid process

Opacified parotid gland

Mandibular ramus

Fig. 14-13. Tangential parotid gland showing opacification.

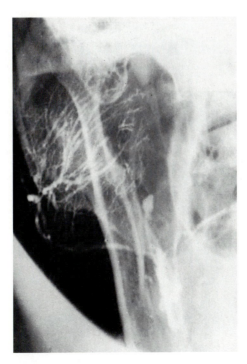

Fig. 14-14. Tangential parotid gland showing opacification.

Parotid and Submandibular Glands
LATERAL PROJECTION
R or L position

Film: 8 × 10 in (18 × 24 cm) lengthwise.

Position of patient

- Place the patient in a semiprone or seated-upright position.

Position of part

Parotid gland

- With the affected side closest to the film, extend the patient's neck so that the space between the cervical area of the spine and the mandibular rami is cleared.
- Center the film to a point approximately 1 inch (2.5 cm) superior to the mandibular angle.
- Adjust the head so that the median sagittal plane is rotated approximately 15 degrees toward the cassette from a true lateral position.

Submandibular gland

- Center the film to the inferior margin of the angle of the mandible.
- Adjust the patient's head in a true lateral position (Fig. 14-15).
- Iglauer[1] suggested depressing the floor of the mouth to displace the submandibular gland below the mandible. When the patient's throat is not too sensitive, accomplish this by having the patient place an index finger on the back of the tongue on the affected side.
- *Shield gonads.*
- Ask the patient to suspend respiration for the exposure.

Central ray

- Direct the central ray perpendicular to the center of the cassette at a point (1) 1 inch (2.5 cm) superior to the mandibular angle to demonstrate the parotid gland or (2) at the inferior margin of the mandibular angle to demonstrate the submandibular gland.

---

[1]Iglauer S: A simple maneuver to increase the visibility of a salivary calculus in the roentgenogram, Radiology 21:297, 1933.

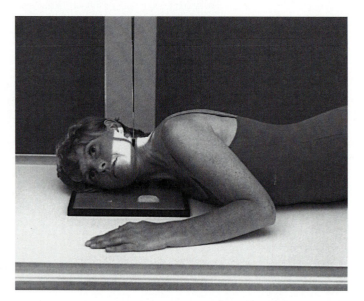

Fig. 14-15. Lateral submandibular gland.

Structures shown

A lateral image demonstrates the bony structures and any calcific deposit or swelling in the unobscured areas of the parotid (Figs. 14-16 and 14-17) and submandibular glands (Fig. 14-18). The glands and their ducts are well outlined when an opaque medium is used.

□ Evaluation criteria

The following should be clearly demonstrated:

- Mandibular rami free of overlap from the cervical vertebrae to best show the parotid gland superimposed over the ramus.
- Superimposed mandibular rami and angles, if no tube angulation or head rotation is used for the submandibular gland.
- Oblique position for the parotid gland.

NOTE: To obtain an image of the deeper portions of the parotid and submandibular glands, it is often necessary to obtain an oblique projection. Any of the axiolateral projections of the mandible can be used for this purpose as described in Chapter 21.

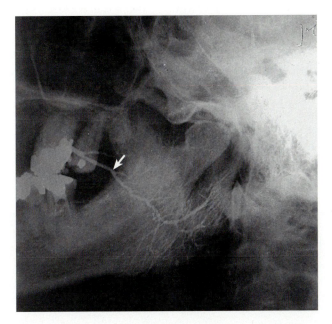

Fig. 14-16. Lateral parotid gland showing opacified gland and parotid (Stensen's) duct *(arrow)*.

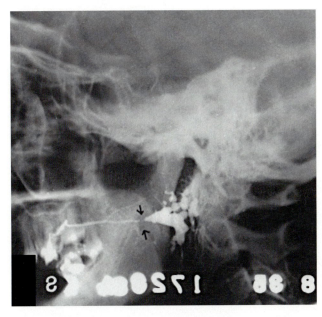

Fig. 14-17. Lateral parotid gland showing opacification and blockage of parotid (Stensen's) duct *(arrows)*.

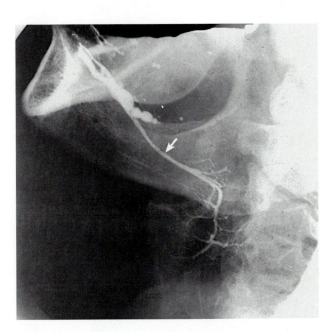

Fig. 14-18. Lateral submandibular (submaxillary) gland showing opacification and submandibular (Wharton's) duct *(arrow)*.

Submandibular and Sublingual Glands
AXIAL PROJECTION
INTRAORAL TECHNIQUE

Film: Occlusal: 2¼ × 3 in (57 × 76 mm).

Position of patient

- Elevate the patient's thorax on several firm pillows.
- Flex the patient's knees to relax the abdominal muscles and thereby allow full extension of the neck.
- Adjust the shoulders to lie in the same transverse plane.
- After placement of the occlusal film, fully extend the neck and rest it on the vertex with the median sagittal plane vertical (Figs. 14-19 and 14-20).
- *Shield gonads.*

Film placement

- Tape a side marker *(R or L)* onto one corner of the exposure surface of the occlusal film packet.
- Place the film in the mouth with the long axis directed transversely.
- Center the packet to the median sagittal plane and gently insert it far enough so that it is in contact with the anterior borders of the mandibular rami.
- Instruct the patient to gently close the mouth (to hold the packet in position).
- Ask the patient to suspend respiration for the exposure.

Central ray

- With the central ray perpendicular to the plane of the film, direct it to the intersection of the median sagittal plane and a coronal plane passing through the second molars.

Structures shown

An axial image of the floor of the mouth is demonstrated, showing the entire sublingual gland areas and the duct and anteromedial part of the submandibular gland areas (Fig. 14-21).

☐ Evaluation criteria

The following should be clearly demonstrated:
- Soft tissue density of the floor of the mouth.
- Both sides of the mandible and dental arches symmetric.
- Sublingual glands in their entirety along with a portion of the submandibular glands when the film includes the lower molars.

NOTE: This is the only projection that gives an unobstructed image of the sublingual gland regions. It is sometimes necessary to use the verticosubmental projection for the submandibular gland regions to demonstrate tumor masses or lesions that lie posterior or lateral to the floor of the oral cavity as seen in Fig. 14-22.

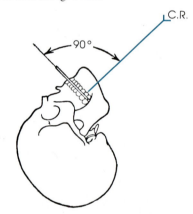

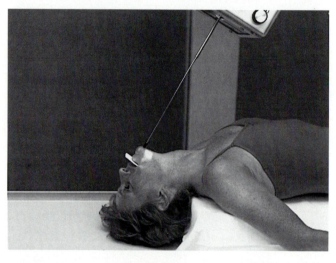

Fig. 14-19. Axial submandibular and sublingual glands.

Fig. 14-20. Intraoral method.

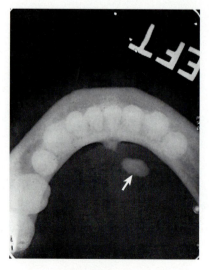

Fig. 14-21. Axial submandibular (submaxillary) and sublingual glands. Calcification *(arrow)* in sublingual region.

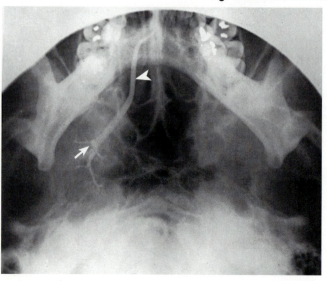

Fig. 14-22. Verticosubmental submandibular (submaxillary) gland *(arrow)* and duct *(arrowhead)*.

Chapter 15

ANTERIOR PART OF NECK

Pharynx
Larynx
Thyroid Gland

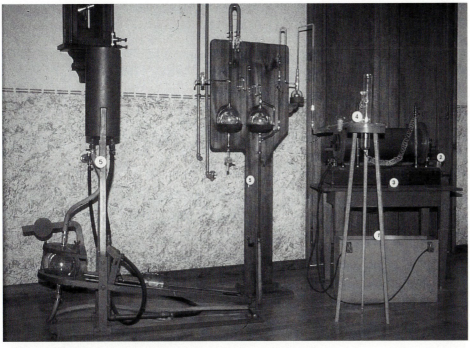

The equipment Dr. Roentgen used while discovering x-rays: *1*, lead battery, *2*, mechanical interrupter (15 to 20 interruptions per second), *3*, Ruhmkorff sparked generator, *4*, electrical discharge tube, *5*, vacuum pump to evacuate gas from the tube.

The neck occupies the region between the skull and the thorax. Its upper limit is defined by an imaginary line extending from the inferior border of the symphysis menti to the external occipital protuberance. Its lower limit is defined by a line extending from the jugular notch to the superior border of the first thoracic vertebra (Figs. 15-1 and 15-2). For radiographic purposes, the neck is divided into posterior and anterior portions in accordance with the tissue composition and function of the contained structures. The several procedures that are required to demonstrate the osseous structures occupying the posterior division of the neck are described in the discussion on the cervical vertebrae in Chapter 8 in Volume 1 of this text. The portions of the central nervous system and of the circulatory system passing through the neck are described under the respective Chapters 25 and 26 in Volume 2.

The portion of the neck lying in front of the vertebrae is composed largely of soft tissues, the upper parts of the respiratory and digestive systems being the principal structures and the ones under consideration in this discussion. The thyroid and parathyroid glands, as well as the larger part of the submandibular glands, are also located in the anterior portion of the neck.

The *thyroid gland* consists of two lateral lobes connected at their lower thirds by a narrow median portion called the *isthmus* (Fig. 15-3). The lobes are approximately 2 inches (5 cm) long, 1¼ inches (3 cm) wide, and ¾ inch (2 cm) thick. The isthmus lies at the front of the upper part of the trachea, and the lobes lie at the sides. The lobes reach from the lower third of the thyroid cartilage to the level of the first thoracic vertebra. Although the thyroid gland is normally suprasternal in position, occasionally it presents a retrosternal extension into the superior aperture of the thorax. The *parathyroid glands* are small ovoid bodies and are normally four in number—two on each side. They are situated, one above the other, on the posterior aspect of the adjacent lobe of the thyroid gland.

The *pharynx,* serving as a passage for both air and food, is common to the respiratory and digestive systems (Fig. 15-2). The pharynx is a musculomembranous, tubular structure situated in front of the vertebrae and behind the nose, the mouth, and the larynx. Approximately 5 inches (13 cm) in length, the pharynx extends from the undersurface of the body of the sphenoid bone and the basilar part of the occipital bone inferiorly to the level of the disk between the sixth and seventh cervical vertebrae, where it becomes continuous with the esophagus. The pharyngeal cavity is subdivided into nasal, oral, and laryngeal portions. The nasopharynx lies above the soft palate, the upper part of which forms its floor, and anteriorly communicates with the posterior apertures of the nose, the *choanae,* and laterally with the *auditory* (pharyngotympanic or eustachian) *tubes.* The choanae communicate with the nasal cavity. On the roof and posterior wall of the nasopharynx, between the orifices of the auditory (pharyngotympanic or eustachian) tubes, the mucosa contains a mass of lymphoid tissue known as the *pharyngeal tonsil* (or ade-

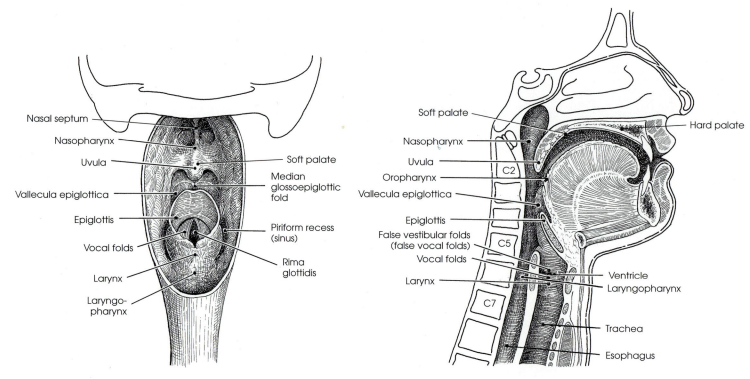

Fig. 15-1. Interior posterior view of neck.

Nasal septum
Nasopharynx
Uvula
Vallecula epiglottica
Epiglottis
Vocal folds
Larynx
Laryngo-pharynx
Soft palate
Median glossoepiglottic fold
Piriform recess (sinus)
Rima glottidis

Fig. 15-2. Sagittal section of face and neck.

Soft palate
Nasopharynx
Uvula
Oropharynx
Vallecula epiglottica
Epiglottis
False vestibular folds (false vocal folds)
Vocal folds
Larynx
Hard palate
C2
C5
C7
Ventricle
Laryngopharynx
Trachea
Esophagus

noids when enlarged). Hypertrophy of this tissue interferes with nasal breathing and is common in children. This condition is well demonstrated in a lateral radiograph of the nasopharynx. The *oropharynx* is the portion extending from the soft palate to the level of the hyoid bone. It communicates with the mouth through the faucial isthmus and contains the *palatine tonsils,* which are located on its lateral walls between the two palatine, or faucial, arches. The base, or root, of the tongue forms the anterior wall of the oropharynx. The *laryngeal pharynx* (hypopharynx) lies posterior to the larynx, its anterior

wall being formed by the posterior surface of the larynx. The two structures communicate by means of the upper laryngeal aperture. The laryngopharynx extends inferiorly to the level of *cricoid cartilage* and is continuous with the esophagus. The air-containing nasal and oral pharynges are well visualized in lateral images, except during the act of phonation, when the soft palate contracts and tends to obscure the nasal pharynx. An opaque medium is required for the demonstration of the lumen of the laryngeal pharynx, although it can be distended with air during the *Valsalva maneuver* (an increase in intratho-

racic pressure produced by forcible exhalation effort against the closed glottis).

The *larynx* (Figs. 15-1 through 15-5) is the organ of voice. Serving as the air passage between the pharynx and the trachea, the larynx is also one of the divisions of the respiratory system.

The larynx is a movable, tubular structure, is broader above than below, and is approximately 1½ inches (4 cm) in length. Situated below the root of the tongue and in front of the laryngeal pharynx, the larynx is suspended from the hyoid bone and extends from the level of the superior margin of the fourth cervical ver-

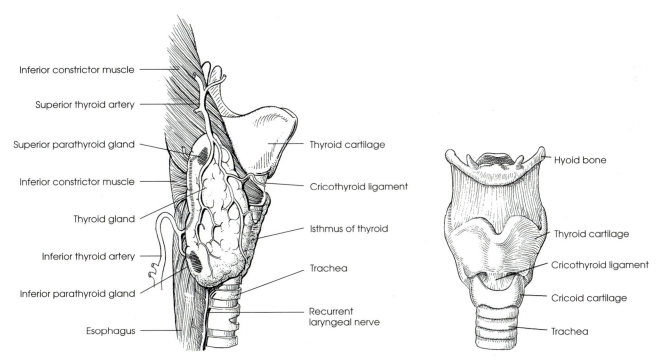

Fig. 15-3. Lateral aspect of laryngeal area.

Fig. 15-4. Anterior aspect of larynx.

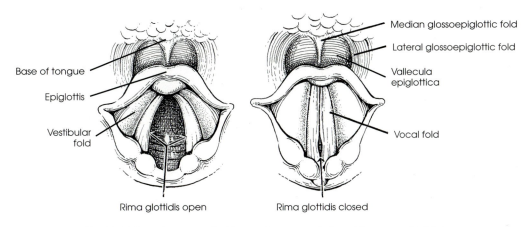

Fig. 15-5. Superior aspect of larynx (open and closed true vocal folds.)

tebra to its junction with the trachea at the level of the inferior margin of the sixth cervical vertebra. The framework of the larynx is composed of nine cartilages— three single (epiglottis, thyroid, cricoid) and three paired (arytenoid, corniculate, cuneiform). These cartilages are connected together with ligaments, are moved by muscles, and are clothed in a mucous membrane that is drawn into folds over certain of these structures. The thin, leaf-shaped *epiglottis* is situated behind the root of the tongue and the hyoid bone and above the laryngeal entrance. The *thyroid cartilage,* the largest of the group, forms the laryngeal prominence, or "Adam's apple." The lower border of the *cricoid cartilage,* the second largest of the group, is connected to the first ring of the trachea.

The inlet of the larynx is oblique, slanting posteriorly as it descends. A pouchlike fossa, called the *piriform recess* (sinus of the hypopharynx), is located on each side of the larynx and external to its orifice. The piriform recesses are well shown as triangular areas on frontal projections when insufflated with air (Valsalva maneuver) or when filled with an opaque medium.

The anterior surface of the free superior part of the epiglottis is attached to the root of the tongue by a median and two lateral folds of mucous membrane that bound two depressions called the *valleculae epiglottica*. The *median glossoepiglottic fold* extends between the front of the epiglottis and the base of the tongue. The *lateral glossoepiglottic folds* extend laterally and anteriorly from the margin of the epiglottis to the junction of the side walls of the pharynx and the tongue. It has been stated that the epiglottis and valleculae serve as a trap to prevent leakage into the larynx between acts of swallowing.

The entrance of the larynx is guarded superiorly and anteriorly by the epiglottis and laterally and posteriorly by folds of mucous membrane called the *aryepiglottic* and *interarytenoid folds*. These folds, extending around the margin of the laryngeal inlet (orifice) from their junction with the epiglottis, function as a sphincter during deglutition (swallowing).

The laryngeal cavity is subdivided into three compartments by two pairs of mucosal folds, which, extending anteroposteriorly, project from its lateral walls. The superior pair of folds, separated from each other by a median interval called the *rima vestibuli* (vestibular slit), are the *vestibular folds,* or false vocal cords. The space above them is called the *laryngeal vestibule,* or simply vestibule. The lower two folds are separated from each other by a median fissure called the *rima glottidis.* They are known as the vocal folds, or *true vocal folds* (Fig. 15-5). The "vocal cords" are vocal ligaments, which are covered by the vocal folds. The ligaments and the rima glottidis make up the vocal apparatus of the larynx and are collectively referred to as the *glottis*. The middle compartment, the space between the upper and lower mucosal folds, expands into a space on each side called the *laryngeal ventricle,* or simply ventricle. The lower space or compartment is continuous with the cavity of the trachea. The position and contour of the laryngeal structures vary considerably during speech and deglutition.

Soft Palate, Pharynx, and Larynx
METHODS OF EXAMINATION

The throat structures may be examined with or without an opaque contrast medium; the technique employed depends on the abnormality being investigated. Computed tomography (CT) studies are often performed for the areas of the palate, pharynx, and larynx to radiographically demonstrate the part with little or no discomfort to the patient. Magnetic resonance imaging (MRI) is also used to evaluate the larynx. The radiologic modality selected is often determined by the institution and physician. The following radiologic examinations are not performed as often as in the past.

Palatography

Bloch and Quantrill[1] investigated suspected tumors of the soft palate by a positive-contrast technique using the following steps:

- Seat the patient laterally before a vertical grid device with the nasopharynx centered to the cassette.
- For the first palatogram, have the patient swallow a small amount of a thick, creamy barium sulfate suspension to coat the inferior surface of the soft palate and the uvula.
- Obtain a second lateral image after the injection of 0.5 ml of the creamy barium suspension into each nasal cavity to coat the superior surface of the soft palate and the posterior wall of the nasopharynx.

Morgan et al.[2] described a technique for evaluating abnormalities of chewing and swallowing in children. These examiners record the chewing and swallowing function with cineradiography as the child chews barium-impregnated chocolate fudge (the recipe for which they include in their article).

Cleft palate studies are taken in the following manner:

- Seat the patient laterally upright with the image receptor centered to the nasopharynx.
- Make the exposures during phonation to demonstrate the range of movement of the soft palate and the position of the tongue during each of the following sounds[3,4]: "d-a-h," "m-m-m," "s-s-s," and "e-e-e."

[1]Bloch S and Quantrill JR: The radiology of nasopharyngeal tumors, including positive contrast nasopharyngography, S Afr Med J 42:1030-1036, 1968.

[2]Morgan JA et al: Barium-impregnated chocolate fudge for the study of chewing mechanism in children, Radiology 94:432-433, 1970.
[3]Randall P, O'Hara AE, and Bakes FP: A simple roentgen examination for the study of soft palate function in patients with poor speech, Plast Reconstr Surg 21:345-356, 1958.
[4]O'Hara AE: Roentgen evaluation of patients with cleft palate, Radiol Clin North Am 1:1-11, 1963.

Soft palate, pharynx, and larynx

Nasopharyngography

Hypertrophy of the pharyngeal tonsil, or adenoids, is clearly delineated in a direct lateral projection centered to the nasopharynx (¾ inch [2 cm] directly anterior to the external acoustic [auditory] meatus) as seen in Fig. 15-6. To ensure filling of the nasopharynx with air, the film must be exposed during the intake of a deep breath through the nose. Mouth breathing moves the soft palate posteriorly to near approximation with the posterior wall of the nasopharynx and thus causes the air intake to bypass the nasopharynx as it is directed inferiorly into the larynx.

Positive-contrast nasopharyngography is performed to assess the extent of nasopharyngeal tumors (Fig. 15-7). Some examiners recommend an iodized oil for this examination.[1] Others prefer finely ground barium sulfate, either mixed in paste form[2] or applied dry with a pressure blower.

Preliminary filming commonly consists of a submentovertical (SMV) projection of the skull and an upright lateral projection centered to the nasopharynx (¾ inch

[1]Johnson TH, Green AE, and Rice EN: Nasopharyngography: its technique and uses, Radiology 88:1166-1169, 1967.
[2]Khoo FY, Chia KB, and Nalpon J: A new technique of contrast examination of the nasopharynx with cinefluorography and roentgenography, AJR 99:238-248, 1967.

[2 cm] directly anterior to the external acoustic [auditory] meatus). When an iodized oil or a barium paste is used, the following steps are observed:
- Place the patient on the examining table in the supine position after local anesthetization.
- Elevate the shoulders to extend the neck enough to permit the orbitomeatal line to be adjusted at an angle of 40 to 45 degrees to the horizontal.
- Keep the head in this position throughout the examination.
- Both before and after the instillation of the contrast medium into the nasal cavities, obtain the basal projections with the central ray directed midway between the mandibular angles at an angle of 15 to 20 degrees cephalad.
- Obtain lateral projections by using a horizontal central ray centered to the nasopharynx.
- On completion of this phase of the examination, have the patient sit up and blow the nose. This act evacuates most of the contrast medium, and the remainder will be swallowed. It is reported that none of the contrast medium is aspirated because the swallowing mechanism is triggered before the contrast medium reaches the larynx.

Additional studies in the upright position are then made as directed by the examining physician. (See patient cases in Figs. 15-8 to 15-11.)

Chittinand et al.[1] described an opaque-contrast nasopharyngographic procedure wherein the patient is not required to keep the neck in an uncomfortable extended position for the entire examination. The following steps are observed:
- Seat the patient before a vertical grid device.
- Obtain preliminary lateral and submentovertical projections.
- According to the authors, topical anesthetization is not required for their method of examination.
- Using a standard spray bottle, spray each nasal cavity with water as a wetting agent, after which spray Micropaque powder through each nostril with a powder blower connected to a pressure unit.
- Take two SMV projections—one at rest and one during a modified Valsalva maneuver—and a lateral projection.
- Have the patient blow the nose; any of the medium not expelled is swallowed. The authors state that immediate chest radiographs should not reveal barium in the lungs, and 24-hour follow-up radiographs should reveal complete clearing of the nasopharynx.

[1]Chittinand S, Patheja SS, and Wisenberg MJ: Barium nasopharyngography, Radiology 98:387-390, 1971.

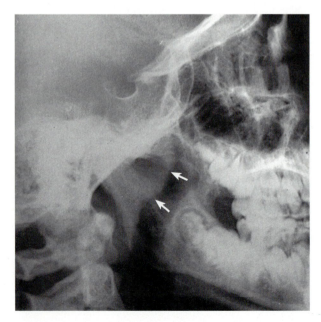

Fig. 15-6. Lateral pharyngeal tonsil demonstrating hypertrophy *(arrows).*

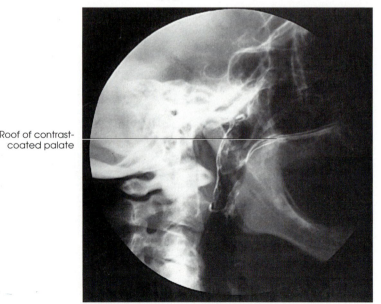

Roof of contrast-coated palate

Fig. 15-7. Lateral nasopharyngogram.

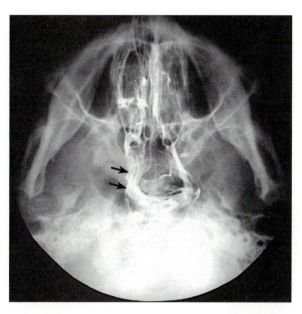

Fig. 15-8. SMV nasopharyngography. Right ninth nerve sign. There is asymmetry of nasopharynx with flattening on right and an irregularity *(arrows).*

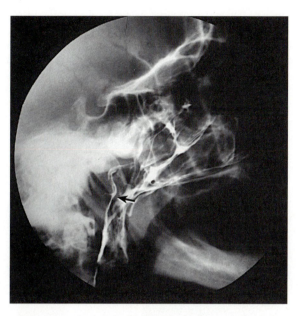

Fig. 15-9. Lateral nasopharyngography. Right ninth nerve sign. Lateral projection shows a mass in posterior aspect of nasopharynx *(arrow)* with an umbilication (same patient as in Fig. 15-8).

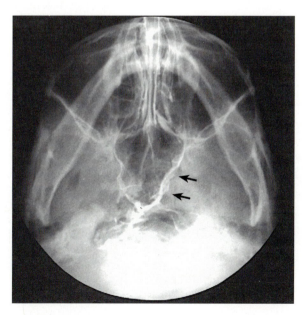

Fig. 15-10. SMV nasopharyngography. Sixty-nine-year-old female with a long history of decreased hearing on left side and left facial paresthesia (burning, prickling). Nasopharynx is asymmetric with blunting of cartilage at opening of auditory tube *(arrows).*

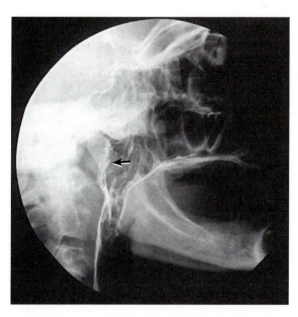

Fig. 15-11. Lateral nasopharyngography showing a shallow niche at C1 level, which may represent an ulcer *(arrow).*

Pharyngography

Opaque studies of the pharynx are made with an ingestible contrast medium, usually a thick, creamy mixture of water and barium sulfate. This examination is frequently carried out using fluoroscopy with spot-film images only. These or conventional projections are made during deglutition.

Deglutition

The act of swallowing is performed by the rapid and highly coordinated action of many muscles. The following points are important in radiography of the pharynx and upper esophagus:

1. The mid-area of the tongue becomes depressed to collect the mass, or bolus, of material to be swallowed.

2. The base of the tongue forms a central groove to accommodate the bolus and then moves superiorly and inferiorly along the roof of the mouth to propel the bolus through the faucial isthmus into the pharynx.

3. Simultaneously with the posterior thrust of the tongue, the larynx moves anteriorly and superiorly under the root of the tongue, the sphincteric folds nearly closing the laryngeal inlet (orifice).

4. The epiglottis divides the passing bolus and drains the two portions laterally into the piriform recesses as it lowers over the laryngeal entrance.

The bolus is projected into the pharynx at the height of the anterior movement of the larynx (Figs. 15-12 to 15-14). One has only to swallow a few times to study the process of deglutition and to understand the need to synchronize a rapid exposure with the peak of the act.

The shortest exposure time possible must be used for studies made during deglutition. The following steps should be observed:

• Ask the patient to hold the barium sulfate bolus in the mouth until signaled and then to swallow the bolus in one movement.

• Request that the patient refrain from swallowing again if a mucosal study is to be attempted.

• Take the mucosal study during the modified Valsalva maneuver for double-contrast delineation.

Fluoroscopic equipment is available that is capable of exposing up to 12 frames per second using the 100 mm or 105 mm cut or roll film. Many institutions with such equipment use it to spot radiograph the patient in rapid sequence during the act of swallowing. Another technique is to record the fluoroscopic image on videotape or cine film. The recorded image may then be studied to identify any abnormalities during the active progress of deglutition.

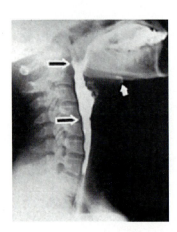

Fig. 15-12. Lateral projection. Exposure made at peak of laryngeal elevation. Hyoid bone *(white arrow)* is almost at level of mandible. Pharynx *(between large arrows)* is completely distended with barium.

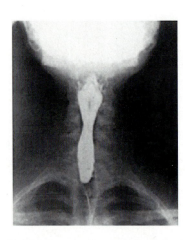

Fig. 15-13. AP projection. Same patient as in Fig. 15-12. Epiglottis divides bolus into two streams, filling piriform recess below. Barium can also be seen entering upper esophagus.

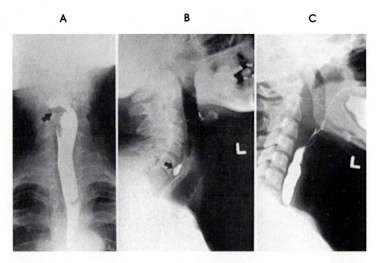

A   B   C

Fig. 15-14. AP projection of pharynx and upper esophagus with barium. **A,** Head has been turned to right, with resultant asymmetric filling of pharynx. Bolus is passing through left piriform recess, leaving right side unfilled *(arrow)*. **B,** Lateral projection after swallowing barium, showing a diverticulum *(arrow)*. **C,** Lateral projection made slightly late shows only filling of upper esophagus.

(Courtesy Edward F. Gunson.)

Gunson method

Gunson[1] offered a practical suggestion for synchronizing the exposure with the height of the swallowing act in deglutition studies of the pharynx and superior esophagus. Gunson's method consists of tying a dark-colored shoestring (metal tips removed) snugly around the patient's throat above the thyroid cartilage (Fig. 15-15). The anterior and superior movement of the larynx is then shown by the elevation of the shoestring as the thyroid cartilage moves anteriorly and, immediately thereafter, by the displacement of the shoestring as the cartilage passes superiorly.

[1]Gunson EF: Radiography of the pharynx and upper esophagus: shoestring method, Xray Techn 33:1-8, 1961.

It is desirable to have the exposure coincide with the peak of the anterior movement of the larynx, the instant at which the bolus of contrast material is projected into the pharynx, but, as stated by Templeton and Kredel,[2] the action is so rapid that satisfactory filling is usually obtained if the exposure is made as soon as the anterior movement is noted.

[2]Templeton FE and Kredel RA: The cricopharyngeal sphincter, Laryngoscope 53:1-12, 1943.

A   B   C

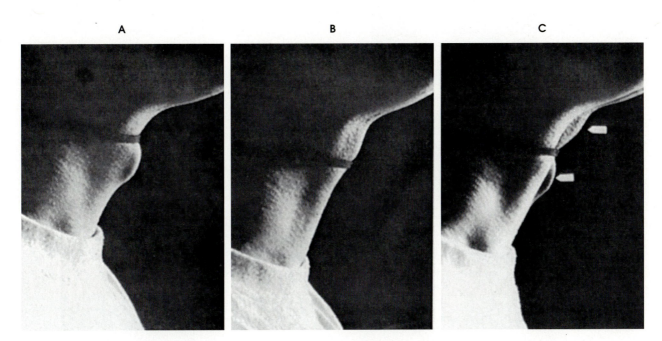

Fig. 15-15. A, Ordinary dark shoelace has been tied snugly around patient's neck above Adam's apple. **B,** Exposure was made at peak of superior and anterior movement of larynx during swallowing. At this moment, pharynx is completely filled with barium, representing ideal instant for making x-ray exposure. **C,** Double-exposure photograph emphasizing movement of Adam's apple during swallowing. Note extent of anterior as well as superior excursion *(arrows).*

(Courtesy Edward F. Gunson.)

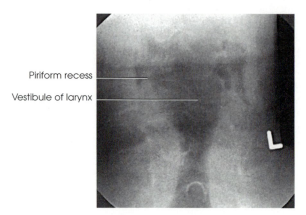

Piriform recess

Vestibule of larynx

L

Fig. 15-16. AP projection during inspiration.

(Courtesy Dr. Judah Zizmor.)

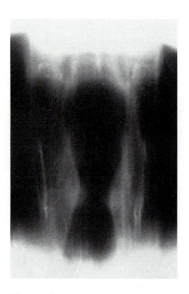

Fig. 15-17. AP projection linear tomogram during inspiration.

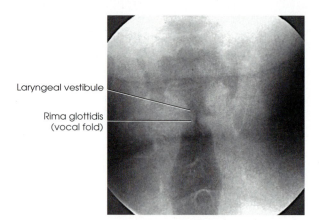

Laryngeal vestibule

Rima glottidis
(vocal fold)

Fig. 15-18. AP projection during phonation of "e-e-e."

(Courtesy Dr. Judah Zizmor.)

Laryngopharyngography

Stationary or tomographic negative-contrast studies of the air-containing laryngopharyngeal structures are made in both AP and lateral projections, the latter in the upright position with a soft tissue radiographic technique. AP projections are made with the patient in either the supine or the seated-upright position, with the head extended enough to prevent superimposition of the mandibular shadow on that of the larynx.

Negative-contrast studies of the laryngopharyngeal structures provide considerable information concerning any alteration in the normal anatomy and function of these organs. Both negative- and positive-contrast AP projections are made during the following respiratory and stress maneuvers.

Quiet inspiration

Quiet inspiration tests abduction of the vocal cords. The resultant radiograph should show the cords open (abducted), with an uninterrupted column of air extending from the laryngeal vestibule inferiorly into the trachea (Figs. 15-16 and 15-17).

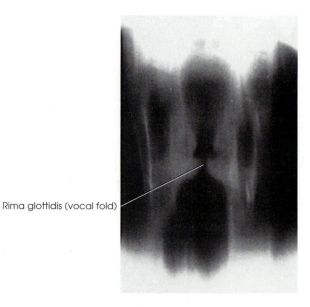

Rima glottidis (vocal fold)

Fig. 15-19. AP projection linear tomogram during phonation of "e-e-e."

Normal (expiratory) phonation

Normal (expiratory) phonation tests adduction of the vocal cords.

Instruct the patient to take a deep breath and then, exhaling slowly, to phonate either a high-pitched "e-e-e" or a low-pitched "a-a-h." The resultant image should show the closed (adducted) vocal cords just above the break in the air column at the closed rima glottidis (Figs. 15-18 and 15-19).

Phonation is normally performed during expiration. This test is now generally referred to as normal or expiratory phonation to distinguish it from the following test.

Inspiratory phonation

Powers et al.[1] introduced the use of inspiratory phonation (also called reverse phonation and aspirate or aspirant maneuver) for the demonstration of the laryngeal ventricle.

Instruct the patient to exhale completely. Then, have the patient slowly inhale while making a harsh, stridulous sound with the phonation of "e" or another high-pitched sound. This test adducts the vocal cords, moves them inferiorly, and balloons the ventricle for clear delineation (Fig. 15-20).

[1]Powers WE, Holtz S, and Ogura J: Contrast examination of the larynx and pharynx: inspiratory phonation, AJR 92:40-42, 1964.

Valsalva maneuver

Valsalva maneuver shows complete closure of the glottis. This maneuver tests the elasticity and functional integrity of the glottis (Fig. 15-21).

For the true Valsalva maneuver, ask the patient to take a deep breath. Then, have the patient hold the breath in while bearing down as if trying to move the bowels. This act forces the breath against the closed glottis, and it increases both intrathoracic and intra-abdominal pressure.

Modified Valsalva maneuver

Modified Valsalva maneuver tests the elasticity of the laryngeal pharynx (hypopharynx) and the piriform recesses. The resultant radiograph should show the glottis closed and the laryngeal pharynx and piriform recesses distended with air (Fig. 15-22).

For the modified Valsalva maneuver, ask the patient to pinch the nostrils together with the thumb and forefinger of one hand. Then, have the patient keep the mouth closed while making and sustaining a slight effort to blow the nose. Another way is to have the patient blow the cheeks outward against the closed nostrils and mouth as if blowing into a horn or balloon.

Each maneuver to be employed must be carefully explained and demonstrated just before its use and the patient required to perform the maneuver one or more times until able to perform it correctly.

Tomolaryngography

Tomographic studies of the laryngopharyngeal structures, either before or after the introduction of a radiopaque contrast medium, are made in the frontal plane. One set is usually made during quiet inspiration (Fig. 15-17) and one during normal (expiratory) phonation (Fig. 15-19), but the stress maneuvers are used as indicated. The rapid-travel linear sweep is generally considered to be the technique of choice for these studies, and the exposures are made during the first half of a wide arc (40 to 50 degrees) to prevent overlap streaking by the facial bones and teeth.

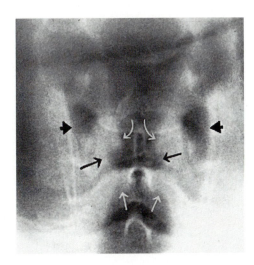

Fig. 15-20. AP projection. Inspiratory phonation showing laryngeal ventricle *(horizontal black arrows)*, false vocal cords *(curved white arrows)*, true vocal folds *(straight white arrows)* and piriform recesses *(black arrowheads)*.

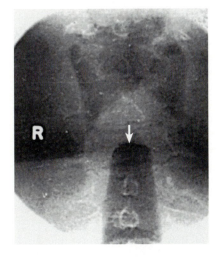

Fig. 15-21. AP projection. True Valsalva maneuver showing closed glottis *(arrow)*.

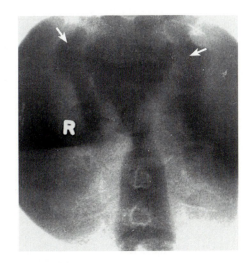

Fig. 15-22. AP projection. Modified Valsalva maneuver showing air-filled piriform recesses *(arrows)*.

Positive-contrast laryngopharyngography

Positive-contrast examinations of the larynx and laryngopharynx (hypopharynx) are usually performed to determine the exact site, size, and extent of tumor masses of these structures. The examination is carried out using fluoroscopy with the use of spot radiographs and/or cineradiographic recordings.

An iodized oil, in conjunction with the examination procedure described by Powers et al.,[1] is the medium most commonly used, although other radiopaque media are employed (see bibliography). In this procedure a mild sedative may be administered before the examination. The following steps are then observed:

- After satisfactory preliminary radiographs, and with the patient seated upright, anesthetize the laryngopharyngeal structures with a topical anesthetic to inhibit the gag, cough, and deglutition reflexes if needed.

- Give the patient explicit instructions on each of the test maneuvers to be used.
- Caution the patient to avoid coughing and swallowing after the introduction of the radiopaque medium (Figs. 15-23 to 15-25).
- A syringe loaded with the specified amount of iodized oil is attached to a curved metal cannula for the administration of the medium. With the patient seated upright, the radiologist slowly drips the iodized oil over the back of the tongue or directly into the larynx, coating all structures of the larynx and laryngopharynx. The patient is then examined fluoroscopically, and spot radiographs are exposed at the height of each of the various test maneuvers. Some examiners obtain cineradiographic recordings with a continuous catheter drip of thin barium or iodized oil into the larynx.

[1]Powers WE, McGee HH, and Seaman WB: Contrast examination of the larynx and pharynx, Radiology 68:169-178, 1957.

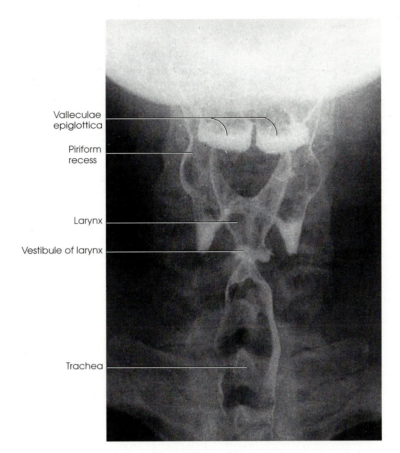

Valleculae
epiglottica

Piriform
recess

Larynx

Vestibule of larynx

Trachea

Fig. 15-23. Normal AP laryngogram.

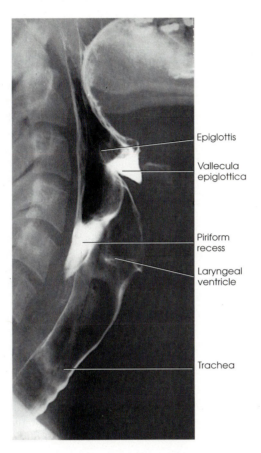

Epiglottis

Vallecula
epiglottica

Piriform
recess

Laryngeal
ventricle

Trachea

Fig. 15-24. Normal lateral laryngogram.

A

B

C

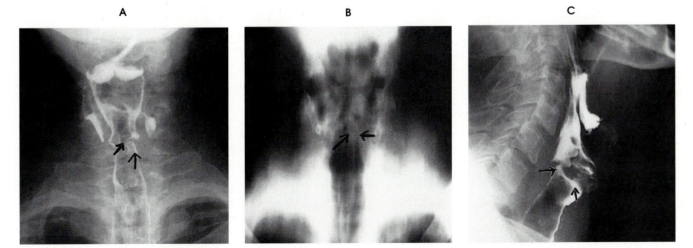

Fig. 15-25. A, AP projection. **B,** Tomogram showing rounded soft tissue mass involving two-thirds of left cord hanging down into subglottic larynx *(arrows).* **C,** On lateral projection this is best demonstrated with Valsalva maneuver.

Thyroid Gland
METHODS OF EXAMINATION

Radiographic examination of the thyroid gland is not performed regularly at most health care facilities. The thyroid gland is effectively evaluated using CT, nuclear medicine, or ultrasound.

The thyroid gland is enclosed within a capsule and is situated in the middle portion of the neck surrounding the front and sides of the superior area of the trachea. It normally extends from the lower third of the thyroid cartilage inferiorly for a distance of 2 inches (5 cm) to about the level of the first thoracic vertebra. The thyroid gland is subject to a variety of abnormalities, the most frequently observed change being enlargement, which results in swelling (called a *goiter*) in the front aspect of the neck. The enlargement may be either diffuse or nodular, depending on the nature of the abnormality present. It may be confined to the neck, or a portion of the enlarged gland may protrude into the superior thoracic cavity behind the sternum, in which case it is called an intrathoracic, retrosternal, or substernal goiter. The normal thyroid gland is not discernible on AP projections of the neck, and only the narrow median portion, the isthmus, is visualized on lateral projections (Figs. 15-26 and 15-27).

Diffuse enlargement of the thyroid gland usually requires no more than AP and lateral projections of the neck and chest. These radiographs generally demonstrate any intrathoracic extension of the gland, any compression or displacement of the trachea by the enlarged gland, the presence of any calcium deposits, and the need for further evaluation. Following are some guidelines for their use:

- Use the lateral projection of the neck for the demonstration of an intrathoracic extension of the goiter when the shoulders cannot otherwise be rotated posteriorly enough to clear the superior mediastinum.
- When nodular enlargement is present, obtain oblique studies of the neck.
- For these, adjust the patient to place the thyroid mass tangent to the film.

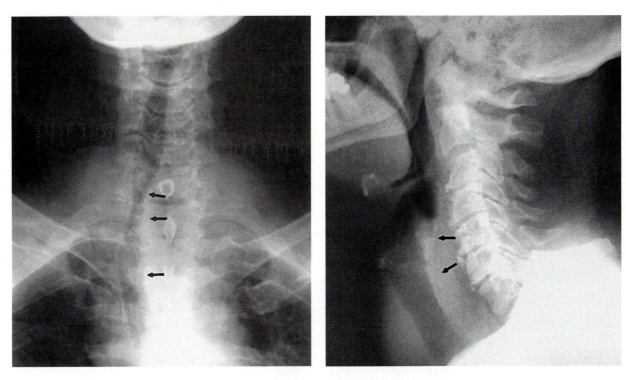

Fig. 15-26. AP and right lateral projections demonstrating benign suprasternal and substernal enlargement of thyroid gland, showing compression, narrowing, and displacement of trachea to right *(arrows)*.

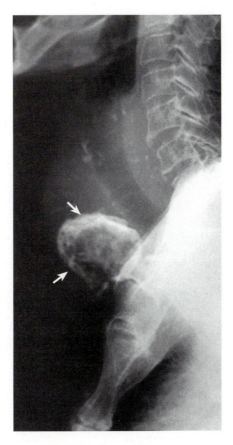

Fig. 15-27. Lateral projection. Calcified hematoma of thyroid gland *(arrows)*.

Pharynx and Larynx
AP PROJECTION

Radiographic studies of the pharyngolaryngeal structures are made during breathing, phonation, stress maneuvers, and swallowing. To minimize the incidence of motion, the shortest possible exposure time must be used in the examinations. For the purpose of obtaining improved contrast on the AP projections, the use of a grid is recommended.

Film: 8 × 10 in (18 × 24 cm) or 10 × 12 in (24 × 30 cm) lengthwise.

Position of patient

- Except for tomographic studies, which require a recumbent body position (Fig. 15-28), place the patient in the upright position, either seated or standing, whenever possible.

Position of part

- Center the median sagittal plane of the body to the midline of the vertical grid device.
- Ask the patient to sit or stand straight; in the latter position, have the patient distribute the weight of the body equally on the feet.
- Adjust the patient's shoulders to lie in the same horizontal plane to prevent rotation of the head and neck, with resultant obliquity of the throat structures.
- Center the cassette at the level of or just below the laryngeal prominence.
- Extend the patient's head only enough to prevent the mandibular shadow from obscuring the laryngeal area.
- *Shield gonads.*
- *Respiration:* Make preliminary radiographs, both AP and lateral, during the inspiratory phase of quiet nasal breathing to ensure filling the throat passages with air. To easily determine the optimum time for the exposure, watch the breathing movements of the chest. Make the exposure *just before* the chest comes to rest at the end of one of its inspiratory expansions (Figs. 15-29 and 15-30).

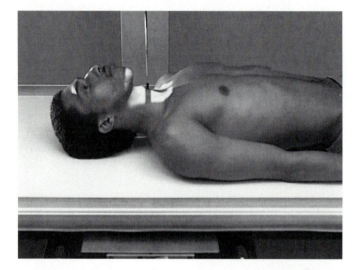

Fig. 15-28. AP pharynx and larynx. Supine position for tomography.

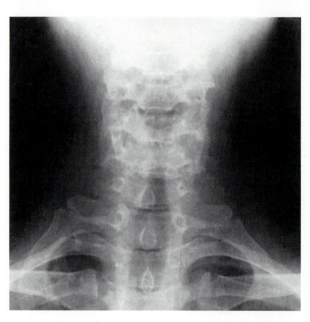

Fig. 15-29. AP pharynx and larynx. Quiet breathing.

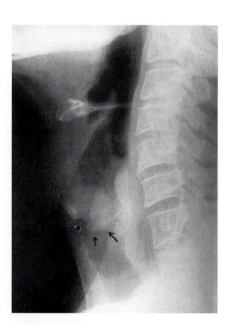

Fig. 15-30. Lateral pharynx and larynx. Polypoid mass of right false fold hanging into subglottic larynx *(arrows).*

Central ray

- Direct the central ray perpendicular to the laryngeal prominence.

Further studies of the pharynx and larynx (the procedure or procedures to be employed usually determined fluoroscopically) may be made at the following times:

1. During the Valsalva and/or the modified Valsalva stress maneuvers (Fig. 15-31). (See the initial descriptions of the Valsalva and modified Valsalva effects under "Laryngography" in the previous section of this chapter.)
2. At the height of the act of swallowing a bolus of 1 tablespoon of creamy barium sulfate suspension. Ask the patient to hold the barium sulfate bolus in the mouth until signaled and then to swallow it in one movement. Then ask the patient to refrain from swallowing again if a double-contrast study is to be attempted.
3. During the modified Valsalva maneuver immediately after the barium swallow for double-contrast delineation of the piriform recesses.
4. During phonation and/or with the larynx in the rest position after its opacification with an iodinated contrast medium.

Tomographic studies of the larynx are made during the phonation of a high-pitched "e-e-e." Following these tomographic studies of the larynx, one or more sectional studies may be made at the selected level or levels with the larynx at rest (Figs. 15-32 and 15-33).

□ Evaluation criteria

The following should be clearly demonstrated:

- Area from the superimposed mandible and base of the skull to the lung apices and superior mediastinum.
- No overlap of the laryngeal area by the mandible.
- No rotation of neck.
- Throat filled with air in preliminary studies.
- Radiographic density permitting visualization of the pharyngolaryngeal structures.

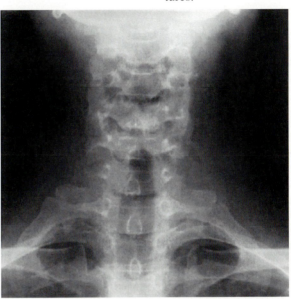

Fig. 15-31. AP pharynx and larynx. Valsalva maneuver.

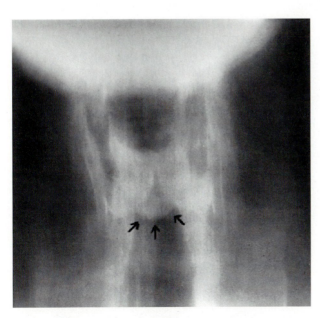

Fig. 15-32. AP pharynx and larynx. Tomogram showing polypoid laryngeal mass (arrows).

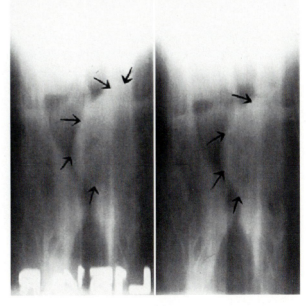

Fig. 15-33. AP pharynx and larynx. Tomograms showing large cyst of left aryepiglottic fold and piriform recess (arrows).

(Courtesy Dr. Judah Zizmor.)

Soft Palate, Pharynx, and Larynx
LATERAL PROJECTION
R or L position

Film: 8 × 10 in (18 × 24 cm) lengthwise.

Position of patient

- Ask the patient to sit or stand laterally before the vertical grid device.
- Adjust the patient so that the coronal plane that passes through or just anterior to the temporomandibular joints is centered to the midline of the film.

Position of part

- Ask the patient to sit or stand straight, with the adjacent shoulder resting firmly against the stand for support.
- Adjust the body so that the median sagittal plane is parallel with the plane of the film.
- Depress the shoulders as much as possible, and adjust them to lie in the same transverse plane; if needed, have the patient clasp the hands in back to posteriorly rotate the shoulders.
- Extend the patient's head slightly.
- Immobilize the head by having the patient fix his or her gaze on an object in line with the patient's visual axis.

Central ray

- With the central ray adjusted to be perpendicular to the film, center the cassette (1) 1 inch (2.5 cm) below the level of the external acoustic (auditory) meatuses for demonstration of the nasopharynx and for cleft palate studies, (2) at the level of the mandibular angles for the demonstration of the oropharynx, or (3) at the level of the laryngeal prominence for the demonstration of the larynx, the laryngeal pharynx, and the upper end of the esophagus (Fig. 15-34).

Procedure

- Make preliminary studies of the pharyngolaryngeal structures, during the inhalation phase of quiet nasal breathing to ensure filling the passages with air (Fig. 15-35).

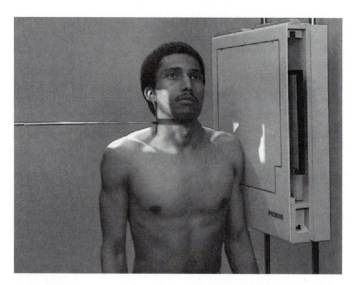

Fig. 15-34. Lateral pharynx and larynx.

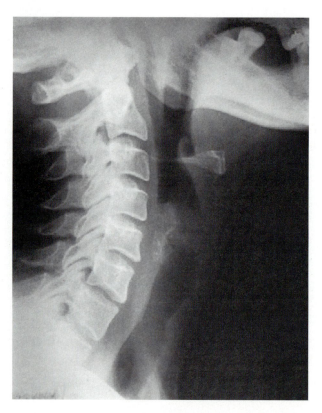

Fig. 15-35. Lateral pharynx and larynx. Normal breathing.

According to the site and nature of the abnormality being investigated, further studies may be made in one or more of the following maneuvers, each of which must be explained to, and practiced by, the patient just before its actual use:

1. During the phonation of specified vowel sounds for the demonstration of the vocal cords and for cleft palate studies (Fig. 15-36).
2. During the Valsalva maneuver to distend the subglottic larynx and trachea with air (Fig. 15-37). (See the initial description of the Valsalva maneuver under "Laryngography" earlier in this chapter.)
3. During the modified Valsalva maneuver to distend the supraglottic larynx and the laryngeal pharynx with air. (See the initial description of the modified Valsalva maneuver under "Laryngography" earlier in this chapter.)

4. At the height of the act of swallowing a bolus of 1 tablespoon of creamy barium sulfate suspension for the demonstration of the pharyngeal structures.
5. Of the larynx at rest or during phonation following its opacification with an iodinated medium.
6. During the act of swallowing a tuft or pledget of cotton (or food) saturated with a barium sulfate suspension for the demonstration of nonopaque foreign bodies located in the pharynx or upper esophagus.

□ **Evaluation criteria**

The following should be clearly demonstrated:

- Soft tissue density of the pharyngolaryngeal structures.
- Area from the nasopharynx to the uppermost part of the lungs in preliminary studies.
- Specific area of interest centered in detailed examinations.
- No superimposition of the trachea by the shoulders.
- Closely superimposed mandibular shadows.
- Throat filled with air in preliminary studies.

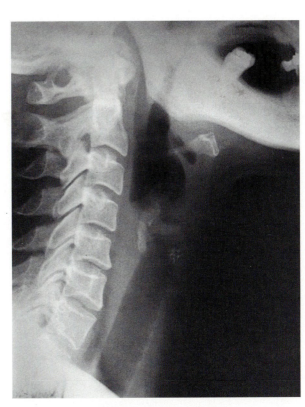

Fig. 15-36. Lateral pharynx and larynx. Phonating "e-e-e."

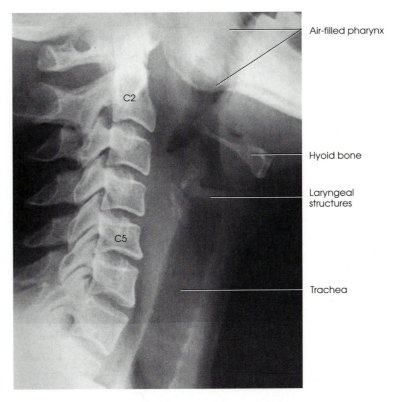

Fig. 15-37. Lateral pharynx and larynx. Valsalva maneuver.

C2

C5

Air-filled pharynx

Hyoid bone

Laryngeal structures

Trachea

Chapter 16
DIGESTIVE SYSTEM

Abdomen, Liver, Spleen, Biliary Tract

Patient positioned for an AP abdomen; 1940s.

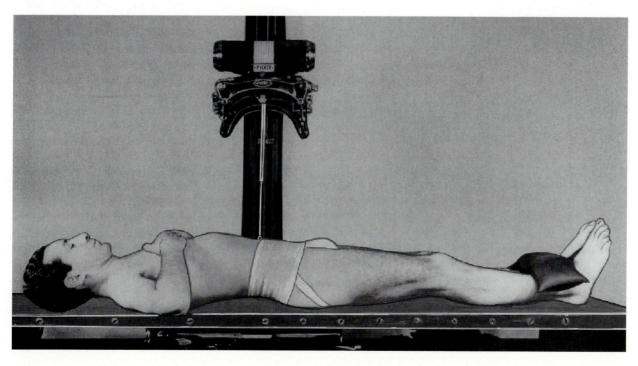

The digestive system consists of the alimentary tract (described in Chapter 17) and certain accessory organs that contribute to the digestive process.

The radiologically important accessory organs of the digestive system are the teeth, which serve to masticate the food; the salivary glands, which secrete fluid into the mouth for the salivation of food; and the liver and pancreas, which secrete specialized digestive juices into the small intestine.

The anatomy and positioning of the oral, cervical, and thoracic portions of the digestive system are described in Chapters 14, 15, and 10, respectively.

Peritoneum

The abdominopelvic cavity encloses a double-walled, seromembranous sac called the *peritoneal sac*. The outer, or parietal, layer of the peritoneum closely adheres to the abdominal and greater (false) pelvic walls and to most of the undersurface of the diaphragm. The inner, or visceral, layer is reflected over or around the contained organs and forms folds called the *mesentery* and *omenta,* which serve to support the viscera in position. The narrow space between the two layers, or walls, of the peritoneum is called the *peritoneal cavity*. The peritoneum does not adhere to the walls of the lesser (true, or minor) pelvis, except at its superior reaches. This nonadhering peritoneum allows pelvic surgery to be performed without entry into the peritoneal cavity.

Liver and Biliary System

The *liver,* a massive, irregularly wedge-shaped gland, is situated with its base on the right and its apex directed anteriorly and to the left (Fig. 16-1). The adult liver measures approximately 8½ inches (21.5 cm) transversely at its widest point, 6½ inches (16.5 cm) vertically at its longest point, and 4½ inches (11 cm) anteroposteriorly at its deepest point. The deepest point of the liver is the inferior aspect just above the right kidney. The diaphragmatic surface of the liver is convex, conforms to the undersurface of the diaphragm and the anterior wall of the abdomen, and is attached to a fold of peritoneum called the *falciform ligament*. This diaphragmatic surface is extensive and is divided into the superior, anterior, right, and posterior parts. The posterior surface slants inferiorly and anteriorly to the visceral surface. The visceral surface is concave and molded over the subjacent viscera on which it rests. Almost all of the right hypochondrium and a large part of the epigastrium are occupied by the liver. The right portion extends inferiorly into the right lateral region as far as the fourth lumbar vertebra, and the left extremity extends across the left hypochondrium as far as the mammary line.

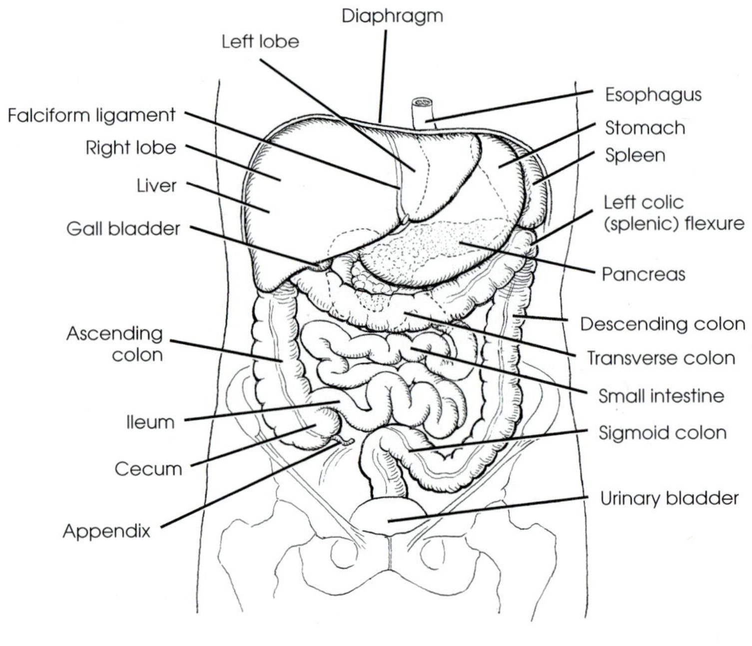

Anatomically, the liver is divided into two major lobes at the falciform ligament: a large right lobe and a much smaller left lobe. Two minor lobes are located on the medial side of the right lobe (the *caudale lobe* on the posterior surface and the *quadrate* lobe on the inferior surface, Figs. 16-1 to 16-3). The hilum of the liver, called the porta hepatis (porta), is situated transversely between the two minor lobes. The porta hepatis transmits the hepatic artery, the portal vein, and the hepatic bile ducts; the branches of these three vessels accompany each other in their ramifications through the liver. The sulcus, a deep groove through which the inferior vena cava passes, is located on the posterior surface of the liver and separates the caudate lobe from the right lobe proper. The hepatic veins empty into the inferior vena cava. The fossa for the gall bladder lies on the posteroinferior surface of the right lobe, just below the porta hepatis (porta) and beside the quadrate lobe.

The liver is composed of minute lobules held together by a delicate connective tissue. The terminal branches of the hepatic artery and the portal vein and the beginning branches of the hepatic veins and the bile ducts are transmitted through the liver. Each lobule contains a mass of hepatic cells arranged in irregular columns between blood capillaries and capillary-like blood channels called *sinusoids*. The sinusoids pass from the periphery to the center of the lobule, where they empty into a central vein. The central vein, extending the length of the lobule, opens into a beginning branch of the hepatic vein. The bile capillaries arise from the cells and converge toward the periphery of the lobule, where they unite to form the beginning branches of the bile ducts.

The *portal vein* and the *hepatic artery,* both of which convey blood to the liver, enter the porta hepatis (porta) and branch out through the liver substance. The portal vein ends in the sinusoids, and the hepatic artery ends in capillaries that communicate with sinusoids. Thus, in addition to the usual arterial blood supply, the liver receives blood from the portal system. The portal system, of which the portal vein is the main trunk, consists of the veins arising from the walls of the stomach, from the greater part of the intestinal tract and the gall bladder, and from the pancreas and the spleen. The blood circulating through these organs is rich in nutrients and is carried to the liver for modifi-

Fig. 16-1. Anterior aspect of abdominal viscera in relation to surrounding structures.

Labels: Diaphragm, Left lobe, Falciform ligament, Right lobe, Liver, Gall bladder, Ascending colon, Ileum, Cecum, Appendix, Esophagus, Stomach, Spleen, Left colic (splenic) flexure, Pancreas, Descending colon, Transverse colon, Small intestine, Sigmoid colon, Urinary bladder

cation before being returned to the heart. The hepatic veins convey the blood from the liver sinusoids to the inferior vena cava.

The liver has numerous physiologic functions. The primary consideration from the radiographic standpoint is the formation of bile. The gland secretes bile at the rate of 1 to 3 pints (½ to 1½ liters) each day. Bile, the channel of elimination for the waste products of red blood cell destruction, is an excretion as well as a secretion. As a secretion, it is an important aid in the emulsification and assimilation of fats. The bile is collected from the liver cells by the ducts and either carried to the gall bladder for temporary storage or poured directly into the duodenum through the common bile duct.

The biliary, or excretory, system of the liver consists of the bile ducts and the gall bladder (Figs. 16-3 and 16-4). Beginning within the lobules as bile capillaries, the ducts unite to form larger and larger passages as they converge, finally forming two main ducts, one leading from each major lobe. The two main hepatic ducts emerge at the porta hepatis (porta) and join to form the *common hepatic duct,* which, in turn, unites with the *cystic duct* to form the *common bile duct.* The hepatic and cystic ducts are each about 1½ inches (4 cm) in length. The common bile duct passes inferiorly for a distance of approximately 3 inches (7.5 cm). The common bile duct joins the pancreatic duct, and they enter together or side by side into an enlarged chamber known as the *hepatopancreatic ampulla* (ampulla of Vater). The ampulla opens into the descending portion of the duodenum through the greater duodenal papilla. In 80% of subjects, the ducts open into the descending portion of the duodenum side by side but remain separated by a thin membrane. The distal end of the common bile duct is controlled by the *bile duct sphincter* (sphincter choledochus) as it enters the duodenum. The hepatopancreatic ampulla is controlled by a circular muscle known as the *sphincter of the hepatopancreatic ampulla* (sphincter of Oddi). During interdigestive periods, the sphincter remains in a contracted state, thus routing most of the bile into the gall bladder for concentration and temporary storage; during digestion, it relaxes to permit the bile to flow from the liver and gall bladder into the duodenum.

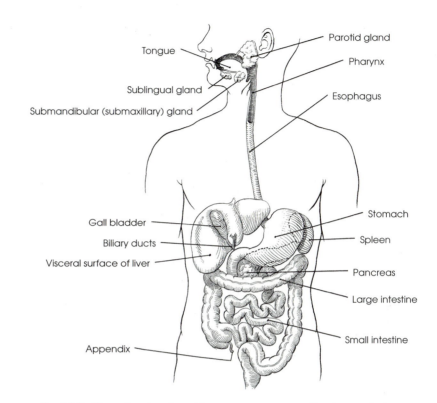

Fig. 16-2. Alimentary tract and its accessory organs. (To demonstrate the position of the gall bladder in relation to the liver, the liver is shown with the inferior portion pulled anteriorly and superiorly, thus placing the liver in an atypical position. The true relationship of the liver and gall bladder is seen in Fig. 16-1.)

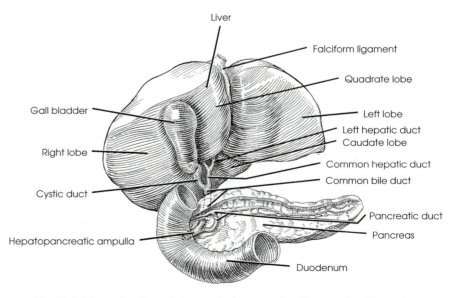

Fig. 16-3. Visceral surface (inferoposterior aspect) of liver and gall bladder.

The *gall bladder* is a thin-walled, more or less pear-shaped musculomembranous sac with a capacity of approximately 2 ounces. The gall bladder functions to concentrate bile by absorption of the water content, to store bile during interdigestive periods, and, by the contraction of its musculature, to evacuate the bile during digestion. The muscular contraction of the gall bladder is activated by a hormone called *cholecystokinin*. This hormone is secreted by the duodenal mucosa and liberated into the blood when fatty or acid chyme passes into the intestine. The organ consists of a narrow neck that is continuous with the cystic duct; of a body, or main portion; and of a fundus, which is its broad lower portion. The gall bladder is usually lodged in a fossa on the visceral (inferior) surface of the right lobe of the liver, where it lies in an oblique plane from above inferiorly and anteriorly. Measuring about 1 inch (2.5 cm) in width at its widest part and 3 to 4 inches (7.5 to 10 cm) in length, it extends from the lower right margin of the porta hepatis (porta) to a variable distance below the anterior border of the liver. The position of the gall bladder varies with bodily habitus, being high and well away from the midline in hypersthenic persons and low and near the spine in asthenic individuals. The gall bladder is sometimes embedded in the liver and frequently hangs free below the inferior margin of the liver.

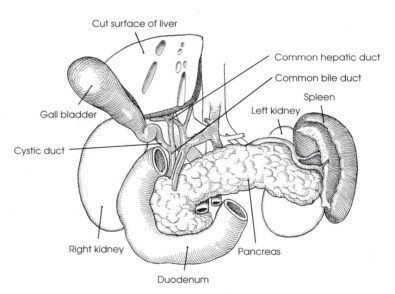

Fig. 16-4. Visceral (inferoposterior) surface of gall bladder and bile ducts.

Pancreas and Spleen

The *pancreas* is an elongated, racemose gland situated across the posterior abdominal wall. Reaching from the duodenum to the spleen (Fig. 16-5), the pancreas is about 5½ inches (14 cm) in length and consists of a head, a neck, a body, and a tail. The head, which is the broadest portion of the organ, extends inferiorly and is enclosed within the curve of the duodenum at the level of the second or third lumbar vertebra. The neck is the slightly constricted portion connecting the head and the body; it lies immediately below the pylorus, which rests on its upper anterior surface. The body and tail of the pancreas pass transversely behind the stomach and in front of the left kidney, the narrow tail terminating near the spleen. The pancreas cannot be visualized on plain radiographic studies.

The pancreas is both an exocrine and an endocrine gland. The exocrine cells of the pancreas are arranged in lobules with a highly ramified duct system. This exocrine portion of the gland produces *pancreatic juice,* which acts on proteins, fats, and carbohydrates. The endocrine portion of the gland consists of the *islet cells* (islets of Langerhans), which are randomly distributed throughout the pancreas. Each islet consists of clusters of cells surrounding small groups of capillaries. These cells produce the hormones *insulin* and *glucagon,* which are responsible for sugar metabolism. The islet cells do not communicate directly with the ducts but release their secretions directly into the blood through a rich capillary network.

The digestive juice secreted by the exocrine cells of the pancreas is conveyed into the *pancreatic duct* (duct of Wirsung) and from there into the duodenum. The pancreatic duct often unites with the common bile duct to form a single passage via the hepatopancreatic ampulla (ampulla of Vater), which opens directly into the descending duodenum. However, this arrangement varies. The two ducts (common bile and pancreatic) sometimes remain divided until their common termination at the sphincter of the hepatopancreatic ampulla (sphincter of Oddi). The pancreatic duct then opens directly into the duodenum instead of communicating with the common bile duct through the ampulla of the biliary duct. An accessory pancreatic duct (duct of Santorini) is sometimes present; it opens into the duodenum independently.

The *spleen* is included in this section only because of its location; it belongs to the lymphatic system. The spleen is a glandlike but ductless organ that functions to produce lymphocytes and to store and remove dead or dying red blood cells. The spleen is more or less bean-shaped and measures about 5 inches (14 cm) in length, 3 inches (7.5 cm) in width, and 1½ inches (4 cm) in thickness. Situated obliquely in the left upper quadrant, the spleen is just below the diaphragm and behind the stomach. It is in contact with the abdominal wall laterally, with the left suprarenal (adrenal) gland and left kidney medially, and with the left colic (splenic) flexure of the colon inferiorly. The spleen is visualized both with and without contrast media.

To review the location of the gall bladder and stomach as they change with body habitus, see Volume 1, Chapter 3 of this atlas.

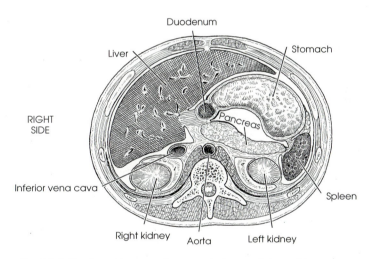

ANTERIOR SURFACE

Duodenum
Liver
Stomach
RIGHT SIDE
Pancreas
Inferior vena cava
Spleen
Right kidney
Aorta
Left kidney

Fig. 16-5. Sectional image of upper abdomen (viewed from the patient's feet) showing relationship of digestive system components.

Digestive system

A complete radiologic investigation of gastrointestinal disorders may include an examination of (1) the paranasal sinuses and teeth for the detection of lesions or localized infections, (2) the abdomen as a whole for the detection of any condition such as renal stones and tumor masses that might cause referred symptoms, (3) the liver and gall bladder, and (4) the several portions of the alimentary tract for the detection of any local lesion. The extent of the examination of each patient, however, depends on the site, type, and extent of pathologic involvement. A patient usually receives a complete examination, that is, an examination of each of the regions listed above, only when the symptoms are obscure—when the cause of the digestive disturbance has not been localized.

Radiologists differ somewhat on certain details of the procedures employed in examining the different parts of the gastrointestinal tract and its accessory organs; however, the various techniques are similar. For an optimal examination of the abdomen, the intestinal tract should be evacuated of gas and fecal material to obtain an unobstructed image of the contained viscera. The technique employed to clear the intestinal tract depends on whether the survey radiographs are preliminary to a specialized examination and on the condition of the patient.

Demonstration of the gastrointestinal tract requires the use of a contrast medium as well as specific preliminary preparation, both of which vary according to the region being investigated. Each physician has an established routine covering the preparation of the patient under varying circumstances, the selected contrast medium, and the radiographic procedure employed in examinations of the gall bladder and other gastrointestinal organs.

The procedures generally employed in examinations of the alimentary tract and its accessory organs will be considered under the following headings:

1. Abdomen
2. Liver and spleen
3. Biliary tract
   a. Gall bladder
4. Pancreas
5. Alimentary tract (Chapter 17)
   a. Esophagus
   b. Stomach
   c. Small intestine
   d. Large intestine

Abdomen
PRELIMINARY PROCEDURES AND POSITIONS

Preparation

Careful preliminary preparation of the intestinal tract is important in radiologic investigations of the abdominal viscera. In the presence of nonacute conditions, the preparation can consist of any combination of controlled diet, laxative, or enemas. The preparation ordered is generally determined by the medical facility in which the examination is to be performed.

Although many patients referred for an examination of the abdomen are well enough to undergo routine preparation, a number have, or are suspected of having, some condition that removes them from the "routine" classification even though they are not acutely ill. In such cases, the referring physician is consulted as to the presumptive diagnosis, and the procedure is varied as needed. Preliminary preparation is never administered to acutely ill patients, to those who have a condition such as intestinal obstruction or perforation, or to those who have a visceral rupture.

Exposure technique

In examinations of the abdomen without a contrast medium, it is imperative to obtain maximum soft tissue differentiation throughout its different regions. Because of the wide range in the thickness of the abdomen and the delicate differences in physical density between the contained viscera, it is necessary to use a more critical exposure technique than is required to demonstrate the difference in density between an opacified organ and the structures adjacent to it. The exposure factors should therefore be adjusted to produce a radiograph with moderate gray tones and less black-and-white contrast. If the kVp is too high, the possibility of not demonstrating small or semiopaque gallstones increases. Some individuals suggest the kVp for the sthenic patient be held to approximately 70 kVp (Fig. 16-6).

A sharply defined outline of the psoas muscles, the lower border of the liver, the kidneys, the ribs, and the transverse processes of the lumbar vertebrae are the best criteria for judging the quality of an abdominal radiograph.

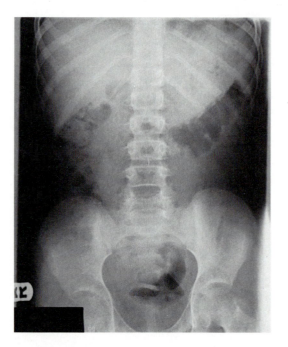

Fig. 16-6. AP abdomen projection showing proper positioning and collimation.

(Courtesy Elizabeth Zaffuto, R.T.)

Immobilization

One of the prime requisites in abdominal examinations is the prevention of movement, both voluntary and involuntary. The following steps are observed:

- To prevent muscle contraction caused by tenseness, adjust the patient in a comfortable position so that he or she can relax.
- Explain the breathing procedure and make sure the patient understands exactly what is expected.
- If needed, apply a compression band across the abdomen for *immobilization* but not compression.
- Do not start the exposure for 1 to 2 seconds after the suspension of respiration, to allow the patient to come to rest and to allow involuntary movement of the viscera to subside.

Voluntary motion produces a blurred outline of the structures that do not have involuntary movement, such as the liver, psoas muscles, and the spine. Involuntary motion caused by peristalsis may produce either a localized or a generalized haziness of the image. Involuntary contraction of the abdominal wall or of the muscles around the spine may cause movement of the entire abdominal area and produce generalized radiographic haziness.

Radiographic projections

Radiography of the abdomen may include one or more radiographic projections. The most commonly performed is the supine AP projection, often called a KUB because it includes the *k*idneys, *u*reters, and *b*ladder. Projections used to complement the supine AP may include an upright AP abdomen and/or an AP projection in the lateral decubitus position (the left lateral decubitus is most often preferred). Both radiographs are useful in assessing the abdomen in cases of visceroptosis (prolapse or falling down of the abdominal viscera) and in determining air-fluid levels. Other abdominal projections may include a lateral or a lateral projection in the supine (dorsal decubitus) body position. Many institutions also obtain a PA chest to include the upper abdomen and diaphragm. The PA chest is indicated since any air escaping from the gastrointestinal tract into the peritoneal space will rise to the highest level, usually just beneath the diaphragm.

Radiation protection

General radiation protection techniques must be used. Whether gonadal shielding is used depends on three considerations:

1. Gonadal shielding is desirable if the gonads lie within close proximity (2 inches [5 cm]) to the primary x-ray field despite proper beam limitation.
2. Gonadal shielding should be used if the clinical objectives of the examination will not be compromised. The concern is whether the use of gonadal shielding will cover an area of interest on the radiograph.
3. Gonadal shielding should be used if the patient has a reasonable reproductive potential.

After considering the above criteria and irrespective of the decision reached, all patients must receive close and accurate collimation to limit the x-ray beam. In addition to reducing the amount of radiation exposure to an unnecessary area of the patient, this practice also results in a radiograph with improved quality.

ABDOMINAL RADIOGRAPHY PROCEDURES

Radiographs obtained to evaluate the patient's abdomen vary considerably depending on the institution and physician. For example, some consider the preliminary evaluation radiograph to consist of only the AP (supine) projection. Others take two projections: a supine and an upright AP abdomen (often called a flat and an upright). When evaluating the abdomen to rule out free air and infections, a three-way or acute abdomen series may be requested. The three projections usually include (1) an AP with the patient supine, (2) an AP upright, and (3) a PA chest. If the patient is unable to stand for the upright AP projection, the projection is performed using the left lateral decubitus position. (The PA chest projection can be used to detect free air that may accumulate under the diaphragm as demonstrated in Figs. 16-13 and 16-14.)

Positioning for the above abdomen radiographs is described on the following pages. For a description of positioning for the PA chest, see Chapter 10 in Volume 1 of this atlas.

Abdomen

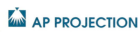

AP PROJECTION

Film: 14 × 17 in (35 × 43 cm) lengthwise.

Position of patient

- For the AP abdomen, or KUB, projection, place the patient either in the supine or upright position. The supine position is preferred for most initial examinations of the abdomen.

Position of part

- Center the median sagittal plane of the body to the midline grid device.
- If the patient is upright, distribute the weight of the body equally on the feet.
- Adjust the shoulders to lie in the same transverse plane, and place the arms where they will not cast shadows on the film.
- With the patient supine, place a support under the knees to relieve strain.
- For the *supine position,* center the cassette at the level of the crests of the ilia (Fig. 16-7).

- For the *upright position,* center the film 2 to 3 inches (5 to 7.5 cm) above the level of the crests of the ilia or high enough to include the diaphragm (Fig. 16-8).
- If the bladder is to be included on the upright radiograph, center at the level of the crests of the ilia.
- If a patient is too tall to include the entire pelvic area, take a second radiograph to include the bladder on a 10 × 12 in (24 × 30 cm) film if needed. The 10 × 12 in (24 × 30 cm) cassette is placed crosswise and centered 2 to 3 inches (5 to 7.5 cm) above the upper border of the symphysis pubis.
- If needed, apply a compression band across the abdomen with moderate pressure for immobilization.
- *Shield gonads*: Use local gonad shielding for examinations of male patients (not shown for illustrative purposes).
- Ask the patient to suspend respiration at the end of exhalation.

Central ray

- Direct the central ray perpendicular to the film at the level of the crests of the ilia for the supine radiograph, or 2 to 3 inches (5 to 7.5 cm) above the level of the crests to include the diaphragm for the upright radiograph.

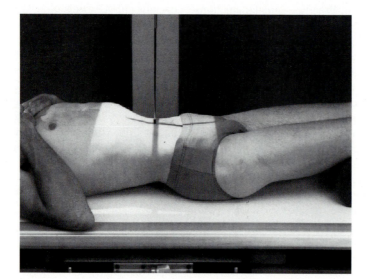

Fig. 16-7. AP abdomen, supine.

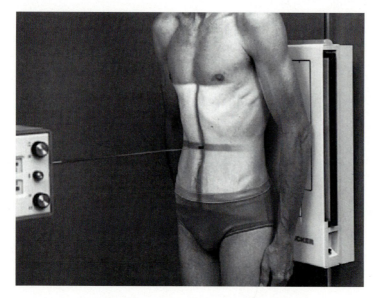

Fig. 16-8. AP abdomen, upright.

Structures shown

An AP projection of the abdomen shows the size and shape of the liver, the spleen and the kidneys, and intra-abdominal calcifications or evidence of tumor masses (Fig. 16-9). (See additional examples of a supine and upright abdomen in Figs. 16-15 and 16-16.)

□ Evaluation criteria

The following should be clearly demonstrated:

■ The area from the symphysis pubis to the upper abdomen. Two radiographs may be needed if the patient is tall.
■ Proper patient alignment ensured by:
  □ Centered vertebral column.
  □ Ribs, pelvis, and hips equidistant to the edge of the radiograph on both sides.
■ No rotation of patient, as indicated by:
  □ Spinous processes in the center of the lumbar vertebrae.
  □ Ischial spines of the pelvis symmetric, if visible.
  □ Alae or wings of the ilia symmetric.
■ Soft tissue gray tones should demonstrate:
  □ Lateral abdominal wall and the properitoneal fat layer.
  □ Psoas muscles, lower border of the liver, and the kidneys.
  □ The inferior ribs.
  □ Transverse processes of the lumbar vertebrae.
■ "RIGHT" or "LEFT" marker visible, but not lying over the abdominal contents.
■ Diaphragm without motion on upright abdomen examinations. Crosswise cassette placement is appropriate if the patient is very large.
■ Density on upright abdomen examination similar to supine examination.
■ Upright abdomen identified with an appropriate marker.

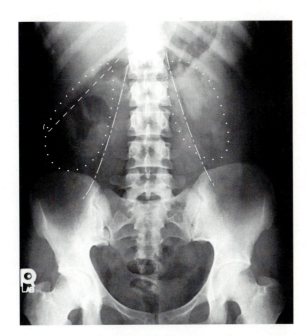 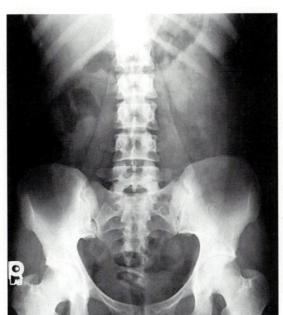

Fig. 16-9. AP abdomen showing kidney shadows *(dotted line)*, margin of liver *(dashed line)*, and psoas muscles *(dot-dash lines)*.

(Courtesy Lois Baird, R.T.)

Abdomen

PA PROJECTION
Upright

When the kidneys are not of primary interest, the upright PA projection should be considered. The PA projection greatly reduces patient gonadal dose compared with the AP projection of the abdomen.

Film: 14 × 17 in (35 × 43 cm) lengthwise.

Position of patient

- With the patient in the upright position, place the anterior abdominal surface in contact with the vertical grid device.
- Center the abdominal midline to the midline of the film.
- Center the film 2 to 3 inches (5 to 7.5 cm) above the level of the crests of the ilia (Fig. 16-10) as previously described for the upright AP projection. The central ray, structures shown, and evaluation criteria are the same as for the upright AP projection.

Abdomen

AP PROJECTION
Left lateral
decubitus position

Film: 14 × 17 in (35 × 43 cm).

Position of patient

- When the patient is too ill to stand, place the patient in a lateral recumbent position lying on a radiolucent pad on a transportation cart.
- A left lateral decubitus position is usually used in place of an upright.
- If possible, have the patient lie on the side for several minutes before the exposure to allow any air to rise to its highest level within the abdomen.
- Place the arms above the level of the diaphragm so that they are not projected over any abdominal contents.
- Flex the patient's knees slightly to provide stabilization.
- Exercise care to ensure that the patient will not fall from the cart and that the wheels of the cart are securely locked in position.

Position of part

- Adjust the height of the vertical grid device so that the long axis of the film is centered to the median sagittal plane.
- Position the patient so that the level of the crests of the ilia are centered to the film. A slightly higher centering point may be needed to ensure that the diaphrams are included on the image (Fig. 16-11).
- Adjust the patient to ensure that a true lateral position is attained.
- *Shield gonads.* (Not shown for illustrative purposes.)
- Ask the patient to suspend respiration at the end of exhalation.

Central ray

- Direct the central ray *horizontal* and perpendicular to the midpoint of the film to enter at the level of the crests of the ilia.

NOTE: A right lateral decubitus position is often requested or it may be required when the patient cannot lie on the left side.

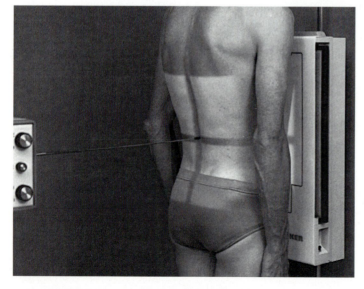

Fig. 16-10. PA abdomen in upright position. Suggested for survey examination of abdomen when kidneys are not of primary interest.

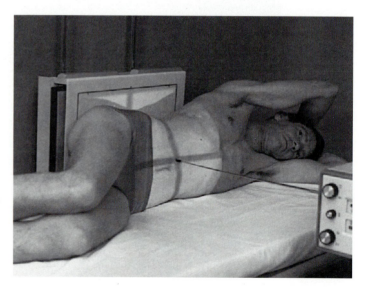

Fig. 16-11. AP abdomen, left lateral decubitus position.

Structures shown

In addition to showing the size and shape of the liver, spleen, and kidneys, the AP abdomen with the patient placed in the left decubitus position is most valuable for demonstrating air-fluid levels when an upright abdomen projection cannot be obtained (Fig. 16-12).

□ Evaluation criteria

The following should be clearly demonstrated:

- Diaphragm without motion.
- Both sides of the abdomen. If not possible:
  - □ Elevate and demonstrate the side down when fluid is suspected.
  - □ Demonstrate the side up when free air is suspected.
- Abdominal wall, flank structures, and the diaphragm.
- No rotation of patient.
- Proper identification visible including patient side and marking to indicate which side is up.

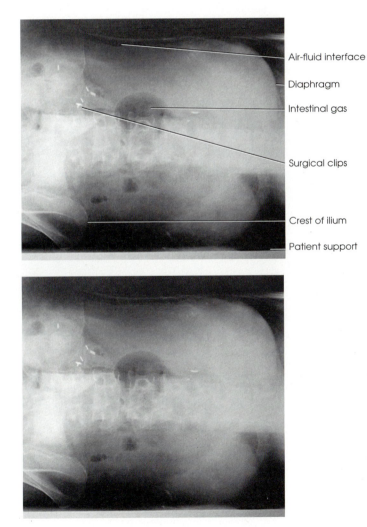

Air-fluid interface

Diaphragm

Intestinal gas

Surgical clips

Crest of ilium

Patient support

Fig. 16-12. AP abdomen, left lateral decubitus position resulting in air marked by the air-fluid interface.

(Courtesy Darla Kaikis, R.T.)

Abdominal sequencing

To demonstrate small amounts of intraperitoneal gas in acute abdominal cases, Miller[1,2] recommends that the patient be kept in the left lateral position on a stretcher for 10 to 20 minutes before performing abdominal radiographs. This position allows the gas to rise into the area under the right hemidiaphragm where the image will not be superimposed by the gastric gas bubble. For larger amounts of free air, many departments suggest the patient lie on the side for a minimum of 5 minutes before the radiograph is produced. Projections of the abdomen are then taken as follows:

- Perform an AP or PA projection of the chest and upper abdomen in the left lateral decubitus position.
- Use chest exposure technique for this radiograph (Fig. 16-13).
- Maintain the patient in the left lateral decubitus position while being moved onto a horizontally placed table. Tilt the table and patient to the upright position.
- Turn the patient to obtain AP or PA projections of the chest and abdomen (Figs. 16-14 and 16-15).
- Return the table back to the horizontal position for a supine AP or PA projection of the abdomen (Fig. 16-16).

---

[1]Miller RE and Nelson SW: The roentgenologic demonstration of tiny amounts of free intraperitoneal gas: experimental and clinical studies, AJR 112:574-585, 1971.

[2]Miller RE: The technical approach to the acute abdomen, Semin Roentgenol 8:267-279, 1973.

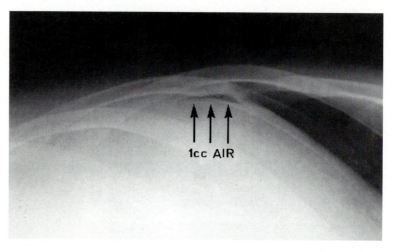

Fig. 16-13. Enlarged portion of an AP abdomen left lateral decubitus position on a patient who was injected with 1 cc of air into the abdominal cavity.

(Courtesy Dr. Roscoe E. Miller.)

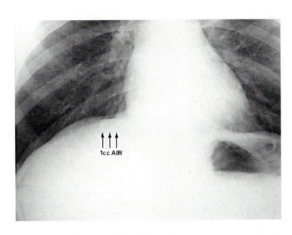

Fig. 16-14. Enlarged portion of an upright AP chest showing free air on same patient as in Fig. 16-13.

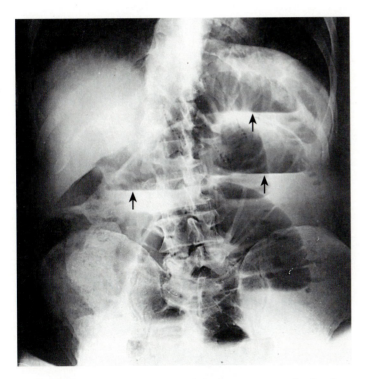

Fig. 16-15. AP abdomen. Upright study on same patient as in Fig. 16-16 showing air-fluid levels *(arrows)* in intestine.

(Courtesy Dr. Hugh M. Wilson.)

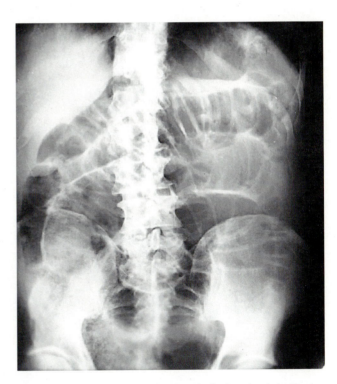

Fig. 16-16. AP abdomen. Supine study showing intestinal obstruction on same patient as in Fig. 16-15.

Abdomen

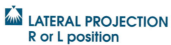

LATERAL PROJECTION
R or L position

Film: 14 × 17 in (35 × 43 cm) length-wise.

Position of patient

- Turn the patient to a lateral recumbent position on either the right or left side.

Position of part

- Flex the patient's knees to a comfortable position, and adjust the body so that the median coronal plane is centered to the midline of the grid.
- Place supports between the knees and the ankles.
- Flex the elbows, and place the hands under the patient's head (Fig. 16-17).
- Center the cassette at the level of the crests of the ilia or high enough to include the diaphragm.
- Place a compression band across the pelvis for stability if needed.
- *Shield gonads.* (Not shown for illustrative purposes.)
- Ask the patient to suspend respiration at the end of exhalation.

Central ray

- Direct the central ray perpendicular to the film, entering the median coronal plane at the level of the crest of ilium.

Structures shown

A lateral projection of the abdomen demonstrates the prevertebral space occupied by the abdominal aorta, as well as any intra-abdominal calcifications or tumor masses (Fig. 16-18).

□ Evaluation criteria

The following should be clearly demonstrated:
- Abdominal contents visible with soft tissue gray tones.
- No rotation of patient, indicated by:
  - □ Superimposed ilia.
  - □ Superimposed lumbar vertebrae pedicles and open intervertebral foramina.
- As much of the remaining abdomen as possible when diaphragm is included.

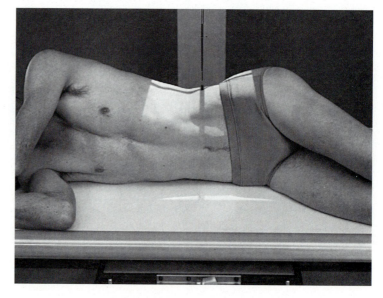

Fig. 16-17. Right lateral abdomen.

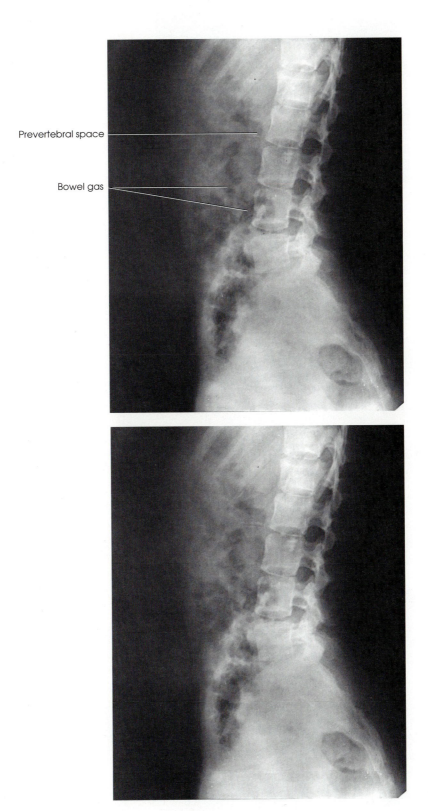

Prevertebral space

Bowel gas

Fig. 16-18. Lateral abdomen.

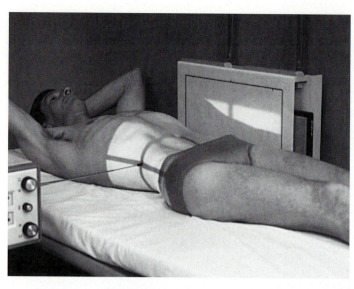

Fig. 16-19. Lateral abdomen, left dorsal decubitus position.

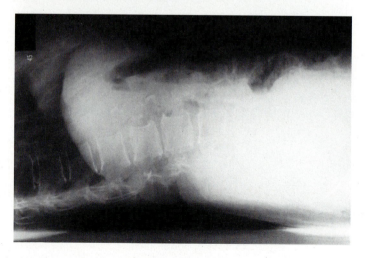

Gas filled colon

Gas level in colon

Diaphragm

Posterior ribs

Support elevating
patient

Fig. 16-20. Lateral abdomen, left dorsal decubitus position. Calcified aorta *(arrows).*

Abdomen

 LATERAL PROJECTION
R or L dorsal
decubitus position

Film: 14 × 17 in (35 × 43 cm).

Position of patient

- When the patient cannot stand or lie on the side, place the patient in the supine position lying on a transportation cart or other suitable support with either the patient's right or left side in contact with the vertical grid device.
- Place the arms across the upper chest to ensure they are not projected over any abdominal contents, or place them behind the head.
- Flex the patient's knees slightly to relieve strain on the back.
- Exercise care to ensure that the patient does not fall from the cart or table.
- If a cart is used, *securely lock all wheels.*

Position of part

- Adjust the height of the vertical grid device so that the long axis of the film is centered to the median coronal plane.
- Then, position the patient so that a point approximately 2 inches (5 cm) above the level of the crests of the ilia is centered to the film (Fig. 16-19).
- Adjust the patient to make sure there is no rotation from the supine position.
- *Shield gonads.* (Not shown for illustrative purposes.)
- Ask the patient to suspend respiration at the end of exhalation.

Central ray

- Direct the central ray *horizontal* and perpendicular to the center of the film, entering the median coronal plane 2 inches (5 cm) above the level of the crests of the ilia.

Structures shown

The lateral projection of the abdomen is valuable in demonstrating the prevertebral space and is quite useful in determining air-fluid levels in the abdomen (Fig. 16-20).

☐ Evaluation criteria

The following should be clearly demonstrated:

- Diaphragm without motion.
- Abdominal contents visible with soft tissue gray tones.
- Patient elevated so that entire abdomen is demonstrated.

Abdominal Fistulae and Sinuses

For radiographic demonstration of the origin and extent of fistulae (abnormal passages, usually between two internal organs) and sinuses (abnormal channels leading to abscesses), the following steps are observed:

- Fill the tract with a radiopaque contrast medium, usually under fluoroscopic control.
- Obtain right-angle projections.
- Oblique projections are occasionally required to demonstrate the full extent of a sinus tract.
- For the exploration of fistulae and sinuses in the abdominal region, have the intestinal tract as free of gas and fecal material as possible.
- Unless the injection is made under fluoroscopic control, take a scout radiograph of the abdomen to check the condition of the intestinal tract before beginning the examination.
- When more than one sinus opening is present, occlude each accessory opening with a sterile gauze packing to prevent reflux of the contrast substance, and identify it by a specific lead marker placed over the dressing (Figs. 16-21 to 16-23).
- Dress and identify the primary sinus opening in a similar manner if the catheter is removed after the injection.
- When a reflux of the contrast medium occurs, cleanse the skin thoroughly before making an exposure.

- When fluoroscopy is not employed, place the patient in position for the first projection before the physician makes the injection, to prevent drainage of the opaque substance by unnecessary movement. The initial radiograph is taken and evaluated before proceeding or changing the patient's position.

A modified gastrointestinal procedure is usually employed to detect the origin of colonic fistulae. An iodized oil is frequently used in conjunction with a thin suspension of barium sulfate because the oil breaks up into clearly visible globules as soon as it reaches the watery barium suspension in the lumen of the intestine. For the demonstration of a colonic fistula, the colon is filled with an enema consisting of the full amount of water but only about a third the amount of barium ordinarily used. The physician then injects an iodized oil through the fistulous tract and localizes its origin at the intestinal wall by the globulation of the oil. For the demonstration of a fistula of the small intestine, the patient ingests a thin barium suspension, which the physician observes fluoroscopically or radiographically until it reaches the suspected region. The fistulous tract is then injected with the iodized oil. These examinations are performed using fluoroscopic control, with films being exposed as indicated.

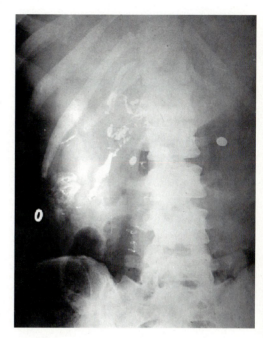

Fig. 16-21. AP abdomen showing contrast-filled sinus tract with lead "O" on body surface.

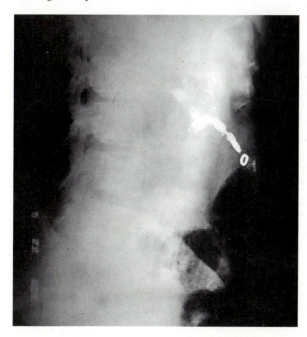

Fig. 16-22. Lateral abdomen showing sinus tract.

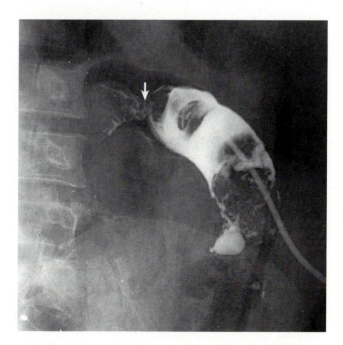

Fig. 16-23. Oblique abdomen, LPO position, showing fistula (arrow).

Liver and Spleen
AP PROJECTION

Advances in nuclear medicine, diagnostic sonography, computed tomography, and magnetic resonance have greatly reduced the frequency of performing the radiologic procedures that follow. When radiographs are taken, they are generally done to identify calcifications or gas collections from an abscess. It is, therefore, important to use correct technique.

Film: 14 × 17 in (35 × 43 cm) crosswise or lengthwise, depending on the build of the patient.

Position of patient

- Place the patient in the supine position for a general survey examination and for determination of the size and shape of the liver and the spleen.

Position of part

- Center the median sagittal plane of the body to the midline of the grid.
- Adjust the shoulders to lie in the same transverse plane.
- Flex the elbows and abduct the arms enough to clear the film area.
- Flex the knees to relieve strain.
- With the cassette placed crosswise in the Bucky tray, adjust its position so that approximately 1 inch of the iliac bone is included on the lower border of the film (Fig. 16-24).
- If the patient is too tall for this centering to include the diaphragm, place the cassette lengthwise.
- For exceptionally broad subjects who are also tall, make two exposures: one with the film placed crosswise to include the entire diaphragm and one with the film placed lengthwise to include the crests of the ilia.
- To prevent contour distortion, do not apply compression in liver and spleen examinations.
- *Shield gonads.* (Not shown for illustrative purposes.)
- Ask the patient to suspend respiration at the end of exhalation.

Central ray

- Direct the central ray perpendicular through the xiphoid process to the center of the film.

Structures shown

An AP projection shows the size and shape of the liver, the spleen, and the kidneys (Fig. 16-25).

☐ Evaluation criteria

The following should be clearly demonstrated:
- Diaphragm to the crests of the ilia.
- Upper abdomen visible with soft tissue gray tones.
- No rotation of patient, indicated by:
  - ☐ Crests of the ilia symmetric.
  - ☐ Ribs symmetric.
  - ☐ Spinous processes centered within the vertebral bodies.
- Vertebral column centered to the radiograph.

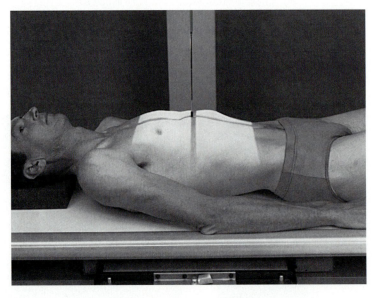

Fig. 16-24. AP liver and spleen.

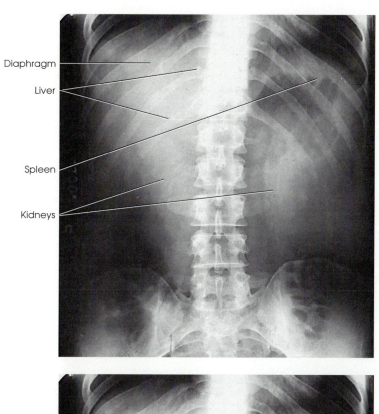

Diaphragm

Liver

Spleen

Kidneys

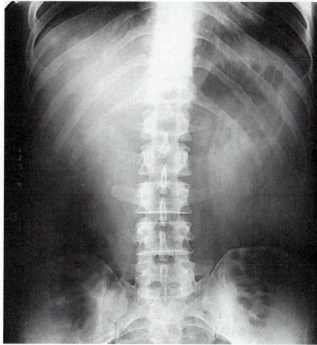

Fig. 16-25. AP liver and spleen.

Liver

PA AXIAL PROJECTIONS
BENASSI METHOD

Film: Two 14 × 17 in (35 × 43 cm).

Position of patient

- Place the patient prone so that the broad anterior surface of the liver is nearer the film.

Position of part

- Center the median sagittal plane of the body to the midline of the grid.
- Flex the patient's elbows, and adjust the arms in a comfortable position.
- Adjust the shoulders to lie in the same transverse plane.
- With the cassette placed crosswise or lengthwise, according to the patient's build, adjust the position of the Bucky tray so that the midpoint of the cassette will coincide with the central ray (Fig. 16-26).
- Do not apply compression.
- *Shield gonads.* (Not shown for illustrative purposes.)
- Ask the patient to suspend respiration at end of exhalation.

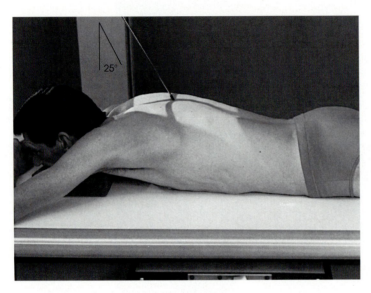

Fig. 16-26. PA axial liver with 25-degree caudal angulation.

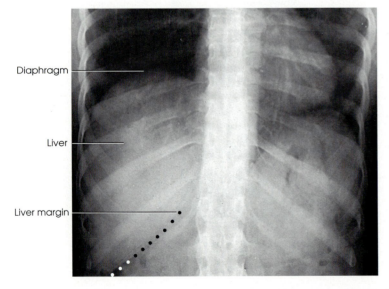
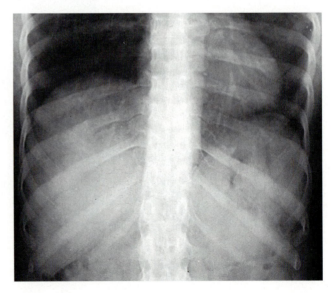

Diaphragm

Liver

Liver margin

Fig. 16-27. PA axial liver with 25-degree caudal angulations.

Central ray

- Direct the central ray through the xiphoid process (1) at an angle of 25 degrees caudad for the first radiograph (Figs. 16-27 and 16-28) and (2) at an angle of 10 degrees cephalad for the second radiograph (Figs. 16-28 and 16-29).
- For a general survey examination, direct the central ray perpendicular.

Structures shown

The two axial images demonstrate the greater surface of the liver.

□ **Evaluation criteria**

The following should be clearly demonstrated:

- ■ Diaphragm.
- ■ Liver outline.
- ■ Center of film at the level of the liver region.
- ■ Vertebral column centered to the radiograph.
- ■ No rotation of the patient.

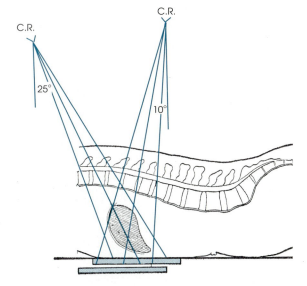

Fig. 16-28. PA axial projections showing both the 25-degree caudal and 10-degree cephalad angulations.

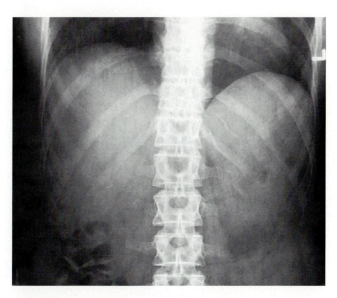

Fig. 16-29. PA axial liver with 10-degree cephalic angulation.

Spleen

AP OLIQUE PROJECTION
LPO position

Film: 11 × 14 in (30 × 35 cm) lengthwise.

Position of patient

• Place the patient in the supine position so that the spleen is nearer the film.

Position of part

• Elevate the right side of the patient's body about 40 to 45 degrees, and center the left side to the midline of the grid.
• Support the elevated shoulder and hip on sandbags or firm pillows.
• Place the arms in a comfortable position.

• With the cassette in the Bucky tray, adjust its position so that the cassette is centered at or just below the level of the xiphoid process (Fig. 16-30).
• Do not apply compression.
• *Shield gonads.* (Not shown for illustrative purposes.)
• Ask the patient to suspend respiration at the end of exhalation.

Central ray

• Direct the central ray perpendicular, approximately 2 inches (5 cm) left of the midline at the level of the xiphoid process.

Structures shown

An oblique image demonstrates the greater surface of the spleen (Fig. 16-31).

□ **Evaluation criteria**

The following should be clearly demonstrated:
■ Diaphragm.
■ Splenic region centered on the radiograph.
■ Lateral border of abdomen without excessive density.

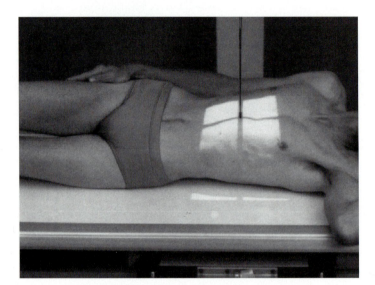

Fig. 16-30. AP oblique spleen, LPO position.

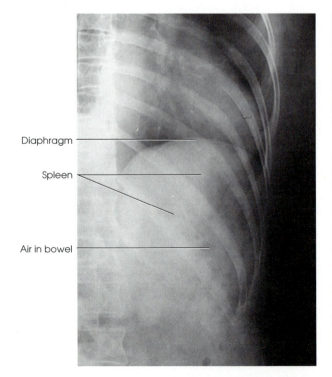
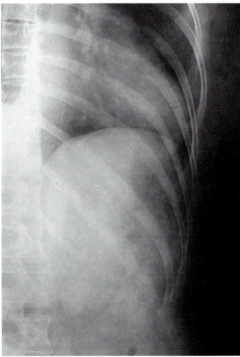

Diaphragm

Spleen

Air in bowel

Fig. 16-31. AP oblique spleen, LPO position.

Biliary Tract and Gall Bladder

There are several techniques for examining the gall bladder and the biliary ductal system. In many institutions, sonography is the modality of choice. This section of the atlas discusses the radiographic techniques currently available.

Table 16-1 lists some of the medical combining forms associated with the biliary system. *Cholegraphy* is the general term for a radiographic study of the biliary system. More specific terms can be used to describe the portion of the biliary system under investigation: *cholecystography* is the radiographic investigation of the gall bladder; *cholangiography* is the radiographic study of the biliary ducts; radiography of both the gall bladder and the biliary ducts is *cholecystangiography* or *cholecystocholangiography*.

Cholecystography was developed by Graham et al. in 1924 and 1925.[1] The oral cholegraphic contrast media were developed in the sequence listed in Table 16-2. Before Telepaque, the first of the three-iodinated compounds, preoperative visual-

---

[1]Graham EA, Cole WH, and Copher GH: Cholecystography: the use of sodium tetraiodophenolphthalein, JAMA 84:1175-1177, 1925.

ization of the biliary tract was limited to the gall bladder. In addition to permitting visualization of the bile ducts, the three-iodinated compounds resulted in a decrease in side reactions.

The contrast agent selected for use in the direct injection techniques to be discussed later (percutaneous transhepatic, operative, T tube) may be any one of the water-soluble, iodinated compounds employed for intravenous urography.

Table 16-1. Biliary system combining forms

Root forms	Meaning
chole-	Relationship with bile
cysto-	Bag, or sac
choledocho-	Common bile duct
cholangio-	Bile ducts
cholecyst-	Gall bladder

Table 16-2. Oral cholegraphic contrast media

	Contrast media	Visualization
Two-iodinated compounds		
1924-1925	Tetrabromophenolphthalein	Gall bladder
	Tetraiodophenolphthalein	Gall bladder
1940	Priodax	Gall bladder
1944	Monophen	Gall bladder
Three-iodinated compounds		
1949	Telepaque	Gall bladder and ducts
1952	Teridax	Gall bladder and ducts
1960	Biloptin	Gall bladder and ducts
	Oragrafin	Gall bladder and ducts
1962	Bilopaque	Gall bladder and ducts
Six-iodinated compounds		
1952-1953	Biligrafin forte	Gall bladder and ducts
	Cholografin	Gall bladder and ducts
1956	Duografin (Cholografin methylglucamine plus Renografin)	Gall bladder and ducts Urinary tract

The radiographic study of the biliary system requires the introduction of a contrast medium. The contrast medium may be administered (1) by mouth *(oral)* (Figs. 16-32 and 16-33), (2) by injection into a vein in a single bolus or by drip infusion *(intravenous)* (Fig. 16-34), or (3) by direct injection into the ducts (a) through *percutaneous transhepatic puncture* (Fig. 16-35), (b) during biliary tract surgery *(operative* or immediate) (Fig. 16-36), or (c) through an indwelling drainage tube (postoperative, delayed, or *T tube)* (Fig. 16-37). Each technique of examination is named according to (1) the route of entry of the medium (italicized above) and (2) the portion of the biliary tract examined.

The contrast medium can be delivered to the liver by either the oral or the venous route because of the double blood supply to this organ. When given by mouth, the contrast medium is absorbed through the intestines and carried to the liver through the portal vein. Contrast medium administered intravenously is most commonly injected into one of the antecubital veins and thus passes through the heart and into the arterial circulation. The contrast agent circulates to the liver via the hepatic artery and the portal vein. In the hepatic cells, the contrast substance is biochemically changed and then excreted with the bile and conveyed to the gall bladder by the system of ducts. The contrast-carrying bile is stored and concentrated in the gall bladder, rendering it radiopaque.

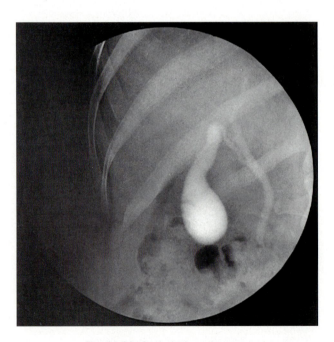

Fig. 16-32. Oral cholecystogram.

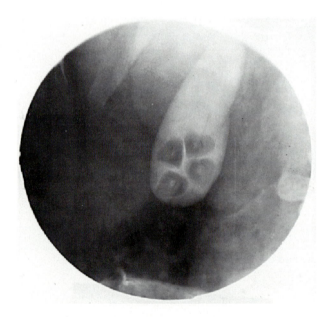

Fig. 16-33. Oral cholecystogram showing cholesterol stones.

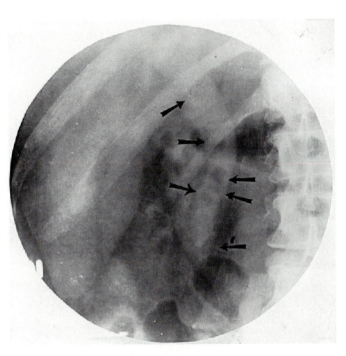

Fig. 16-34. Intravenous cholangiogram showing stones in common bile duct *(arrows).*

(Courtesy Dr. William H. Shehadi.)

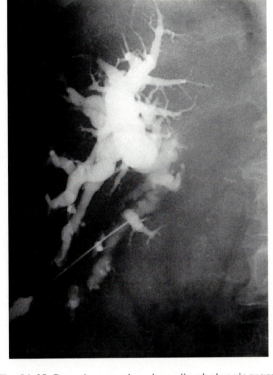

Fig. 16-35. Percutaneous transhepatic cholangiogram.

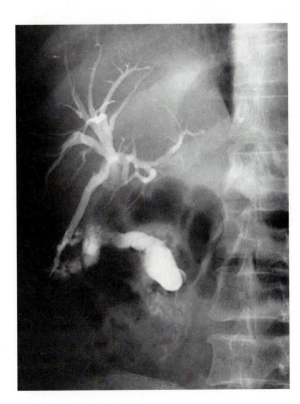

Fig. 16-36. Operative cholangiogram.

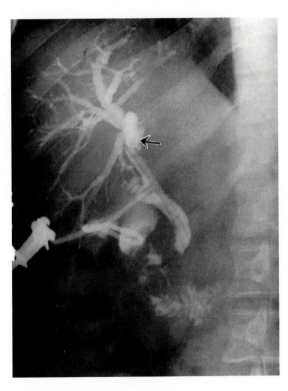

Fig. 16-37. Postoperative cholangiogram showing retained stone *(arrow).*

EVALUATION OF BILIARY TRACT

Biliary tract examinations are performed to determine (1) the function of the liver—its ability to remove the contrast medium from the bloodstream and excrete it with the bile, (2) the patency and condition of the biliary ducts, and (3) the concentrating and emptying power of the gall bladder.

The greatest number of biliary tract examinations are probably performed in quest of gall stones. The calculi, or stones, formed in the biliary tract vary widely in composition, size, and shape. Pure cholesterol stones appear as negative filling defects within the opacified bile (Fig. 16-33). Calcium-containing deposits, either as solitary calculi or in the form of milk of calcium, can be readily detected on the plain radiograph (Fig. 16-38).

Technical requirements

For optimal technical quality, use the following guidelines:
- Ensure that the focal spot of the x-ray tube is *small* and in good condition.
- Ensure that the intensifying screens are clean, and in perfect contact.
- Ensure that the grid is in perfect operating condition.
- Closely collimate the area of patient irradiation.
- Make the patient comfortable to decrease the risk of motion.
- Stabilize elevated parts and place radiolucent pads under pressure points.
- Employ immobilization with a broad compression band to aid in the control of movement if needed.
- Teach the patient to relax as well as to suspend respiration during the exposures.

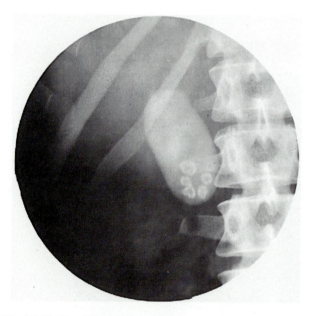

Fig. 16-38. Opacified gall bladder with radiopaque stones.

- Utilize a short exposure time to eliminate blurring of the gall bladder and ducts as a result of vibratory movement caused by peristaltic action in the adjacent segments of the intestine.
- Adjust the exposure factors to produce maximum soft tissue differentiation (70 to 80 kVp recommended). The image must show a sharp outline of the lower border of the liver, the right kidney, and the margin of the right psoas muscle, as well as a degree of intrastructural detail of the included bony parts.
- Ensure that the scout radiograph of patients of asthenic habitus is dark enough to demonstrate the shadow of the gall bladder through the vertebral shadow.
- Make exposures at the end of exhalation because this phase of respiration places the patient under less strain.
- Do not ask the patient either to exhale or to inhale to the point of strain because spasmodic contraction of the abdominal muscles will occur.
- Give the breathing instructions carefully.

According to the body habitus of the patient and the degree of body fat present, the gall bladder moves laterally and superiorly 1 to 3 inches (2.5 to 7.5 cm) on full exhalation, and conversely, it moves medially and inferiorly 1 to 3 inches (2.5 to 7.5 cm) on full inhalation (Figs. 16-39 and 16-40). This information should be utilized when the gall bladder image on the scout radiograph is partially obscured by the rib or by small amounts of gas. When cholecystograms are made at the end of inhalation, they should be so marked.

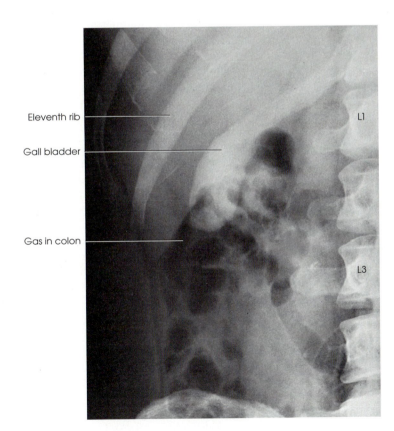

Fig. 16-39. AP gall bladder. Suspended exhalation.

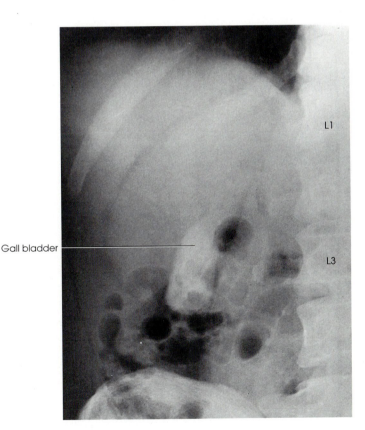

Fig. 16-40. AP gall bladder. Suspended inhalation.

Oral Cholecystography
Indications and contraindications

Hundreds of thousands of people in the United States are evaluated or hospitalized each year for symptoms related to gall bladder disease. The most common radiographic procedure used to study the gall bladder is cholecystography following the oral administration of contrast medium. Oral cholecystography, commonly abbreviated *OCG*, can be used to demonstrate a number of abnormal conditions. It is frequently used because the oral contrast medium currently available is generally well tolerated and permits satisfactory visualization of the extrahepatic bile ducts as well as the gall bladder in a large percentage of patients examined.

Common indications for oral cholecystography include but are not limited to:

1. *Cholelithiasis*, the presence of stones or calculi in the gall bladder (*choledocholithiasis* refers to calculi in the common bile duct).
2. *Cholecystitis*, an acute or chronic inflammation of the gall bladder and a common complication of cholelithiasis.
3. *Biliary neoplasia*, any unusual growth of, or within, the gall bladder.
4. *Opacities* or *masses* of the right upper quadrant.
5. *Biliary stenosis*, the narrowing or occlusion of the common bile duct. This condition may be congenital or caused by gall stones or an external neoplasm surrounding the common bile duct (e.g., a tumor of the head of the pancreas).

The success of oral cholecystography depends on the integrative function (1) of the intestinal mucosa in receiving and absorbing the contrast substance and liberating it into the portal bloodstream for conveyance to the liver, (2) of the liver in removing the opaque substance from the blood and excreting it with the bile, and (3) of the gall bladder (a) in concentrating the inflowing opacified bile by removing a large part of its approximately 90% water content and (b) in storing the concentrated bile during the interdigestive period.

The patient's allergic response to iodine compounds should be determined prior to the procedure. Oral cholecystography is generally contraindicated for patients with vomiting or diarrhea; pyloric obstruction; malabsorption syndrome; severe jaundice, liver dysfunction, or hepatocellular disease; or hypersensitivity to iodinated contrast media.

Instructions to patient

Prior to the procedure, the following steps are observed:

- To secure full cooperation, explain to the patient the purpose of the preliminary preparation and the procedure to be followed.
- Tell the patient the approximate time required for the examination, allowing for the possibility of delay should the colon require further cleansing or the emptying time of the gall bladder be delayed.
- Give the patient clearly printed instructions covering (1) preliminary preparation of the intestinal tract, (2) preliminary diet, (3) exact time to ingest the oral medium, (4) avoidance of laxatives for 24 hours before the ingestion or injection of the medium, (5) avoidance of all food, both solid and liquid, after receiving an oral medium (water may be taken as desired before the oral examination), and (6) the time to report for the examination.
- When the patient reports for the examination, question him or her as to how each step of the preparation procedure was followed.
- For the oral technique, ask the patient whether any reaction such as vomiting or diarrhea occurred. Vomiting may be important if it occurs within 2 hours after ingestion of the contrast medium. Mild catharsis may do no harm, but diarrhea can result in egestion of a majority of the contrast substance, so that only a faint shadow, if any, of the gall bladder will be visualized.
- Because prolonged fasting causes the formation of gas, as well as a possible headache, give patients early-morning appointments if at all possible.

Preparation of intestinal tract

Much of the success of biliary tract examinations depends on attaining a clear image of the right upper quadrant of the abdomen (Fig. 16-41). In some cases a scout radiograph may be taken on the day prior to the oral cholecystogram. This radiograph serves a dual purpose. The fecal content of the bowel can be assessed to determine the extent of cleansing enemas required and to identify possible small radiopaque stones which might otherwise be camouflaged by the contrast medium (Figs. 16-42 and 16-43).

Based on the scout radiograph, the bowel content may be judged to be light to moderate, so that it can be eliminated with one or two cleansing enemas, or it may be so heavy that it requires a laxative. Often, no preparation is needed. If used, laxatives are administered 24 hours preceding the ingestion or injection of a contrast agent to allow irritation of the intestinal mucosa to subside and, in the oral technique, to prevent egestion of the contrast medium with the fecal material.

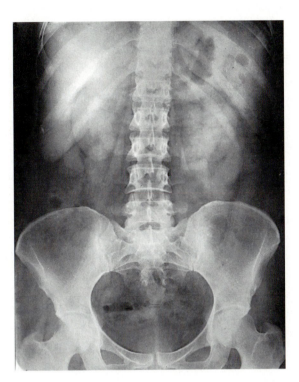

Fig. 16-41. AP abdomen. Prepared intestinal tract.

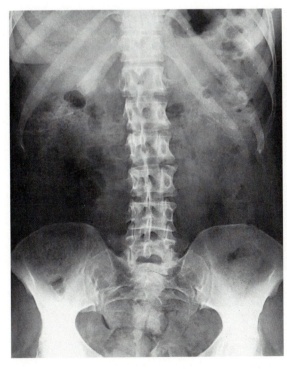

Fig. 16-42. AP abdomen. Unprepared intestinal tract.

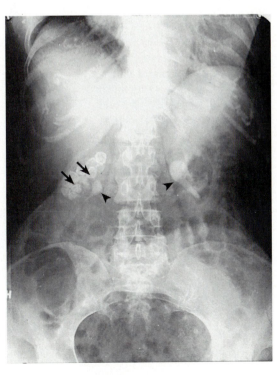

Fig. 16-43. AP abdomen. Multiple biliary stones (arrows) and bilateral renal stones (arrowheads).

Preliminary diet

Medical opinion varies on the subject of the preliminary diet. Some physicians believe the patient should be given a noon meal rich in simple fats on the day before the examination. This fat causes the gall bladder to contract; theoretically, the contrast-filled bile will then be more concentrated and clearly visible when the OCG is performed. All medical personnel agree, however, that the patient should receive a fat-free evening meal to prevent the gall bladder from contracting and expelling the opacified bile. Breakfast is usually withheld in all techniques.

In many institutions, the oral cholecystogram is often scheduled to be performed at the same time as an upper gastrointestinal examination. In that case, the patient is kept *NPO (non per os*; i.e., nothing should be taken in through the mouth) until the completion of both procedures. On the day of the examination, the oral cholecystogram is performed before the GI procedure.

Contrast administration

The contrast medium available for oral cholecystography is normally given to the patient in a single dose approximately 2 to 3 hours after the evening meal on the night preceding the examination. The usual single dosage is 3 gm and is administered in the form of 4 to 6 tablets. Breakfast is usually withheld on the morning of the procedure.

The contrast media used in oral cholecystography differ in their rate of absorption and liberation into the portal bloodstream. The absorption time varies from 10 to 12 hours for most present-day oral agents. The administration of the contrast agent is scheduled to allow enough time to elapse for maximum concentration of the contrast agent in the gall bladder. An exception to this is the administration of ipodate calcium, which is rapidly absorbed and allows visualization of the biliary ducts in an average of 1.5 hours, with visualization of the gall bladder in 3 to 4 hours.

Scout radiographs

To determine if the contrast material was absorbed and concentrated in the gall bladder, one or more scout (preliminary) radiographs are often obtained. The decision regarding whether to continue the OCG is often based on if, and how well, the gall bladder is visualized on the scout radiographs.

Anatomic descriptions of the gall bladder are based on the average. They usually state that the gall bladder is a pear-shaped organ situated in an oblique plane in the right upper quadrant of the abdomen, where, from the neck end, its long axis slants inferiorly and slightly anteriorly. In practice many deviations from this arrangement are encountered. The shape of the gall bladder varies considerably from the classic pyriform configuration. Depending on bodily habitus and the arrangement of its attachment to the liver, the gall bladder may, in its usual right-sided position, be located anywhere from the level of the eighth rib down to well within the iliac fossa and anywhere from the median sagittal plane to near the lateral wall of the abdomen. It is sometimes found in the left side of the abdomen (Fig. 16-44) even though the liver is in the normal position. Because of the possibility of the latter location, the initial study may include a 14 × 17 in (35 × 43 cm) radiograph of the abdomen in addition to a 10 × 12 in (24 × 30 cm) or an 8 × 10 in (18 × 24 cm) image of the right side. The wide range in the right-sided location of the gall bladder can be covered with the 10 × 12 in (24 × 30 cm) or smaller film by centering at the level of the ninth costal cartilage for patients of average build, about 2 inches (5 cm) higher for those approaching the hypersthenic type, and 2 inches (5 cm) lower for asthenic patients.

The scout radiographs may be taken with the patient supine or prone. The prone position is generally preferred because it places the structures of the biliary system closer to the film.

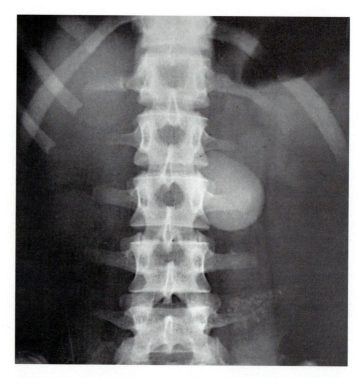

Fig. 16-44. AP upper abdomen showing left-sided gall bladder.

Initial procedure

Patient instructions and preparation validation

Prior to performing the procedure, the radiographer observes the following steps:

- When the patient reports for the procedure, determine that each step of the preparation was followed.
- Ask the patient if the contrast medium was administered and if any reaction such as vomiting or diarrhea occurred. Vomiting may be important if it occurs within 2 hours after ingestion of the contrast medium. Mild catharsis may do no harm, but diarrhea can result in egestion of a majority of the contrast substance, so that only a faint shadow, if any, of the gall bladder will be visualized.
- Determine whether the patient has remained NPO.
- Finally, ensure that the patient has not had a cholecystectomy. If the gall bladder has been removed, there is no reason to continue with the procedure.

- If the patient has correctly followed the preparation, discuss the procedure with the patient. Taking the time to review the procedure and answer any questions will gain the patient's respect and cooperation.
- Once the patient understands the procedure, have the patient change into an examination gown if not properly dressed.

Inspection of scout radiographs

As soon as the scout radiographs have been processed, they are carefully inspected for the following information: (1) the presence or absence of the gall bladder (Fig. 16-45) and (2) if present, (a) whether the concentration of the contrast medium is sufficient for adequate visualization, (b) whether it is overlapped by intestinal and/or bony shadows (Fig. 16-46), (c) its exact location, and (d) whether a change in the exposure factors is needed for proper demonstration of the organ.

When the gall bladder is not visualized, the entire abdomen should be evaluated if that procedure has not already been performed. A 14 × 17 in (35 × 43 cm) scout radiograph is recommended to evaluate the patient for possible transposition of the abdominal organs and to check the iliac fossa of patients with asthenic body habitus. It is also possible that the gall bladder may be obscured by fecal material in the colon. If such is the case, it may be necessary to administer an enema to clean the colon to the region of the right colic flexure. It may be necessary to question the patient again about the preparation. It is possible that the patient did not fast or did not take all of the contrast medium.

When the gall bladder does not visualize on the first attempt, the patient may be kept on the fat-free diet for an additional 24 hours. An additional, or reinforced, dose of contrast material may be given that evening and the examination repeated the next day. Another option is to schedule the patient for an ultrasonic examination of the gall bladder, especially when the patient experiences vomiting or diarrhea. If the gall bladder is opacified on the scout radiographs, the radiographer should proceed with the examination.

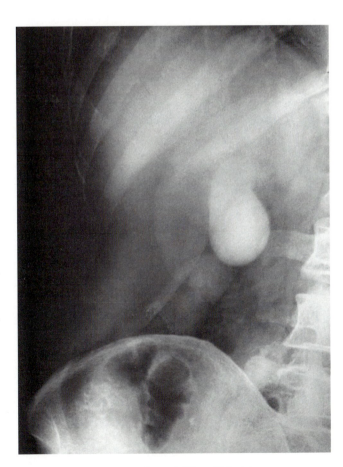

Fig. 16-45. Normal AP gall bladder.

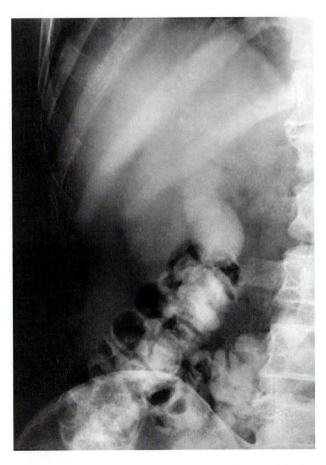

Fig. 16-46. AP gall bladder superimposed over residual contrast medium in colon.

The opacified gall bladder

Evaluation of the opacified gall bladder may include either radiographic and/or fluoroscopic techniques. When radiographic evaluation is used, the patient may be examined in any combination of the following positions: supine (Fig. 16-47), prone (Fig. 16-48), prone oblique (Fig. 16-49), upright (Fig. 16-50), and/or lateral decubitus (Fig. 16-51). The upright or decubitus radiographs are helpful in detecting small stones that may layer or gravitate to the fundus of the gall bladder. Following inspection of the radiographs, fluoroscopy may be performed and spot radiographs taken, if indicated.

Because of the variability in the position of the gall bladder, institutional routines are often supplemented to visualize the organ. For example, if the fundus is superimposed by intestinal contents or the spine, recumbent PA oblique projections are often helpful in separating these structures. Should the ribs lie over the gall bladder, the exposure may be made at the end of full inspiration since inspiration displaces the abdominal organs inferiorly (see Figs. 16-39 and 16-40). Radiographs taken with the patient standing (or decubitus positions for the patient unable to stand) are often beneficial because gravity changes the position of the abdominal viscera, which may free the gall bladder from superimposition. For exceptionally thin patients, it is sometimes necessary to use the lateral projection (Fig. 16-52) and, for oblique studies, the supine position. When the gall bladder is located in the iliac fossa, it is necessary to use the supine position to draw the organ superiorly. In extreme cases, use of a cephalic angulation of either the table or the central ray is necessary. The right lateral decubitus position is used for stratification studies of the low-placed gall bladder.

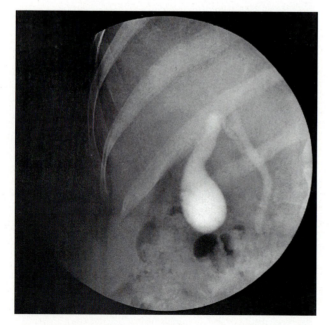

Fig. 16-47. AP gall bladder, patient supine.

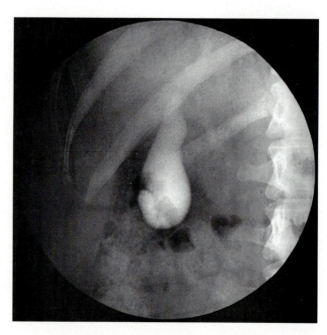

Fig. 16-48. PA gall bladder, patient prone.

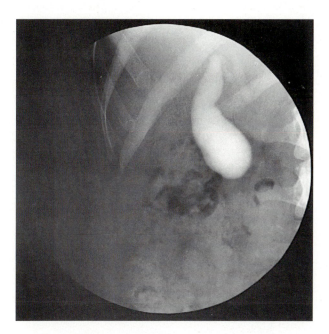

Fig. 16-49. PA oblique gall bladder, LAO position.

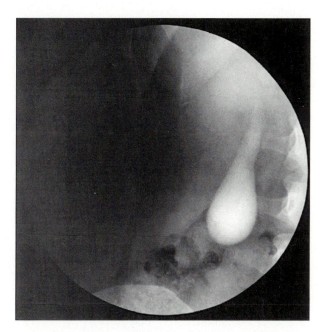

Fig. 16-50. AP gall bladder, upright. (Note how level of gall bladder has moved inferiorly.)

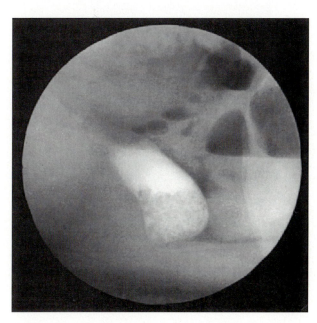

Fig. 16-51. Lateral gall bladder, right lateral decubitis position showing multiple small stones that have settled to bottom of gall bladder.

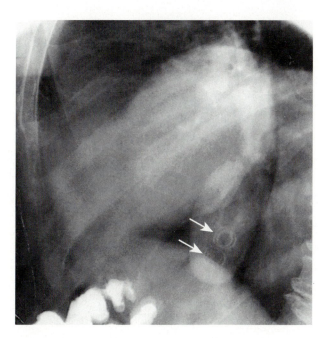

Fig. 16-52. Right lateral gall bladder showing intra-hepatic gall bladder with stones *(arrows).*

Fatty meal

In the earlier years of radiology, patients were often given a fatty meal after satisfactory visualization of the gall bladder. The fatty meal consisted of a commercially available bar, eggs and milk, or eggnog. The meal caused the gall bladder to contract, and additional diagnostic information was seldom obtained (Figs. 16-53 and 16-54). An injection of the hormone cholecystokinin will also cause the gall bladder to contract. The fatty meal is seldom used today because of the diagnostic capability of ultrasonography.

Post-procedure instructions

Once the gall bladder has been adequately visualized, the patient can go home or to return to the hospital room. Currently available contrast material is eliminated mainly via the alimentary canal, so the patient should be instructed to eat and drink normally.

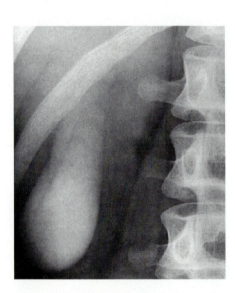

Fig. 16-53. PA oblique gall bladder, LAO position; prefatty meal.

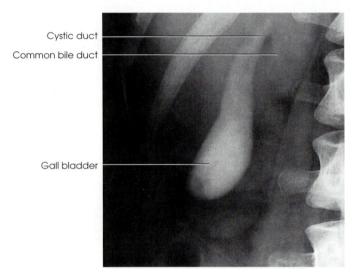

Cystic duct

Common bile duct

Gall bladder

Fig. 16-54. Postfatty meal in same patient as in Fig. 16-53.

(Courtesy Dr. Marcy L. Sussman.)

Biliary Tract and Gall Bladder

⚜ PA PROJECTION

Film: 10 × 12 in (24 × 30 cm) for scout radiograph, 8 × 10 in (18 × 24 cm) for subsequent exposures.

Position of patient

- Place the patient in the prone position with a pillow under the head.
- If the patient is thin, place the pillow lengthwise, and adjust it so that it extends inferiorly as far as or a little below the transmamillary line.

Position of part

- Adjust the body so that the right side of the abdomen is centered to the midline of the grid.
- Rest the left cheek on the pillow to rotate the vertebrae slightly toward the left side.
- Flex the right elbow, and adjust the arm in a comfortable position.
- Place the left arm alongside the body if needed.
- Elevate the ankles to relieve pressure on the toes.
- Center the cassette according to the habitus of the patient (Fig. 16-55).
- When examining a woman with pendulous breasts, have the patient spread the breasts superior and laterally to ensure clearing the gall bladder region.
- Immobilize with a compression band.
- *Shield gonads.* (Not shown for illustrative purposes.)
- Ask the patient to suspend respiration at the end of exhalation in the routine procedure. Watch for an indication of tenseness and allow about 2 seconds to elapse after the cessation of respiration before making the exposure. This interval is to permit any peristaltic action to subside and to give the patient time to relax.

Central ray

- Direct the central ray perpendicular and centered to the gall bladder at a level appropriate to the patient's habitus.

Upright position

- Adjust the body so that the previously localized gall bladder is centered to the midline of the grid (Fig. 16-56).

- Elevate the gall bladder to, or almost to, the location it assumed in the prone position by instructing the patient to fully extend the arms. Otherwise, depending on the habitus of the patient, center the film 2 to 4 inches (5 to 10 cm) below the prone level to allow for the change in gall bladder position. The remainder of the procedure is the same as for the prone position.

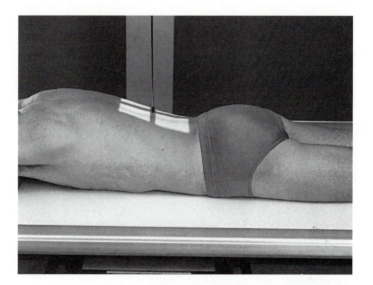

Fig. 16-55. PA gall bladder.

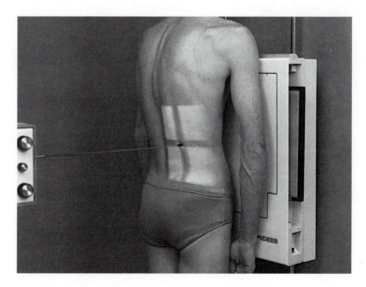

Fig. 16-56. PA gall bladder, upright position.

Structures shown

The upright PA projection presents a somewhat axial representation of the opacified gall bladder. The foreshortening in the PA projection is caused by the angle between the long axis of the obliquely placed gall bladder and the plane of the film. The degree of angulation and consequently the amount of foreshortening vary according to body habitus and are influenced by body position, being less in the upright position (Figs. 16-57 and 16-58).

The gall bladder is directed anteriorly at an inferior angle that ranges from an almost horizontal position in the hypersthenic patient to an almost vertical position in the asthenic patient. As a result, foreshortening of the gall bladder is negligible in asthenic patients. On the other hand, in patients of the hypersthenic type, the neck, body, and fundus of the gall bladder are superimposed and thus cast an irregularly circular or triangular shadow, the shape depending on the degree of lateral displacement (Fig. 16-59). In the sthenic patient, the gall bladder casts a pear-shaped shadow that is somewhat foreshortened but does not show actual superimposition of the different regions of the gall bladder (Fig. 16-60).

In the upright position the gall bladder assumes a more vertical angle as it moves inferiorly, posteriorly, and medially. The extent of the change in both angle and location depends on habitus and abdominal fat. The upright body position is used to demonstrate the mobility of the gall bladder, to detect the presence of stones that are too small to cast an image, and to differentiate papilloma or other tumors shadows from cholesterol calculi shadows, as determined by the mobility of the latter. Small stones that are heavier than bile gravitate to the fundic portion of the gall bladder, where the aggregate has either sufficient radiopacity or sufficient radiolucency to cast an image. Because the opacified bile layers out according to concentration, that is, according to specific gravity, or weight, minute stones will float at the surface of a certain bile layer, depending on the relative specific gravity, and cast an image that has the appearance of a horizontal band (Fig. 16-58).

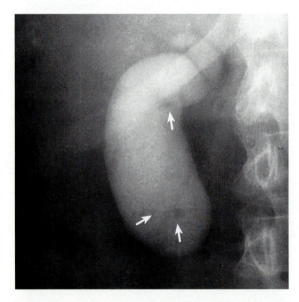

Fig. 16-57. PA gall bladder, prone position showing innumerable small negative shadows filling greater portion of gall bladder and representing bile pigment calculi *(arrows)*.

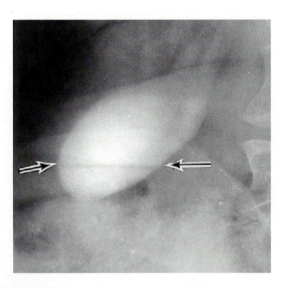

Fig. 16-58. Same patient as in Fig. 16-57 in upright position. Note linear stratification of bile pigment calculi *(arrows)* in lower portion of gall bladder.

□ Evaluation criteria

The following should be clearly demonstrated:

- Entire gall bladder and area of the cystic duct.
- Gall bladder with a short scale of contrast.
- No motion visible on the gall bladder.
- No rotation of patient.
- Centering in upright position lower and more medial to include entire gall bladder.
- Compensation for abdominal thickness in upright position so that density is similar to that in recumbent position.
- Improved visibility in the upright position if the gall bladder was superimposed by bowel contents in the recumbent position.
- Upright position identified with an appropriate marker.

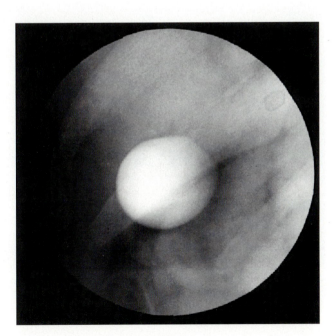

Fig. 16-59. PA gall bladder, hypersthenic patient. Note almost horizontal position of gall bladder.

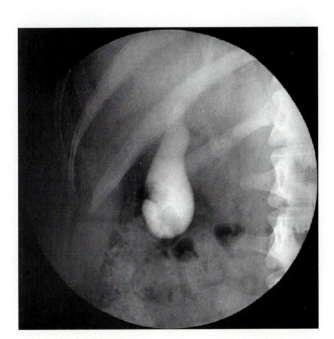

Fig. 16-60. PA gall bladder on sthenic patient.

Biliary Tract and Gall Bladder

 PA OBLIQUE PROJECTION LAO position

 LATERAL PROJECTION R lateral position

Film: 8 × 10 in (18 × 24 cm) lengthwise.

Position of patient

- For the radiographic procedure, place the patient in the recumbent position for oblique and lateral projections of the gall bladder.

Position of part

LAO position

The degree of rotation necessary for a satisfactory demonstration of the gall bladder depends on the location of the organ with reference to the vertebrae (thin subjects require more rotation than do heavier patients), on the angulation of the long axis of the organ, and on whether the right colic (hepatic flexure) is clear.

- With the patient in the prone position, elevate the right side to the desired degree of obliquity (15 to 40 degrees).
- Instruct the patient to support self on the flexed knee and elbow.
- Adjust the body to center the previously localized gall bladder to the midline of the grid.
- Place a foam sponge against the anterior surface of the abdomen (Fig. 16-61).

Right lateral position

With the patient lying on the right side, use the right lateral position to differentiate gallstones from renal stones or calcified mesenteric lymph nodes if needed. The lateral position is also required to separate the superimposition of the gall bladder and the vertebrae in exceptionally thin patients and to place the long axis of a transversely placed gall bladder parallel with the plane of the film.

- Center the patient to the cassette at the point where the gall bladder has been previously localized (Fig. 16-62).
- *Shield gonads.* (Not shown for illustrative purposes.)
- Ask the patient to suspend respiration at the end of exhalation, unless the scout radiograph indicates otherwise.

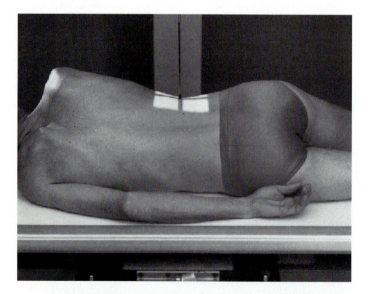

Fig. 16-61. PA oblique gall bladder, LAO position.

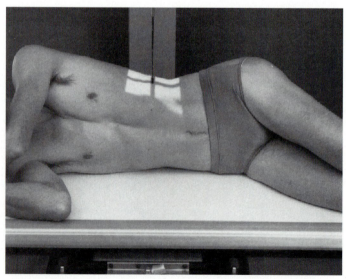

Fig. 16-62. Right lateral gall bladder.

Central ray

- Direct the central ray perpendicular to the midpoint of the film at a level appropriate for the body habitus of the patient for both the oblique and lateral projections.

Structures shown

The oblique and lateral projections show the opacified gall bladder free from self-superimposition or foreshortening and from the structures adjacent to the gall bladder (Figs. 16-63 to 16-65).

☐ Evaluation criteria

The following should be clearly demonstrated:

- Entire gall bladder and area of the cystic duct.
- Gall bladder with a short scale of contrast.
- No motion visible on the gall bladder.
- Improved visibility in the oblique projection if the gall bladder was superimposed over bowel contents or bony shadows in other projections.
- Compensation for increased thickness in lateral projection so that density is similar to that in other projections.

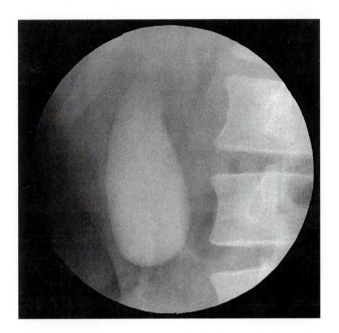

Fig. 16-63. PA oblique gall bladder, LAO position.

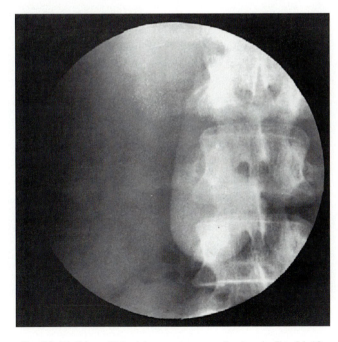

Fig. 16-64. PA gall bladder on same patient as in Fig. 16-63.

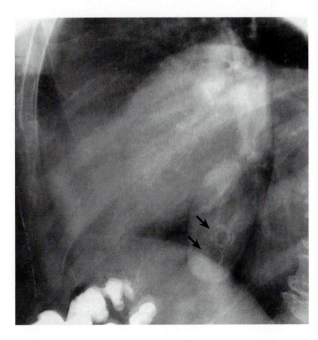

Fig. 16-65. Right lateral gall bladder demonstrating stones *(arrows)*.

Biliary Tract and Gall Bladder

▲ AP PROJECTION
Right lateral
decubitus position

The use of the right lateral decubitus body position for demonstration of the gall bladder was developed by Whelan.[1]

Film: 8 × 10 in (18 × 24 cm) or 10 × 12 in (24 × 30 cm) placed vertically.

Position of patient

- Place the patient on a stretcher or a moveable table before a vertical grid device.
- With a grid, position the patient on the horizontal table.

---

[1]Whelan FJ: Special cholecystographic technique, Xray Techn 19:230-234, 1948.

Position of part

- Place the patient on the right side with the body elevated 2 to 3 inches (5 to 7.5 cm) on a suitable radiolucent support to center the gall bladder region to a vertically placed cassette.

Central ray

- Direct the central ray *horizontal* to enter the localized area of the gall bladder (Fig. 16-66).

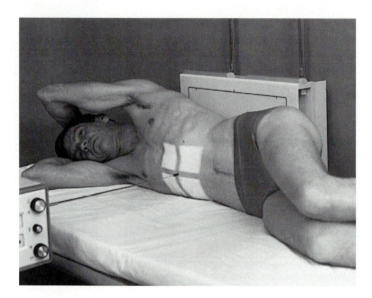

Fig. 16-66. AP gall bladder, right lateral decubitus position.

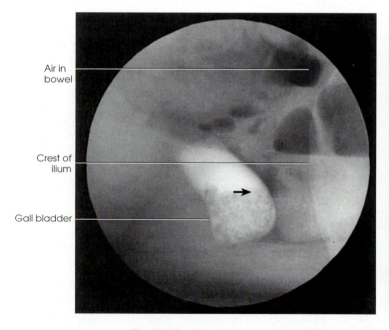
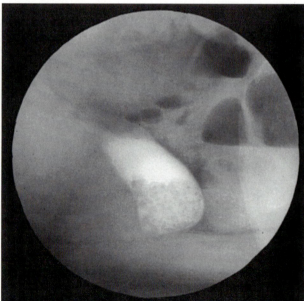

Air in bowel

Crest of ilium

Gall bladder

Fig. 16-67. AP gall bladder, right lateral decubitus position on same patient as in Fig. 16-69 showing layering of multiple small stones (*arrow*).

Structures shown

The right lateral decubitus position, as well as the upright position, is used to demonstrate (1) stones that are heavier than bile and that are too small to be visible other than when accumulated in the dependent portion of the gall bladder and (2) stones that are lighter than bile and that are visualized only by stratification (Fig. 16-67). This position has the further advantage of permitting the gall bladder to gravitate toward the dependent right side, where it will lie below any adjacent gas-containing loops of the intestine and away from bony superimposition when it occupies a low and/or medial position. The decubitus position is also used for patients who cannot stand for an upright PA or AP projection (Figs. 16-68 and 16-69).

□ Evaluation criteria

The following should be clearly demonstrated:
• Entire gall bladder and area of the cystic duct.
• Gall bladder with a short scale of contrast.
• No motion visible on the gall bladder.
• If included, vertebrae visible, indicating that the patient was not rotated.
• Gall bladder lying below any gas.
• Decubitus marker.

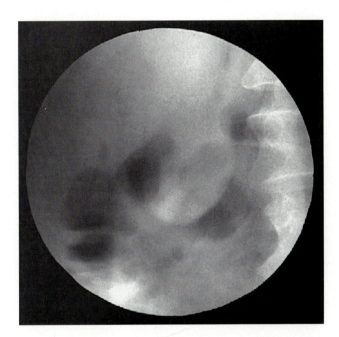

Fig. 16-68. PA gall bladder, prone position.

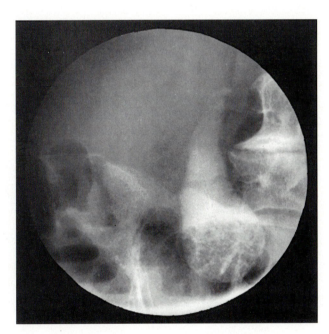

Fig. 16-69. PA gall bladder, upright position.

INTRAVENOUS CHOLANGIOGRAPHY

The intravenous cholangiogram (IVC) is seldom performed because of a relatively higher incidence of reactions to the contrast medium and the availability of other diagnostic procedures. For a more complete description of the IVC, see earlier editions of this atlas. When used, the intravenous technique of cholangiography is employed in the investigation of (1) the biliary ducts of cholecystectomized patients and (2) the biliary ducts and gall bladder of noncholecystectomized patients (a) in cases of nonvisualization by the oral technique and (b) in cases in which, because of vomiting or diarrhea, the patient cannot retain the orally administered medium long enough for its absorption. In cases of nonvisualization, the intravenous procedure may be instituted at once to save time for the radiology department as well as the patient and to spare the patient the rigors of having the intestinal tract prepared again.

Position of patient

- Place the patient in the supine position for a preliminary radiograph of the abdomen.
- Place the patient in the RPO position (15 to 40 degrees) for an AP oblique projection of the biliary ducts (Figs. 16-70 and 16-71).
- Make a scout (localization) radiograph and/or tomogram (Fig. 16-72) to check for centering and exposure factors.
- Advise the patient that when the contrast medium is injected, the patient may experience a hot flush.

Timed from the completion of the injection, duct studies are ordinarily made at 10-minute intervals until satisfactory visualization is obtained. Maximum opacification usually requires 30 to 40 minutes.

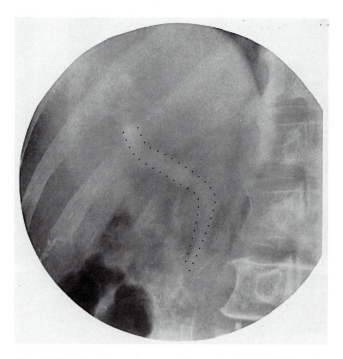

Fig. 16-70. AP oblique showing biliary duct *(dots)*. RPO position.

Contraindications

Intravenous cholangiography is not generally indicated for patients who have liver disease or for those whose biliary ducts are not intact. The probability of obtaining radiographs of diagnostic value greatly decreases when the patient's bilirubin is increasing or when it exceeds 2 mg/dl. In cases of obstructive jaundice and post-cholecystectomy, ultrasonography has become the preferred technique for demonstrating the biliary system.

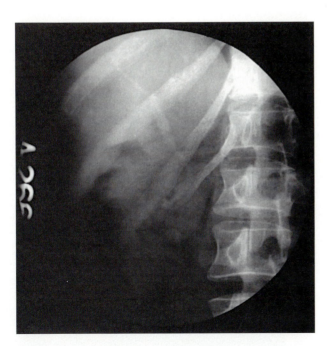

Fig. 16-71. AP oblique biliary duct 10 minutes after injection. RPO position.

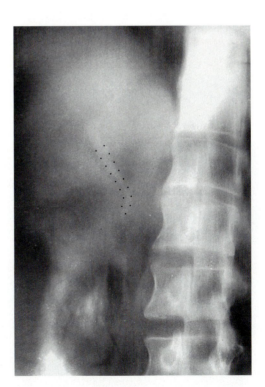

Fig. 16-72. AP oblique biliary duct tomogram at 11 cm level showing duct *(dots)*. RPO position.

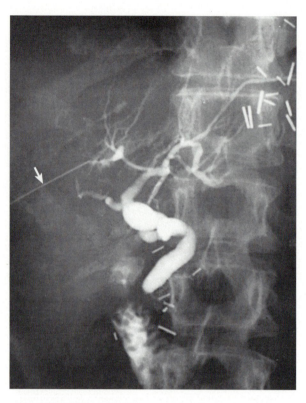

Fig. 16-73. PTC with Chiba needle *(arrow)* in position showing dilated biliary ducts.

(Courtesy Carol Drobik, R.T.)

Percutaneous transhepatic cholangiography

Percutaneous transhepatic cholangiography (PTC)[1] is another technique employed for preoperative radiologic examination of the biliary tract. This technique is used for patients with jaundice when the ductal system has been shown to be dilated by computed tomography or ultrasonography but the etiology of the obstruction is unclear. The performance of this examination has greatly increased because of the availability of the Chiba, or "skinny," needle. In addition to its diagnostic ability, PTC is often used to place a drainage catheter for treatment of obstructive jaundice rather than for diagnosis. When a drainage catheter is used, both diagnostic and drainage techniques are performed at the same time. (Biliary drainage is discussed in the following section.)

[1]Evans JA, Glenn F, Thorbjarnarson B, and Mujahed Z: Percutaneous transhepatic cholangiography, Radiology 78:362-370, 1962.

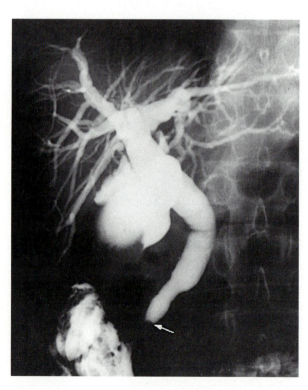

Fig. 16-74. PTC demonstrating obstruction caused by impacted stone at ampulla *(arrow)*.

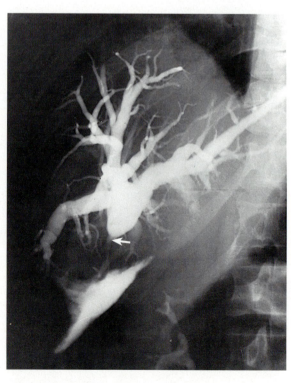

Fig. 16-75. PTC demonstrating stenosis *(arrow)* of common hepatic duct caused by trauma.

PTC is performed by placing the patient on the radiographic table in the supine position. The patient's right side is surgically prepared and appropriately draped. Following a local anesthetic, the "skinny" needle is held parallel to the floor and inserted through the right lateral intercostal space and advanced toward the liver hilum. The stylet of the needle is withdrawn and a syringe filled with contrast medium is attached to the needle. Under fluoroscopic control, the needle is slowly withdrawn until the contrast medium is seen to fill the biliary ducts. The biliary tree is most often readily located since the patient's ducts are generally dilated. Following filling of the biliary ducts, the needle may be completely withdrawn and serial or spot AP projections of the biliary area are taken (Figs. 16-73 to 16-75).

BILIARY DRAINAGE PROCEDURE AND STONE EXTRACTION

If dilated biliary ducts are identified by computed tomography, PTC, or ultrasonography, the radiologist, after consultation with the referring physician, may elect to place a drainage catheter in the biliary duct.[1,2] A needle larger than the Chiba needle used in the PTC procedure is inserted through the lateral abdominal wall and into the biliary duct. A guide wire is then passed through the lumen of the needle, and the needle is removed. A catheter is passed over the guide wire, and the guide wire is then removed, leaving the catheter in place.

---

[1]Molnar W and Stockum AE: Relief of obstructive jaundice through percutaneous transhepatic catheter—a new therapeutic method, AJR 122:356-357, 1974.
[2]Hardy CH, Messmer JM, and Crawley LC: Percutaneous transhepatic biliary drainage, Radiol Technol 56:8-12, 1984.

The catheter can be left in place for prolonged drainage, or it can be used for attempts to extract retained stones if they are identified. Retained stones are extracted by use of a wire basket and a small balloon catheter under fluoroscopic control. This extraction procedure is usually attempted after the catheter has been in place for some time (Figs. 16-76 and 16-77).

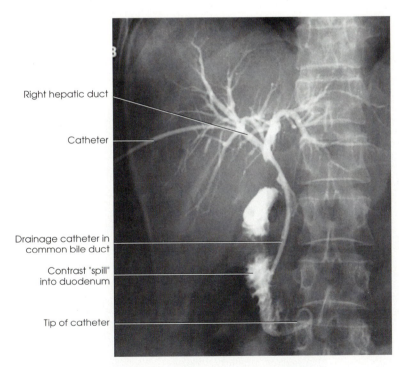

Right hepatic duct

Catheter

Drainage catheter in common bile duct

Contrast "spill" into duodenum

Tip of catheter

Fig. 16-76. PTC with drainage catheter in place.

(Courtesy Carol Drobik, R.T.)

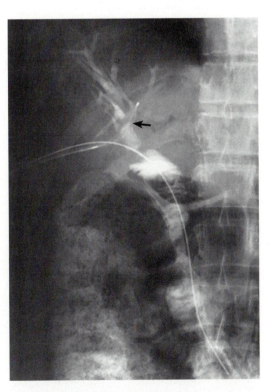

Fig. 16-77. Post-PTC image showing wire basket *(arrow)* around retained stone.

(Courtesy Carol Drobik, R.T.)

OPERATIVE (IMMEDIATE) CHOLANGIOGRAPHY

Operative cholangiography, introduced by Mirizzi[1] in 1932, is carried out during biliary tract surgery, as its title indicates. Following drainage of the bile, and in the absence of obstruction, this technique permits contrast filling of the major intrahepatic ducts as well as of the extrahepatic ducts. The value of operative cholangiography is such that it has become an integral part of biliary tract surgery. It is used in the investigation of the patency of the bile ducts and of the functional status of the sphincter of the hepatopancreatic ampulla to reveal the presence of calculi that cannot be detected by palpation and to demonstrate such conditions as small intraluminal neoplasms and stricture or dilation of the ducts. When the pancreatic duct shares a common channel with the distal common bile duct before emptying into the duodenum, it is sometimes seen on operative cholangiograms because it has been partially filled by reflux.

[1]Mirizzi PL: La colangiografía durante las operaciones de las vías bilares, Bol Soc Cir B Air 16:1133-1161, 1932.

During the preparation of the operating room and in cooperation with the nursing staff, the radiographer performs the following steps:

- Adjust the grid on the operating table.
- Clean the mobile unit with a damp (not wet) cloth, and place the machine in a convenient and easily maneuverable position.
- Connect and test the machine, and adjust the controls according to predetermined exposure factors.
- Make an adequate number of cassettes for immediate processing of the films.
- Adjust the patient on the operating table so that the right upper quadrant of the abdomen is centered to the grid.
- Elevate the left side of the body 15 to 20 degrees if needed to prevent the possibility of superimposing the bile ducts on the vertebrae.

After exposing, draining, and exploring the biliary tract, and frequently after excising the gall bladder, the surgeon injects the contrast medium. This solution is usually introduced into the common bile duct, through a needle, a small catheter, or, after cholecystectomy, through an inlying T tube. When the latter route is used, the procedure is referred to as *delayed operative* or *operative T-tube cholangiography.*

The exposure time used for operative cholangiography must be as short as possible, and the exposures must be made during temporary respiratory arrest, which the anesthetist controls. AP or AP oblique (RPO position) films are exposed at the direction of the surgeon. The total volume of contrast medium is usually introduced in small amounts in two to four stages, with one or more films being exposed after each injection (Figs. 16-78 to 16-82).

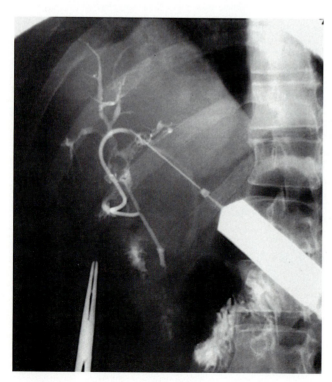

Fig. 16-78. Operative cholangiography. Injection of 5 ml contrast medium.

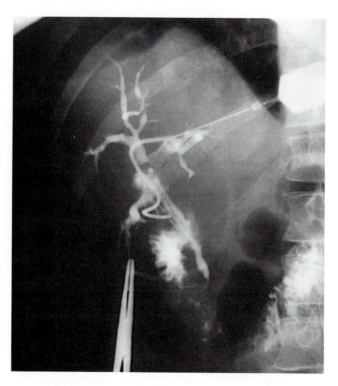

Fig. 16-79. Injection of 10 ml contrast medium.

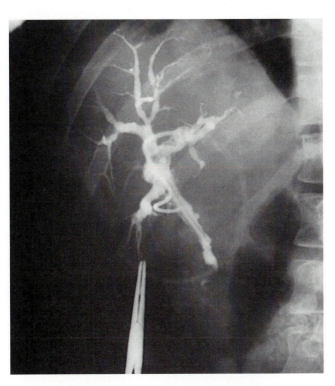

Fig. 16-80. Injection of 15 ml contrast medium.

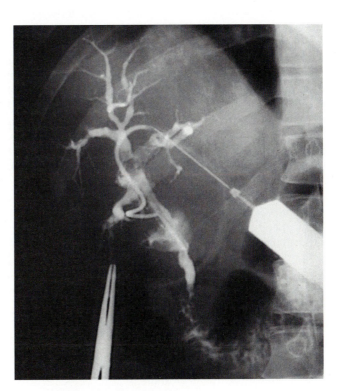

Fig. 16-81. Injection of 20 ml contrast medium.

(Courtesy Dr. Robert L. Pinck.)

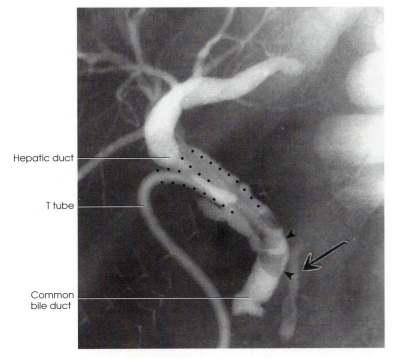

Hepatic duct

T tube

Common
bile duct

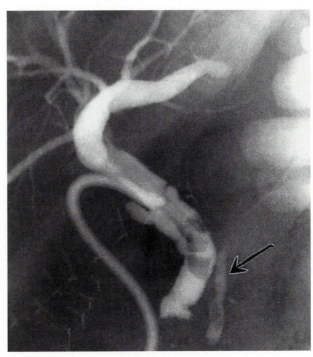

Fig. 16-82. Delayed operative cholangiogram showing T tube *(dots)* and residual stones *(arrowheads)* in common duct and markedly dilated bile ducts. Reflux into pancreatic duct *(arrow)*.

POSTOPERATIVE CHOLANGIOGRAPHY

Postoperative, delayed, and *T-tube chol-angiography* are radiologic terms applied to the biliary tract examination that is performed by way of the T-shaped tube left in the common bile duct for postoperative drainage. This examination is performed to demonstrate the caliber and patency of the ducts, the status of the sphincter of the hepatopancreatic ampulla, and the presence of residual or previously undetected stones or other pathologic conditions.

Postoperative cholangiography is performed in the radiology department. Preliminary preparation usually consists of the following:

1. The drainage tube is clamped the day preceding the examination to let the tube fill with bile as a preventive measure against air bubbles entering the ducts, where they would simulate cholesterol stones.
2. The preceding meal is withheld.
3. When indicated, a cleansing enema is administered about 1 hour before the examination. Premedication is not required.

The contrast agent used is one of the water-soluble, organic contrast media. The density of the contrast medium used in postoperative cholangiograms is recommended to be no more than 25% to 30% because small stones may be obscured in a higher concentration.

After a preliminary radiograph of the abdomen has been obtained, the patient is adjusted in the RPO position (AP oblique projection) with the right upper quadrant of the abdomen centered to the midline of the grid (Figs. 16-83 and 16-84).

Using universal precautions, the contrast medium is injected under fluoroscopic control, with spot and conventional radiographs exposed as indicated. Otherwise, 10×12 in (24×30 cm) films are exposed serially after each of several fractional injections of the medium and then at specified intervals until most of the contrast solution has entered the duodenum.

Stern et al.[1] stress the importance of obtaining a lateral projection to demonstrate the anatomic branching of the hepatic ducts in this plane and to detect any abnormality not otherwise demonstrated (Fig. 16-85). (See p. 68 for description of lateral positioning.) The clamp is generally not removed from the T-tube before completion of the examination, so the patient may be turned onto the right side for this study.

[1]Stern WZ, Schein CJ, and Jacobson HG: The significance of the lateral view in T-tube cholangiography, AJR 87:764-771, 1962.

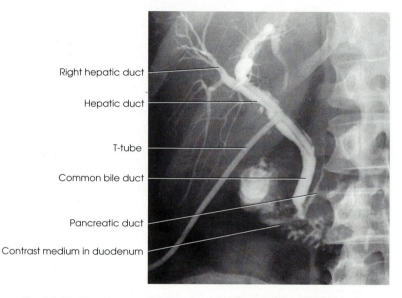

Right hepatic duct
Hepatic duct
T-tube
Common bile duct
Pancreatic duct
Contrast medium in duodenum

Fig. 16-83. AP oblique postoperative cholangiogram, RPO position.

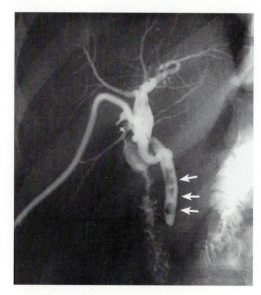

Fig. 16-84. AP oblique postoperative cholangiogram showing multiple stones in common bile duct *(arrows)*. RPO position.

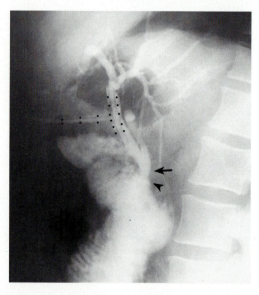

Fig. 16-85. Right lateral cholangiogram showing anteroposterior location of T-tube *(dots)*, common bile duct *(arrow)* and hepatopancreatic ampulla (of Vater) *(arrowhead)*.

(Courtesy Dr. William Z. Stern.)

Pancreas
OPERATIVE PANCREATOGRAPHY

Because of the introduction of endoscopic retrograde cholangiopancreatography (the next procedure to be discussed), intraoperative ultrasonography, and computed tomography, operative pancreatography is performed less frequently. For a more complete description, see the fourth edition of this atlas, Volume 3.

Operative (direct) *pancreatography* is the surgicoradiologic procedure wherein a water-soluble, iodinated contrast medium is introduced into the main pancreatic duct (duct of Wirsung) for the investigation of abnormalities of the pancreas. This may be done (1) by reflux filling from an injection made into the common bile duct when these two passages share a common channel before emptying into the duodenum or (2) by direct injection through transduodenal catheterization of the duct (Figs. 16-86 and 16-87).

The radiographer should be present when the operating room is being prepared so that, in cooperation with the nursing staff, he or she can perform the following steps:
- Center the grid or the cassette to the median sagittal plane of the patient's body at the level of the xiphoid process.
- Clean the mobile unit, and place it in a convenient and easily movable position.

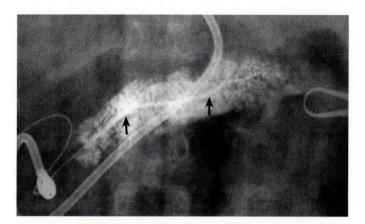

Fig. 16-86. Operative transampullary AP pancreatogram showing pancreatic duct *(arrows)* and extravasation of contrast material into parenchymal pancreatic tissue caused by inflammation.

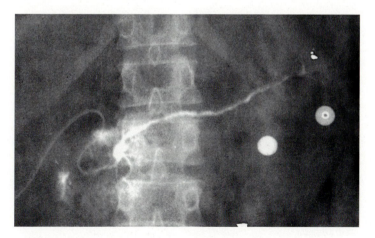

Fig. 16-87. Postoperative AP pancreatogram on same patient as in Fig. 16-86 made 16 days later, showing dramatic reduction in extravasation as result of recovery from pancreatitis.

ENDOSCOPIC RETROGRADE CHOLANGIOPANCREATOGRAPHY (ERCP)

Endoscopic retrograde cholangiopancreatography (ERCP) is a procedure used to diagnose biliary and pancreatic pathologic conditions. ERCP is useful in diagnosis when the biliary ducts are not dilated and when there is no obstruction at the ampulla.

ERCP is performed by passing a fiberoptic endoscope through the mouth into the duodenum under fluoroscopic control.

To ease passage of the endoscope, the patient's throat is sprayed with a local anesthetic. Since this causes temporary pharyngeal paresis, food and drink are usually prohibited for at least 1 hour after the examination. Food may be withheld for up to 10 hours after the procedure to minimize irritation to the stomach and small bowel.

After the endoscopist locates the hepatopancreatic ampulla (ampulla of Vater), a small cannula is passed through the endoscope and directed into the ampulla (Fig. 16-88). Following proper placement of the cannula, the contrast medium is injected into the common bile duct. The patient may then be moved, fluoroscopy performed, and spot radiographs taken (Figs. 16-89 and 16-90). Oblique spot radiographs may be taken to prevent overlap of the common bile duct and the pancreatic duct. The injected contrast material should drain from normal ducts within approximately 5 minutes, so radiographs must be exposed immediately.

The contrast medium used may vary, depending on the preference of the radiologist or gastroenterologist. Dense contrast agents opacify small ducts very well, but the dense contrast material may obscure small stones. If small stones are suspected, a more dilute contrast medium is suggested.[1] A history of patient sensitivity to iodinated contrast medium in another examination (e.g., intravenous urogram) does not necessarily contraindicate its use during ERCP. Caution must be exercised to watch for a reaction to the contrast medium during ERCP.

ERCP is often indicated when both clinical and radiographic findings indicate abnormalities in the biliary system or the pancreas. An oral cholecystogram, ultrasound examination, or intravenous cholangiogram is usually performed before ERCP. Ultrasonography of the upper part of the abdomen before endoscopy is often recommended to assure the physician that no pseudocysts are present. This step is important because contrast medium injected into pseudocysts may lead to inflammation or rupture of the pseudocysts.

[1]Cotton P and William C: Practical gastrointestinal endoscopy, Oxford, England, 1980, Blackwell Scientific Publications, Ltd, p 64.

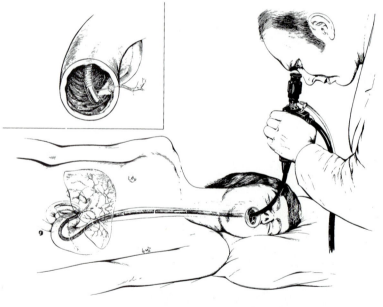

Fig. 16-88. Cannulation procedure. Procedure is begun with patient in left lateral position. This schematic diagram gives overview of location of examiner, position of scope, and its relationship to various internal organs during cannulation. Side-viewing duodenoscope is pointed toward papilla. *Inset,* Magnified view of appearance of the tip of scope with cannula in papilla.

(From Stewart ET, Vennes JA, and Gennen JE: Atlas of endoscopic retrograde cholangiopancreatography, St Louis, 1977, Mosby, p 6.)

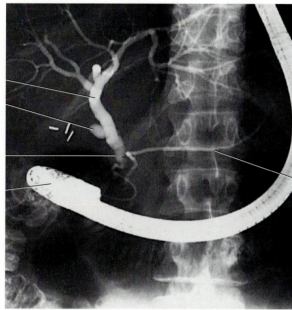

Common hepatic duct

Cystic stump

Common bile duct

Endoscope

Pancreatic duct

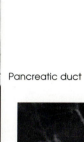

Fig. 16-89. ERCP spot radiograph, PA projection.

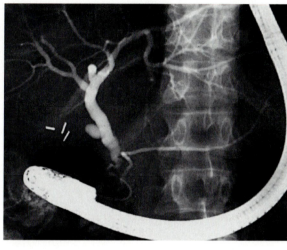

Pancreatic duct

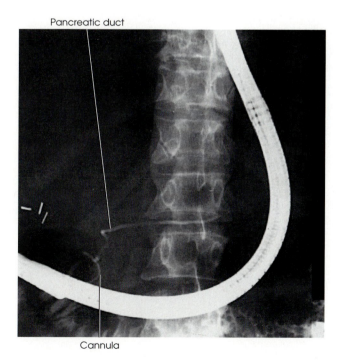

Cannula

Fig. 16-90. ERCP spot radiograph, PA projection.

Chapter 17

DIGESTIVE SYSTEM

Alimentary Tract

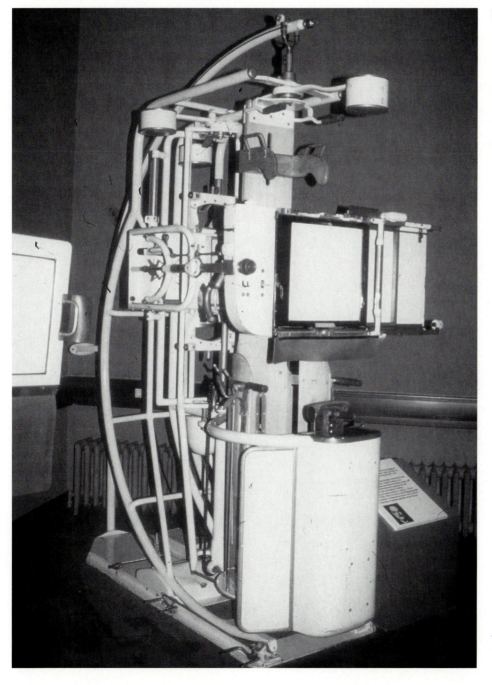

A radiographic and fluoroscopic table from the 1930s.

The digestive system includes several anatomic areas and organs, some of which (abdomen, liver, spleen, and biliary tract) are described in Chapter 16. The digestive system also includes the alimentary tract, which is a musculomembranous tubelike structure. The regions of the alimentary tract vary in diameter according to functional requirements. The greater part of the tract, which is about 29 to 30 feet (8.6 to 8.9 m) in length, lies in the abdominal cavity. The component parts of the alimentary tract (Fig. 17-1) are the mouth, in which the food is masticated and converted into a bolus by insalivation; the pharynx and esophagus, which are the organs of deglutition (swallowing); the stomach, in which the digestive process begins; the small intestine, in which the digestive process is completed; and the large intestine, or colon, an organ of egestion and water absorption, which terminates at the anus.

ESOPHAGUS

The *esophagus* is a long muscular tube which extends from the inferior border of the cricoid cartilage to the stomach (Fig. 17-1). The adult esophagus is approximately 10 inches (25 cm) in length and ¾ inch (2 cm) in diameter. Its wall is composed of 4 layers, similar to the rest of the alimentary canal. Beginning with the outermost layer and going in, the layers are (1) a fibrous layer, (2) a muscular layer, (3) a submucosa layer, and (4) a mucosa layer. The muscular layer has internal circular fibers and external longitudinal fibers.

The *cervical esophagus* originates at the level of the inferior margin of the cricoid cartilage, the level of the sixth cervical vertebra. At its origin the esophagus lies in the median sagittal plane. The *thoracic esophagus* enters the thorax from the distal portion of the neck, where it deviates slightly toward the left side. In the thorax, the esophagus passes through the posterior mediastinum and returns to the midline. The esophagus lies posterior to and to the right of the aortic arch, posterior to the left main bronchus, and between the posterior pericardium and the descending thoracic aorta. In the lower thorax, the esophagus again deviates slightly to the left of the midline, crosses the descending aorta, and passes through the diaphragm at the tenth thoracic vertebra to become the *abdominal esophagus*. Inferior to the diaphragm the esophagus curves sharply left, increases in diameter, and joins the stomach at the *esophagogastric* (gastro-esophageal) *junction* at the level of the xiphoid tip (Tll). The expanded portion of the terminal esophagus is called the *cardiac antrum*.

Several normal areas of narrowing are found in the esophagus. The most superior of these is located at the junction of the pharynx and the esophagus. In the thorax the esophagus is normally compressed as it is crossed by the aortic arch and the left main bronchus. The lower esophagus shows a marked narrowing as it passes through the esophageal hiatus of the diaphragm.

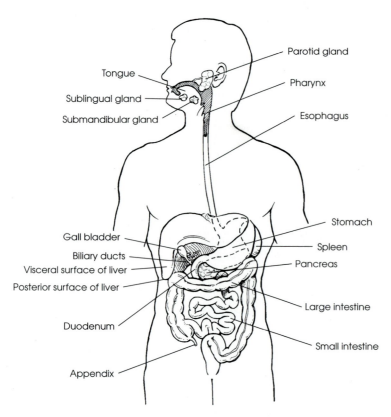

Tongue
Sublingual gland
Submandibular gland
Parotid gland
Pharynx
Esophagus

Gall bladder
Biliary ducts
Visceral surface of liver
Posterior surface of liver
Duodenum
Appendix
Stomach
Spleen
Pancreas
Large intestine
Small intestine

Fig. 17-1. Alimentary tract and its accessory organs. To demonstrate the position of the gall bladder in relation to the liver, the liver is shown with the inferior portion pulled anteriorly and superiorly, thus flipping the liver in an atypical position.

STOMACH

The *stomach* is the dilated, saclike portion of the digestive tract extending between the esophagus and the small intestine (Figs. 17-2 and 17-3). Its wall is composed of four layers. Beginning with the outermost layer and going in, they are (1) a covering layer, the serosa; (2) a muscular layer consisting of oblique, circular, and longitudinal fibers; (3) a submucous layer; and (4) a thick, soft mucosal lining, which is thrown into numerous *gastric folds* (rugae) when the organ is contracted.

The stomach is divided into four parts: (1) the cardia, (2) the fundus, (3) the body, and (4) the pyloric portion. The *cardia* of the stomach is the section immediately surrounding the esophageal opening. The *fundus* of the stomach is the superior portion of the stomach that expands superiorly and fills the dome of the left hemidiaphragm. When the patient is in the upright position the fundus is usually filled with gas and is referred to in radiography as the gas bubble. Descending from the fundus and beginning at the level of the cardiac notch is the *body* of the stomach. The body ends at a vertical plane passing through the angular notch. Distal to this plane is the *pyloric portion* of the stomach. The pyloric portion of the stomach consists of the *pyloric antrum* and the narrow *pyloric canal* to the immediate right of the angular notch and a constricted terminal *pylorus*. The pylorus is a greatly thickened muscular wall surrounding the pyloric canal.

The stomach has an anterior and a posterior surface. The right border of the stomach is marked by the *lesser curvature*. The lesser curvature begins at the esophagogastric junction (esophageal orifice), is continuous with the right border of the esophagus, and is a concave curve ending at the pylorus. Two-thirds of the distance along the lesser curvature is a sharp indentation called the *angular notch*. The left and inferior borders of the stomach are marked by the *greater curvature*. The greater curvature begins at the sharp angle at the esophagogastric junction, the *cardiac notch*, and follows the superior curvature of the fundus and then the convex curvature of the body down to the pylorus. The greater curvature is four to five times longer than the lesser curvature. Sometimes present in the greater curvature is the *sulcus intermedius,* a less defining notch opposite the angular notch of the lesser curvature.

The stomach has two openings, each of which is controlled by a muscular sphincter. The esophagus joins the stomach at the esophagogastric junction through an opening termed the *cardiac orifice.* The muscles controlling the cardiac orifice are called the *cardiac sphincter*. The opening between the stomach and the small intestine is the *pyloric orifice,* and the muscles controlling the pyloric orifice are called the *pyloric sphincter.*

The size, shape, and position of the stomach depend on bodily habitus and vary with posture and with the amount of stomach contents (see illustrations in Volume 1, Chapter 3, Figs. 3-7 to 3-10). In persons of the hypersthenic habitus, the stomach is almost horizontal and is high, with its most dependent portion well above the umbilicus. In persons of the opposite extreme, the asthenic habitus, the stomach is vertical and occupies a low position, its most dependent portion extending well below the transpyloric or interspinous line. Between these two extremes are the many intermediate types of bodily habitus, with corresponding variations in the shape and position of the stomach.

The stomach has several functions in the digestive process. The stomach serves as a storage area for food until it can be further digested. Acids, enzymes, and other chemicals are secreted to chemically break down food. Through churning and peristalsis, food is mechanically broken down. Food which has been mechanically and chemically altered in the stomach is transported to the duodenum as a material called *chyme*.

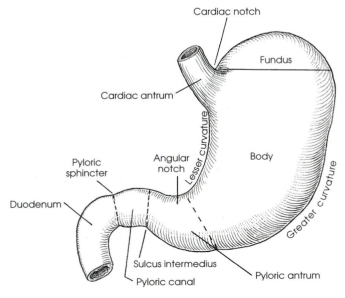

Fig. 17-2. Anterior surface of stomach.

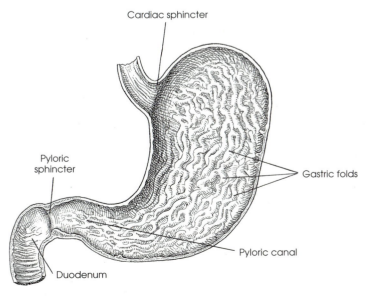

Fig. 17-3. Section of stomach showing rugae.

SMALL INTESTINE

The *small intestine* extends from the pyloric sphincter of the stomach to the ileocecal valve, where it joins the large intestine at a right angle. The length of the adult small intestine averages about 22 feet (6½ m), and its diameter gradually diminishes from approximately 1½ inches (4 cm) in the proximal part to approximately 1 inch (2.5 cm) in the distal part. The wall of the small intestine is composed of four coats: serous (outermost layer), muscular, submucous, and mucous (innermost layer). The muscular coat consists of an inner layer of circular fibers and an outer layer of longitudinal fibers. The mucous layer is thrown into circular folds from which small processes called *villi* project. The small intestine is divided into three portions: the duodenum, the jejunum, and the ileum.

The *duodenum* is 8 to 10 inches (20 to 25 cm) in length and is the widest portion of the small bowel (Fig. 17-4). It is retroperitoneal and relatively fixed in position. Beginning at the pylorus, the duodenum follows a C-shaped course, its several regions being described as first (superior), second (descending), third (horizontal or inferior), and fourth (ascending) portions. The segment of the first (superior) portion is called the *duodenal bulb* because of its radiographic appearance when filled with an opaque medium. The second (descending) portion is about 3 or 4 inches (7 to 10 cm) in length. This segment passes inferiorly along the head of the pancreas and in close relation to the undersurface of the liver. The common bile duct and the pancreatic duct usually unite to form the hepatopancreatic ampulla (ampulla of Vater), which opens on the summit of the *greater duodenal papilla* in the duodenum. The third (horizontal) portion passes toward the left at a slight superior inclination for a distance of about 2½ inches (6 cm) and continues as

the fourth (ascending) portion on the left side of the vertebrae. This portion joins the jejunum at a sharp curve called the *duodenojejunal flexure* and is supported by the suspensory muscle of the duodenum (ligament of Treitz). Although the duodenal loop is the most fixed part of the small bowel and normally lies in the upper part of the umbilical region of the abdomen, its position varies with bodily habitus and with the amount of gastric and intestinal contents.

The remainder of the small intestine is arbitrarily divided into two portions, the upper two-fifths being referred to as the *jejunum* and the lower three-fifths as the *ileum*. The jejunum and the ileum are gathered into freely movable loops, or convolutions, and are attached to the posterior wall of the abdomen by the mesentery. The loops lie in the central and lower part of the abdominal cavity within the arch of the large intestine. The main functions of the small bowel are digestion and absorption.

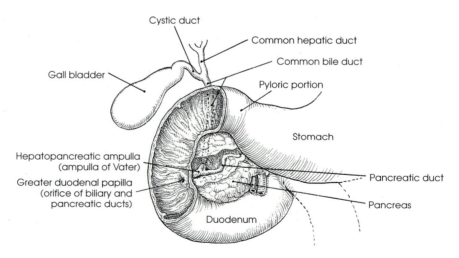

Fig. 17-4. Duodenal loop in relation to biliary and pancreatic ducts.

LARGE INTESTINE

The *large intestine* begins in the right iliac region when it joins the ileum of the small intestine, forms an arch surrounding the loops of the small intestine, and ends at the anus (Fig. 17-5). The large intestine is about 5 feet (1.5 m) long and is greater in diameter than the small bowel. The large intestine is subdivided into the cecum, the colon, the rectum, and the anal canal. The wall of the intestine is composed of serous (outermost), muscular, submucous, and mucous (innermost) coats. The muscular coat consists of an inner layer of circular fibers and an outer layer of longitudinal fibers arranged in three bands over the greater part of the intestine and in two bands over the remaining part. The bands, called *teniae coli,* are shorter than the other layers, with the result that between the teniae coli the wall of the large intestine is pouched, or sacculated. The recesses of the sacculations are called *haustra.* The main functions of the large intestine are reabsorption of fluids and elimination of waste products.

The *cecum* is the pouchlike portion of the large intestine and is situated below the junction of the ileum and the colon. The cecum is approximately 2½ inches (6 cm) in length and 3 inches (7.5 cm) in diameter. The *appendix,* or vermiform process, is attached to the posteromedial side of the cecum. The appendix is a narrow, wormlike tube and averages about 3 inches (7.5 cm) in length. The wall of the appendix is similar to that of the intestine. The *ileocecal valve* is situated just below the junction of the ascending colon and the cecum. The valve projects into the lumen of the cecum and guards the opening between the ileum and the cecum.

The colon is subdivided into ascending, transverse, descending, and sigmoid portions. The *ascending portion* passes superiorly from its junction with the cecum to the undersurface of the liver, where it joins the transverse portion at an angle called the *right colic* (hepatic) *flexure.* The *transverse portion,* which is the longest and most movable part of the colon, crosses the abdomen to the undersurface of the spleen. The transverse portion then makes a sharp curve, called the *left colic* (splenic) *flexure,* and ends in the descending portion. The *descending portion* passes inferiorly and medially to its junction with the sigmoid portion at the superior aperture of the lesser pelvis. The *sigmoid portion* curves on itself to form an S-shaped loop and ends in the rectum at the level of the third sacral segment.

The *rectum* extends from the sigmoid to the anal canal. The *anal canal* terminates at the anus, which is the external aperture of the intestine (Fig. 17-6). The rectum is approximately 6 inches (15 cm) in length. The distal portion, about 1 inch (2.5 cm) long, is constricted to form the anal canal. Just above the anal canal is a dilation called the *rectal ampulla.* Following the sacrococcygeal curve, the rectum passes inferiorly and posteriorly to the level of the pelvic floor and then bends sharply anteriorly and inferiorly into the anal canal that extends to the anus. The rectum and anal canal thus have two anteroposterior curves, a fact that must be remembered when an enema tube is inserted.

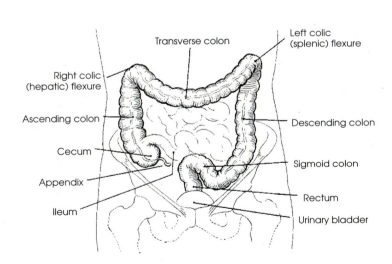

Fig. 17-5. Anterior aspect of large bowel.

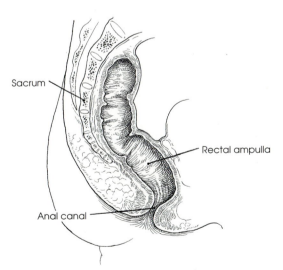

Fig. 17-6. Sagittal section showing direction of anal canal and rectum.

Digestive system

TECHNICAL CONSIDERATIONS: GASTROINTESTINAL TRANSIT

Peristalsis is the term applied to the contraction waves by which the digestive tube propels its contents toward the rectum. Normally three or four waves per minute occur in the filled stomach. The waves begin in the upper part of the organ and travel toward the pylorus. The average emptying time of the normal stomach is from 2 to 3 hours.

Peristaltic action in the intestines is greatest in the upper part of the tract, showing a gradual decrease toward the lower portion. The duodenum and the jejunum undergo, in addition to the peristaltic waves, localized contractions, which usually occur at intervals of 3 to 4 seconds during digestion. The first part of a barium meal normally reaches the ileocecal valve in 2 to 3 hours, the last portion in 4 to 5 hours. The barium usually reaches the rectum within 24 hours.

The specialized procedures frequently employed in radiologic examinations of the esophagus, the stomach, and the intestines will be discussed in this section. The esophagus extends between the pharynx and the cardiac end of the stomach and occupies a constant position in the posterior part of the mediastinum, where its radiographic demonstration presents little difficulty with use of contrast media. On the other hand, the stomach and intestines vary in size, shape, position, and muscular tonus according to the patient's habitus. In addition to the normal structural and functional differences, there is an extensive variety of gastrointestinal abnormalities, many of which cause further changes in location and motility. These variations make the investigation of each gastrointestinal patient an individual study, and meticulous attention must be given to each detail in the examination procedure.

Examinations of the alimentary tract usually consist of a combination of fluoroscopy and radiography. The fluoroscopic examination enables observation of the tract in motion, special mucosal studies, and determination of the subsequent procedure required for a complete examination. Films are exposed, as indicated, during and after the fluoroscopic examination for a permanent record of the findings.

Contrast media

Since the thin-walled alimentary tract does not have sufficient density to cast its shadow through those of the surrounding structures, its radiographic demonstration requires the use of an artificial contrast medium. *Barium sulfate,* which is a water-insoluble salt of the metallic element barium, is the contrast medium universally employed in examinations of the alimentary tract (Fig. 17-7). The barium sulfate used for this purpose is a specially prepared, chemically pure product to which various chemical substances have been added. Barium sulfate is available either in a dry powder or liquid form. The powdered barium is mixed with plain water in different concentrations. The concentration used depends on the part to be examined and the preference of the physician.

A number of special barium sulfate products are also available. Those with finely divided barium sulfate particles tend to resist precipitation and remain in suspension longer than the regular barium preparations. Some barium preparations contain gums or other suspending or dispersing agents and are referred to as suspended or flocculation-resistant preparations.

The speed with which the barium mixture passes through the alimentary tract depends on the suspending medium, the temperature, and the consistency of the preparation as well as on the motile function of the alimentary tract.

In addition to barium sulfate, *water-soluble, iodinated contrast media* suitable for opacification of the alimentary tract are also available (Fig. 17-8). These preparations are modifications of basic intravenous urographic media such as diatrizoate sodium and diatrizoate methylglucamine.

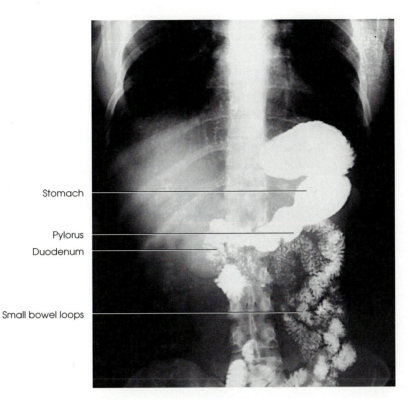

Stomach

Pylorus
Duodenum

Small bowel loops

Fig. 17-7. Barium sulfate suspension in the stomach.

(Courtesy Nina Kowalczyk, R.T.)

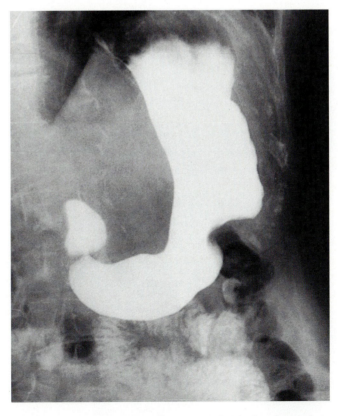

Fig. 17-8. Water-soluble iodinated solution in the stomach.

(Courtesy Dr. William H. Shehadi.)

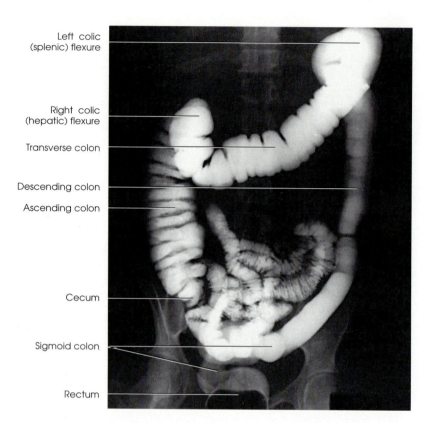

Left colic (splenic) flexure

Right colic (hepatic) flexure

Transverse colon

Descending colon

Ascending colon

Cecum

Sigmoid colon

Rectum

Fig. 17-9. Barium sulfate suspension administered by rectum.

(Courtesy Betsy Delzeith, R.T.)

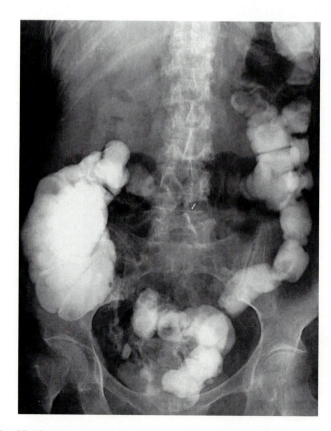

Fig. 17-10. Water-soluble iodinated solution administered by mouth.

The iodinated solutions move through the gastrointestinal tract more quickly than do barium sulfate suspensions (Figs. 17-9 and 17-10). The iodinated solution normally clears the stomach in 1 to 2 hours, and the entire iodinated contrast column reaches and outlines the colon in about 4 hours. An orally administered iodinated medium differs from barium sulfate in the following ways:

1. It outlines the esophagus, although it does not adhere to the mucosa as well as does a barium sulfate suspension.

2. It affords an entirely satisfactory examination of the stomach and duodenum, including mucosal delineation.

3. It permits rapid survey of the entire small bowel, although the medium fails to provide clear anatomic detail of this portion of the alimentary tract. This failure results from the dilution of the contrast medium with a considerable decrease in opacification.

4. Because of the normal function of rapid water absorption through the colonic mucosa, the medium once again becomes densely concentrated, with the result that it delineates the entire large bowel almost as well as does a retrograde filling with a barium sulfate suspension. Because of this result and its accelerated transit time, a reasonably rapid investigation of the large bowel by the oral route can be performed when a patient cannot cooperate for a satisfactory enema study.

A great advantage of water-soluble media is that they are easily removed by aspiration either before or during surgery. Further, if a water-soluble, iodinated medium escapes into the peritoneum through a pre-existing perforation of the stomach or intestine, no ill effects will result, and the medium is readily absorbed from the peritoneal cavity and excreted by the kidneys. This is a definite advantage when investigating perforated ulcers.

A disadvantage of the iodinated preparations is their strongly bitter taste, which can be masked only to a limited extent. The patient should be forewarned so that he or she will be better able to tolerate the bitter taste.

Radiologic apparatus

Advances in the design of modern radiographic and fluoroscopic equipment have led to virtual replacement in most medical facilities of the older system of dark room fluoroscopy by image intensification. Image intensification systems (Fig. 17-11) do not require adaptation of the eye to night vision, and the unit is capable of being connected to accessory units such as cine film recorders, television systems, spot-film cameras, and video recorders. Remote control fluoroscopic rooms are also available and are used by the fluoroscopist located in an adjacent control area (Fig. 17-12).

Although conventional cassette-loaded spot-film devices are still used with image intensification in the majority of fluoroscopic installations, developments in spot-film cameras have resulted in an increase in the number of spot-film cameras and a slight decline in the number of conventional cassette-loaded spot-filming units. Current spot-film cameras require neither as much radiation exposure of the patient nor as great a time of interruption to expose the spot film during the fluoroscopic examination. The reduced radiation to the patient also results in less of a heat load placed on the x-ray tube compared with conventional spot filming. The most common spot-film camera sizes available are for film widths of 100 and 105 mm. Modern fluoroscopic systems now produce the spot-film images on laser printers. Digital fluoroscopic units are also available which permit the recording of multiple fluoroscopic images on one film.

During an examination of the alimentary tract, compression and palpation of the abdomen are often used. Many types of compression devices are available; the fluoroscopic unit pictured in Fig. 17-11 shows a compression cone in contact with the patient's abdomen. This device is often used during general fluoroscopic examinations. Other types of commercial compression devices are available, such as the pneumatic compression paddle shown in Fig. 17-13. This device is often placed under the duodenal bulb and then inflated to place pressure on the abdomen. The air is then slowly released and the compression on the body part eliminated.

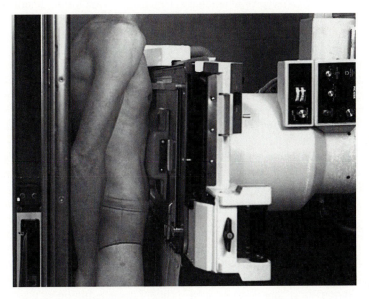

Fig. 17-11. Image intensification system: compression cone in contact with abdomen.

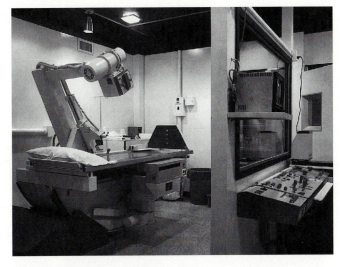

Fig. 17-12. Remote control fluoroscopic room showing patient fluoroscopic table *(left)* and fluoroscopist's control console *(right)*. Patient is viewed by fluoroscopist through the large window.

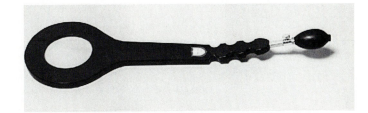

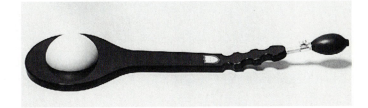

Fig. 17-13. Compression paddle: *above,* noninflated; *below,* inflated.

Preparation of examining room

The examining room should be completely prepared before the patient enters. In preparing the room, the radiographer should observe the following steps:

- Adjust the equipment controls to the appropriate settings.
- Have the footboard and shoulder support available.
- Check the mechanism of the spot-film device and/or spot-film camera and see that sufficient films are available.
- Prepare the required type and amount of contrast medium.

Before commencing the examination, the radiographer should do the following:

- Explain to the patient that the barium sulfate mixture may taste a little chalky.
- Inform the patient that the room may be somewhat darkened during fluoroscopy.
- When the fluoroscopist enters the examining room, introduce the patient and the fluoroscopist to each other.

Radiation protection

During fluoroscopy, spot filming (Figs. 17-14 and 17-15), and radiographic filming for either a partial or a complete gastrointestinal examination, the patient will receive radiation. It is taken for granted that properly added filtration is in place at all times in every x-ray tube in the radiology department. It is further assumed that, based on the capacity of the machines and the best available accessory equipment,

the exposure factors are adjusted to deliver the least possible radiation to the patient.

Protection of the patient from unnecessary radiation is a professional responsibility of the radiographer. (See Chapter 1 of this atlas for specific guidelines.) In this chapter, the *"Shield gonads"* statement at the end of the *"Position of part"* section indicates that the patient is to be protected from unnecessary radiation by restricting the radiation beam using proper collimation. Additionally, placing lead shielding between the gonads and the radiation source is appropriate when the clinical objectives of the examination are not compromised.

Exposure time

One of the most important considerations in gastrointestinal radiography is the elimination of motion. The highest degree of motor activity is normally found in the stomach and the proximal part of the small intestine, the activity gradually decreasing along the intestinal tract until it becomes fairly slow in the distal part of the large bowel. Peristaltic speed also depends on the individual patient's habitus and is influenced by the presence of pathologic changes, by body position, and by respiration. The choice of the exposure time for each region must be based on these factors.

In esophageal examinations the radiographer should observe the following guidelines:

- Use an exposure time of 0.1 second

or less for upright radiographs. The time may be slightly longer for recumbent images because the barium descends more slowly.

- Remember that the rate of passage of the barium through the esophagus is fairly slow if the barium is swallowed at the end of full inhalation. The rate of passage is increased if the barium is swallowed at the end of moderate inhalation where it passes through the upper esophagus rapidly. However, it is delayed in the lower part for several seconds if the barium is swallowed at the end of full exhalation.
- Respiration is inhibited for several seconds after the beginning of deglutition, which allows sufficient time for the exposure to be made without instructing the patient to hold his or her breath after swallowing.

In examinations of the stomach and small intestine, the radiographer should observe the following guidelines:

- Use an exposure time for patients who have normal peristaltic activity of no longer than 0.2 second and in no case more than 0.5 second; the exposure time should be 0.1 second or less for those with hypermotility.
- In examinations of the large bowel, use exposure times of 0.5 to 1 second for frontal and oblique images of the entire colon and exposure times of 1.5 to 2 seconds for lateral and axial images of the rectosigmoid region.
- *Respiration:* Exposures of the stomach and intestines are made at the end of exhalation in the routine procedure.

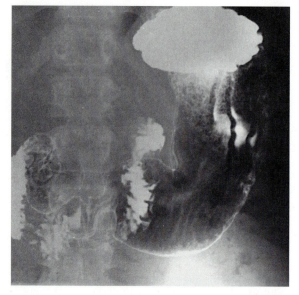

Fig. 17-14. AP spot radiograph of barium-filled fundus of stomach.

(Courtesy Beth Changet, R.T.)

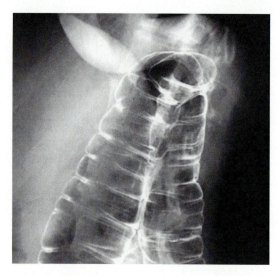

Fig. 17-15. Spot radiograph of air-contrast colon showing left colic (splenic) flexure.

(Courtesy Beth Changet, R.T.)

Esophagus

The esophagus may be examined by performing a *full-column, single-contrast* study in which only barium or another radiopaque contrast agent is used to fill the esophageal lumen. A *double-contrast* procedure also may be used in which barium and carbon dioxide crystals (which liberate carbon dioxide) are the two contrast agents. No preliminary preparation of the patient is necessary.

Barium sulfate mixture

For the full-column, single-contrast technique, a 30% to 50% weight/volume suspension[1] is useful. For a double-contrast examination, a low-viscosity, high-density barium developed for double-contrast gastric examinations may be used. Whatever the weight/volume concentration of the barium, the most important criterion of the barium is that it must flow sufficiently to coat the walls of the esophagus. It is also important to closely follow the barium manufacturer's mixing instructions to attain optimum performance of the contrast medium.

---

[1]Skucas J: Contrast media. In Margulis AR and Burhenne HJ, editors: Alimentary tract radiology, vol 1, ed 4, St Louis, 1989, Mosby, pp 90-91.

Examination procedures

For a *single-contrast* examination (Figs. 17-16 to 17-18), the following steps are observed:

- Start the fluoroscopic and spot-film examination with the patient in the upright position whenever possible.
- Use the horizontal and Trendelenburg positions as indicated.
- After the fluoroscopic examination of the heart and lungs, and when the patient is upright, instruct the patient to take the cup containing the barium suspension in the left hand and to drink it on request.

The fluoroscopist asks the patient to swallow several mouthfuls of the barium so that the act of deglutition can be observed to determine whether there is any abnormality. The fluoroscopist instructs the patient to perform various breathing maneuvers under fluoroscopic observation so that the fluoroscopist can take spot radiographs of areas or lesions not otherwise demonstrated.

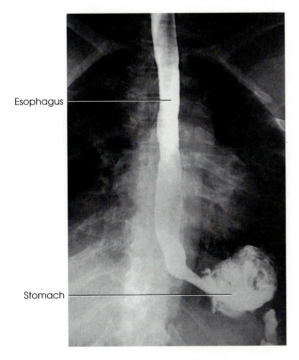

Fig. 17-16. AP esophagus, single-contrast.

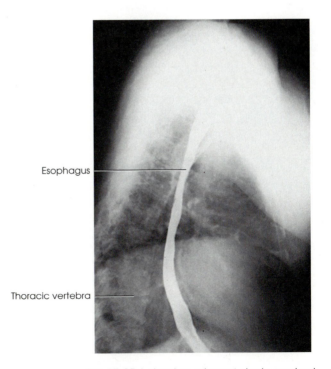

Fig. 17-17. Lateral esophagus, single-contrast.

The performance of the *double-contrast* esophageal examination (Fig. 17-19) is similar to that of a single-contrast fluoroscopic examination. For a double-contrast examination, a free-flowing, high-density barium must be used. A gas-producing substance, usually carbon dioxide crystals, can be added to the barium mixture or can be given by mouth immediately *before* the barium suspension is given. Spot radiographs are exposed during the examination, and delayed images may be taken on request.

Opaque foreign bodies lodged in the pharynx or in the upper part of the esophagus can usually be demonstrated without the use of a contrast medium. A soft tissue neck or a lateral projection of the retrosternal area may be taken for this purpose. The following steps are observed:

• Take a lateral neck radiograph at the height of deglutition for the delineation of opaque foreign bodies in the upper end of the intrathoracic esophagus.

• Deglutition elevates this portion of the esophagus a distance of two cervical segments, which places it above the level of the clavicles.

Tufts or pledgets of cotton saturated with a thin barium suspension are sometimes used to demonstrate an obstruction and also for the detection of nonopaque foreign bodies in the pharynx and upper esophagus.

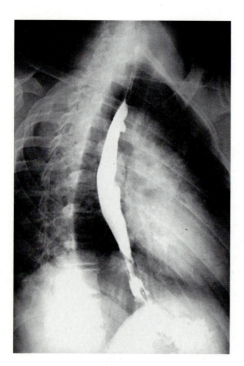

Fig. 17-18. PA oblique esophagus, single-contrast. RAO position.

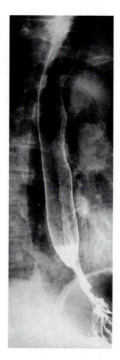

Fig. 17-19. PA oblique distal esophagus, double-contrast spot-film. RAO position.

(Courtesy Deborah Saunders, R.T.).

Esophagus

AP/PA, OBLIQUE, AND LATERAL PROJECTIONS

Film: 14 × 17 in (35 × 43 cm) placed lengthwise and centered at the level of T5 or T6 for the inclusion of the entire esophagus.

Position of patient

• Positioning used for chest radiographs (PA, oblique, and lateral; see Volume 1, Chapter 10) is employed in examinations of the esophagus. Because it is possible to obtain a wider space for an unobstructed image of the esophagus between the vertebrae and the heart with an RAO position of 35 to 40 degrees (Fig. 17-20), this is usually used in preference to the LAO position. The LPO position has also been recommended.[1]

---

[1]Cockerill EM et al: Optimal visualization of esophageal varices, AJR 126:512-523, 1976.

• Unless the upright position is specified (Fig. 17-21), place the patient in the recumbent position for esophageal studies (Figs. 17-22 and 17-23). The recumbent body position is used to obtain more complete contrast filling of the esophagus, especially of the proximal part, by having the barium column flow against gravity. The recumbent position is routinely used for the demonstration of variceal distentions of the esophageal veins because the best filling of the varices (Fig. 17-24) is obtained by having the blood flow against gravity. Variceal filling is more complete during increased venous pressure, which may be applied by full exhalation or by the Valsalva maneuver (see Glossary and Chapter 3, Volume 1).

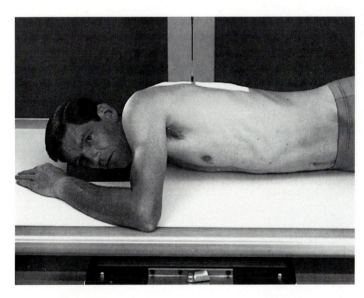

Fig. 17-20. PA oblique esophagus, RAO position.

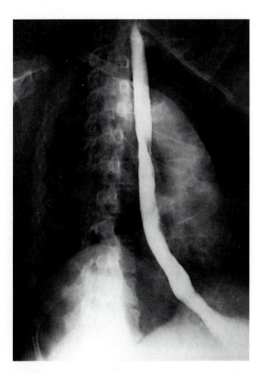

Fig. 17-21. Upright PA oblique esophagus, RAO position.

(Courtesy Betsy Delzeith, R.T.)

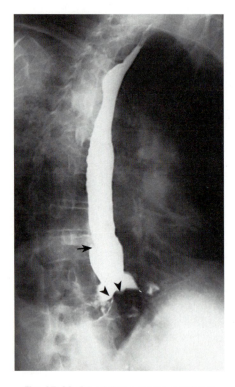

Fig. 17-22. PA oblique single-contrast esophagus showing tear in esophageal lumen *(arrow)* and lesion partially obstructing esophagus *(arrowheads).* RAO position.

Fig. 17-23. PA oblique double-contrast proximal esophagus on spot-film. RAO position.

(Courtesy Deborah Saunders, R.T.)

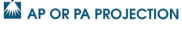

AP OR PA PROJECTION

- Place the patient in the supine or prone position with the arms at the side and the shoulders and hips equidistant from the table.
- Center the median sagittal plane to the grid.
- Turn the head slightly if needed to facilitate drinking of the barium mixture.
- *Shield gonads.*

PA OBLIQUE PROJECTION
RAO or LPO position

- Position the patient in the RAO or LPO position with the median sagittal plane forming an angle of 35 to 45 degrees from the grid device.
- Adjust the arms in a comfortable position with the shoulders lying in the same plane.
- Center the elevated side to the grid through a plane approximately 2 inches lateral to the median sagittal plane (Figs. 17-22 and 17-23).
- *Shield gonads.*

LATERAL PROJECTION
R or L position

- Place the patient in the lateral body position facing the radiographer.
- Place the patient's arms forward.
- Center the median coronal plane to the grid.
- *Shield gonads.*

Central ray

- Direct the central ray perpendicular to the midpoint of the film at the level of T5 or T6.

Structures shown

The contrast-medium–filled esophagus should be demonstrated from the lower part of the neck to the esophagogastric junction, where the esophagus joins the stomach.

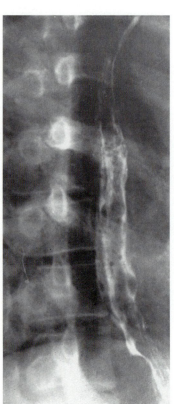

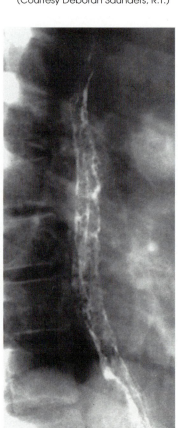

Fig. 17-24. Spot-film studies showing esophageal varices.

□Evaluation criteria

The radiograph should demonstrate:

General

■ Esophagus from the lower part of the neck to its entrance into the stomach.

■ Esophagus filled with barium.

■ Penetration of the barium.

AP or PA

■ Esophagus through the superimposed thoracic vertebrae.

■ No rotation of the patient.

Oblique

■ Esophagus between the vertebrae and heart when the patient is properly obliqued.

Lateral

■ No interference with visualization of the proximal esophagus from the patient's arms.

■ Ribs posterior to the vertebrae superimposed to show that the patient was not rotated.

NOTE: The general criteria apply to all three projections: AP/PA, oblique, and lateral.

Barium administration

• Feed the barium sulfate suspension to the patient either by spoon, by cup, or through a drinking straw, depending on its consistency.

• Ask the patient to swallow several mouthfuls of the suspension in rapid succession and then to hold a mouthful until immediately before the exposure.

• For the demonstration of esophageal varices, instruct the patient (1) to exhale fully and then to swallow the barium bolus and avoid inhaling until the exposure has been made or (2) to take a deep breath and, while holding the breath, to swallow the bolus and then perform the Valsalva maneuver (Fig. 17-24).

• For other conditions, instruct the patient simply to swallow the barium bolus, which is normally done during moderate inhalation. Because respiration is inhibited for about 2 seconds after deglutition, it is not necessary to instruct the patient to hold his or her breath for the exposure. Make two or three exposures in rapid succession before the contrast medium passes into the stomach if it is swallowed at the end of full inhalation. On the other hand, the demonstration of the entire esophagus sometimes requires that the exposure be made while the patient is drinking the barium suspension through a straw in rapid and continuous swallows.

Stomach: Gastrointestinal Series

Upper gastrointestinal tract radiographs are employed to evaluate the distal esophagus, stomach, and some or all of the small intestine. An upper gastrointestinal examination (Fig. 17-25), usually called a GI series or a UGI, may include the following:

1. A preliminary radiograph of the abdomen to delineate the liver, the spleen, the kidneys, the psoas muscles, and bony structures and to detect any abdominal or pelvic calcifications or tumor masses. The detection of calcifications and tumor masses requires that the survey radiograph of the abdomen be taken after any preliminary cleansing of the intestinal tract but before administration of the contrast medium.

2. An examination consisting of fluoroscopic and serial radiographic studies of the esophagus and the stomach and duodenum with an ingested opaque mixture, usually barium sulfate.

3. When requested, a small intestine study consisting of radiographs obtained at frequent intervals during the passage of the contrast column through the small bowel, at which time the appendix and the ileocecal region may be examined.

Ambulatory outpatients or acutely ill patients, such as those with a bleeding ulcer, are usually examined in the supine position by a fluoroscopic and spot-film procedure. Everything possible should be done to expedite the procedure. Any contrast preparation must be ready, and the examination room must be fully prepared before the patient is brought into the radiology department.

Preparation of patient

Before being assigned an appointment for an examination as time-consuming as a gastrointestinal series, the patient should be told the approximate time required for the procedure so that his or her schedule can be arranged accordingly. It is also important that the patient understand the reason for preliminary preparation so that full cooperation can be given.

The stomach must be empty for an examination of the upper gastrointestinal tract (the stomach and the small intestine). It is also desirable to have the colon free of gas and fecal material. When the patient is constipated, a non-gas-forming laxative may be administered the day before the examination. The preparation usually consists of administering to the patient a soft, low-residue diet for 2 days to prevent gas formation as a result of excessive fermentation of the intestinal contents. Cleansing enemas may be given to ensure a properly prepared colon. To ensure an empty stomach, both food and water are withheld after midnight, for a period of 8 to 9 hours before the examination. When a small intestine study is to be made, food and fluid are withheld after the evening meal.

Because it is believed that nicotine and chewing gum stimulate gastric secretion as well as salivation, some physicians instruct the patient not to smoke or chew gum after midnight. This restriction is made to prevent excessive accumulation of fluid in the stomach from diluting the barium suspension enough to interfere with its coating property.

Barium sulfate suspension

The contrast medium that is generally used in routine gastrointestinal examinations is barium sulfate and water. The preparation must be thoroughly mixed according to the manufacturer's instructions. Specially formulated, high-density barium is also available. Advances in the production of barium have all but eliminated the use of a single barium formula as sufficient for most gastrointestinal examinations performed in the department.

Most physicians use one of the many commercially prepared barium suspensions. These products are available in several flavors, and some are conveniently packaged in individual cups containing the dry ingredients. To these, the radiographer merely has to add water, recap the cup, and shake it to obtain a smooth suspension ready for use. Other barium suspensions are completely mixed and ready to use.

Two general gastrointestinal examination procedures are routinely used to examine the stomach: the *single-contrast* method and the *double-contrast* method. A *biphasic* examination is a combination of the single- and double-contrast methods on the same day. *Hypotonic duodenography* is another less frequently used examination.

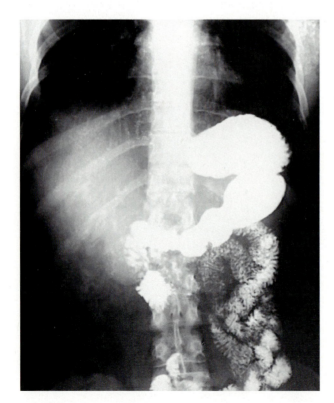

Fig. 17-25. Barium-filled AP stomach and small bowel.

(Courtesy Nina Kowalczyk, R.T.)

SINGLE-CONTRAST EXAMINATION

In the single-contrast method (Fig. 17-26), the barium sulfate suspension is administered during the initial fluoroscopic examination. The barium suspension used for this study is usually in the 30% to 50% weight/volume range.[1]

Whenever possible, the examination is begun with the patient in the upright position. The fluoroscopist may first examine the heart and lungs fluoroscopically and observe the abdomen to determine whether food or fluid is in the stomach. The patient is then given a glass of barium and instructed to drink it as requested by the fluoroscopist. If the patient is in the recumbent position, the suspension is administered through a drinking straw.

The fluoroscopist asks the patient to swallow two or three mouthfuls of the barium, during which time the fluoroscopist examines and exposes any indicated spot films of the esophagus. By manual manipulation of the stomach through the abdominal wall, the fluoroscopist then coats the gastric mucosa. Compression films may be taken with the spot-film device or other compression devices to demonstrate a mucosal lesion of the stomach or duodenum. After the study of the rugae and as the patient drinks the remainder of the barium suspension, the fluoroscopist observes the filling of the stomach and further examines the duodenum. He or she is able to determine the size, shape, and position of the stomach; to examine its changing contour during peristalsis; to observe the filling and emptying of the duodenal bulb; to detect any abnormal alteration in the function or contour of these organs; and to take spot films as indicated. The contrast medium normally begins to pass into the duodenum almost immediately. A delay may be caused by nervous tension of the patient.

[1]Skucas J: Contrast media. In Margulis AR and Burhenne HJ, editors: Alimentary tract radiology, vol 1, ed 4, St Louis, 1989, Mosby.

Fluoroscopy is performed with the patient in the upright and the recumbent positions, while the body is rotated and the table is angled so that all aspects of the esophagus, stomach, and duodenum are demonstrated. Spot films are exposed as indicated. If esophageal involvement is suspected, a study is usually made with a thick barium suspension.

The subsequent radiographs of the stomach and duodenum should be made immediately after fluoroscopy before any considerable amount of the barium suspension passes into the jejunum.

Positions of patient

The stomach and the duodenum may be examined using PA, AP, oblique, and lateral projections, with the patient in the upright and the recumbent positions, as indicated by the fluoroscopic findings.

Variations of the supine positions are (1) an LPO position, (2) lowering the head end of the table 25 to 30 degrees to demonstrate a hiatal hernia, and (3) lowering the head end of the table 10 to 15 degrees and rotating the patient slightly toward the right side to place the esophagogastric (gastroesophageal) junction in profile to the right of the spine. The latter position is used to demonstrate esophageal regurgitation and hiatal hernias. The medical significance of diagnosing hiatal hernias is a topic that has received much attention in recent years. Some authors state that there is little correlation between the presence of a hiatal hernia and gastrointestinal symptoms. If little correlation exists, radiographic evaluation of hiatal hernias is of little value in the majority of cases.

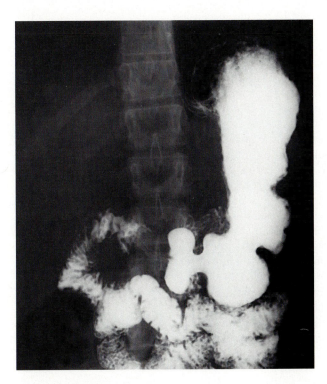

Fig. 17-26. Barium-filled AP stomach, single-contrast method.

(Courtesy Timothy, Hill, R.T.)

DOUBLE-CONTRAST EXAMINATION

A second approach to the examination of the gastrointestinal tract is the *double-contrast* technique (Fig. 17-27). The principal advantages of this method over the single-contrast method are that small lesions are not as easily obscured and the mucosal lining of the stomach can be more clearly visualized. However, for successful results, the patient must be able to move with relative ease throughout the examination.

The following steps are observed:
- To begin the examination, place the patient on the fluoroscopic table in the upright position.
- Give the patient a gas-producing substance in the form of a powder, crystals, pills, or carbonated beverage. (An older technique involved placing pinholes in the sides of a drinking straw so that the patient ingested air while drinking the barium suspension during the course of examination.)
- Then give the patient a small amount of commercially available high-density barium suspension. To obtain even coating of the stomach walls, the barium must flow freely and have a low viscosity. Many high-density barium products are available with weight/volume ratios of up to 250%.
- After the patient drinks the barium, place the patient in the recumbent position and instruct him or her to turn from side to side or to roll over a few times. This movement serves to coat the mucosal lining of the stomach as the carbon dioxide continues to expand. The patient may feel the need to belch but should refrain from doing so until the examination is finished to ensure that optimum contrast will remain for the duration of the examination.

Glucagon or other anticholinergic medications may be intravenously or intramuscularly given to the patient just before the examination to relax the gastrointestinal tract. This medication allows for greater distention of the stomach and bowel for improved visualization. The physician must consider such factors as side effects, contraindications, availability, and cost of the medication before administration.

Radiographic filming procedure

The radiographs taken after the fluoroscopic examination may be the same images obtained for the single-contrast examination as described previously. Often the radiographs with the greatest amount of diagnostic information are the spot films taken during fluoroscopy. Therefore the fluoroscopist will, in most cases, have already obtained most of the necessary diagnostic radiographs.

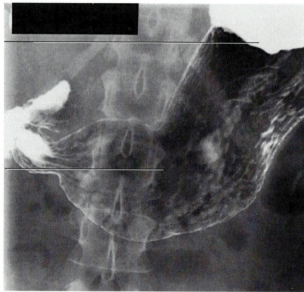

Barium in fundus

Air-filled, barium-coated stomach

A

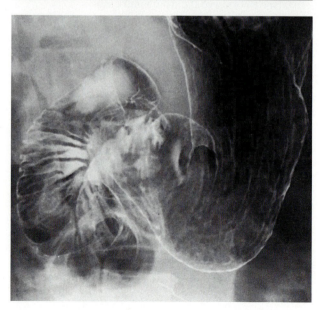

B

Fig. 17-27. Double-contrast stomach, spot films.

(Courtesy Dr. James Jerele.)

BIPHASIC EXAMINATION

The *biphasic* gastrointestinal examination incorporates the advantages of both the single- and double-contrast upper gastrointestinal examinations with both examinations being performed on the same day. The patient is first examined by performing a double-contrast examination of the upper gastrointestinal tract. On completion, the patient is given an approximate 15% weight/volume barium suspension and a single-contrast examination is then performed. This biphasic approach increases the accuracy of diagnosis while not significantly increasing the cost of the examination.

HYPOTONIC DUODENOGRAPHY

The use of *hypotonic duodenography* as a primary diagnostic tool has decreased in recent years. When lesions lying beyond the duodenum are suspected, the double-contrast gastrointestinal examination described previously can aid in the diagnosis. When pancreatic disease is suspected, computed tomography or needle biopsy can also be used for diagnosis. Thus the need to perform hypotonic duodenography has been reduced.

Hypotonic duodenography, first described by Liotta,[1] and requiring intubation (Figs. 17-28 and 17-29), is used for the evaluation of postbulbar duodenal lesions and for the detection of pancreatic disease. The tubeless technique requires temporary drug-induced duodenal paralysis so that a double-contrast examination can be performed without interference from peristaltic activity. During the atonic state, when the duodenum is distended with the contrast medium to two or three times its normal size, it presses against and outlines any abnormality in the contour of the head of the pancreas.

[1]Liotta D: Puor le diagnostic des tumeurs du pancréas: la duodénografie hypotonique, Lyon Chir 50:445-460, 1955.

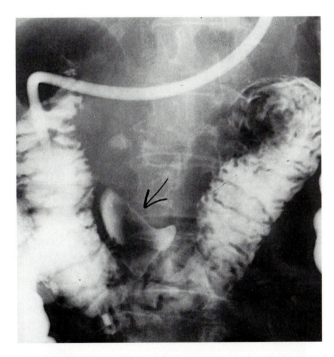

Fig. 17-28. Hypotonic duodenogram showing deformity of duodenal diverticulum by small carcinoma of head of pancreas *(arrow)*.

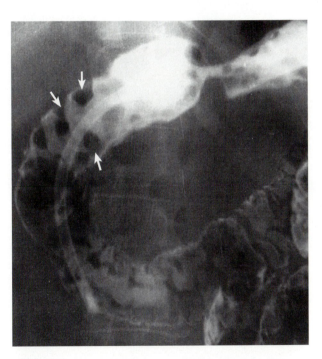

Fig. 17-29. Hypotonic duodenogram showing multiple defects *(arrows)* in duodenal bulb and proximal duodenum caused by hypertrophy of Brunner glands.

(Courtesy Dr. Arthur R. Clemett.)

Stomach and Duodenum

PA PROJECTION

Film: 10 × 12 in (24 × 30 cm) or 14 × 17 in (35 × 43 cm) lengthwise for recumbent projections of the average subject; 11 × 14 in (30 × 35 cm) or 14 × 17 in (35 × 43 cm) lengthwise for upright study.

Position of patient

- Radiographic studies of the stomach and duodenum are made with the patient in the recumbent position. An upright PA projection is sometimes obtained to demonstrate the relative position of the stomach.

- In adjusting thin patients in the prone position, support the weight of the body on pillows or other suitable pads positioned under the thorax and pelvis. This adjustment prevents the stomach or duodenum from pressing against the vertebrae, with resultant pressure-filling defects.

Position of part

- Adjust the patient's position, either recumbent or upright so that the midline of the grid will coincide (1) with a sagittal plane passing halfway between the midline and the lateral border of the abdominal cavity at the level of L1/L2 when a 10 × 12 in (24 × 30 cm) film is used or (2) with the median sagittal plane of the body centered when a 14 × 17 in (35 × 43 cm) film is used (Fig. 17-30).

- Center the film longitudinally at the estimated level of L1/L2 when the patient is prone for the PA projection (Figs. 17-31 and 17-32).

- Center the film 3 to 6 inches (7.5 to 15 cm) lower for upright images. The greatest visceral movement between the prone and the upright positions occurs in asthenic patients.

- Do not apply an immobilization band for standard radiographic projections of the stomach and intestines because the pressure is likely to cause filling defects and because it interferes with the emptying and filling of the duodenal bulb, which is important in serial studies.

- *Shield gonads.* (Not shown for illustrative purposes.)

- Ask the patient to suspend respiration at the end of exhalation unless otherwise requested.

Central ray

- Direct the central ray perpendicular to the film at the level of L1/L2.

Structures shown

A PA projection of the contour of the barium-filled stomach and the duodenal bulb is demonstrated. The upright projection shows the size, shape, and relative position of the filled stomach, but it does not give an adequate demonstration of the un-

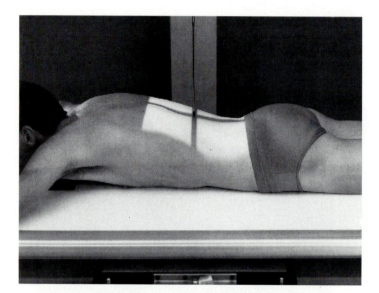

Fig. 17-30. PA stomach and duodenum.

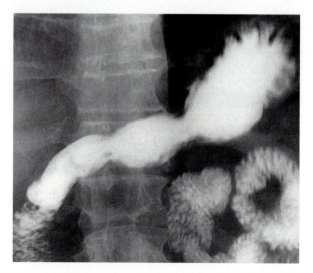

Fig. 17-31. Single-contrast PA stomach and duodenum.

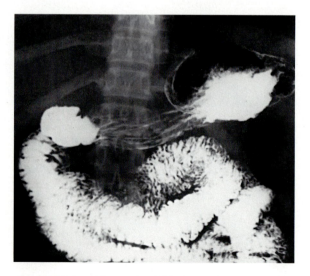

Fig. 17-32. Double-contrast PA stomach and duodenum.

(Courtesy Sharon Peterson, R.T.)

filled fundic portion of the organ. In the prone position, the stomach moves superiorly 1½ to 4 inches (3.7 to 10 cm) according to the patient's habitus (Figs. 17-33 to 17-36). At the same time, it spreads horizontally, with a comparable decrease in its length. An exception to this occurrence is that the fundus usually fills in asthenic patients.

The pyloric canal and the duodenal bulb are well demonstrated in patients ranging from the asthenic to the hyposthenic type. They are often partially obscured in patients of the sthenic type, and, except in the angled position, are completely obscured in those of the hypersthenic type by the prepyloric portion of the stomach.

□ **Evaluation criteria**

The radiograph should demonstrate:
- Entire stomach and duodenal loop.
- Stomach centered at the level of the pylorus for 10 × 12 in (24 × 30 cm) and 11 × 14 in (30 × 34 cm) films.
- Lower lung fields on 14 × 17 in (35 × 43 cm) radiographs for demonstration of a possible hiatal hernia.
- No rotation of the patient.
- Penetration of the barium.

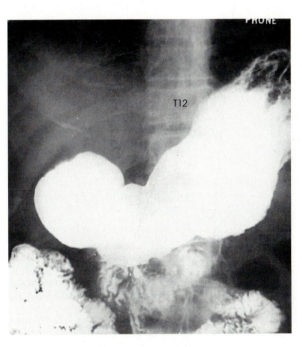

Fig. 17-33. Hypersthenic patient.

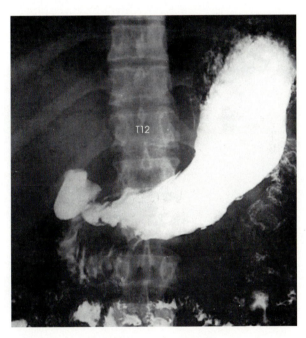

Fig. 17-34. Sthenic patient.

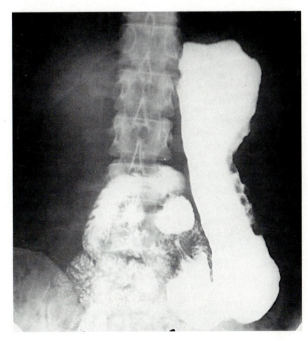

Fig. 17-35. Hyposthenic patient.

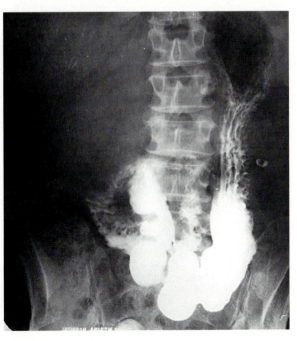

Fig. 17-36. Asthenic patient.

Stomach and Duodenum
PA AXIAL PROJECTION

Film: 14 × 17 in (35 × 43 cm) length-wise.

Position of patient
- Place the patient in the prone position.

Position of part
- Adjust the patient's position so that the median sagittal plane is centered to the grid.
- For the sthenic patient, center the cassette at the level of L2 (Fig. 17-37); center it somewhat higher for the hypersthenic patient and somewhat lower for the asthenic patient.
- *Shield gonads.* (Not shown for illustrative purposes.)
- Ask the patient to suspend respiration at the end of exhalation unless otherwise requested.

Central ray
- Direct the central ray to the midpoint of the film at an angle of 35 to 45 degrees cephalad. Gugliantini[1] recommends a cephalic angulation of 20 to 25 degrees for the demonstration of the stomach in infants.

Structures shown

Gordon[2] developed the PA axial projection to "open up" the high, horizontal (hypersthenic type) stomach for the demonstration of the greater and lesser curvatures, the antral portion of the stomach, the pyloric canal, and the duodenal bulb. The resultant image gives this type of stomach much the same configuration as the average sthenic type of stomach (Fig. 17-38).

☐**Evaluation criteria**

The radiograph should demonstrate:
- Entire stomach and proximal duodenum.
- Stomach centered at the level of the pylorus.
- Penetration of the barium.

[1]Gugliantini P: Utilitá delle incidenze oblique caudocraniali nello studio radiologico della stenosi congenita ipertrofica del piloro, Ann Radiol [Diagn] 34:56-69, 1961. Abstract, AJR 87:623, 1962.
[2]Gordon SS: The angled posteroanterior projection of the stomach: an attempt at better visualization of the high transverse stomach, Radiology 69:393-397, 1957.

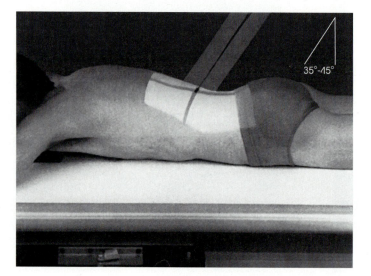

Fig. 17-37. PA axial stomach.

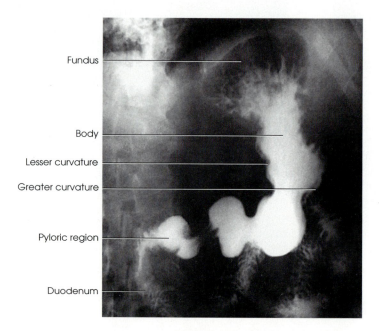

Fundus

Body

Lesser curvature

Greater curvature

Pyloric region

Duodenum

Fig. 17-38. PA axial stomach.

Stomach and Duodenum

PA OBLIQUE PROJECTION
RAO position

Film: 10 × 12 in (24 × 30 cm) lengthwise.

Position of patient

- Place the patient in the recumbent position.

Position of part

- After the PA projection, instruct the patient to rest the head on the right cheek and to place the right arm along the side of the body.
- Have the patient turn toward the left and support self on the left forearm and the flexed left knee.
- Before making the final adjustment in body rotation, adjust the patient's position so that a longitudinal plane passing approximately midway between the vertebrae and the lateral border of the elevated side will coincide with the midline of the grid (Fig. 17-39).

- The approximate 40 to 70 degrees of rotation required to give the best image of the pyloric canal and the duodenum depends on the size, shape, and position of the stomach. In general, hypersthenic patients require a greater degree of rotation than do sthenic and asthenic patients.
- The RAO position is used for serial studies of the pyloric canal and the duodenal bulb because gastric peristalsis is usually more active when the patient is in this position.
- *Shield gonads.* (Not shown for illustrative purposes).
- Ask the patient to suspend respiration at the end of exhalation unless otherwise requested.

Central ray

- Direct the central ray perpendicularly midway between the vertebral column and the elevated lateral border of the abdomen at the approximate level of L1/L2.

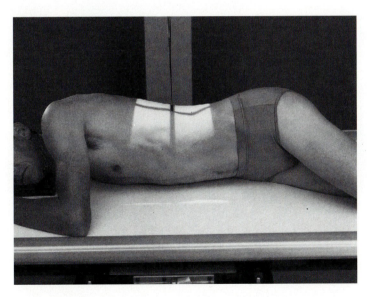

Fig. 17-39. PA oblique stomach and duodenum, RAO position.

Structures shown

A PA oblique projection of the stomach and the entire duodenal loop is presented. This position gives the best image of the pyloric canal and the duodenal bulb in patients whose habitus approximates the sthenic type (Figs. 17-40 and 17-41).

Since gastric peristalsis is generally more active with the patient in the RAO position, a serial study of several exposures is sometimes obtained at intervals of 30 to 40 seconds for the delineation of the pyloric canal and duodenal bulb.

☐ Evaluation criteria

The radiograph should demonstrate:
- Entire stomach and duodenal loop.
- No superimposition of the pylorus and duodenal bulb.
- Duodenal bulb and loop in profile.
- Stomach centered at the level of the pylorus.
- Penetration of the barium.

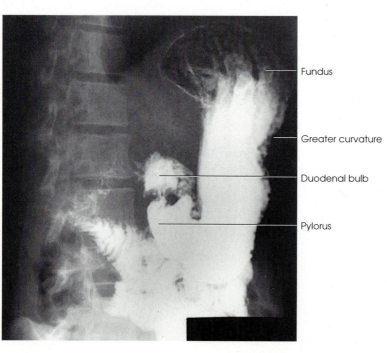

Fundus

Greater curvature

Duodenal bulb

Pylorus

Fig. 17-40. Single-contrast PA oblique stomach, RAO position.

(Courtesy Timothy Hill, R.T.)

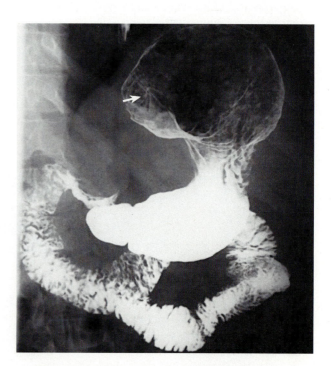

Fig. 17-41. Double-contrast PA oblique stomach and duodenum. Note esophagus entering stomach (arrow).

(Courtesy Betsy Delzeith, R.T.)

Stomach and Duodenum

AP OBLIQUE PROJECTION
LPO position

Film: 10 × 12 in (24 × 30 cm) lengthwise.

Position of patient

- Place the patient in the supine position.

Position of part

- Have the patient abduct the left arm and place the hand near the head or place the extended arm alongside the body.
- Place the right arm alongside the body or across the upper chest, as preferred.
- Have the patient turn toward the left resting on the left posterior body surface.
- Flex the patient's right knee and rotate the knee toward the left for support.
- Place a positioning sponge against the patient's elevated back for immobilization.

- Adjust the patient's position so that a longitudinal plane passing approximately midway between the vertebrae and the left lateral margin of the abdomen is centered to the film.
- Adjust the center of the cassette at the level of the body of the stomach at approximately the L1/L2 level (Fig. 17-42).
- The degree of rotation required to best demonstrate the stomach depends on the patient's body habitus. An average angle of 45 degrees should be sufficient for the sthenic patient but the degree of angulation can vary from 30 to 60 degrees.
- *Shield gonads.* (Not shown for illustrative purposes.)
- Ask the patient to suspend respiration at the end of exhalation unless otherwise instructed.

Central ray

- Direct the central ray perpendicular midway between the vertebral column and the dependent lateral border of the abdomen at the approximate level of L1/L2.

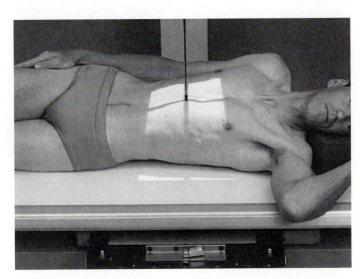

Fig. 17-42. AP oblique stomach and duodenum, LPO position.

Structures shown

The PA oblique projection demonstrates the fundic portion of the stomach (Fig. 17-43). Because of the effect of gravity, the pyloric canal and duodenal bulb are not as filled with barium as they are in the opposite and complementary position (the RAO position, as previously seen in Figs. 17-39 to 17-41).

The radiograph should demonstrate:
- Entire stomach and duodenal loop.
- Fundic portion of stomach.
- No superimposition of the pylorus and duodenal bulb.
- Body of the stomach centered to the radiograph.
- Penetration of the barium.
- Body and pylorus with double-contrast visualization.

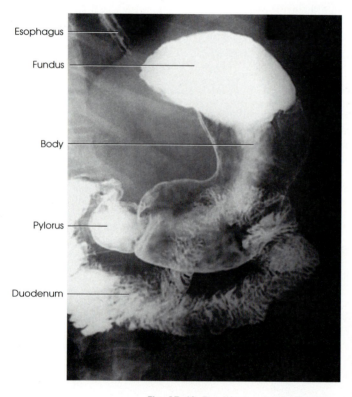 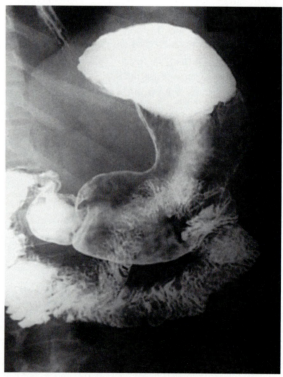

Fig. 17-43. Double-contrast AP oblique stomach and duodenum, LPO position.

(Courtesy Betsy Delzeith, R.T.)

Stomach and Duodenum

 LATERAL PROJECTION
R position

Film: 10×12 in $(24 \times 30$ cm) or 11×14 in $(30 \times 35$ cm) lengthwise, the longer film being required for the upright position.

Position of patient

- Place the patient in the *upright left lateral position* for demonstration of the left retrogastric space and in the *recumbent right lateral position* for demonstration of the right retrogastric space, the duodenal loop, and the duodenojejunal junction.

Position of part

- With the patient in either the upright or the recumbent position, adjust the body so that a plane passing midway between the median coronal plane and the anterior surface of the abdomen will coincide with the midline of the grid.
- Center the cassette at the level of the pylorus or at a level midway between the xiphoid process and the umbilicus.
- Adjust the body in a true lateral position (Fig. 17-44).
- *Shield gonads.* (Not shown for illustrative purposes.)
- Ask the patient to suspend respiration at the end of exhalation unless otherwise requested.

Central ray

- Direct the central ray perpendicular midway between the median coronal plane and the anterior surface of the abdominal cavity, at the L1/L2 level for the recumbent patient and at L3 when the patient is upright. The stomach moves superiorly when the patient is in the recumbent position.

Structures shown

A lateral projection shows the anterior and posterior aspects of the stomach, the pyloric canal, and the duodenal bulb (Figs. 17-45 and 17-46). The right lateral projection frequently affords the best image of the pyloric canal and the duodenal bulb in patients of hypersthenic habitus.

□ Evaluation criteria

The radiograph should demonstrate:

- Entire stomach and duodenal loop.
- No rotation of the patient, as demonstrated by the vertebrae.
- Stomach centered at the level of the pylorus.
- Penetration of the barium.

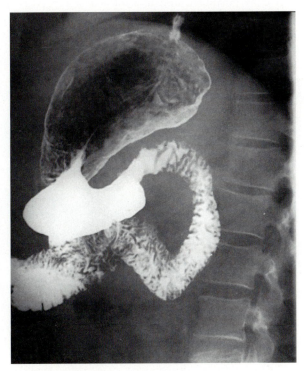

Fig. 17-44. Right lateral stomach and duodenum.

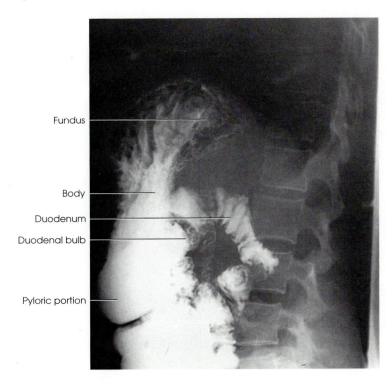

Fig. 17-45. Single-contrast right lateral stomach.

(Courtesy Timothy Hill, R.T.)

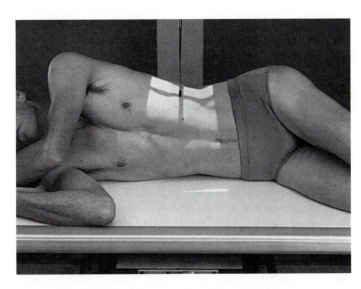

Fig. 17-46. Double-contrast right lateral stomach, and duodenum.

(Courtesy Betsy Delzeith, R.T.)

Stomach and Duodenum

 AP PROJECTION

Film: 11 × 14 in (30 × 35 cm) crosswise for stomach and duodenum, lengthwise for small hiatal hernias; 14 × 17 in (35 × 43 cm) lengthwise for large diaphragmatic herniations.

Position of patient

• Place the patient in the supine position. The stomach moves superiorly and to the left in this position, and, except in thin subjects, its pyloric end is elevated so that the barium suspension flows into and fills its cardiac and/or fundic portions. The filling of the fundus displaces the gas bubble into the pyloric end of the stomach, where it affords double-contrast delineation of posterior wall lesions when a single-contrast examination is performed. If the patient is thin, the intestinal loops do not move superior enough to tilt the stomach for fundic filling. It is therefore necessary to rotate the body toward the left or to angle the head end of the table downward.

• Tilt the table to full or partial Trendelenburg angulation for the demonstration of diaphragmatic herniations (Fig. 17-47). In the Trendelenburg position, the involved organ or organs, which may appear to be normally located in all other body positions, shift upward and protrude through the hernial orifice (most frequently through the esophageal hiatus).

Position of part

• Adjust the position of the patient so that the midline of the grid will coincide (1) with the midline of the body when a 14 × 17 in (35 × 43 cm) film is used (Figs. 17-47 and 17-48) or (2) with a sagittal plane passing midway between the midline and the left side of the body when an 11 × 14 in (30 × 35 cm) film is used. Longitudinal centering of the large film depends on the extent of the hernial protrusion into the thorax and is determined during fluoroscopy.

• For the stomach and duodenum, center the smaller film at the estimated level of the pylorus (approximately L1/L2). The greatest difference in superior movement of the viscera between the prone and supine positions occurs in hypersthenic subjects.

• *Shield gonads.* (Not shown for illustrative purposes.)

• Ask the patient to suspend respiration at the end of exhalation unless otherwise requested.

Central ray

• Direct the central ray perpendicular to (1) the midline at the level of L1/L2 for 14 × 17 in (35 × 43 cm) film or (2) midway between the midline and the left lateral border of the abdomen at the level of L1/L2 for a smaller film.

Structures shown

Stomach

An AP projection of the stomach shows a well-filled fundic portion and, usually, double-contrast delineation of the body, the pyloric portion, and the duodenum (Fig. 17-49). Because of the elevation and superior displacement of the stomach, this position affords the best AP projection of the retrogastric portion of the duodenum and jejunum.

Diaphragm

An AP projection of the abdominothoracic region demonstrates the organ or organs involved in, and the location and extent of, any gross hernial protrusion through the diaphragm as seen in Figs. 17-50 and 17-51.

□ Evaluation criteria

The radiograph should demonstrate:

■ Entire stomach and duodenal loop.
■ Double-contrast visualization of the body, pylorus, and duodenal bulb.
■ Retrogastric portion of the duodenum and jejunum.
■ Lower lung fields on 14 × 17 in (35 × 43 cm) radiographs for demonstration of diaphragmatic hernias.
■ Stomach centered at the level of the pylorus on 10 × 12 in (24 × 30 cm) and 11 × 14 in (30 × 35 cm) radiographs.
■ No rotation of the patient.
■ Penetration of the barium.

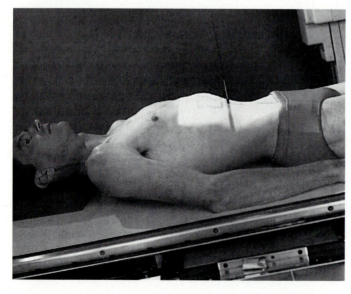

Fig. 17-47. AP stomach and duodenum with table in partial Trendelenburg position.

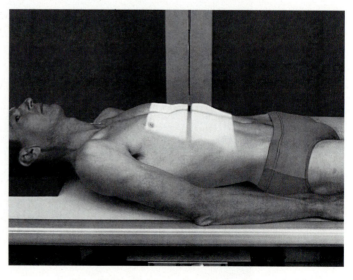

Fig. 17-48. AP stomach and duodenum.

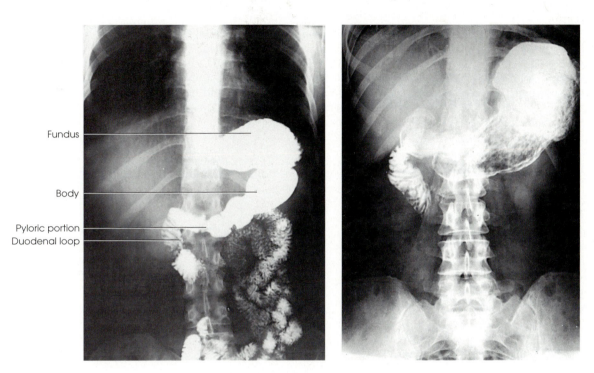

Fundus

Body

Pyloric portion
Duodenal loop

Fig. 17-49. AP stomach and duodenum.

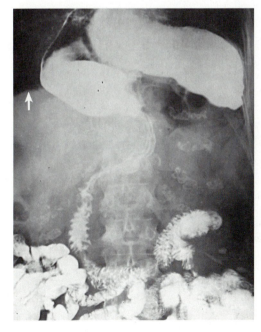

Fig. 17-50. AP stomach and duodenum showing hiatal hernia above the level of the diaphragm (*arrow*).

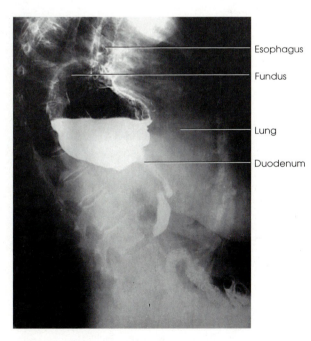

Esophagus

Fundus

Lung

Duodenum

Fig. 17-51. Upright left lateral stomach showing hiatal hernia. (Comparison lateral radiographs can be seen in Figs. 17-45 and 17-46.)

Minimal Hiatal Hernia
PA OBLIQUE PROJECTION
RAO position
WOLF METHOD[1]

Film: 14 × 17 in (35 × 43 cm) lengthwise.

The Wolf method is a modification of the Trendelenburg position. The technique was developed for the purpose of applying greater intra-abdominal pressure than is provided by body angulation alone and thereby ensuring more consistent results in the radiographic demonstration of small, sliding gastroesophageal herniations through the esophageal hiatus.

The Wolf method requires the use of a semicylindrical radiolucent compression device measuring 22 inches in length, 10 inches in width, and 8 inches in height. (The compression sponge depicted in Fig. 17-52 is slightly smaller than the one described by Wolf.)

---

[1]Wolf BS and Guglielmo J: Method for the roentgen demonstration of minimal hiatal herniation, J Mt Sinai Hosp NY 23:738, 741, 1956.

Wolf and Guglielmo[2] state that this device not only provides Trendelenburg angulation of the patient's trunk but also increases intra-abdominal pressure enough to permit adequate contrast filling and maximum distention of the entire esophagus. A further advantage of this device is that it does not require angulation of the table; thus the patient is able to hold the barium container and to ingest the barium suspension through a straw with comparative ease.

---

[2]Wolf BS and Guglielmo J: The roentgen demonstration of minimal hiatus hernia, Med Radiogr Photogr 33:90-92, 1957.

Position of patient

- Place the patient in the prone position on the radiographic table.

Position of part

- Instruct the patient to assume a modified knee-chest position during the placement of the compression device.
- Place this device horizontally under the abdomen and just below the costal margin.
- Adjust the patient in a 40- to 45-degree RAO position, with the thorax centered to the midline of the grid.
- Instruct the patient to ingest the barium suspension in rapid, continuous swallows.
- To allow for complete filling of the esophagus, make the exposure during the third or fourth swallow (Fig. 17-52).
- *Shield gonads.* (Not shown for illustrative purposes.)
- Ask the patient to suspend respiration at the end of exhalation.

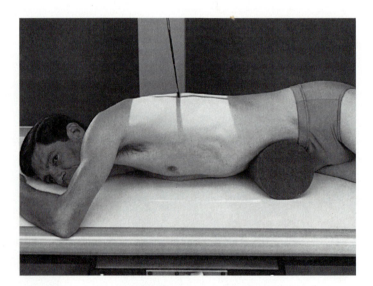

Fig. 17-52. PA oblique stomach with compression sponge, RAO position.

Tom McMahon

Central ray

- Direct the central ray perpendicular to the long axis of the patient's back and center it at the level of either T6 or T7. This position usually results in an angulation of the central ray between 10 and 20 degrees caudad.

Structures shown

The Wolf method demonstrates the relationship of the stomach to the diaphragm and is useful in diagnosing a hiatal hernia (Fig. 17-53).

□ Evaluation criteria

The radiograph should demonstrate:
- The middle or distal aspects of the esophagus and the upper aspect of the stomach.
- The esophagus visible between the vertebral column and the heart.

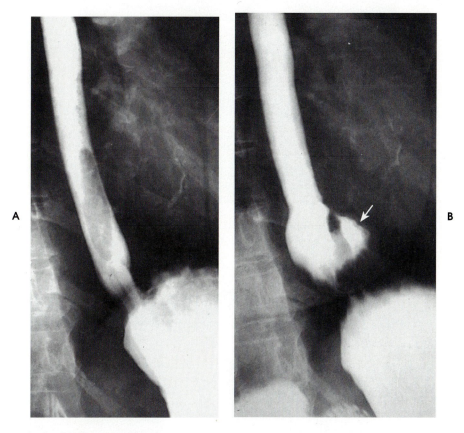

A   B

Fig. 17-53. Comparison PA axial oblique images on one patient. **A,** Without abdominal compression; no evidence of hernia. **B,** With abdominal compression; large sliding hernia obvious *(arrow)*.

Stomach and Duodenum
PA OBLIQUE PROJECTION
RAO position
Serial and mucosal studies

Some institutions obtain radiographs specifically to demonstrate the gastric mucosa after the fluoroscopic examination. A pneumatic paddle may be used as pictured. The paddle is fluoroscopically positioned under the area of the pyloric sphincter and the duodenal bulb. A radiograph is taken with the pneumatic bulb inflated, and additional radiographs are taken as the paddle is deflated.

Position of patient

- Place the patient in the prone and slightly RAO positions, and center the region to be studied to approximately the midline of the grid.
- Place an inflatable paddle under the area of interest.

Position of part

- Under fluoroscopic control, adjust the patient so that the area of the duodenal bulb is centered to the paddle.
- For a mucosal study, inflate the compression bladder of the paddle to provide the desired degree of pressure (Figs. 17-54 and 17-55).
- *Shield gonads.* (Not shown for illustrative purposes.)
- Ask the patient to suspend respiration at the end of exhalation unless otherwise requested.

Central ray

- After the fluoroscopic adjustments, position the x-ray tube over the patient and expose postfluoroscopic films.
- Place the cassette in the Bucky tray and center it to the paddle.
- Direct the central ray perpendicular to the cassette.
- For subsequent exposures, change the cassette.

Structures shown

This method demonstrates a compression and a noncompression study of the pyloric end of the stomach and the duodenal bulb at different stages of filling and emptying. A compression study of the mucosa of a localized area of the gastrointestinal tract is also shown (Fig. 17-56).

□ Evaluation criteria

The radiograph should demonstrate:
- ■ Pylorus and duodenal bulb centered, free of superimposition, and in profile.

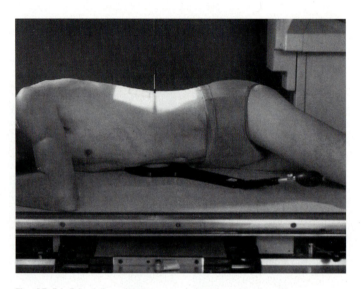

Fig. 17-54. PA oblique pylorus and duodenal bulb with compression paddle, RAO position.

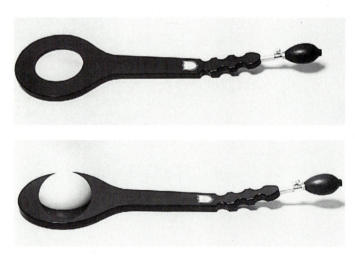

Fig. 17-55. Compression paddle: *above,* noninflated; *below,* inflated.

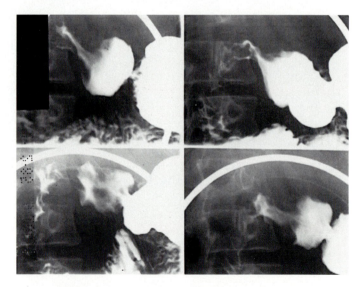

Fig. 17-56. Serial compression study showing varying degrees of compression and the value of compression paddle in demonstrating duodenal bulb.

(Courtesy Dr. John C. Spellmeyer.)

Small Intestine

Radiologic examinations of the small bowel are performed by administering a barium sulfate preparation (1) by *mouth*, (2) by complete *reflux filling* with a large-volume barium enema, or (3) by direct injection into the bowel through an intestinal tube, which is called *enteroclysis*, or small intestine enema. The two latter methods are usually employed only when the oral method fails to provide conclusive information.

Preparation for examination

In preparation for the small intestine study, it is preferable that the patient be given a soft or low-residue diet for 2 days preceding the examination. Often, however, because of economics it is not possible to delay the examination for 2 days. Food and fluid therefore are usually withheld after the evening meal, and breakfast is withheld. A cleansing enema may be administered to clear the colon; however, an enema is not always recommended for enteroclysis, since enema fluid may be retained in the small bowel. The barium formula varies depending on the method of examination. The patient's bladder should be empty before and during the procedure to avoid displacing or compressing the ileum.

ORAL METHOD OF EXAMINATION

The oral examination is usually preceded by a preliminary radiograph of the abdomen. Each small bowel radiograph is identified by a time marker indicating the interval between its exposure and the ingestion of barium. These studies are made with the patient adjusted in either the supine or prone position. The supine position is used (1) to take advantage of the superior and lateral shift of the barium-filled stomach for visualization of the retrogastric portions of the duodenum and jejunum and (2) to prevent possible compression overlapping of loops of the bowel. The prone position is also used to compress the abdominal contents, yielding increased radiographic quality. For examination of thin subjects, it may be necessary to angle the table to the Trendelenburg position for the later radiographs to "unfold" low-lying and superimposed loops of the ileum.

The first small bowel radiograph is usually taken 15 minutes after the patient drinks the barium. The basic routine established for the following interval exposure varies from 15 to 30 minutes, according to the average transit time peculiar to the barium sulfate preparation employed. Regardless of the barium preparation used, however, the fluoroscopist inspects the radiographs as they are processed and varies the procedure according to the requirements of the individual patient. Fluoroscopic and radiographic studies, spot or conventional, may be made of any segment of the bowel as the loops become opacified.

Some radiologists administer a glass of ice water (or other routinely used food stimulant) to the patient with hypomotility after 3 or 4 hours to accelerate peristalsis. Others will give water-soluble gastrointestinal contrast medium, tea, or coffee to stimulate peristalsis. Still others administer peristaltic stimulants every 15 minutes through the transit time. By these methods, the transit of the medium is followed fluoroscopically, with spot and conventional radiographs exposed as indicated, and the examination is usually completed in 30 to 60 minutes.

Small Intestine

 PA OR AP PROJECTION

Film: 14 × 17 in (35 × 43 cm) length-wise.

Position of patient

- Place the patient in the prone or supine position.

Position of part

- Adjust the patient so that the median sagittal plane is centered to the grid.
- For the sthenic patient, center the cassette at the level of L2 (about 2 inches above the iliac crest) for radiographs taken within 30 minutes of contrast administration (Fig. 17-57).
- For delayed radiographs, center at the level of the crests of the ilia.
- *Shield gonads.* (Not shown for illustrative purposes.)
- Ask the patient to suspend respiration at the end of exhalation unless otherwise requested.

Central ray

- Direct the central ray perpendicular to the midpoint of the film (L2) for early radiographs or at the level of the crests of the ilia for delayed sequence exposures.

Structures shown

The PA or AP projection demonstrates the small bowel progressively filling until the barium reaches the iliocecal valve (Figs. 17-58 to 17-65).

When the barium has reached the ileocecal region, fluoroscopy may be performed and compression radiographs obtained (Fig. 17-66).

The examination is usually completed when the barium is visualized in the cecum.

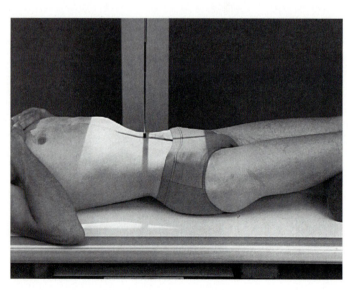

Fig. 17-57. AP small intestine.

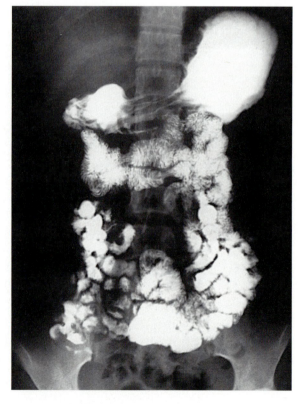

Fig. 17-58. Immediate AP small intestine.

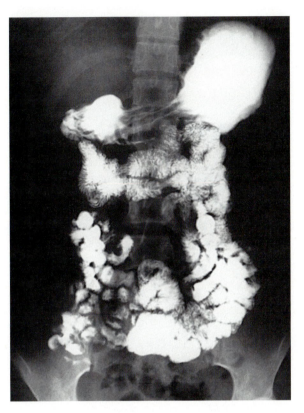

Fig. 17-59. AP small intestine at 15 minutes.

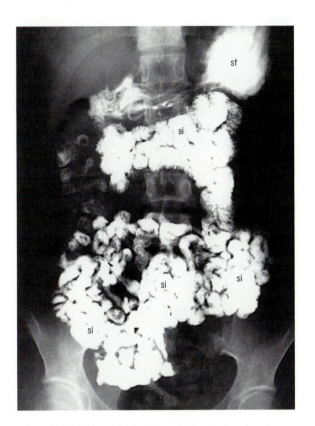

Fig. 17-60. AP small intestine at 30 minutes showing stomach *(st)* and small intestine *(si)*.

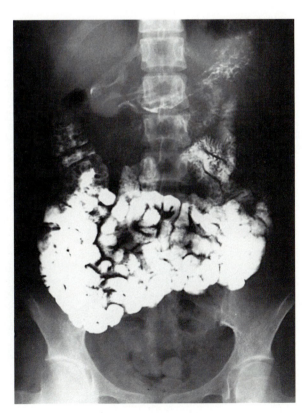

Fig. 17-61. AP small intestine at 1 hour.

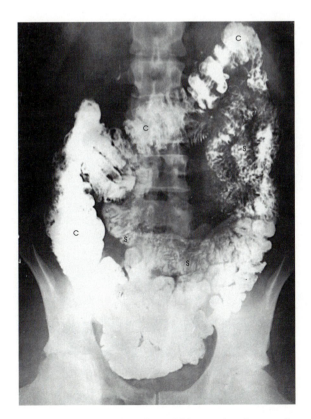

Fig. 17-62. AP small intestine at 2 hours showing small intestine *(s)* and colon *(c)*.

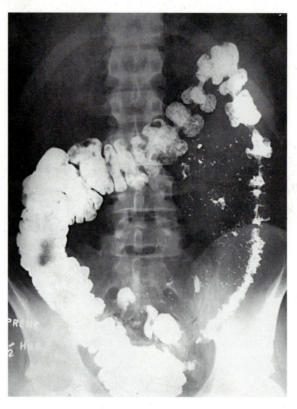

Fig. 17-63. AP small intestine at 3½ hours with barium in colon.

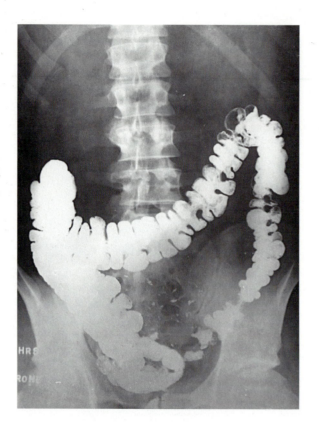

Fig. 17-64. AP small intestine at 4½ hours.

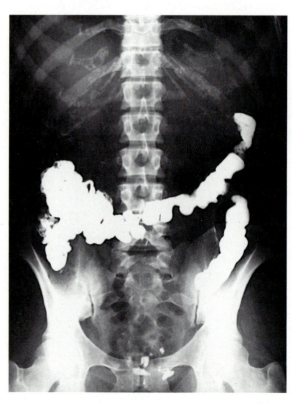

Fig. 17-65. AP small intestine at 24 hours.

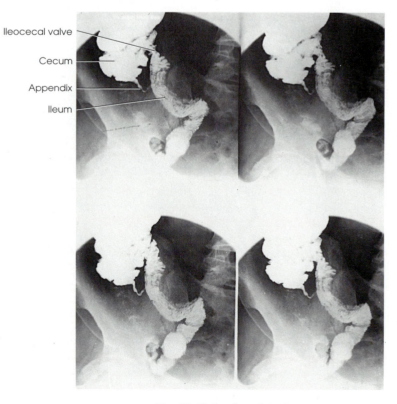

Ileocecal valve
Cecum
Appendix
Ileum

Fig. 17-66. Ileocecal studies.

COMPLETE REFLUX EXAMINATION[1,2]

For a complete reflux examination of the small bowel, the patient's colon and small bowel are filled by administering an enema to demonstrate the colon and small bowel. Prior to commencing the examination, glucagon may be administered to the patient to relax the intestine. Diazepam (Valium) may also be given to diminish discomfort during the initial portion of the filling of the bowel. A 15% ± 5% weight/volume barium suspension is often used, and a large amount of suspension (about 4500 ml) is required to fill the colon and small intestine.

A retention enema tip is used, and the patient is placed in the supine position for the examination. The barium suspension is allowed to flow until it is observed in the duodenal bulb. The enema bag is then lowered to the floor to drain the colon before obtaining radiographs of the small bowel (Fig. 17-67).

[1]Miller RE: Complete reflex small bowel examination, Radiology 84:457-462, 1965.
[2]Miller RE: Localization of the small bowel hemorrhage; complete reflex small bowel examination, Am J Dig Dis 17:1019-1023, 1972.

ENTEROCLYSIS PROCEDURE

Enteroclysis (the injection of nutrient or medicinal liquid into the bowel) is a radiographic procedure in which the contrast medium is injected into the duodenum under fluoroscopic control to examine the small bowel. The contrast medium is injected through a Bilbao or Sellink tube.

Before the procedure is begun, it is imperative that the colon of the patient be thoroughly cleansed. Enemas are not recommended as preparation for enteroclysis, since some fluid may be retained in the small bowel. Under fluoroscopic control, a Bilbao or Sellink tube with a stiff guide wire is advanced to the end of the duodenum at the duodenojejunal flexure, near the ligament of Treitz. Barium is given to the patient through the tube at a rate of approximately 100 ml/min (Fig. 17-68). Spot radiographs, with and without compression, are taken as required. In some patients, air or methylcellulose is injected into the small bowel after the contrast fluid has reached the cecum (Fig. 17-69).

Following fluoroscopic examination of the patient's small bowel, radiographs to demonstrate the small bowel may be requested. The projections most often requested include the AP, PA, obliques, and lateral. Both recumbent and upright images may be requested. For information on positioning the patient, see the positioning descriptions involving the abdomen in Chapter 16 of this atlas.

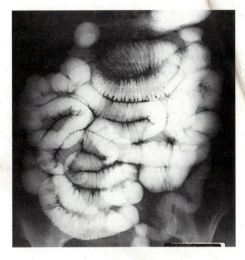

Fig. 17-67. Normal retrograde reflux examination of the small intestine.

(Courtesy Dr. Roscoe E. Miller.)

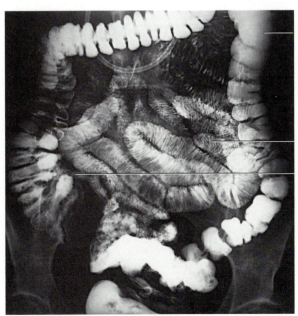

Fig. 17-68. Enteroclysis procedure with barium visualized in colon.

(Courtesy Dr. Roscoe E. Miller.)

Barium in colon

Small intestine

Terminal ileum

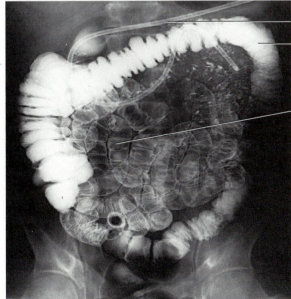

Fig. 17-69. Air-contrast enteroclysis.

Sellink tube

Barium in colon

Barium/air in small intestine

INTUBATION EXAMINATION PROCEDURES

Gastrointestinal intubation is the procedure in which a long, specifically designed tube is inserted through the nose and passed into the stomach, from whence the tube is carried inferiorly by peristaltic action. Gastrointestinal intubation is employed for both therapeutic and diagnostic purposes.

When used therapeutically, the intestinal tube is connected to a suction system for continuous siphoning of the gas and fluid contents of the gastrointestinal tract. The purpose of the measure is to prevent or relieve postoperative distention or to deflate or decompress an obstructed small bowel.

Although used much less frequently than in the past, a *Miller-Abbott* (M-A) double-lumen, single balloon tube (or one similar) can be used to intubate the small intestine. Just above the tip of the tube is a small, thin rubber balloon. Marks on the tube, beginning at the tip, or distal end, indicate the extent of its passage as read from the edge of the nostril. The marks are graduated in centimeters to 85 and in feet thereafter. The lumen of the tube is asymmetrically divided into the following lumina, or channels: (1) a small balloon lumen that communicates with the balloon only and that is used for the inflation and deflation of the balloon and for the injection of mercury to weight the balloon and (2) a large aspiration lumen that communicates with the gastrointestinal tract through perforations near and at the distal end of the tube. Gas and fluids are withdrawn and liquids injected by way of the aspiration lumen.

The introduction of an intestinal tube is an unpleasant experience for the patient, especially one who is acutely ill. Depending on the condition of the patient, the tube is more readily passed if the patient can sit erect and lean slightly forward or if the patient can be elevated almost to a sitting position.

With the intestinal tube in place, the patient is turned to an RAO position, a syringe is connected to the balloon lumen, and the mercury is poured into the syringe and is allowed to flow into the balloon. The air is then slowly withdrawn from the balloon. The tube is secured with an adhesive strip beside the nostril to prevent regurgitation or advance. The stomach is aspirated, either by syringe or by attaching the large arm of the lumen to the suction apparatus.

With the tip of the tube in approximation to the pyloric sphincter and the patient in the RAO position, where gastric peristalsis is usually more active, the tube should pass into the duodenum in a reasonably short time. Without intervention, however, this process sometimes takes many hours. Having the patient drink ice water to stimulate peristalsis frequently is successful. When this measure fails, the examiner guides the tube into the duodenum by manual manipulation under fluoroscopic observation. After the tube enters the duodenum, it is again inflated to provide a bolus, which the peristaltic waves can more readily move along the intestine.

When the tube is inserted for decompression of an intestinal obstruction and possible later radiologic investigation, the adhesive strap is removed and replaced with an adhesive loop attached to the forehead. The tube can slide through the loop without tension as it advances toward the obstructed site. The patient is then returned to the room. Radiographs of the abdomen may be taken to check the progress of the tube and the effectiveness of decompression. Simple obstructions are sometimes relieved by suction; others require surgical intervention.

If the passage of the intestinal tube is arrested, the suction is discontinued and the patient is returned to the radiology department for an M-A tube study. The contrast medium employed for studies of a localized segment of the small bowel may be either a water-soluble iodinated solution (Fig. 17-70) or a thin barium sulfate suspension. Under fluoroscopic observation, the contrast agent is injected through the large lumen of the tube with a syringe. Spot and conventional radiographs are exposed as indicated.

When the intestinal tube is introduced for the purpose of performing a small intestine enema, the tube is advanced into the proximal loop of the jejunum and then secured at this level with an adhesive strap beside the nose. Medical opinion varies as to the quantity of barium suspension required for this examination (Fig. 17-71). The medium is injected through the aspiration lumen of the tube in a continuous, low-pressure flow. Spot and conventional radiographs are exposed as indicated. Except for the presence of the tube in the upper jejunum, the resultant radiographs resemble those obtained by the oral method.

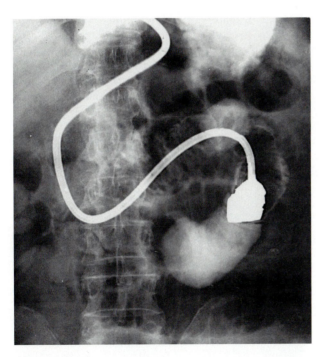

Fig. 17-70. Miller-Abbott (M-A) tube study with water-soluble medium.

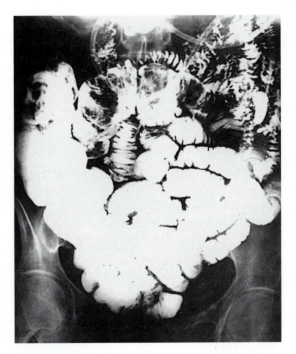

Fig. 17-71. Small bowel examination via M-A tube by injecting barium sulfate.

Large Intestine

There are two basic radiologic methods of examining the large intestine by means of diagnostic or contrast enemas: (1) the *single-contrast* method (Fig. 17-72), in which the colon is examined with a barium sulfate suspension only, and (2) the *double-contrast* method (Fig. 17-73), which may be performed in a two-stage or a single-stage procedure. In the *two-stage double-contrast procedure,* the colon is examined first with a barium sulfate suspension and then, immediately after evacuation of the barium suspension, with an air enema or another gaseous enema. In the *single-stage double-contrast procedure,* the fluoroscopist selectively injects the barium suspension and the gas.

The contrast medium demonstrates the anatomy and tonus of the colon and most of the abnormalities to which it is subject. The gaseous medium serves to distend the lumen of the bowel and to render visible, through the transparency of its shadow, all parts of the barium-coated mucosal lining of the colon and any small intraluminal lesions, such as polypoid tumors.

Following a description of the technique of administering the different types of barium enemas, the positioning required to obtain the radiographs is described and illustrated.

Contrast media

Commercially prepared barium sulfate products comprise the contrast media in general use for routine retrograde examinations of the large bowel. Some are referred to as colloidal preparations because they have finely divided barium particles that resist precipitation, whereas others are referred to as suspended or flocculation-resistant preparations because they contain some form of suspending or dispersing agent.

The newest barium products available are referred to as *high-density barium sulfate.* These high-density barium products absorb a greater percentage of radiation, similar to the older, "thick" barium products. The primary advantage of the high-density barium is that it is excellent for use in double-contrast studies of the alimentary tract in which uniform coating of the lumen is required.

Air is the gaseous medium usually used in double-contrast enema studies; thus the procedure is generally called an *air-contrast study.* Carbon dioxide may also be used because it is more rapidly absorbed than is the nitrogen of air when evacuation of the gaseous medium is incomplete.

In selected cases, specifically prepared, water-soluble, iodinated contrast agents are administered orally to the patient to study the colon when retrograde filling of the colon with barium is not possible or is contraindicated. A disadvantage of the iodinated solutions is that evacuation often is insufficient for satisfactory double-contrast visualization of the mucosal pattern. A great advantage of these agents is that, if a patient is unable to cooperate for a successful enema study, the colon can be satisfactorily examined with an ingested dose of an oral iodinated medium because (1) the transit time from ingestion to colonic filling is fast (averaging 3 to 4 hours); (2) being practically nonabsorbable from the gastrointestinal mucosa, the oral dose reaches and outlines the entire large bowel; and (3) unlike an ingested barium sulfate suspension, this medium is not subject to drying, flaking, and unequal distribution in the colon, so that the oral dose frequently delineates the colon almost as well as does a barium enema.

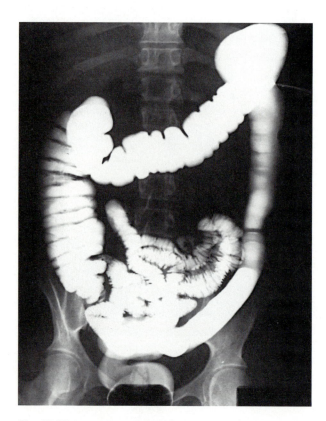

Fig. 17-72. Large intestine, single-contrast examination.

(Courtesy Betsy Delzeith, R.T.)

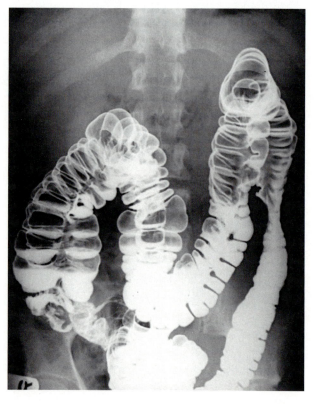

Fig. 17-73. Large intestine double-contrast examination.

(Courtesy Betsy Delzeith, R.T.)

Preparation of intestinal tract

Medical opinion varies about preparation measures. However, members of the medical profession usually agree that the large bowel must be completely emptied of its contents to render all portions of its inner wall visible for inspection. When coated with a barium sulfate suspension, retained fecal masses are likely to simulate the appearance of polypoid or other small tumor masses (Fig. 17-74). This makes thorough cleansing of the entire colon a matter of prime importance. Any preliminary preparation of the intestinal tract of patients who have a condition such as severe diarrhea, gross bleeding, or symptoms of obstruction is, of course, limited. Other patients are prepared, with modification where indicated, according to the specifications established by the examining physician. In the usual procedure, the preliminary preparation includes dietary restrictions as well as a laxative. Cleansing enemas are also used, as are commercially available complete colon cleansing kits designed for easy use by outpatients or hospital nursing personnel.

Standard barium enema apparatus

Disposable soft-plastic enema tips and enema bags are commercially available in different sizes. For patients who have inflamed hemorrhoids, fissures, a stricture, or other abnormalities of the anus, a soft rubber rectal catheter of small caliber should be used.

Disposable rectal *retention tips* (Fig. 17-75) have replaced the older retention catheters such as the Bardex or Foley. Retention tips are used with patients who have a relaxed anal sphincter, as well as others who cannot retain an enema. Some fluoroscopists routinely use retention enema tips and inflate if needed. The retention tip is a double-lumen tube with a thin balloon at its distal end. Because of the danger of intestinal rupture, retention tips must be inserted with extreme care.

The disposable rectal retention tip has a balloon that fits snugly against the enema nozzle both before and after deflation so that it can be inserted and removed with little discomfort to the patient. A reusable squeeze inflator is recommended to limit the air capacity to approximately 90 cc. One complete squeeze of the inflator provides adequate distention of the retention balloon without danger of overinflation. These disposable retention tips are available for both double-contrast and single-contrast enemas. To provide the greatest safety to the patient, inflation of any retention balloon is recommended to be made with caution, using fluoroscopy, just before the examination.

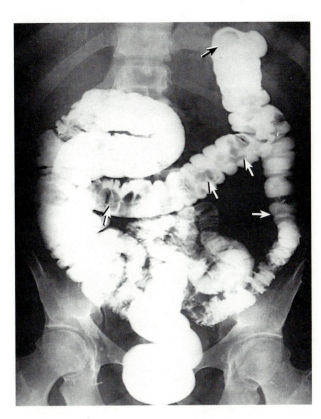

Fig. 17-74. Single-contrast barium-filled colon showing fecal material that simulates or masks pathologic condition *(arrows)*.

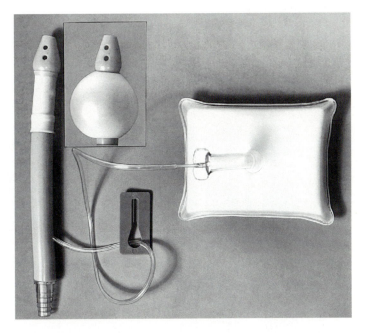

Fig. 17-75. Disposable retention enema tip. Uninflated balloon fits snugly. *Inset,* Balloon inflated with 90 cc of air, one complete squeeze of inflator.

For the performance of a double-contrast barium enema examination, a special rectal tip is needed in order to instill air in the colon (Fig. 17-76), or air can simply be pumped in using a sphygmomanometer bulb. Double-contrast retention tips are also available.

Most enema bags have a capacity of 3 quarts (3000 ml) when fully distended and have graduated quantity markings on the side. A filter may be incorporated within the bag to prevent the passage of any unmixed lumps of barium. The tubing is approximately 6 feet in length, and the soft plastic enema tips are available in several sizes.

Preparation of barium suspensions

The concentration of the barium sulfate suspensions employed for a single-contrast colonic enema varies considerably; the often recommended range is between 12% to 25% for weight to volume. For double-contrast examinations, a relatively high-density barium product is used; a 75% to 95% weight/volume ratio is common.

Commercial barium enema preparations are available as premixed liquids that can be poured into the disposable enema kit bag. Powdered barium is also available in single-contrast disposable kit bags; all that is needed is to add water and then mix the solution by shaking the bag.

Instructions for mixing the barium preparation vary according to the manufacturer and the type of barium used. The best recommendation regarding the accurate mixing of the barium is to precisely follow the manufacturer's instructions.

If warm barium enemas are administered, the temperature should be somewhat below body temperature, about 85° to 90° F (29° to 30° C). In addition to being unpleasant and debilitating, an enema that is too warm is injurious to the tissues and produces so much irritation that it is difficult, if not impossible, for the patient to retain the enema long enough for a satisfactory examination.

Cold barium enema suspensions (41° F [5° C]) have been recommended[1] on the basis that the colder temperature produces less irritation, has a mild anesthetic effect that relaxes the colon, and stimulates tonic contraction of the anal sphincter. These effects result in greater comfort and ease of retention for the patient and permit less difficult and more rapid filling of the colon. The patient not only has no sensation of chill but also finds the cold suspension soothing and easy to retain. The cold temperature is most easily obtained by preparing the barium suspension a day in advance and refrigerating it overnight.

---

[1]Levene G: Low temperature barium-water suspensions for roentgenologic examination of the colon, Radiology 77:117-118, 1961.

Preparation and care of patient

In no radiologic examination is the full cooperation of the patient more essential to success than in retrograde examinations of the colon. Few patients who are physically able to do so fail to retain the enema when they understand the procedure and realize that in large measure the success of the examination depends on them. The radiographer should observe the following guidelines in preparing the patient for the examination:

- Take time to explain the procedural differences between an ordinary cleansing enema and a diagnostic enema: (1) the fluoroscopist examines all portions of the bowel as it is being filled with the contrast medium under fluoroscopic observation; (2) this part of the examination involves palpation of the abdomen, rotation of the body as required to visualize the different segments of the colon, and the taking of spot radiographs without and, where indicated, with compression; and (3) a series of large radiographs are then taken before the colon can be evacuated (Fig. 17-77).
- Assure the patient that retention of the diagnostic enema will be comparatively easy because its flow is controlled under fluoroscopic observation.
- Instruct the patient (1) to keep the anal sphincter tightly contracted against the rectal tube to hold it in position and to prevent leakage, (2) to relax the abdominal muscles to prevent intra-abdominal pressure, and (3) to concentrate on deep oral breathing to reduce the incidence of colonic spasm and resultant cramps.
- Assure the patient that the flow of the enema will be stopped for the duration of any cramping.

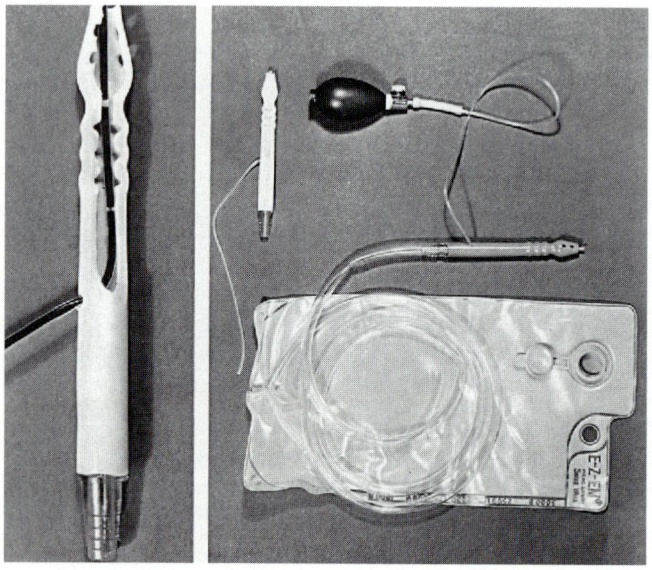

Fig. 17-76. Air-contrast enema tip shown with air tube filled with ink to demonstrate position.

The patient who has not had a previous colonic examination is usually fearful of being embarrassed by inadequate draping as well as by failure to retain the enema for the required time. The radiographer can dispel or greatly relieve the anxieties by observing the following steps:

- Assure the patient that he or she will be properly covered.
- Assure the patient that, although there is little chance of mishap, he or she will be well protected so that there is no need to feel embarrassment should one occur.
- Keep a bedpan in the examining room for patients who cannot or may not be able to make the trip to the toilet.

The preliminary preparation required for a retrograde study of the colon is strenuous. The examination itself further depletes the patient's strength. Feeble patients, particularly elderly persons, are likely to become weak and faint from the exertion of the preparation, the examination, and the effort made to expel the enema. An emergency call button should be available in each lavatory so that patients can summon help if needed. Although the patient's privacy must be respected, the radiographer or an aide should frequently make inquiry to ensure that the patient is all right.

Insertion of enema tip

In preparation for the insertion of the enema tip, the following steps are observed:

- Instruct the patient to turn onto the left side, lean forward about 35 to 40 degrees, and rest the flexed right knee on the table, above and in front of the slightly flexed left knee (Sims' position). This position relaxes the abdominal muscles, which decreases intra-abdominal pressure on the rectum and makes relaxation of the anal sphincter less difficult.

- Adjust the IV pole so that the enema contents are 18 to 24 inches (45 to 60 cm) above the level of the anus.
- Adjust the overlapping back of the gown or other draping to expose the anal region only, keeping the patient otherwise well covered. The anal orifice is frequently partially obscured by distended hemorrhoids or by a fringe of undistended hemorrhoids. Sometimes there is a contraction or other abnormality of the orifice. It is therefore necessary that the anus be exposed and sufficiently well lighted for the orifice to be clearly visible so that the enema tip can be inserted without injury or discomfort.
- Run a little of the barium mixture into a waste basin to free the tubing of air, and then lubricate the rectal tube well with a water-soluble lubricant.
- Advise the patient to relax and take deep breaths so that there will be no feeling of discomfort when the tube is inserted.
- Push the right buttock laterally to open the gluteal fold.
- As the abdominal muscles and anal sphincter are relaxed during the exhalation phase of a deep breath, insert the rectal tube gently and slowly into the anal orifice: (1) following the angle of the anal canal, direct the tube anteriorly 1 to 1½ inches (2.5 to 3.8 cm) and (2) following the curve of the rectum, direct the tube slightly superiorly.
- Insert the tube for a total distance of no more than 3½ to 4 inches (8.7 to 10 cm); a greater distance is not only unnecessary but involves possible injury to the rectum.
- If the tube does not enter easily, ask the patient to assist if capable.
- *Never* forcibly insert a rectal tube; the patient may have distended internal hemorrhoids or another condition that would make a forced insertion dangerous.
- After the enema tip is inserted, hold it in position to prevent it from slipping while the patient turns to the supine or prone position for fluoroscopy, according to the preference of the fluoroscopist.
- Adjust the protective underpadding and relieve any pressure on the tubing so that the enema mixture will flow freely.

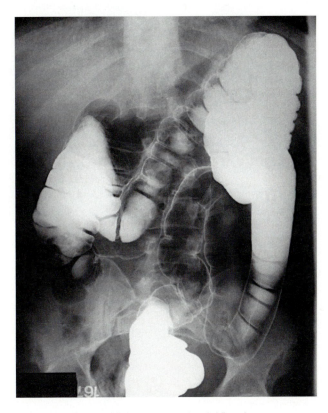

Fig. 17-77. Double-contrast AP colon.

(Courtesy Jonathan Miller, R.T.)

SINGLE-CONTRAST BARIUM ENEMA
Administration of contrast medium

After preparing the patient for the examination, the radiographer observes the following steps:

- Notify the fluoroscopist as soon as everything is ready for the examination.
- If the patient has not been introduced to the fluoroscopist, make the introduction at this time.
- At the fluoroscopist's request, release the control clip and ensure the enema flow.
- When occlusion of the enema tip occurs, displace soft fecal material by withdrawing the rectal tube about 1 inch (2.5 cm) and, before reinserting it, temporarily elevate the enema bag to increase fluid pressure.

The rectal ampulla fills slowly. Unless the flow is stopped for a few seconds at this point, the barium suspension then flows through the sigmoid and descending portions of the colon at a fairly rapid rate, frequently causing a severe cramp and acute stimulation of the defecation impulse. The flow of the enema is usually stopped for several seconds at frequent intervals during the fluoroscopically controlled filling of the colon.

During the fluoroscopic procedure, the examiner rotates the patient to inspect all segments of the bowel. The fluoroscopist takes spot radiographs as indicated and determines the positions to be used for the subsequent radiographic studies. On completion of the fluoroscopic examination, the enema tip is usually removed to more easily maneuver the patient and to prevent accidental displacement of the tip during the filming procedure. A retention tube is not removed until the patient is placed on a bedpan or on the toilet.

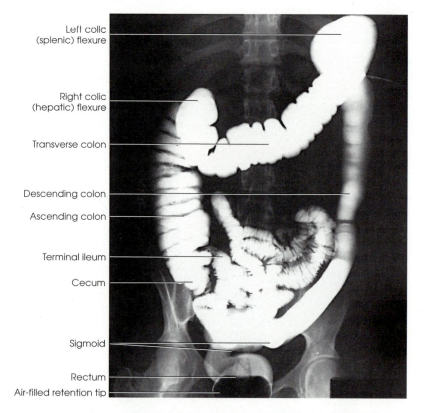

Fig. 17-78. Single-contrast barium enema image.

After the immediate films have been exposed (Fig. 17-78), the patient is escorted to a toilet or placed on a bedpan and instructed to expel as much of the enema as possible. A postevacuation radiograph is then taken (Fig. 17-79). When this radiograph shows evacuation to be inadequate for satisfactory delineation of the mucosa, the patient may be given a hot beverage (tea or coffee) to stimulate further evacuation.

Positioning of opacified colon

The most commonly obtained projections for the single-contrast barium enema are the PA or AP, PA obliques, axial projection for the sigmoid, and a lateral for demonstration of the rectum. (See positioning descriptions which follow.)

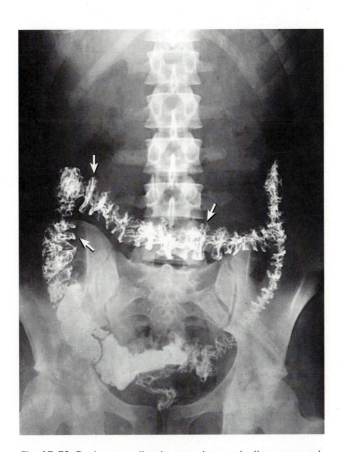

Fig. 17-79. Postevacuation image demonstrating mucosal pattern *(arrows)*.

(Courtesy Dr. Francis H. Ghiselin.)

DOUBLE-CONTRAST BARIUM ENEMA

Two approaches to administering double-contrast barium enemas are currently in use. The first technique is a *two-stage procedure* described by Welin in which the entire colon is filled with a barium suspension. Following the enema administration, the patient evacuates the barium and immediately returns to the fluoroscopic table for injection of air or another gaseous medium into the colon. The second approach is the *single-stage double-contrast examination,* the popularity of which has primarily resulted from recent advancements in the manufacturing of high-density barium sulfate.

Single-stage procedure

Performance of a single-stage double-contrast enema involves certain requirements to ensure an adequate examination. The most important requirement is that the colon of the patient be exceptionally clean. Residual fecal material can often obscure small polyps or tumor masses. A second requirement is that a suitable barium suspension be used. A barium mixture that clumps or flakes will neither clearly demonstrate the lumen nor properly drain from the colon.

Currently available premixed liquid barium products are more consistently mixed by the manufacturer and are generally more uniform for radiographic use than most barium suspensions mixed in the health care institution. A high-density barium product, as high as 200% weight/volume, may be used for a single-stage, double-contrast examination of the colon. The most important criterion of the barium is that it flow sufficiently to coat the walls of the colon.

With advances in the manufacturing of high-density barium, high-quality double-contrast colon radiographs can be consistently obtained during one filling of the colon. In the single-stage procedure, the barium and the air are instilled in a single procedure, compared with the two-step procedure to be discussed in the following section. Miller[1] reported a *7-pump* method for performing single-stage double-contrast examinations, which reduces cost, saves time, and reduces radiation exposure to the patient. For a more complete description of the 7-pump method, see the seventh or earlier editions of this atlas.

---

[1]Miller RE: Barium pneumocolon: technologist-performed "7-pump" method, AJR 139(6):1230-1232, 1982.

Fluoroscopy is performed to check the location of the barium and additional air is given under fluoroscopic control. The patient is slowly rotated 360 degrees and placed in the supine position, following which spot radiography occurs and overhead radiographs are then taken (Figs. 17-80 and 17-81).

In addition to the 7-pump method described, a single-stage double-contrast examination can also be performed without the use of a special air-contrast enema tip. With this technique, the barium and air are instilled in the patient through the closed enema bag system as diagrammed in Fig. 17-82.

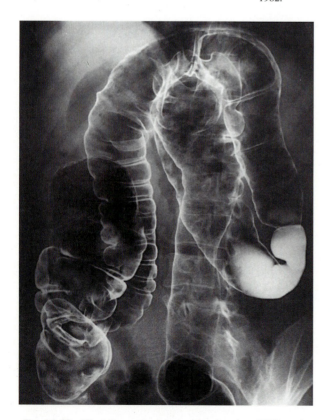

Fig. 17-80. AP oblique double-contrast colon, RPO position.

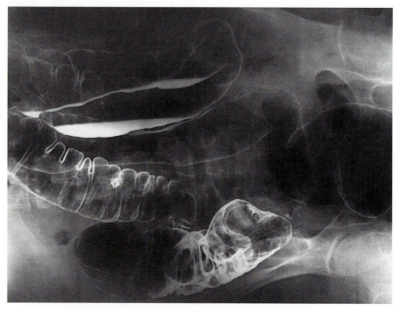

Fig. 17-81. AP colon, right lateral decubitus position.

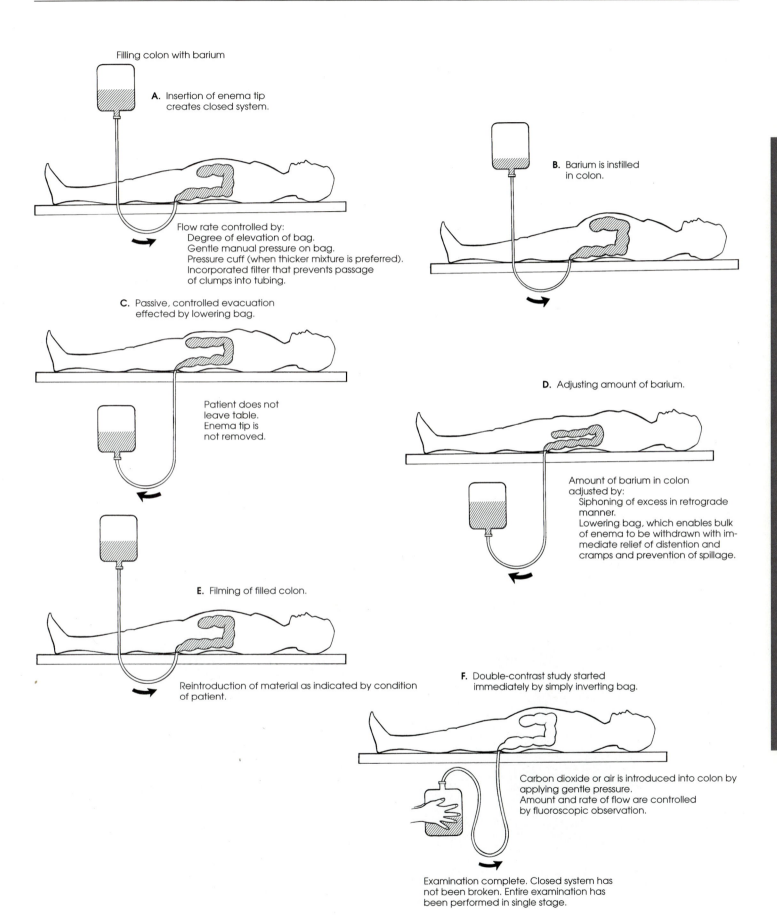

Filling colon with barium

A. Insertion of enema tip creates closed system.

Flow rate controlled by:
Degree of elevation of bag.
Gentle manual pressure on bag.
Pressure cuff (when thicker mixture is preferred).
Incorporated filter that prevents passage of clumps into tubing.

B. Barium is instilled in colon.

C. Passive, controlled evacuation effected by lowering bag.

Patient does not leave table. Enema tip is not removed.

D. Adjusting amount of barium.

Amount of barium in colon adjusted by:
Siphoning of excess in retrograde manner.
Lowering bag, which enables bulk of enema to be withdrawn with immediate relief of distention and cramps and prevention of spillage.

E. Filming of filled colon.

Reintroduction of material as indicated by condition of patient.

F. Double-contrast study started immediately by simply inverting bag.

Carbon dioxide or air is introduced into colon by applying gentle pressure.
Amount and rate of flow are controlled by fluoroscopic observation.

Examination complete. Closed system has not been broken. Entire examination has been performed in single stage.

Fig. 17-82. Conduction of single-stage, closed-system, double-contrast examination.

(Adapted from Pochaczevsky R and Sherman RS: A new technique for roentgenologic examination of the colon. AJR 89:787-796, 1963.)

Welin method

Welin[1,2] developed a technique for double-contrast enemas that reveals even the smallest intraluminal lesions (Figs. 17-83 and 17-84). Welin states that this method of examination has been extremely valuable in the early diagnosis of such conditions as ulcerative colitis, regional colitis, and polyps.

Welin stresses the importance of preparing the intestine for the examination, stating that (1) the colon must be cleansed as thoroughly as possible and (2) the colonic mucosa must be prepared in such a way as to permit the adhesion of an extremely thin and even coating of barium on the colonic wall. He recommends regulation of evacuation so that the two stages of the examination can be carried out at short intervals to avoid unnecessary waiting time and states that the patient need not be in the examining room more than a total of 20 to 25 minutes.

[1]Welin S: Modern trends in diagnostic roentgenology of the colon, Br J Radiol 31:453-464, 1958.
[2]Welin S: Results of the Malmo technique of colon examination, JAMA 199:369-371, 1967.

Stage one

With the patient in the prone position to prevent possible ileal leak, the colon is filled to the left colic (splenic) flexure, after which a conventional radiograph is taken, a right lateral projection of the barium-filled rectum. The patient is then sent to the lavatory to evacuate. Afterward, if the patient feels the need to do so, he or she is allowed to lie down and rest.

Stage two

When the patient returns to the examining table, the enema tip is inserted, and the patient is again turned to the prone position. The prone position not only prevents ileal leak with resultant opacification and overlap of the small intestine on the rectosigmoid area but also aids in adequate drainage of excess barium from the rectum.

The fluoroscopist allows the barium mixture to run up to the middle of the sigmoid colon (slightly farther if the sigmoid is long). The patient is then turned onto the right side, and air is instilled through the enema tip. The air forces the barium along, distributing it throughout the colon, and the patient is turned as required for even coating of the entire colon. Spot radiographs are made as indicated. If barium has flowed back into the rectum, it is drained out through the enema tip. More air is then instilled. Welin stresses the importance of instilling enough air to obtain proper distention of the colon, from 1800 to 2000 cc or more.

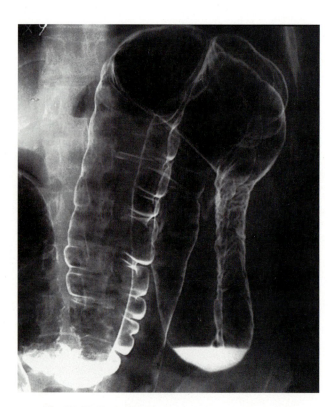

Fig. 17-83. Upright oblique position of splenic flexure, following implementation of Welin method.

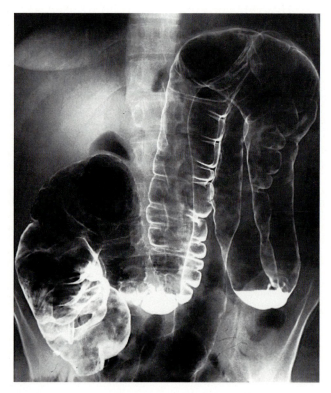

Fig. 17-84. Upright PA colon following implementation of Welin method.

(Courtesy Dr. Sölve Welin.)

When sufficient distention of the colon has been obtained, 14×17 in (35×43 cm) radiographs are obtained (Figs. 17-85 to 17-87) to include the rectum in the following sequence: a PA, PA obliques (LAO and RAO), and a right lateral of the rectum (10×12 in [24×30 cm]). The patient is then turned to the supine position for an AP and two AP obliques (LPO and RPO), all to include the transverse colon and its flexures. These studies are followed by right and left lateral decubitus positions both to include the rectum. Finally, the patient is placed in the erect position for PA and PA obliques (RAO and LAO) of the horizontal colon and the left colic (splenic) and right colic (hepatic) flexures.

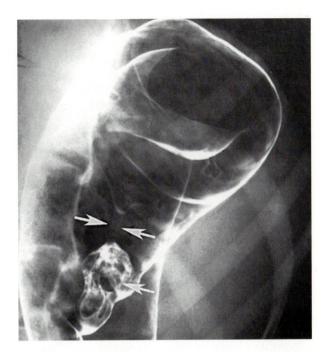

Fig. 17-85. Pedunculated polyps *(arrows)* during stage two of Welin method.

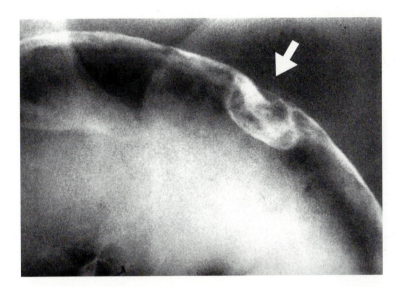

Fig. 17-86. Small carcinoma with intubation *(arrow)* during stage two of Welin method.

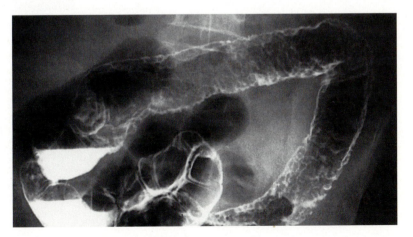

Fig. 17-87. Cobblestone appearance of granulomatous colitis. (Image obtained during stage two of Welin method).

Large Intestine
OPACIFIED COLON

Radiographic studies of the adult colon are made on 14 × 17 in (35 × 43 cm) cassettes. Except for axial projections these films may be centered at the level of the crests of the ilia on patients of sthenic build, somewhat higher for hypersthenic patients and somewhat lower for asthenic patients. The AP and PA projections of the colon in the wide, capacious abdomen may require two exposures, with the films placed crosswise: the first is centered high enough to include the diaphragm and the second low enough to include the rectum. Localized studies of the rectum and rectosigmoid junction are often made on 10 × 12 in (24 × 30 cm) or 11 × 14 in (30 × 35 cm) cassettes centered at or slightly above the level of the symphysis pubis. Pre-evacuation filming of the colon includes one or more images for the demonstration of otherwise obscured flexed and curved areas of the bowel. Depending on the preference of the fluoroscopist, the radiographic projections taken following fluoroscopy vary considerably. Therefore any combination of the following images may be taken to complete the examination.

Large Intestine
PA PROJECTION

Film: 14 × 17 in (35 × 43 cm) lengthwise.

Position of patient
• Place the patient in the prone position.

Position of part
• Center the median sagittal plane to the grid.
• Adjust the center of the cassette at the level of the crest of the ilium (Fig. 17-88).
• In addition to the PA projection, place the fluoroscopic table in a slight Trendelenburg position if needed. This table position helps separate redundant and overlapping loops of the bowel by "spilling" them out of the pelvis.
• *Shield gonads.* (Not shown for illustrative purposes.)
• Ask the patient to suspend respiration for the exposure.

Central ray
• Direct the central ray perpendicular to the film to enter the midline of the body at the level of the crest of the ilium.

Structures shown
The PA projection demonstrates the entire colon with the patient prone (Figs. 17-89 to 17-91).

□ Evaluation criteria
The radiograph should demonstrate:
■ Entire colon including the flexures and the rectum. Two films may be needed for hypersthenic patients.
■ Vertebral column centered so that the ascending and descending colon is included.

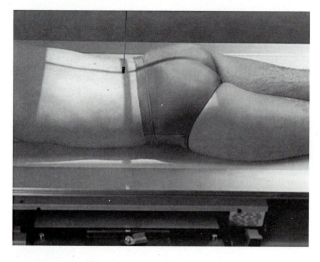

Fig. 17-88. PA large intestine.

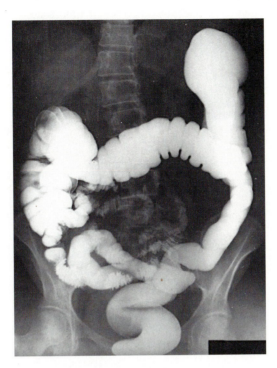

Fig. 17-89. Single-contrast PA large intestine.

(Courtesy Cindy Swords, R.T.)

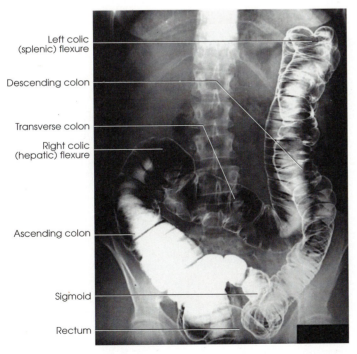

Left colic
(splenic) flexure

Descending colon

Transverse colon

Right colic
(hepatic) flexure

Ascending colon

Sigmoid

Rectum

Fig. 17-90. Double-contrast PA large intestine.

(Courtesy Laurie Davis, R.T.)

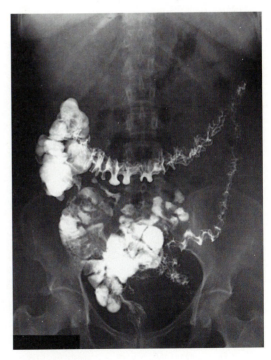

Fig. 17-91. Postevacuation PA large intestine.

(Courtesy Betsy Delzeith, R.T.)

Large Intestine

▧ PA AXIAL PROJECTION

Film: 14 × 17 in (35 × 43 cm) lengthwise or 10 × 12 in (24 × 30 cm) lengthwise.

Position of patient

• Place the patient in the prone position.

Position of part

• Center the median sagittal plane to the grid.
• Adjust the center of the cassette at the level of the crest of the ilium (Fig. 17-92).
• *Shield gonads.* (Not shown for illustrative purposes.)
• Ask the patient to suspend respiration for the exposure.

Central ray

• Direct the central ray 30 to 40 degrees caudad to enter the midline of the body and pass through the level of the anterior superior iliac spines.

Structures shown

The PA axial projection best demonstrates the rectosigmoid area of the colon (Figs. 17-93 and 17-94).

▢ Evaluation criteria

The radiograph should demonstrate:
■ Rectosigmoid area centered to radiograph.
■ Rectosigmoid area with less superimposition than in the PA projection because of the angulation of the central ray.
■ Transverse colon and both flexures not necessarily included.

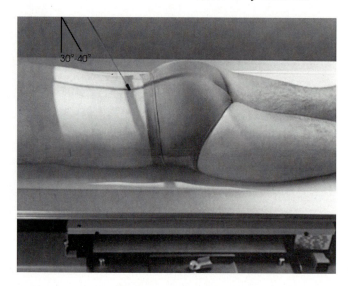

Fig. 17-92. PA axial large intestine.

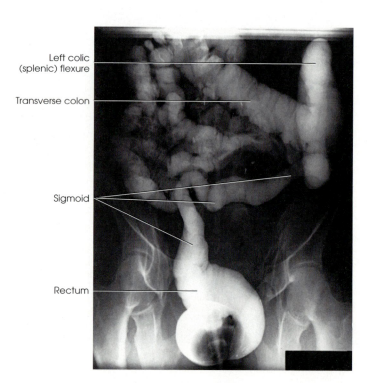

Left colic (splenic) flexure

Transverse colon

Sigmoid

Rectum

Fig. 17-93. Single-contrast PA axial (30-degree angulation) large intestine.

(Courtesy Betsy Delzeith, R.T.)

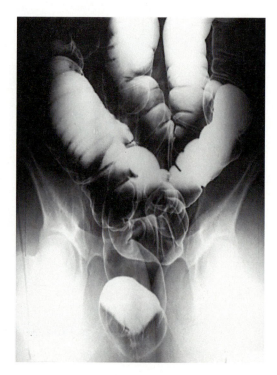

Fig. 17-94. Double-contrast PA axial (40-degree angulation) large intestine.

Large Intestine

PA OBLIQUE PROJECTION
RAO position

Film: 14 × 17 in (35 × 43 cm) lengthwise.

Position of patient

- Place the patient in the prone position.

Position of part

- With the patient's right arm by the side of the body and the left hand by the head, have the patient roll onto the right hip to obtain a 35- to 45-degree rotation from the table.
- Flex the left knee to provide stability.
- Center the body to the midline of the grid.
- Adjust the center of the cassette at the level of the crest of the ilium (Fig. 17-95).
- *Shield gonads.* (Not shown for illustrative purposes.)
- Ask the patient to suspend respiration for the exposure.

Central ray

- Direct the central ray perpendicular to the film to enter approximately 1 to 2 inches (2.5 to 5 cm) lateral to the midline of the body on the elevated side at the level of the crest of the ilium.

Structures shown

The RAO position best demonstrates the right colic (hepatic) flexure, the ascending portion of the colon, and the sigmoid portion of the colon (Figs. 17-96 and 17-97).

The radiograph should demonstrate:
- Entire colon.
- Right colic (hepatic) flexure less superimposed or open when compared with the PA.
- Ascending colon, cecum, and sigmoid colon.

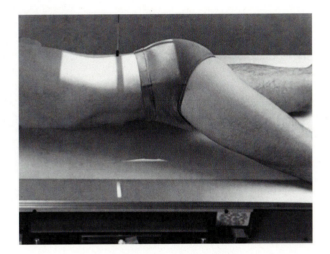

Fig. 17-95. PA oblique large intestine, RAO position.

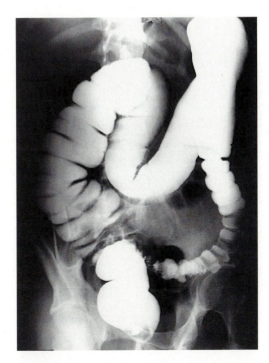

Fig. 17-96. Single-contrast PA oblique large intestine, RAO position.

(Courtesy Dr. Herbert F. Hempel.)

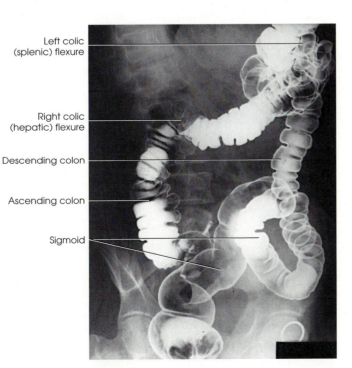

Left colic (splenic) flexure

Right colic (hepatic) flexure

Descending colon

Ascending colon

Sigmoid

Fig. 17-97. Double-contrast PA oblique large intestine, RAO position.

(Courtesy Gail A. Fischer, R.T.)

Large Intestine

PA OBLIQUE PROJECTION
LAO position

Film: 14 × 17 in (35 × 43 cm) lengthwise.

Position of patient

• Place the patient in the prone position.

Position of part

• With the patient's left arm by the side of the body and the right hand by the head, have the patient roll onto the left hip to obtain a 35- to 45-degree rotation from the table.
• Flex the right knee to provide stability.
• Center the body to the midline of the grid.
• Adjust the center of the cassette at the level of the crest of the ilium (Fig. 17-98).
• *Shield gonads.* (Not shown for illustrative purposes.)
• Ask the patient to suspend respiration for the exposure.

Central ray

• Direct the central ray perpendicular to the film to enter approximately 1 to 2 inches (2.5 to 5 cm) lateral to the midline of the body on the elevated side at the level of the crest of the ilium.

Structures shown

The LAO position best demonstrates the left colic (splenic) flexure and the descending portion of the colon (Figs. 17-99 and 17-100).

The radiograph should demonstrate:
■ Entire colon.
■ Left colic (splenic) flexure less superimposed or open when compared with the PA.
■ Descending colon.

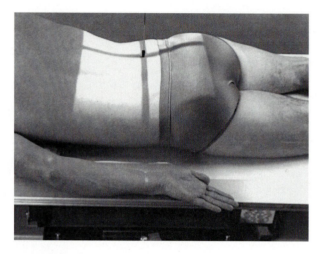

Fig. 17-98. PA oblique large intestine, LAO position.

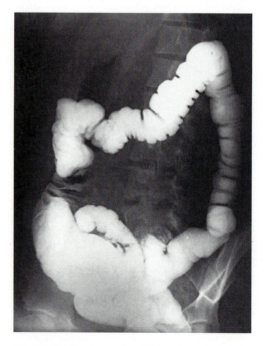

Fig. 17-99. Single-contrast PA oblique large intestine, LAO position.

(Courtesy Cindy Swords, R.T.)

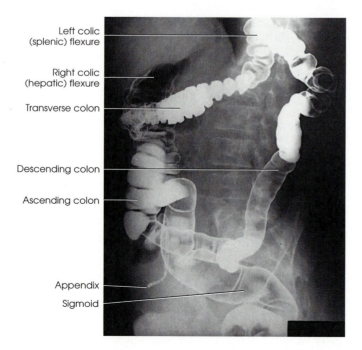

Left colic (splenic) flexure

Right colic (hepatic) flexure

Transverse colon

Descending colon

Ascending colon

Appendix

Sigmoid

Fig. 17-100. Double-contrast PA oblique large intestine, LAO position.

(Courtesy Gail A. Fischer, R.T.)

Large Intestine

 LATERAL PROJECTION
R or L position

Film: 10 × 12 in (24 × 30 cm) lengthwise.

Position of patient

• Place the patient in the lateral recumbent position on either the left or right side.

Position of part

• Center the median coronal plane to the center of the grid.
• Flex the knees slightly for patient stability and place a support between the knees to keep the pelvis lateral.
• Adjust the shoulders and hips to be perpendicular (Fig. 17-101).
• *Shield gonads.* (Not shown for illustrative purposes.)
• Ask the patient to suspend respiration for the exposure.

Central ray

• Direct the perpendicular central ray to enter the median coronal plane at the level of the anterior superior iliac spine.

Structures shown

The lateral projection best demonstrates the rectum and distal sigmoid (Figs. 17-102 and 17-103).

□ Evaluation criteria

The radiograph should demonstrate:
■ Rectosigmoid area in the center of the radiograph.
■ No rotation of the patient.
■ Superimposed hips and femurs.
■ Superior portion of colon not necessarily included when the rectosigmoid region is the area of interest.

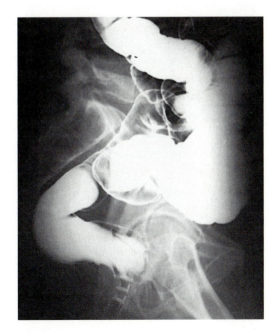

Fig. 17-101. Left lateral rectum.

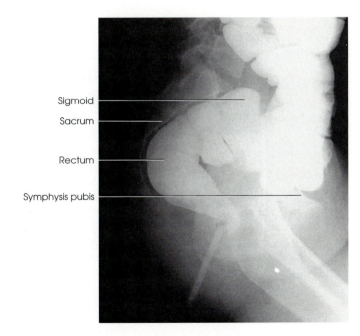

Sigmoid

Sacrum

Rectum

Symphysis pubis

Fig. 17-102. Single-contrast left lateral rectum.

(Courtesy Betsy Delzeith, R.T.)

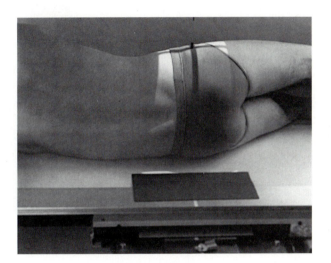

Fig. 17-103. Double-contrast left lateral rectum.

(Courtesy Dr. James Jerele.)

Large Intestine

 AP PROJECTION

Film: 14 × 17 in (35 × 43 cm) lengthwise.

Position of patient

• Place the patient in the supine position.

Position of part

• Center the median sagittal plane to the grid.
• Adjust the center of the cassette at the level of the crest of the ilium (Fig. 17-104).
• *Shield gonads.* (Not shown for illustrative purposes.)
• Ask the patient to suspend respiration for the exposure.

Central ray

• Direct the central ray perpendicular to the film to enter the midline of the body at the level of the crest of the ilium.

Structures shown

The AP projection demonstrates the entire colon with the patient supine (Figs. 17-105 and 17-106).

☐ Evaluation criteria

The radiograph should demonstrate:

■ Entire colon including the splenic flexure and the rectum. Two films may be needed for hypersthenic patients.
■ Vertebral column centered so that the ascending colon and the descending colon are completely included.

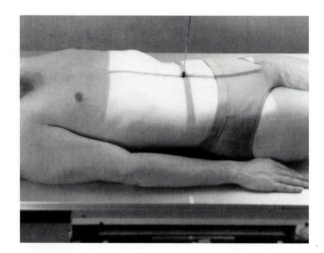

Fig. 17-104. AP large intestine.

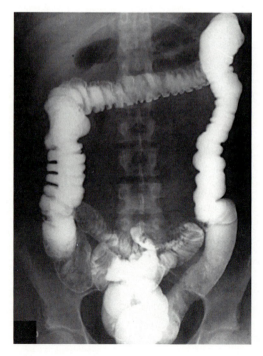

Fig. 17-105. Single-contrast AP large intestine.

(Courtesy Cindy Swords, R.T.)

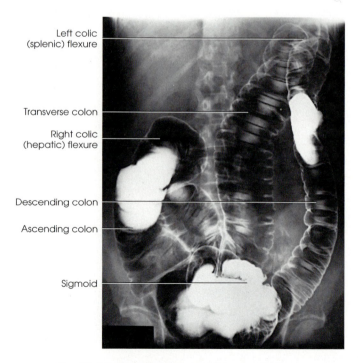

Left colic (splenic) flexure

Transverse colon

Right colic (hepatic) flexure

Descending colon

Ascending colon

Sigmoid

Fig. 17-106. Double-contrast AP large intestine.

(Courtesy Laurie Davis, R.T.)

Large Intestine

 AP AXIAL PROJECTION

Film: 14 × 17 in (35 × 43 cm) lengthwise or 10 × 12 in (24 × 30 cm) lengthwise.

Position of patient

• Place the patient in the supine position.

Position of part

• Center the median sagittal plane to the grid.
• Adjust the center of the cassette at a level approximately 2 inches above the level of the crest of the ilium (Fig. 17-107).
• *Shield gonads.* (Not shown for illustrative purposes.)
• Ask the patient to suspend respiration for the exposure.

Central ray

• Direct the central ray 30 to 40 degrees cephalad to enter the midline of the body approximately 2 inches (5 cm) below the level of the anterior superior iliac spines.
• When a collimated image to demonstrate the rectosigmoid region is desired, direct the central ray to enter the inferior margin of the symphysis pubis.

Structures shown

The AP axial projection best demonstrates the rectosigmoid area of the colon (Figs. 17-108 and 17-109). A similar image is obtained when the patient is prone, as previously illustrated for the PA axial projection in Fig. 17-92.

☐ Evaluation criteria

The radiograph should demonstrate:
■ Rectosigmoid area centered when using a 10 × 12 in (24 × 30 cm) cassette.
■ Rectosigmoid area with less superimposition than in the AP projection because of the angulation of the central ray.
■ Transverse colon and flexures not necessarily included.

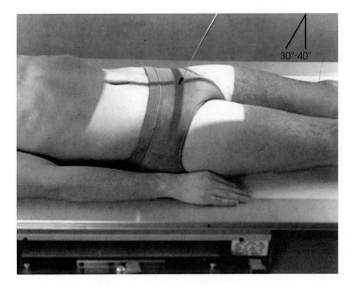

Fig. 17-107. AP axial large intestine.

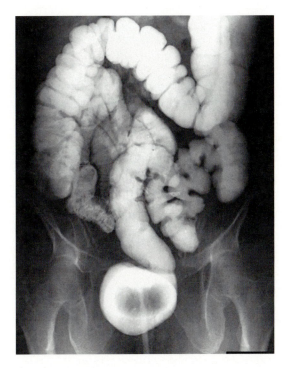

Fig. 17-108. Single-contrast AP axial large intestine.

(Courtesy Betsy Delzeith, R.T.)

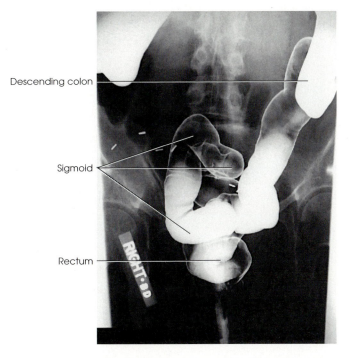

Fig. 17-109. Double-contrast AP axial large intestine.

(Courtesy Barbara Davis, R.T.)

Large Intestine

 AP OBLIQUE PROJECTION
LPO position

Film: 14 × 17 in (35 × 43 cm) lengthwise.

Position of patient

- Place the patient in the supine position.

Position of part

- With the patient's left arm by the side of the body and the right arm across the superior chest, have the patient roll onto the left hip to obtain a 35 to 45 degree rotation from the table.
- Use a positioning sponge and flex the right knee for stability if needed.
- Center the body to the midline of the grid.
- Adjust the center of the cassette at the level of the crest of the ilium (Fig. 17-110).
- *Shield gonads.* (Not shown for illustrative purposes.)
- Ask the patient to suspend respiration for the exposure.

Central ray

- Direct the central ray perpendicular to the film to enter approximately 1 to 2 inches (2.5 to 5 cm) lateral to the midline of the body on the elevated side at the level of the crest of the ilium.

Structures shown

The LPO position best demonstrates the right colic (hepatic) flexure and the ascending and sigmoid portions of the colon (Figs. 17-111 and 17-112).

□ **Evaluation criteria**

The radiograph should demonstrate:
- Entire colon.
- Right colic (hepatic) flexure less superimposed or open when compared with the AP.
- Ascending colon, cecum, and sigmoid colon.

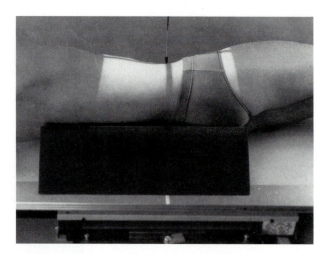

Fig. 17-110. AP oblique large intestine, LPO position.

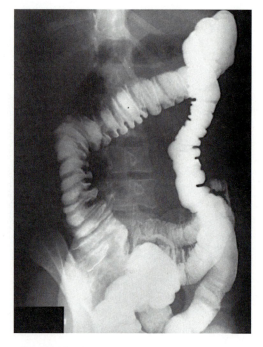

Fig. 17-111. Single-contrast AP oblique large intestine, LPO position.

(Courtesy Cindy Swords, R.T.)

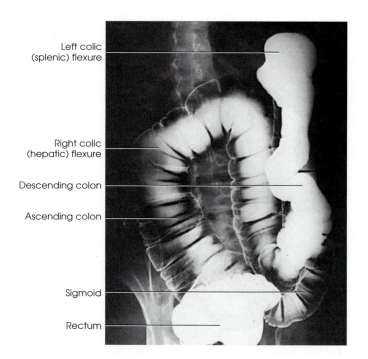

Left colic (splenic) flexure

Right colic (hepatic) flexure

Descending colon

Ascending colon

Sigmoid

Rectum

Fig. 17-112. Double-contrast AP oblique large intestine, LPO position.

Large Intestine

 ### AP OBLIQUE PROJECTION
RPO position

Film: 14 × 17 in (35 × 43 cm) lengthwise.

Position of patient

• Place the patient in the supine position.

Position of part

• With the patient's right arm by the side of the body and the left arm across the superior chest, have the patient roll onto the right hip to obtain a 35 to 45 degree rotation from the table.
• Use a positioning sponge and flex the right knee for stability if needed.
• Center the body to the midline of the grid.
• Adjust the center of the cassette at the level of the crest of the ilium (Fig. 17-113).
• *Shield gonads.* (Not shown for illustrative purposes.)
• Ask the patient to suspend respiration for the exposure.

Central ray

• Direct the central ray perpendicular to the film to enter approximately 1 to 2 inches (2.5 to 5 cm) lateral to the midline of the body on the elevated side at the level of the crest of the ilium.

Structures shown

The RPO position best demonstrates the left colic (splenic) flexure and the descending colon (Figs. 17-114 and 17-115).

The radiograph should demonstrate:
• Entire colon.
• Left colic (splenic) flexure and descending colon.

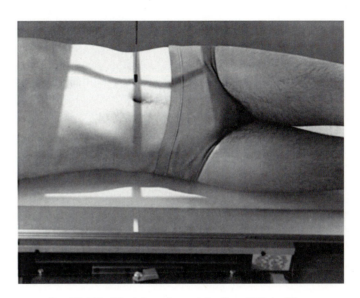

Fig. 17-113. AP oblique large intestine, RPO position.

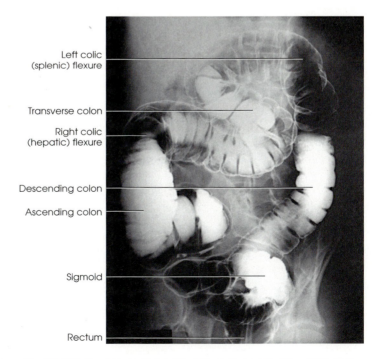

Fig. 17-114. Single-contrast AP oblique large intestine, RPO position.

(Courtesy Cindy Swords, R.T.)

Fig. 17-115. Double-contrast AP oblique large intestine, RPO position.

Left colic (splenic) flexure

Transverse colon

Right colic (hepatic) flexure

Descending colon

Ascending colon

Sigmoid

Rectum

(Courtesy Dr. Robert Harris.)

Decubitus positions

When preparing a patient for an examination in a decubitus position, the following general guidelines are observed:

- Take all decubitus radiographs with the patient lying on the fluoroscopic table with a grid cassette firmly supported behind the patient, with the patient lying on a patient cart with the body against an upright table or chest device, or with a specially designed vertical grid device.
- To ensure that the side of the patient on which the patient is lying is demonstrated, elevate the patient on a suitable radiolucent support. If such is not done, the radiograph will record artifacts from the patient cart mattress or the table edge and superimpose the two images over the portion of the patient's colon on the "down" side.

- For all decubitus procedures, exercise extreme caution to ensure that the wheels on the patient's cart are securely locked so that the patient will not fall.
- For lateral decubitus radiographs, have the patient put the back or abdomen against the vertical grid device. Most patients find it more comfortable to have the back against the vertical grid device than to have the abdomen against the same device.
- If both lateral decubitus radiographs are requested (which is often the case with air-contrast examinations), take one radiograph with the anterior body surface against the vertical grid device and the second radiograph with the patient's posterior body surface against the vertical grid device.

Large Intestine

AP OR PA PROJECTION
Right lateral decubitus position

Film: 14 × 17 in (35 × 43 cm) length-wise.

Position of patient

- Place the patient on the right side with the back or abdomen in contact with the vertical grid device.

Position of part

- With the patient lying on an elevated radiolucent support, center the median sagittal plane to the grid.
- Adjust the center of the cassette at the level of the crest of the ilium (Fig. 17-116).
- *Shield gonads.* (Not shown for illustrative purposes.)
- Ask the patient to suspend respiration for the exposure.

Central ray

- Direct the horizontal central ray perpendicular to the film to enter the midline of the body at the level of the crest of the ilium.

Structures shown

The right lateral decubitus position demonstrates an AP or PA projection of the contrast-filled colon. This position best demonstrates the "up" medial side of the ascending colon and the lateral side of the descending colon when the colon is inflated with air (Figs. 17-117 and 17-118).

☐ Evaluation criteria

The radiograph should demonstrate:
- Area from the left colic (splenic) flexure to the rectum.
- No rotation of the patient as evidenced by the ribs and pelvis.
- For single-contrast examinations, adequate penetration of the barium. For double-contrast examinations, the air-inflated portion of the colon is of primary importance and should not be overpenetrated.

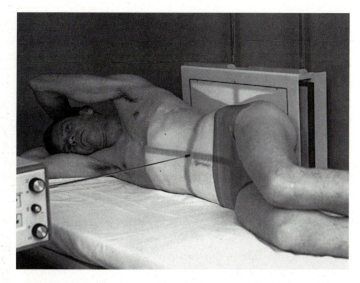

Fig. 17-116. AP large intestine, right lateral decubitus position.

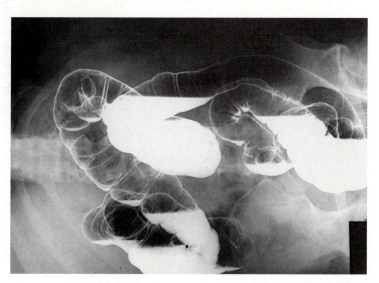

Fig. 17-117. Double-contrast AP large intestine, right lateral decubitus position.

(Courtesy Tracy Taylor, R.T.)

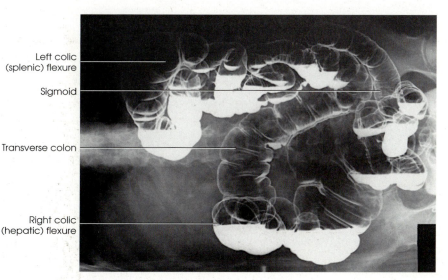

Left colic (splenic) flexure

Sigmoid

Transverse colon

Right colic (hepatic) flexure

Fig. 17-118. Double-contrast AP large intestine, right lateral decubitus position.

(Courtesy Jonathan Miller, R.T.)

Large Intestine

 ### PA OR AP PROJECTION
Left lateral decubitus position

Film: 14 × 17 in (35 × 43 cm) length-wise.

Position of patient

- Place the patient on the left side with the abdomen or back in contact with the vertical grid device.

Position of part

- With the patient lying on an elevated radiolucent support, center the median sagittal plane to the grid.
- Adjust the center of the cassette at the level of the crest of the ilium (Fig. 17-119).
- *Shield gonads.* (Not shown for illustrative purposes.)
- Ask the patient to suspend respiration for the exposure.

Central ray

- Direct the horizontal central ray perpendicular to the film to enter the midline of the body at the level of the crest of the ilium.

Structures shown

The left lateral decubitus position demonstrates a PA or AP projection of the contrast-filled colon. This position best demonstrates the "up" lateral side of the ascending colon and the medial side of the descending colon when the colon is inflated with air (Figs. 17-120 and 17-121).

□ Evaluation criteria

The radiograph should demonstrate:
- Area from the left colic (splenic) flexure to the rectum.
- No rotation of the patient as evidenced by the ribs and pelvis.
- For single-contrast examinations, adequate penetration of the barium. For double-contrast examinations, the air-inflated portion of the colon is of primary importance and should not be overpenetrated.

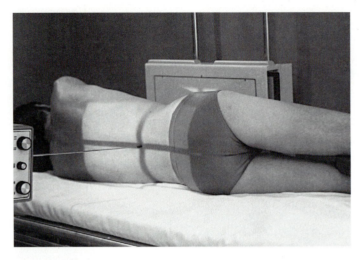

Fig. 17-119. PA large intestine, left lateral decubitus position.

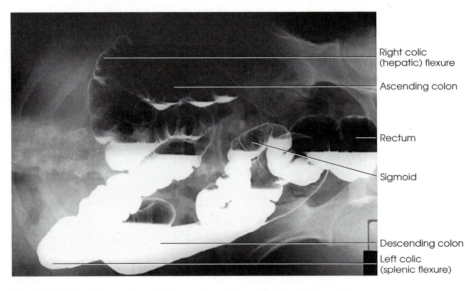

Fig. 17-120. Double-contrast PA large intestine, left lateral decubitus position.

(Courtesy Jonathan Miller, R.T.)

Right colic (hepatic) flexure
Ascending colon
Rectum
Sigmoid
Descending colon
Left colic (splenic flexure)

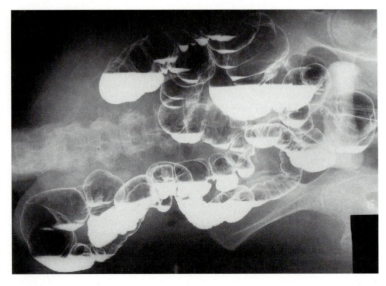

Fig. 17-121. Double-contrast PA large intestine, left lateral decubitus position.

(Courtesy Tracy Taylor, R.T.)

Large Intestine

LATERAL PROJECTION
R or L ventral decubitus position

Film: 14 × 17 in (35 × 43 cm) lengthwise.

Position of patient

- Place the patient in the prone position with either the right or left side against the vertical grid device.

Position of part

- Elevate the patient on radiolucent support and center the median coronal plane to the grid.
- Adjust the center of the cassette at the level of the crest of the ilium.
- *Shield gonads.*
- Ask the patient to suspend respiration for the exposure.

Central ray

- Direct the horizontal central ray perpendicular to the film to enter the median coronal plane of the body at the level of the crest of the ilium.

Structures shown

The ventral decubitus position demonstrates a lateral projection of the contrast-filled colon. This position best demonstrates the "up" posterior portions of the colon and is most valuable in the double-contrast examinations (Fig. 17-122).

□ Evaluation criteria

The radiograph should demonstrate:
- Area from the flexures to the rectum.
- No rotation of the patient.
- For single-contrast examinations, adequate penetration of the barium. For double-contrast examinations, the air-inflated portion of the colon is of primary importance and should not be overpenetrated.
- Enema tip removed for an unobstructed image of the rectum.

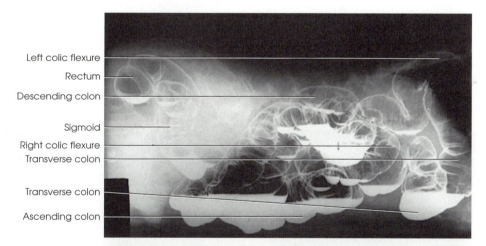

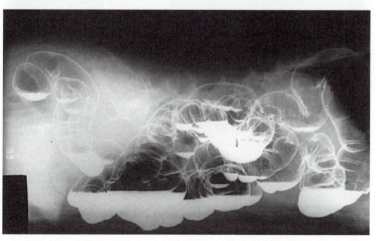

Fig. 17-122. Left lateral projection, ventral decubitus position.

(Courtesy Tracy Taylor, R.T.)

Left colic flexure
Rectum
Descending colon
Sigmoid
Right colic flexure
Transverse colon
Transverse colon
Ascending colon

Large Intestine

AP, PA, OBLIQUE AND LATERAL PROJECTIONS
Upright positions

Upright AP, PA, oblique, and lateral projections may be taken as requested. The positioning and evaluation criteria for upright radiographs are identical to those required for the recumbent positions. However, place the film at a lower level to compensate for the drop of the bowel because of the effect of gravity (Figs. 17-123 to 17-125).

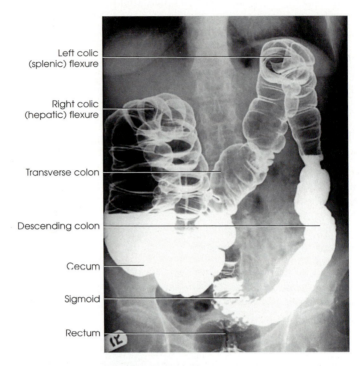

Left colic (splenic) flexure

Right colic (hepatic) flexure

Transverse colon

Descending colon

Cecum

Sigmoid

Rectum

Fig. 17-123. Upright double-contrast AP large intestine.

(Courtesy Betsy Delzeith, R.T.)

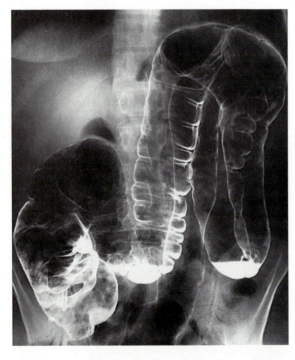

Fig. 17-124. Upright double-contrast PA large intestine.

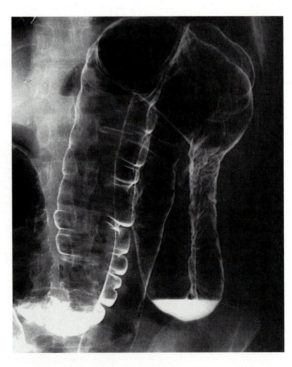

Fig. 17-125. Upright double-contrast AP oblique large intestine, RPO position.

Large Intestine

AXIAL PROJECTION
CHASSARD-LAPINÉ METHOD

The Chassard-Lapiné method is used to demonstrate the rectum, the rectosigmoid junction, and the sigmoid. It has been found[1-3] that this projection, being made at almost a right angle to the AP projection, demonstrates the anterior and posterior surfaces of the lower portion of the bowel and permits the coils of the sigmoid to be projected free from overlapping. This projection may be made after evacuation, although, as Raap[1] states, a pre-evacuation radiograph can be made when the patient has reasonable sphincteric control.

Film: 11 × 14 in (30 × 35 cm) lengthwise.

Position of patient

- Seat the patient on the table.

Position of part

- Instruct the patient to sit well back on the side of the table so that the median coronal plane of the body is as close as possible to the midline of the table.
- If necessary, shift the transversely placed 11 × 14 in (30 × 35 cm) film forward in the Bucky tray so that its transverse axis will coincide as nearly as possible with the median coronal plane of the body.

[1]Raap G: A position of value in studying the pelvis and its contents, South Med J 44:95-99, 1951.
[2]Cimmino CV: Radiography of the sigmoid flexure with the Chassard-Lapiné projection, Med Radiogr Photogr 30:44-45, 1954.
[3]Ettinger A and Elkin M: Study of the sigmoid by special roentgenographic views, AJR 72:199-208, 1954.

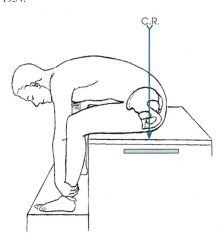

Fig. 17-126. Chassard-Lapiné method.

- Instruct the patient to abduct the thighs as far as the edge of the table permits so that they will not interfere with flexion of the body.
- Center the film to the midline of the pelvis, and ask the patient to lean directly forward as far as possible (Fig. 17-126).
- Direct the patient to grasp the ankles for support.
- Ask the patient to suspend respiration for the exposure.

The exposure required for this projection is approximately the same as that required for a lateral projection of the pelvis.

Central ray

- Direct the central ray perpendicular through the lumbosacral region at the level of the greater trochanters.

Structures shown

The Chassard-Lapiné image demonstrates the rectum, the rectosigmoid junction, and the sigmoid in the axial projection (Fig. 17-127).

☐ Evaluation criteria

The radiograph should demonstrate:

- Rectosigmoid area in the center of the radiograph.
- Rectosigmoid area not obscured by superior area of colon.
- Minimal superimposition of the rectosigmoid area.
- Penetration of the lumbosacral region and the barium.

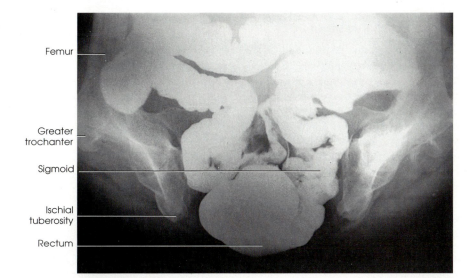

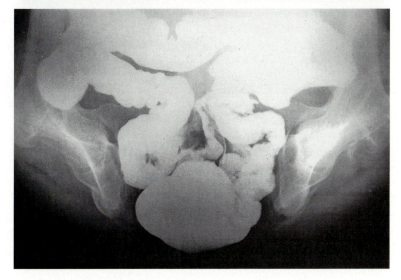

Femur
Greater trochanter
Sigmoid
Ischial tuberosity
Rectum

Fig. 17-127. Axial rectosigmoid, Chassard-Lapiné method.

COLOSTOMY STUDIES

Enterostomy (Gr. *enteron,* intestine + *stoma,* opening) is the general term applied to the surgical procedure of forming an artificial opening to the intestine, usually through the abdominal wall, and to the resultant fecal passage. The regional terms are *colostomy, cecostomy, ileostomy,* and *jejunostomy.*

The colon is the most common site of disease and therefore of operation. Loop colostomy is sometimes performed to divert the fecal column, either temporarily or permanently, from areas of diverticulitis or ulcerative colitis. Most colostomies, however, are performed because of malignancies of the lower bowel and rectum. When a tumor is present, the lower carcinomatous part of the bowel is resected, and the end of the remaining part of the bowel is then brought to the surface through the abdominal wall. This passage, or *stoma,* has no sphincter.

Preparation of intestinal tract

Postoperative contrast enema studies are performed at suitable intervals to determine the efficacy of treatment in cases of diverticulitis and ulcerative colitis and to detect any new or recurrent lesion in the patient who had a tumor. The demonstration of polyps or other intraluminal lesions depends on adequate cleansing of the bowel, which is as important in the presence of colostomy as otherwise. The usual preparation is irrigation of the stoma the night before and again on the morning of the examination.

Colostomy enema equipment

Although all equipment must be scrupulously clean and all nondisposable items must be sterilized after each use, sterile technique is not required because the stoma is part of the intestinal tract. Except for a suitable device to prevent stomal leakage of the contrast material, the equipment employed in the presence of a colostomy is the same as that used in routine contrast enema studies. The same barium sulfate formula is used, and gas studies are made. The opaque and double-contrast studies can be performed in a single-stage examination with the use of a disposable enema kit such as previously described.

Without the use of a device to prevent spillage, the contrast enema may, because of the absence of sphincter control, escape through the colostomy almost as rapidly as it is injected. This would result in unsatisfactory filling of the bowel as well as in obscuring shadows cast by barium soilage of the abdominal wall and the examining table. Abdominal stomas must be effectively occluded for studies made by retrograde injection, and leakage around the stomal catheter must be prevented for studies made by injection into either an abdominal or a perineal colostomy. Numerous devices have been described for this purpose.

Diagnostic enemas may be performed via colostomy with the use of the tips and adhesive disks designed for the patient's use in irrigating the colostomy (Fig. 17-128). The tips are available in four sizes to accommodate the usual sizes of colostomy stomas. These tips usually have a flange to prevent them from slipping through the colostomy opening. An adhesive disk is placed over the flange to minimize reflux soilage. The enema tubing is attached directly to the tip, which the patient holds in position to prevent the weight of the tubing from displacing it to an angled position. In addition to keeping a set of Laird tips on hand, it is recommended that the patient be asked to bring an irrigation device.

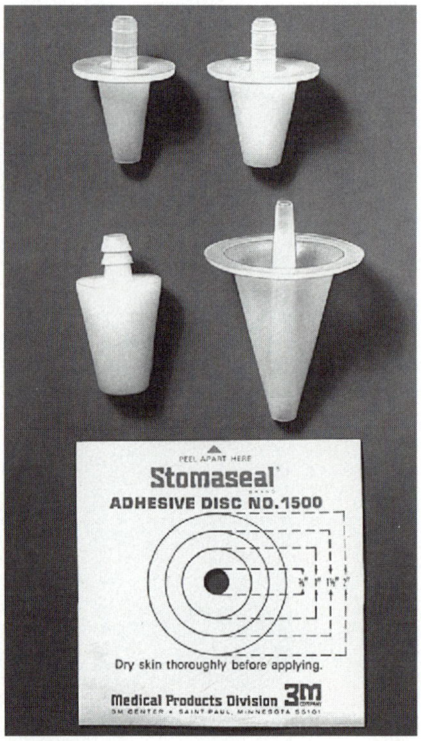

Fig. 17-128. Laird colostomy irrigation tips and Stomaseal disks.

Retention catheters are also used in colostomy examinations. Some examiners use them alone, and others insert them through some device to prevent slipping and to collect leakage. Colostomy stomas are fragile and thus are subject to perforation by any undue pressure or trauma. Perforations have occurred at the insertion of an inflated bulb into a blind pouch and from overdistention of the stoma.

Preparation of patient

If the patient uses a special dressing, a colostomy pouch, or a stomal seal, he or she should be advised to bring a change for use after the examination. When fecal emission is such that a pouch is required, the patient should be given a suitable dressing to place over the stoma after the device has been removed.

The radiographer then observes the following steps:

- Clothe the patient in a kimono type of gown, opening in front or back, according to the location of the colostomy.
- Place the patient on the examining table in the supine position if he or she has an abdominal colostomy and in the prone position if he or she has a perineal colostomy.
- Before taking the preliminary radiograph and while wearing disposable gloves, remove and discard any dressing.
- Cleanse the skin around the stoma appropriately.
- Place a gauze dressing over the stoma to absorb any seepage until the physician is ready to start the examination.
- Lubricate the stomal catheter or tube well (but not excessively) with a water-soluble lubricant. The insertion of the catheter should be performed by the physician or the patient. Perforations of the colon may occur if a catheter is forced through a stoma.

During the performance of the examination, spot radiographs are taken. Postfluoroscopy radiographs are taken as needed. The projections requested depend on the location of the stoma and the anatomy desired to be demonstrated (Figs. 17-129 to 17-132).

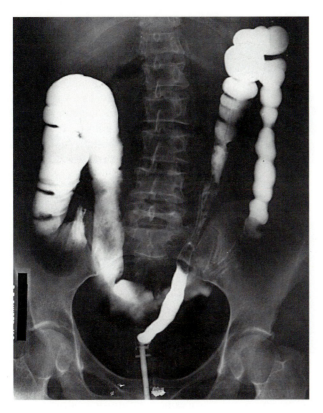

Fig. 17-129. Opaque colon by way of perineal colostomy.

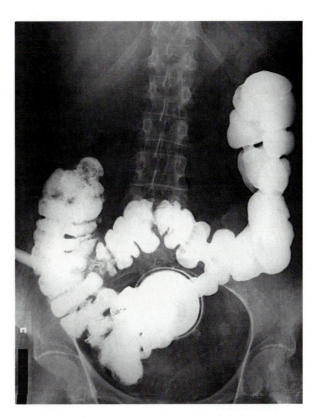

Fig. 17-130. Opaque colon by way of abdominal colostomy.

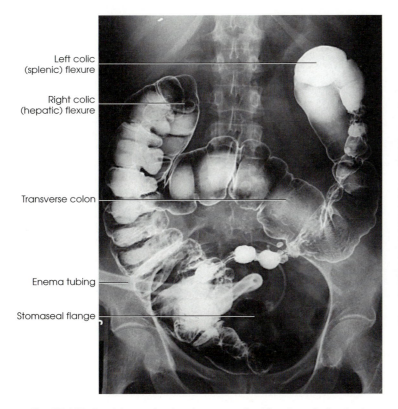

Left colic
(splenic) flexure

Right colic
(hepatic) flexure

Transverse colon

Enema tubing

Stomaseal flange

Fig. 17-131. Double-contrast colon on patient having abdominal colostomy.

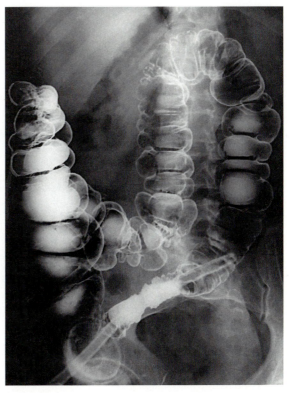

Fig. 17-132. Double-contrast AP oblique colon by way of abdominal colostomy.

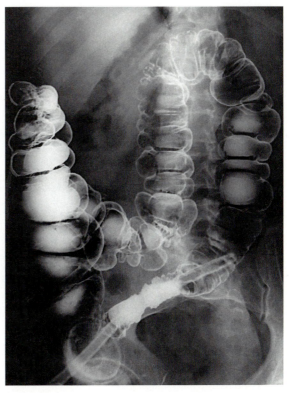

Large intestine

149

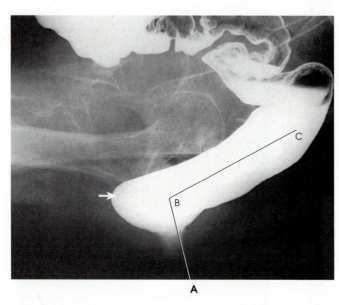

Fig. 17-133. Defecography. Lateral anus and rectum spot film showing the long axis of the anal canal (line *A-B*) and the long axis of the rectal canal (line *B-C*) on a patient with an anorectal angle of 114 degrees. Also demonstrated is an anterior rectocele *(arrow).*

(Courtesy John C. Johnson, M.D., F.A.C.R.)

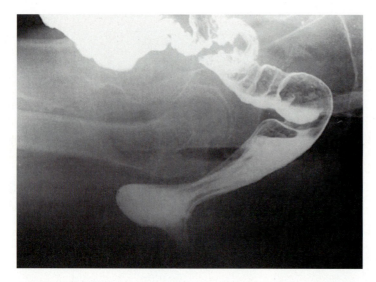

Fig. 17-134. Postevacuation lateral anus and rectum spot film on same patient as in Fig. 17-133.

(Courtesy John C. Johnson, M.D., F.A.C.R.)

DEFECOGRAPHY

Defecography, or *proctography,* is a relatively new radiologic procedure performed on patients with defecational dysfunction. No preparation of the patient is necessary, and cleansing enemas are not recommended because water remaining in the rectum dilutes the contrast medium.

Early investigators[1] mixed a diluted suspension of barium sulfate, heated it, and added potato starch to form a smooth barium paste that was semisolid and malleable.[2,3] Barium manufacturers now package prepared barium products (approximately 100% weight/volume barium sulfate paste) with a special injector mechanism to instill the barium directly into the rectum.

After the barium is instilled, the patient usually is seated in the lateral position on a commercially available radiolucent commode in front of a fluoroscopic unit. A special commode chair is recommended so that the anorectal junction and the zone of interest on the radiograph is not overexposed. Lateral projections are obtained during defecation by spot filming at the approximate rate of 1 to 2 frames per second. Video recording of the defecation process may be used, but the special equipment needed to interpret the images is not always available and a hard copy of the images is also not available.[4] The resulting images are evaluated (Figs. 17-133 and 17-134), measuring the anorectal angle, the angle between the long axes of the anal canal and rectum, and comparing such with normal values.

[1]Burhenne HJ: Intestinal evacuation study: a new roentgenologic technique, Radiol Clin (Basel) 33:79, 1964.
[2]Mahieu P, Pringot J, and Bodart P: Defecography. I. Description of a new procedure and results in normal patients, Gastrointest Radiol 9:247-251, 1984.
[3]Mahieu P, Pringot J, and Bodart P: Defecography. II. Contribution to the diagnosis of defecation disorders, Gastrointest Radiol 9:253-261, 1984.
[4]Mahieu PHG: Defecography. In Margulis AR and Burhenne H: Alimentary tract radiology, vol 1, ed 4, St Louis, 1989, Mosby.

Chapter 18

URINARY SYSTEM

Patient positioned on a cystoscopic table from the 1940s.

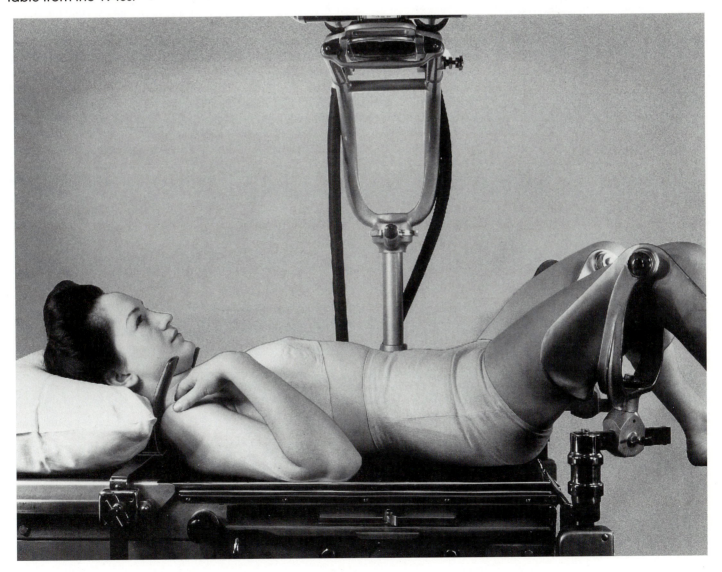

The urinary system comprises a pair of gland-like organs, the kidneys, and a series of musculomembranous excretory ducts (Figs. 18-1 and 18-2). The functions of the *kidneys* include removing waste products from the blood, maintaining fluid and electrolyte balance, and secreting substances that affect blood pressure and other important body functions. The kidneys normally excrete 1 to 2 liters of urine per day. This urine is expelled from the body via the excretory ducts. The excretory ducts consist of (1) a variable number of urine-draining branches called the calyces and an expanded portion called the renal pelvis, which together are known as the pelvicalyceal system; (2) a pair of long tubes, one extending from the pelvis of each kidney, which are called the ureters; (3) a saclike portion, the urinary bladder, which receives the distal portion of the ureters and serves as a reservoir; and (4) a third and smaller tubular portion, the urethra, which conveys the urine to the exterior.

Closely associated with the urinary system are the *suprarenal* (adrenal) *glands.* These glands have no functional relationship with the urinary system but are included in this chapter because of their anatomic relationship with the kidneys. Each of the two suprarenal (adrenal) glands consists of a small, flattened body composed of an internal, medullary portion and an outer, cortical portion. The suprarenal (adrenal) glands are ductless. Each is enclosed in a fibrous sheath and is situated, one on each side, in the retroperitoneal tissue in close contact with the fatty capsule overlying the medial and superior aspects of the upper pole of the kidney. The suprarenal glands (adrenals) furnish important substances: epinephrine, which is secreted by the medulla, and the cortical hormones, which are secreted by the cortex. These glands are subject to malfunction and to a number of diseases. They are not usually demonstrated on preliminary radiographs but are delineated when computed tomography is used. The suprarenal (adrenal) circulation may be demonstrated by selective catheterization of an adrenal artery or vein in angiographic procedures.

The *kidneys* are bean-shaped bodies, the lateral border of each organ being convex and the medial border being concave, and they have slightly convex anterior and posterior surfaces. They are arbitrarily divided into upper and lower poles. The kidneys measure approximately 4½ inches (11.5 cm) in length, 2 to 3 inches (5 to 8 cm) in width, and about 1¼ inches (3 cm) in thickness. The left kidney usually is slightly longer and narrower than the right.

The kidneys are situated behind the peritoneum (retroperitoneal) and are in contact with the posterior wall of the abdominal cavity, one kidney lying on each side of, and in the same coronal plane with, the superior three lumbar vertebrae. They lie in an oblique plane from above inferiorly, anteriorly, and laterally, the anterior slant following the curve of the last thoracic vertebra and the superior three lumbar vertebrae (Fig. 18-3). The kidneys normally extend from the level of the superior border of the twelfth thoracic vertebra to the level of the transverse processes of the third lumbar vertebra in persons of sthenic build; they are somewhat higher in individuals of hypersthenic habitus and somewhat lower in those of asthenic habitus. Because of the large space occupied by the liver, the right kidney is a little lower in position than the left. Each kidney is embedded in a mass of fatty tissue called the adipose capsule, and the whole is enveloped in a sheath of fascia, the *renal fascia,* which is attached to the diaphragm, the lumbar vertebrae, the peritoneum, and other adjacent structures. The kidneys are supported in a fairly fixed position, partially through the fascial attachments and partially by the surrounding organs. They have a respiratory excursion of approximately 1 inch (2.5 cm) and normally drop no more than 2 inches (5 cm) in the change from the supine to the upright position.

The concave medial border of each kidney has a longitudinal slit, or *hilum,* for

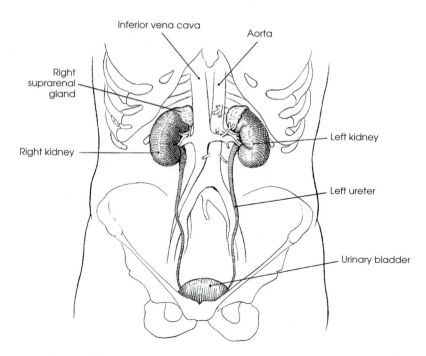

Fig. 18-1. Anterior aspect of urinary system in relation to surrounding structures.

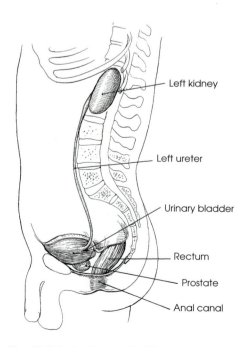

Fig. 18-2. Lateral aspect of the male urinary system in relation to surrounding structures.

transmission of the blood and lymphatic vessels, the nerves, and the ureter (Fig. 18-4). The hilum expands into the body of the gland to form a central cavity called the *renal sinus*. The renal sinus is a fat-filled space surrounding the renal pelvis and vessels. The kidney is composed of an outer, cortical substance and an inner, medullary substance and is covered by a thin layer of fibrous tissue, which is prolonged inward to line the renal sinus.

The medullary substance, composed mainly of the collecting tubules, which give it a striated appearance, consists of 8 to 15 cone-shaped segments called the renal pyramids. The apices of the segments converge toward the renal sinus to drain into the pelvicalyceal system. The more compact cortical substance lies between the periphery of the organ and the bases of the medullary segments and extends medially between the pyramids to the renal sinus. These cortical extensions are called *renal columns*.

The essential microscopic components of the parenchyma of the kidney are called the *nephrons* (Fig. 18-5). There are approximately 1 million of these tubular structures in each kidney. Nephrons are composed of a renal corpuscle and a renal tubule. The proximal nephron consists of a double-walled membranous cup, called the *glomerular capsule* (capsule of Bowman), and a cluster of blood capillaries, called the *glomerulus,* which invaginate the cup of the capsule. The glomerulus and its glomerular capsule are known collectively as the *renal corpuscle.* The glomerulus is formed by a minute branch

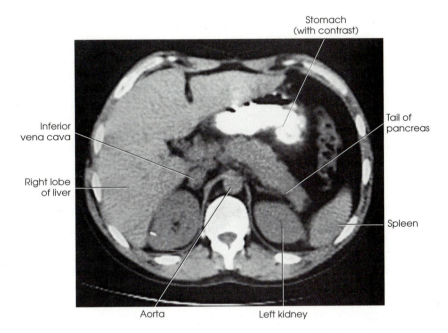

Fig. 18-3. Cross section of abdomen through second lumbar vertebra.

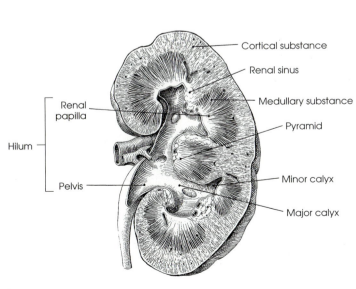

Fig. 18-4. Coronal section of kidney.

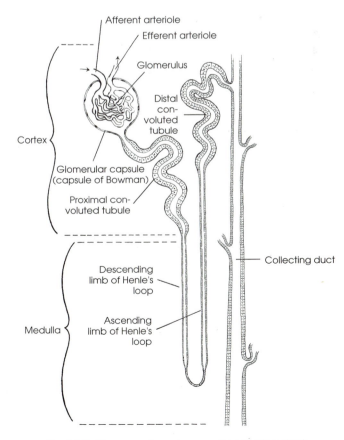

Fig. 18-5. Diagram of nephron and collecting duct.

of the renal artery entering the capsule and dividing into capillaries. The capillaries then turn back and, as they ascend, unite to form a single vessel leaving the capsule. The vessel entering the capsule is called the *afferent arteriole,* and the one leaving, the *efferent arteriole.* After leaving the glomerular capsules, the efferent arterioles pass on to form the capillary network surrounding the straight and convoluted tubules, and these capillaries reunite and continue on to communicate with the renal veins.

The thin inner wall of the capsule closely adheres to the capillary coils and is separated by a comparatively wide space from the outer layer, which is continuous with the beginning of a renal tubule. The glomerulus serves as a filter for the blood, permitting water and finely dissolved substances to pass through the walls of the capillaries into the capsule. This fluid is called the *glomerular filtrate.* The change from filtrate to urine is caused in part by the water and the usable dissolved substances being absorbed through the epithelial lining of the tubules into the surrounding capillary network.

Each *renal tubule* continues from a glomerular capsule in the cortex of the kidney and then travels a circuitous path through the cortical and medullary substances, becoming in turn the *proximal convoluted tubule,* the *straight tubule* (the descending and ascending limbs of the loop of Henle), and the *distal convoluted tubule.* The latter opens into the collecting ducts that begin in the cortex. The collecting ducts converge toward the renal pelvis and unite along their course so that each group within the pyramid forms a central tubule that opens at the *renal papilla* (apex) and drains its tributaries into the minor calyx.

The *calyces* are cup-shaped stems arising at the sides of the papilla (apex) of each renal pyramid, each calyx enclosing one or more papillae (apices), so that there are usually fewer calyces than pyramids. The beginning branches are called the *minor calyces,* numbering from 4 to 13, and they unite to form two or three larger tubes called the *major calyces.* The major calyces unite to form the expanded, funnel-shaped *renal pelvis.* The wide upper portion of the renal pelvis lies within the renal sinus, while its tapering lower part passes through the hilum to become continuous with the ureter.

The *ureter* is 10 to 12 inches (25 to 30 cm) in length. It descends behind the peritoneum and in front of the psoas muscle and the transverse processes of the lumbar vertebrae, passes inferiorly and posteriorly in front of the sacral ala, and then curves anteriorly and medially to enter the posterolateral surface of the urinary bladder at approximately the level of the ischial spine. The ureters convey the urine from the renal pelves to the bladder by slow, rhythmic peristaltic contractions.

The *urinary bladder* is a musculomembranous sac that serves as a reservoir for urine. The bladder is situated immediately posterior and superior to the symphysis pubis, and its fundus (the inferoposterior part of the viscus) is in relation to the rectal ampulla in the male and to the upper part of the vaginal canal in the female. The apex of the bladder is at the anterosuperior aspect and is related to the superior aspect of the symphysis pubis. The most fixed part of the bladder is the neck, which rests on the prostate in the male or on the pelvic diaphragm in the female. The bladder varies in size, shape, and position according to the amount of its content, being approximately tetrahedral in shape and situated entirely within the pelvic cavity when empty. As it fills, the viscus gradually assumes an oval shape while expanding superiorly and anteriorly into the abdominal cavity. The adult bladder can hold approximately 500 cc of fluid when completely full. The desire for *micturition* (urination) occurs when there is about 250 cc of urine in the bladder.

The ureters enter the posterior wall of the bladder at the lateral margins of the superior part of its base, or fundus, and pass obliquely through the wall to their respective internal orifices. These two openings are about 1 inch (2.5 cm) apart when the viscus is empty and about 2 inches (5 cm) apart when it is distended, being an equal distance from the internal urethral orifice, which is placed at the lowest part, called the *neck,* of the bladder. The triangular area between the three orifices is called the *trigone.* The mucosa over the trigone is always smooth, whereas the remainder of the lining is thrown into folds when the viscus is empty.

The *urethra,* which serves to convey the urine to the exterior, is a narrow musculomembranous canal with a sphincter type of muscle at the neck of the bladder. The urethra arises at the internal urethral orifice in the urinary bladder and extends for a distance of about 1½ inches (4 cm) in the female and 7 to 8 inches (17 to 20 cm) in the male.

The female urethra passes along the thick anterior wall of the vagina to the external urethral orifice, which is located in the vestibule about 1 inch (2.5 cm) anterior to the vaginal opening (Fig. 18-6). The male urethra extends from the bladder to the end of the penis and is divided into prostatic, membranous, and spongy (cavernous) portions (Fig. 18-7). The prostatic portion is about 1 inch (2.5 cm) in length, reaches from the bladder to the floor of the pelvis, and is completely surrounded by the prostate. The membranous portion of the canal passes through the urogenital diaphragm; it is slightly constricted and about ½ inch (1.2 cm) long. The spongy (cavernous) portion passes through the shaft of the penis, extending from the floor of the pelvis to the external urethral orifice. The distal prostatic, membranous, and spongy (cavernous) parts of the male urethra also serve as the excretory canal of the reproductive system.

The *prostate* is a small, glandular body surrounding the proximal part of the male urethra and is situated just posterior to the inferior portion of the symphysis pubis. The prostate is considered part of the male reproductive system but, because of its close proximity to the bladder, is commonly described with the urinary system. Conical in shape, the base of the prostate is attached to the inferior surface of the urinary bladder, and its apex is in contact with the pelvic diaphragm. The prostate measures about 1½ inches (4 cm) transversely and ¾ inch (2 cm) anteroposteriorly at its base, and vertically the prostate is approximately 1 inch (2.5 cm) in length.

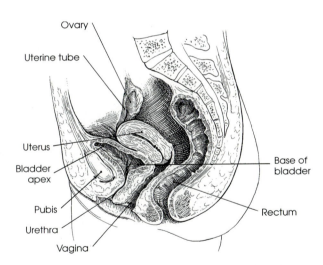

Fig. 18-6. Median sagittal section through female pelvis.

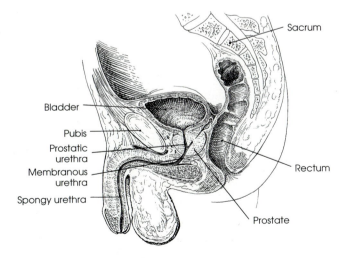

Fig. 18-7. Median sagittal section through male pelvis.

Radiography of the urinary system comprises numerous specialized procedures, each of which requires the use of an artificial contrast medium and each of which was evolved to serve a specific purpose. The specialized procedures are preceded by a plain or scout radiograph of the abdominopelvic areas for the detection of any abnormality demonstrable by this means. The preliminary examination may consist of no more than an AP projection of the abdomen. When indicated, oblique and/or lateral projections are taken to localize calcium and tumor masses, and an upright position may be used to demonstrate the mobility of the kidneys.

The position and mobility of the kidneys and usually their size and shape generally can be demonstrated on preliminary radiographs. This image is possible because of the contrast furnished by the radiolucent fatty capsule surrounding the kidneys. Visualization of the thin-walled drainage or collecting system (the calyces and pelves, the ureters, the urinary bladder, and the urethra) requires that the canals be filled with a contrast medium. The urinary bladder is outlined when it is filled with urine, but it is not adequately demonstrated. The ureters and the urethra cannot be distinguished on preliminary radiographs.

For the delineation and differentiation of cysts and tumor masses situated within the kidney, the renal parenchyma is opacified by an intravenously introduced, organic, iodinated contrast medium and then may be radiographed by tomography or CT. The contrast solution may be introduced into the vein by rapid injection or by infusion. These procedures are respectively called *bolus injection nephrotomography* (Fig. 18-8) and *infusion nephrotomography* (Fig. 18-9). In another technique for investigating cysts and tumor masses of the renal parenchyma, a long needle is inserted through the flank into the cyst or tumor for direct injection of the contrast medium. This procedure is called *percutaneous renal puncture* and is rarely performed today.

Investigations of the blood vessels of the kidneys and of the suprarenal glands are performed by angiographic procedures as described in Volume 2, Chapter 26. An example of the direct injection of contrast medium into the renal artery is seen in Fig. 18-10.

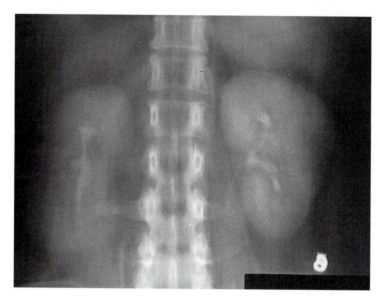

Fig. 18-8. Bolus injection nephrotomogram.

(Courtesy Dr. John A. Evans.)

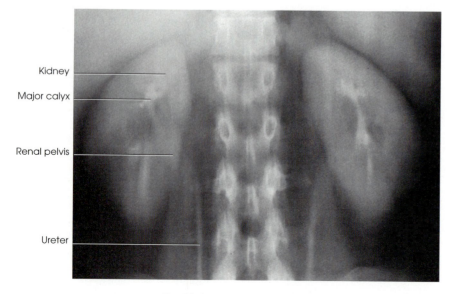

Kidney

Major calyx

Renal pelvis

Ureter

Fig. 18-9. Infusion nephrotomogram.

Radiologic investigations of the renal drainage, or collecting, system are performed by various procedures classified under the general term *urography*. This term embraces two regularly employed techniques of filling the urinary canals with a contrast medium, antegrade or retrograde. *Antegrade* filling techniques allow the contrast to enter the kidney in the normal direction of blood flow. In selective patients this is done by introducing the contrast material directly into the kidney through a percutaneous puncture of the renal pelvis; this technique is called *percutaneous antegrade urography*. Much more frequently employed is the physiologic technique, in which the contrast agent is generally administered intravenously. This technique is called *excretory* or *intravenous urography* and is shown in Fig. 18-11.

The excretory technique of urography is employed in examinations of the upper urinary tracts of infants and children and is generally considered to be the preferred technique for adults unless use of the retrograde technique is definitely indicated. Since the contrast medium is administered intravenously, and all parts of the urinary system are normally demonstrated, the excretory technique is correctly referred to as intravenous urography (IVU). The term *pyelography* refers to the radiographic demonstration of the renal pelves and calyces. For years, the examination has been and continues to be erroneously called an intravenous pyelogram (IVP).

Once the opaque contrast medium enters the bloodstream, it is conveyed to the renal glomeruli and is discharged into the capsules with the glomerular filtrate, which is excreted as urine. With the reabsorption of water, the contrast material becomes sufficiently concentrated to render the urinary canals radiopaque. The urinary bladder is well outlined by this technique, and satisfactory voiding urethrograms may be obtained.

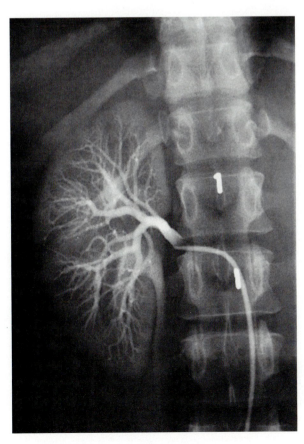

Fig. 18-10. Selective right renal arteriogram.

(Courtesy Dr. Joshua A. Becker.)

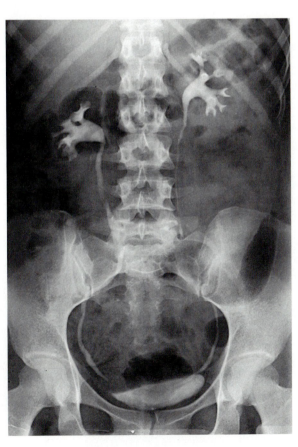

Fig. 18-11. Excretory urogram.

In some procedures involving the urinary system, the contrast is introduced against the normal flow; this is called *retrograde* urography (Fig. 18-12). The contrast medium is injected directly into the canals by means of ureteral catheterization for contrast filling of the upper urinary tract and urethral catheterization for the lower part of the urinary tract. Cystoscopy is required to localize the vesicoureteral orifices for the passage of ureteral catheters.

Retrograde urographic examinations of the proximal urinary tracts are primarily urologic procedures, and the catheterization and contrast filling of the urinary canals are performed by the attending urologist in conjunction with a physical or endoscopic examination. This technique enables the urologist to take catheterized specimens of urine directly from each renal pelvis, and, because the canals can be fully distended by direct injection of the contrast agent, it sometimes gives more

information regarding the anatomy of the different parts of the collecting system than is always possible by the excretory technique. In this procedure an evaluation of kidney function depends on an intravenously administered dye substance to stain the color of the urine subsequently trickling through the respective ureteral catheters. Both techniques of examination are occasionally required for a complete urologic study.

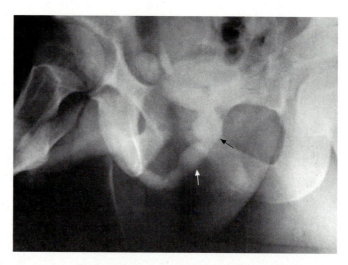

Fig. 18-13. Voiding study following routine injection IVU. Dilation of proximal urethra *(arrows)* is result of urethral stricture.

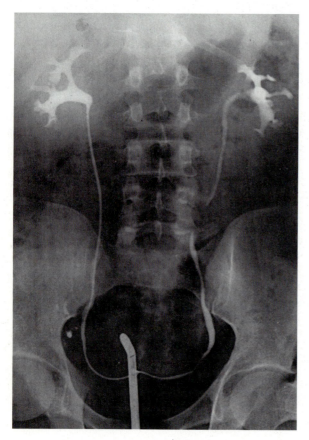

Fig. 18-12. Retrograde urogram.

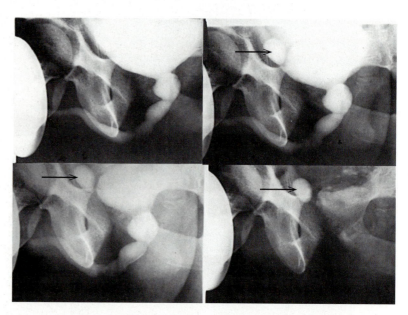

Fig. 18-14. Voiding studies of same patient as in Fig. 18-13 after infusion nephrourography. Note increase in opacification of contrast-filled cavities by this method and bladder diverticulum *(arrows)*.

(Courtesy Dr. Joshua A. Becker.)

Investigations of the lower urinary tract—the bladder, the lower ureters, and the urethra—are usually made by the retrograde technique, which requires no instrumentation beyond the passage of a urethral catheter. However, investigations may also be made by the physiologic technique (Figs. 18-13 and 18-14). Bladder examinations are usually denoted by the general term *cystography* (Fig. 18-15). A procedure understood to include inspection of the lower ureters is *cystoureterography* (Fig. 18-16), and a procedure understood to include inspection of the urethra is *cystourethrography* (Fig. 18-17).

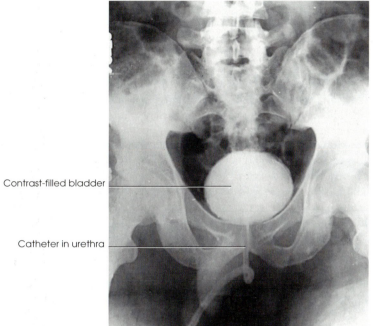

Contrast-filled bladder

Catheter in urethra

Fig. 18-15. Cystogram.

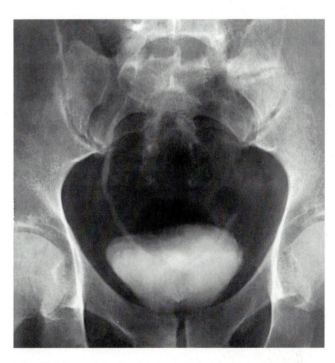

Fig. 18-16. Cystourethrogram, AP bladder showing distal ureters.

(Courtesy John Syring, R.T.)

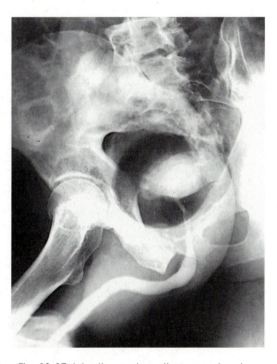

Fig. 18-17. Injection cystourethrogram showing urethra on male patient.

(Courtesy Dr. Oswald S. Lowsley.)

CONTRAST MEDIA

Retrograde urography (Figs. 18-18 and 18-19) began in 1904 by the introduction of air into the urinary bladder. In 1906 retrograde urography as well as cystography was performed with the first opaque medium, a colloidal silver preparation that is no longer used. Silver iodide, which is a nontoxic inorganic compound, was introduced in 1911. Sodium iodide and sodium bromide, also inorganic compounds, came into use for retrograde urography in 1918. The bromides and iodides are no longer in general use for examinations of the renal pelves and ureters because they irritate the mucosa and frequently cause the patient considerable discomfort. Since a large quantity of solution is required to fill the urinary bladder, iodinated salts in concentrations of 30% or less are used in cystography. A large selection of commercially available contrast media may be used for all types of urinary system radiography. The user must review the product insert packaged with all contrast agents.

Excretory urography (Figs. 18-20 and 18-21) was first reported by Rowntree et al in 1923.[1] These investigators employed a 10% solution of chemically pure sodium iodide as the contrast medium. This agent was excreted too slowly to give a satisfactory demonstration of the renal pelves and ureters, and it also proved to be too toxic for functional distribution. Early in 1929 Roseno and Jepkins[2] introduced a compound in which they combined sodium iodide with urea. The latter constituent, which is one of the nitrogenous substances removed from the blood and eliminated by the kidneys, served to accelerate excretion and thus to quickly fill the renal pelves with opacified urine. Although satisfactory renal images were obtained with this compound, the patients experienced considerable distress as a result of its toxicity. Later in 1929 Swick developed the organic compound Uroselectan, which had an iodine content of 42%. The present-day ionic contrast media for excretory urography are the result of extensive research by many investigators. The ionic contrast media are available under various trade names in concentrations ranging from about 50% to 70%. Sterile solutions of the media are supplied in dose-size ampules or vials.

[1]Rowntree LG et al: Roentgenography of the urinary tract during excretion of sodium iodide, JAMA 8:368-373, 1923.
[2]Roseno A and Jepkins H: Intravenous pyelography, Fortschr Roentgenstr 39:859-863, 1929. Abstract: AJR 22:685-686, 1929.

In the early 1970s, work began in developing nonionic contrast media. Development progressed, and several nonionic contrast agents are currently available for urographic, vascular, and intrathecal injection. Although the nonionic contrast agents are generally less likely to cause a reaction in the patient, their cost is several times higher than that of the ionic agents.

Many institutions have developed criteria to determine which patient receives which contrast agent; the choice of whether to use an ionic or nonionic contrast medium therefore remains a decision regarding patient risk and economics.

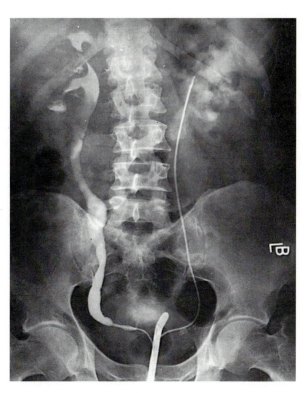

Fig. 18-18. Retrograde urogram with contrast medium-filled right renal pelvis and catheter in left renal pelvis.

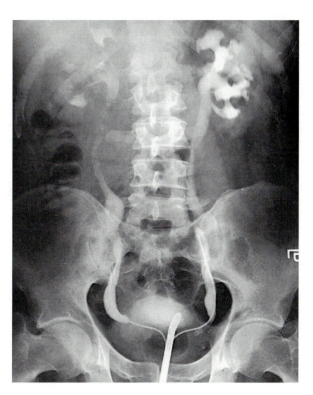

Fig. 18-19. Retrograde urogram.

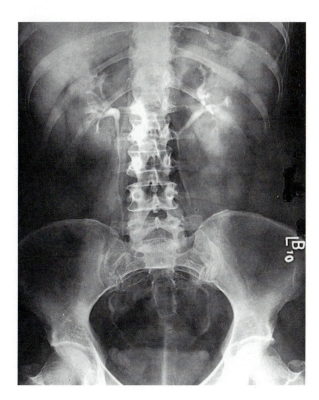

Fig. 18-20. Excretory urogram 10 minutes after contrast medium injection.

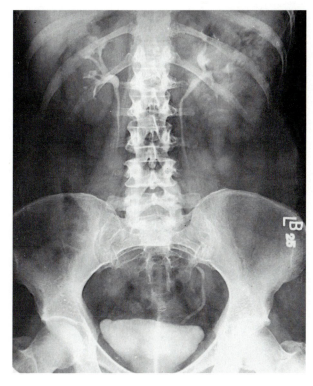

Fig. 18-21. Excretory urogram on same patient as in Fig. 18-20, 25 minutes after contrast medium injection.

(Courtesy Dr. Marcy L. Sussman.)

161

Adverse reactions to iodinated media

The iodinated organic preparations that are compounded for urologic examinations are of low toxicity, with the result that adverse reactions are usually mild and of short duration. The characteristic reactions are a feeling of warmth, flushing, and sometimes a few hives. Occasionally nausea, vomiting, and edema of the respiratory mucous membrane result. Severe and serious reactions occur only rarely, but since they are an ever-present possibility, the clinical history of each patient must be carefully checked and all patients kept under careful observation for any sign of systemic reactions. Emergency equipment and medication to treat any adverse reaction must be readily available.

The vast majority of all reactions to contrast media occur within the first 5 minutes after the injection. Therefore the patient should not be left unattended.

PREPARATION OF INTESTINAL TRACT

Although unobstructed visualization of the urinary tracts requires that the intestinal tract be free of gas and solid fecal material (Fig. 18-22), preparation is not attempted in infants and children, and whether any cleansing measure is possible in adults depends, as always, on the condition of the patient. Gas (particularly swallowed air, which is quickly dispersed through the small bowel) rather than fecal material is usually the offender in these patients.

Hope and Campoy[1] recommend that infants and children be given a carbonated soft drink to distend the stomach with gas. By this maneuver, the gas-containing intestinal loops are usually pushed inferiorly, and the upper urinary tracts, particularly the left, are then clearly visualized through the negative shadow of the gas-filled stomach. Hope and Campoy state that the aerated drink must be given in an amount adequate to fully inflate the stomach: at least 2 ounces are required for a newborn infant and a full 12 ounces for a child 7 or 8 years of age. In conjunction with the carbonated drink, they use a highly concentrated contrast medium. A gas-distended stomach is shown in Fig. 18-23.

---

[1]Hope JW and Campoy F: The use of carbonated beverages in pediatric excretory urography, Radiology 64:66-71, 1955.

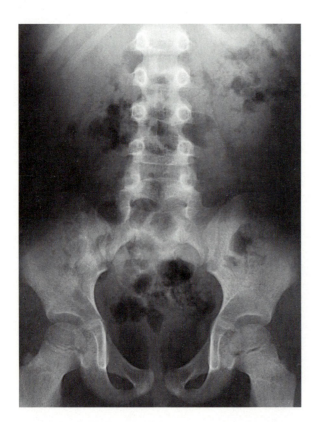

Fig. 18-22. Preliminary AP abdomen for urogram.

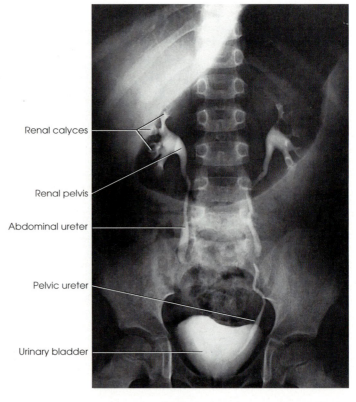

Renal calyces

Renal pelvis

Abdominal ureter

Pelvic ureter

Urinary bladder

Fig. 18-23. Supine urogram at 15-minutes interval with gas-filled stomach.

(Courtesy Dr. David L. Bloom.)

Berdon et al[1] state that the prone position resolves the problem of obscuring gas in a majority of patients (Figs. 18-24 and 18-25). The need to inflate the stomach with air alone or with air as part of an aerated drink is eliminated. By exerting pressure on the abdomen, the prone position shifts the gas laterally away from the pelvicalyceal structures. Gas contained in the antral portion of the stomach is displaced into its fundic portion, that in the transverse colon shifts into the ascending and descending segments, and that in the sigmoid colon shifts into the descending colon and rectum. Berdon et al say that the prone position occasionally fails to produce the desired result in small infants when the small bowel is dilated. Gastric inflation also fails in these patients because the dilated small bowel merely elevates the gas-filled stomach and thus does not improve visualization. They recommend that this group of infants be examined after the intestinal gas has passed.

---

[1]Berdon WE, Baker DH, and Leonidas J: Prone radiography in intravenous pyelography in infants and children, AJR 103:444-455, 1968.

PREPARATION OF PATIENT

Medical opinion varies widely with regard to preparative measures. With modifications as required, the following procedure seems to be in general use:

1. When time permits, a low-residue diet for 1 to 2 days to prevent gas formation caused by excessive fermentation of the intestinal contents.
2. A light evening meal.
3. When indicated by costive bowel action, a non–gas-forming laxative the evening before the examination.
4. NPO after midnight on the day of the examination. However, the patient should *not* be dehydrated. It is important to realize that patients who have multiple myeloma, high uric acid levels, and diabetes must be well hydrated before the IVU is performed. These patients run an increased risk of contrast medium–induced renal failure if they are dehydrated.
5. In preparation for *retrograde urography,* the patient is often requested to force water (4 or 5 glassfuls) for several hours before the examination to ensure excretion of urine in an amount sufficient for bilateral catheterized specimens and renal function tests.
6. Usually no patient preparation is required for examinations of the lower urinary tract.

Outpatients should be given explicit directions regarding any order that the physician gives pertaining to diet, fluid intake, and laxatives or other medication. The patient should also be given a suitable explanation for each preparative measure to ensure cooperation.

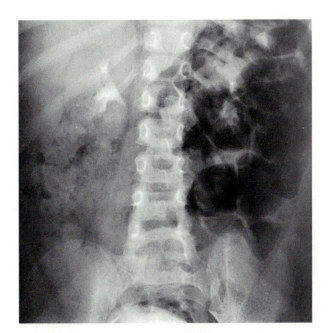

Fig. 18-24. Urogram, supine position.

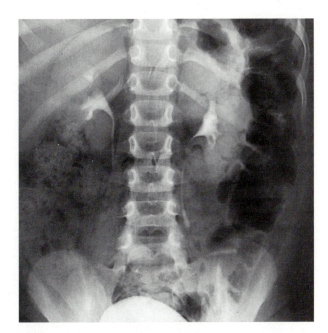

Fig. 18-25. Urogram, prone position. Same patient as in Fig. 18-24 showing markedly improved visualization of left kidney and ureter.

(Courtesy Dr. Walter E. Berdon and Dr. David H. Baker.)

FILM QUALITY AND EXPOSURE TECHNIQUE

Urograms should have the same contrast and density and the same degree of soft tissue density as do abdominal radiographs. The radiographs must show a sharply defined outline of the kidneys, the lower border of the liver, and the lateral margin of the psoas muscles. The amount of bone detail visible in these studies varies according to the thickness of the abdomen (Fig. 18-26).

MOTION CONTROL

An immobilization band usually is not applied over the upper abdomen in urographic examinations because the resultant pressure might interfere with the passage of fluid through the ureters and also might cause distortion of the canals. Thus the elimination of motion in urographic examinations depends on the exposure time and on securing the full cooperation of the patient.

The examination procedure should be explained to the adult patient to prepare him or her for any transitory distress caused by the injection of the contrast solution or by the cystoscopic procedure, and the patient should be assured that everything possible will be done for his or her comfort. Much of the success of these examinations depends on the ability of the radiographer to gain the confidence of the patient.

EQUIPMENT

Retrograde urographic procedures requiring cystoscopy are facilitated if carried out on a combination cystoscopic-radiographic unit. Any standard radiographic table is suitable for preliminary excretory urography and for most retrograde studies of the bladder and urethra. The cystoscopic unit is also used for these procedures, but, for the patient's comfort, it is desirable that it have an extensible leg rest.

For infusion nephrourography, a table that is equipped with tomographic apparatus is necessary. Tomography is desirable when intestinal gas obscures some of the underlying structures or when hypersthenic patients are being examined (Figs. 18-27 to 18-29).

For the patient's comfort as well as to prevent delays during the examination, all preparations for the examination procedure should be made before the patient is placed on the table. In addition to the identification and side marker, when performing excretory urographic studies a time-interval marker is required for each postinjection study. Body-position markers (supine, prone, upright or semiupright, Trendelenburg, decubitus) should also be used. Some institutions perform excretory urograms (proximal urinary tract studies) using 10 × 12 in (24 × 30 cm) or 11 × 14 in (30 × 35 cm) cassettes placed crosswise, but these studies can also be made on 14 × 17 in (35 × 43 cm) cassettes placed lengthwise. The upright study is made on a 14 × 17 in (35 × 43 cm) cassette because it is taken to demonstrate the mobility of the kidneys as well as to outline the lower ureters and bladder. Studies of the bladder before and after voiding are usually taken on 10 × 12 in (24 × 30 cm) films.

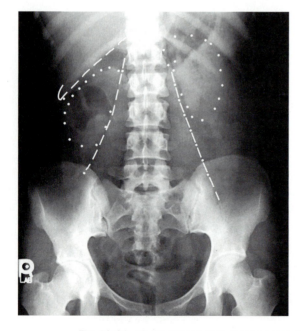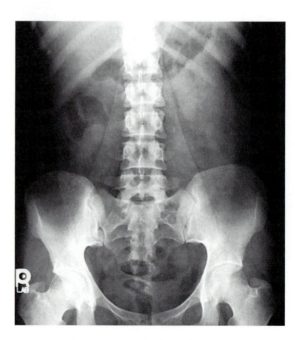

Fig. 18-26. AP abdomen showing margins of the kidney (dots), liver (dashes), and psoas muscles (dot-dash lines).

(Courtesy Lois Baird, R.T.)

The following guidelines are observed in preparing additional equipment for the examination:

- Have an emergency cart fully equipped and conveniently placed.
- Arrange the instrument layout for the injection of the contrast agent on a small, moveable table or on a tray.
- Have the frequently used sterile items readily available. Disposable syringes and needles are available in standard sizes and are widely used in this procedure.
- Have the required nonsterile items available: a tourniquet, a small waste basin, an emesis basin and disposable wipes, one or two bottles of the contrast medium, and a small prepared dressing for application to the puncture site.
- Have alcohol wipes available.
- Provide a folded towel or a small pillow for placement under the elbow to relieve pressure during the injection.

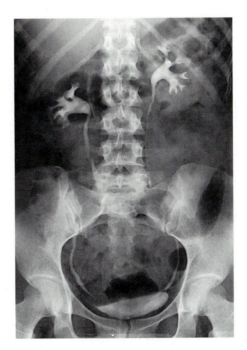

Fig. 18-27. Urogram, AP projection.

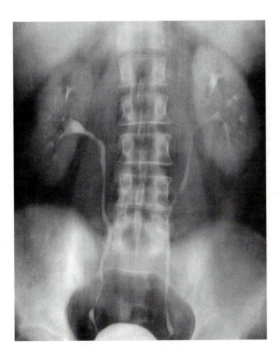

Fig. 18-28. Urogram, AP projection using tomography.

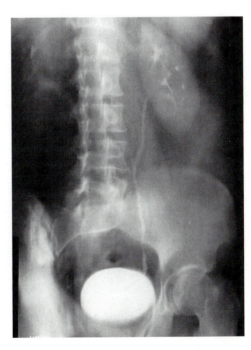

Fig. 18-29. Urogram, AP oblique projection (LPO position) using tomography. Note left kidney is perpendicular to film.

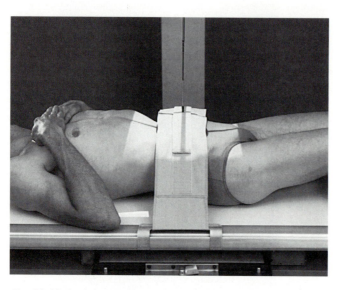

Fig. 18-30. Ureteral compression device in place for urogram.

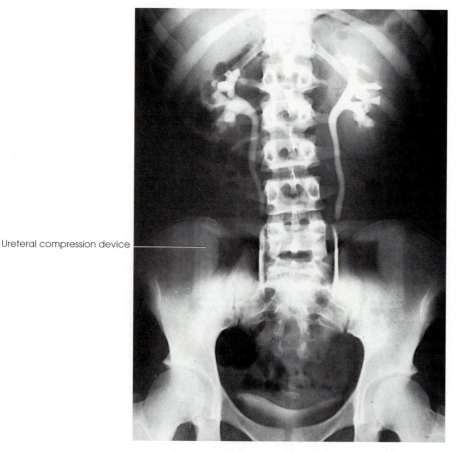

Ureteral compression device

Fig. 18-31. Urogram showing ureteral compression device in proper position over distal ureters.

URETERAL COMPRESSION

In excretory urography, compression is sometimes applied over the distal ends of the ureters. This is done to retard the flow of the opacified urine into the bladder and thus ensures adequate filling of the renal pelves and calyces. If compression is used, it must be placed so that the pressure over the distal ends of the ureters is centered about 2 inches (5 cm) above the superior border of the symphysis pubis; as much pressure as the patient can comfortably tolerate is then applied with the immobilization band (Figs. 18-30 and 18-31). Because of the amount of pressure applied in this procedure, the pressure should be released slowly when the compression device is removed to avoid the possibility of visceral rupture. Compression is generally contraindicated if a patient has urinary stones, an abdominal mass or aneurysm, a colostomy, a suprapubic catheter, or traumatic injury.

As a result of improvements in contrast agents, ureteral compression is not routinely used in most health care facilities. The increased doses of contrast medium now employed usually demonstrate most of the ureteral area over a series of radiographs.

RESPIRATION

For the purpose of comparison, all exposures are made at the end of the same phase of breathing—at the *end of exhalation* unless otherwise requested. Since the normal respiratory excursion of the kidneys varies from ½ to 1½ inches (1.2 to 3.8 cm), differentiation of renal from other shadows is occasionally possible by making an exposure at a different phase of arrested respiration. When an exposure is made at other than the respiratory phase usually employed, the film should be so marked.

PRELIMINARY EXAMINATION

A preliminary examination of the abdomen is made before a specialized investigation of the urinary tract is conducted. This examination sometimes reveals extrarenal lesions that are responsible for the symptoms attributed to the urinary tract and thereby renders the urographic procedure unnecessary. An upright AP projection may also be required to demonstrate the mobility of the kidneys. An oblique and/or lateral projection in the dorsal decubitus position may be required to localize a tumor mass or to differentiate renal stones from gallstones or calcified mesenteric nodes.

The scout radiograph, an AP projection with the patient recumbent, demonstrates the contour of the kidneys, their location in the supine position, and the presence of any renal or other calculi (see Fig. 18-26). This radiograph also serves to check the preparation of the gastrointestinal tract and to enable the radiographer to make any necessary alteration in the exposure factors.

RADIATION PROTECTION

It is the responsibility of the radiographer to observe the following guidelines concerning radiation protection:
- Apply a gonadal shield if it will not overlap the area under investigation.
- Restrict radiation to the area of interest by close collimation.
- Work carefully so that repeat exposures will not be necessary.
- Shield males for all examinations, except those of the urethra, by using a shadow shield or by placing a piece of lead just below the symphysis pubis.
- When excretory urography films are centered to the kidneys, place lead over the female pelvis for shielding. As always, consider radiography of the abdomen and pelvis only if there is no chance of patient pregnancy, unless the procedure is considered an emergency.

INTRAVENOUS UROGRAPHY

Intravenous urography demonstrates both the function and structure of the urinary system. *Function* is demonstrated by the ability of the kidneys to filter the contrast medium from the blood and concentrate it with the urine. Anatomical *structures* are usually visualized as the contrast material follows the excretion route of the urine.

Indications for performing intravenous urography include:
1. Evaluation of abdominal masses, renal cysts, renal tumors.
2. Urolithiasis: calculi or stones of the kidneys or urinary tract.
3. Pyelonephritis: infection of the upper urinary tract which can be acute or chronic.
4. Hydronephrosis: an abnormal dilation of the pelvicalyceal system. Urography is used to help determine the cause of the dilation.
5. Evaluation of the effects of trauma.
6. Preoperative evaluation for function, location, size, and shape of the kidneys and ureters.
7. Renal hypertension. Urography is commonly performed to evaluate functional symmetry of the renal collecting systems.

The most common contraindications for intravenous urography relate to the ability of the kidneys to filter the contrast medium from the blood and the patient's allergic history. Some contraindications can be overcome by the use of nonionic contrast agents. Patients with conditions in which the kidneys are unable to filter waste or excrete urine (renal failure, anuria) should have the kidneys evaluated by some technique other than excretory urography. Elderly patients or patients with any of the following risk factors are strong candidates to receive nonionic contrast medium or should be examined using another modality: asthma, previous contrast media reaction, circulatory or cardiovascular disease, elevated creatinine level, sickle cell disease, diabetes mellitus, or multiple myeloma.

Radiographic procedure

Before the procedure begins, the patient should be instructed to empty the bladder and change into an appropriate radiolucent gown. Emptying the bladder prevents dilution of the contrast medium with urine. The patient's clinical history, allergic history, and blood chemistry levels should be reviewed. Normal *creatinine* level is 0.6 to 1.5 mg/100 ml and normal *BUN* (blood urea nitrogen) level is 8 to 25 mg/100 ml. Any significant elevation of these levels suggests renal dysfunction and should be reviewed by a physician before continuing the procedure. The radiographer then observes the following steps:

- Place the patient on the table in the supine position, and adjust the patient to center the median sagittal plane of the body to the midline of the grid.
- Place a support under the patient's knees to reduce the lordotic curvature of the lumbar spine and to provide more comfort for the patient (Fig. 18-32).
- Attach the footboard in preparation for a possible upright or semiupright position.
- If the head of the table is to be lowered further to enhance pelvicalyceal filling, attach the shoulder support, and adjust it to the patient's height.

- When ureteric compression is to be used, place it so that it is ready for immediate application at the specified time.
- Obtain a preliminary (or scout) radiograph of the abdomen, then prepare for the first postinjection exposure before the contrast medium is injected.
- Place the cassette in the Bucky tray; position identification, side, and time-interval markers; and make any change in centering or exposure technique as indicated by the scout radiograph.
- Have ready a folded towel or other suitable support and the tourniquet for placement under the selected elbow.
- Prepare the contrast medium for injection using aseptic technique.
- According to the preference of the examining physician, 30 to 100 ml of the contrast medium is administered to adult patients of average size. The dosage administered to infants and children is regulated according to age and weight.

- Radiographs are made at specified intervals from the time of the completion of the injection of contrast medium. Depending on whether the patient is partially dehydrated and on the speed of the injection, the contrast agent normally begins to appear in the pelvicalyceal system within 2 to 8 minutes.
- The uptake of contrast medium is seen in the nephrons of the kidney if a radiograph is exposed as the kidneys start to filter the contrast medium from the blood. The initial contrast "blush" of the kidney is termed the *nephrogram phase.* As the kidneys continue to filter and concentrate the contrast medium, it is directed to the pelvicalyceal system. The greatest concentration of contrast medium in the kidneys normally occurs 15 to 20 minutes after injection. Immediately after each film is exposed, it is processed and reviewed to determine, according to the kidney function of the individual patient, the time intervals at which the most intense kidney image will be obtained.

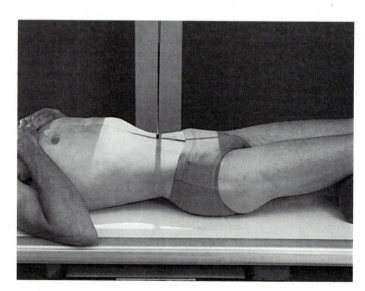

Fig. 18-32. Patient in supine position for urogram, AP projection. Note support under knees.

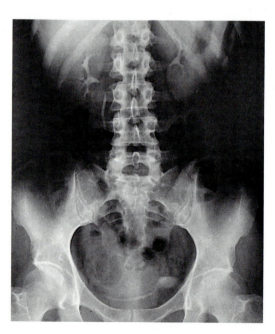

Fig. 18-33. Urogram at 3 minutes.

- The most frequently recommended radiographs for intravenous urography are AP projections at different time intervals ranging from 3 to 20 minutes (Figs. 18-33 to 18-35). Some physicians prefer a bolus injection of the contrast medium followed by a 30-second film to obtain a nephrogram. Thirty-degree AP oblique projections may be taken at 5- to 10-minute intervals. In some cases supplemental radiographs are required to better demonstrate all parts of the urinary system and differentiate normal anatomy from pathology. These may include an AP projection with the patient in the Trendelenburg or upright position; or oblique, or lateral projections; or a lateral projection with the patient in the dorsal or ventral decubitus position.

- Unless further study of the bladder is indicated or voiding urethrograms are to be made, the patient is sent to the lavatory to void. A postvoiding radiograph of the bladder (Figs. 18-36 and 18-37) may be taken to detect, by the presence of residual urine, such conditions as small tumor masses or, in the case of male patients, enlargement of the prostate gland. When all the necessary radiographs have been obtained, the patient is released from the imaging department. Any contrast medium remaining in the body will be filtered from the blood by the kidneys and eventually excreted in the urine. Some physicians suggest having the patient drink extra fluids for a few days to aid in flushing the contrast medium from the system.

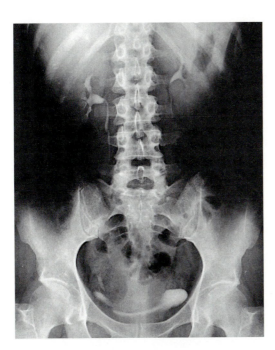

Fig. 18-34. Urogram at 6 minutes.

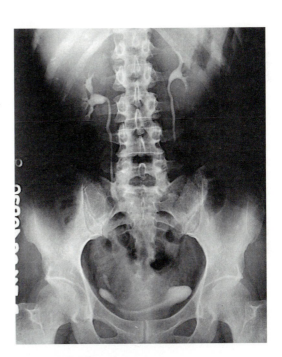

Fig. 18-35. Urogram at 9 minutes.

(Courtesy Dr. William H. Shehadi.)

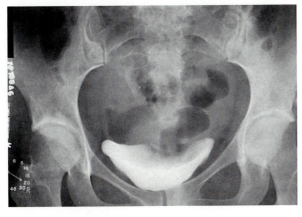

Fig. 18-36. Prevoiding filled bladder.

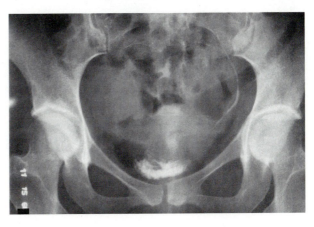

Fig. 18-37. Postvoiding emptied bladder.

Urinary System

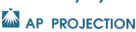

AP PROJECTION

Film: 14 × 17 in (35 × 43 cm) lengthwise.

Position of patient

- Place the patient supine on the radiographic table for the AP projection of the urinary system. Preliminary (scout) and postinjection radiographs are most commonly obtained with the patient supine (Fig. 18-38). The prone position is recommended for the demonstration of the ureteropelvic region and for filling the obstructed ureter in the presence of hydronephrosis. The ureters fill better in the prone position because it reverses the curve of their inferior course. The kidneys are situated obliquely, slanting anteriorly in the transverse plane, so the opacified urine tends to collect in and distend the dependent part of the pelvicalyceal system. The supine position allows the more posteriorly placed upper calyces to fill more readily, and the anterior and inferior parts of the pelvicalyceal system fill more easily in the prone position.

- Place the patient in an upright or semi-upright position for an AP projection to demonstrate the opacified bladder and the mobility of the kidneys (Figs. 18-39). To demonstrate the lower ends of the ureters, it may be helpful to use an AP projection with the head of the table lowered 15 to 20 degrees and with the central ray directed perpendicular to the cassette. In this angled position, the weight of the contained fluid stretches the bladder fundus superiorly, providing an unobstructed image of the lower ureters and the vesicoureteral orifice areas.

- For a description of ureteral compression, see p. 166, of this volume.

Position of part

- Center the median sagittal plane of the body to the midline of the grid device.
- Adjust the shoulders and hips to ensure that they are equidistant from the film.
- Place the arms where they will not cast shadows on the film.
- If the patient is positioned for a supine radiograph, place a support under the knees to relieve strain on the patient's back.

- Center the cassette at the level of the crests of the ilia. If the patient is too tall to include the entire urinary system, obtain a second exposure on a 10 × 12 in (24 × 30 cm) film centered to the bladder. The 10 × 12 in (24 × 30 cm) cassette is placed crosswise and centered 2 to 3 inches (5 to 7.5 cm) above the upper border of the symphysis pubis.
- *Shield gonads.* (Not shown for illustrative purposes.)
- Ask the patient to suspend respiration at the end of exhalation.

Central ray

- Direct the central ray perpendicular to the film at the level of the crests of the ilia.

Structures shown

An AP projection of the urinary system demonstrates the kidneys, ureters, and bladder filled with the contrast medium (Figs. 18-40 to 18-42).

☐ Evaluation criteria

The following should be clearly demonstrated:

AP and PA projections
- Entire renal shadows.
- Bladder and symphysis pubis. A separate radiograph of the bladder area is needed if the bladder was not included.
- No motion.

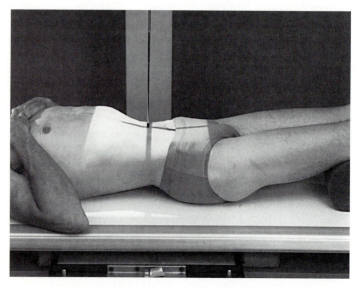

Fig. 18-38. Supine urogram, AP projection.

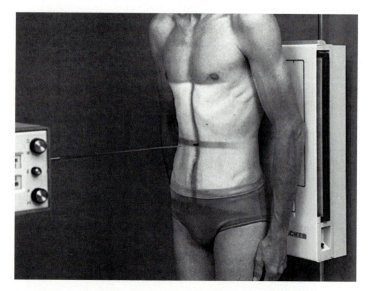

Fig. 18-39. Upright urogram, AP projection.

- Short scale of contrast clearly demonstrating contrast media in the renal area, ureters, and bladder.
- Compression devices, if used, centered over the upper sacrum and resulting in good renal filling.
- Vertebral column centered to the radiograph.
- No artifacts from elastic in the patient's underclothing.
- Prostatic region inferior to the symphysis pubis on older male patients.
- Time marker.
- PA projection demonstrating the lower kidneys and entire ureters. Bladder included if patient size permits. Superimposing intestinal gas in the AP projection moved for the PA projection.

AP bladder

- Bladder.
- No rotation of the pelvis.
- Prostate area on male patients.
- Postvoiding radiographs clearly labeled and demonstrating only residual contrast media.

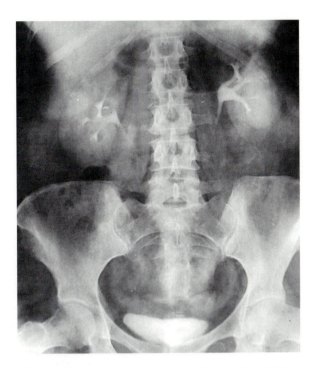

Fig. 18-40. Semiupright urogram, AP projection. Note mobility of kidneys.

(Courtesy Dr. Oswald S. Lowsley.)

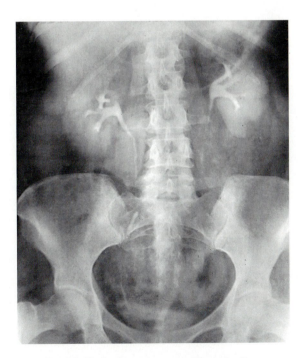

Fig. 18-41. Supine urogram, AP projection.

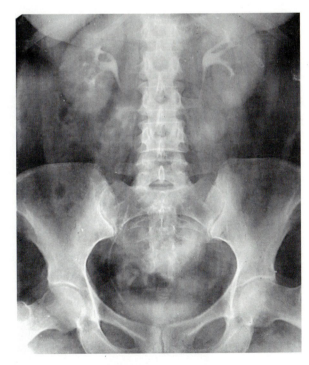

Fig. 18-42. Trendelenburg position urogram, AP projection.

Urinary System

AP OBLIQUE PROJECTIONS
RPO and LPO positions

Film: 14 × 17 in (35 × 43 cm) lengthwise.

Position of patient

• Place the patient supine on the radiographic table for oblique projections of the urinary system. The kidneys are situated obliquely, slanting anteriorly in the transverse plane. When performing AP oblique projections, remember that the kidney closer to the film will be perpendicular and the kidney farther from the film will be parallel with the film plane.

Position of part

• Have the patient turn from the supine position so that the median coronal plane forms an angle of 30 degrees from the film plane.
• Adjust the shoulders and hips so that they are in the same plane, and place suitable supports under the elevated side as needed.
• Place the arms so they will not be superimposed on the urinary system.
• Center the spine to the grid (Fig. 18-43).
• Center the cassette at the level of the crests of the ilia.
• *Shield gonads.* (Not shown for illustrative purposes.

• Ask the patient to suspend respiration at the end of exhalation.

Central ray

• Direct the central ray perpendicular to the film at the level of the crests of the ilia. The central ray enters approximately 2 inches lateral to the midline on the patient's elevated side.

Structures shown

An AP oblique projection of the urinary system demonstrates the kidneys, ureters, and bladder filled with the contrast medium. The elevated kidney will be parallel with the film, and the dependent kidney will be perpendicular with the film (Fig. 18-44).

□Evaluation criteria

The following should be clearly demonstrated:
■ Patient obliqued approximately 30 degrees.
■ No superimposition of the kidney remote from the film on the vertebrae.
■ The entire dependent kidney.
■ Bladder and lower ureters on 14 × 17 in (35 × 43 cm) films if the patient's size permits.
■ Time marker.

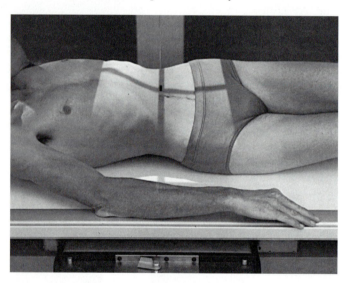

Fig. 18-43. Urogram. AP oblique projection, 30-degree RPO position.

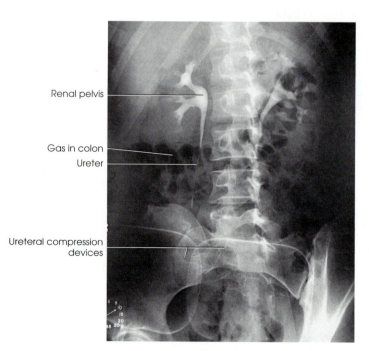
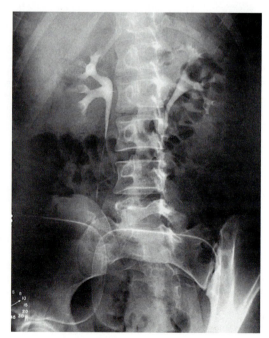

Renal pelvis

Gas in colon
Ureter

Ureteral compression devices

Fig. 18-44. Ten-minute postinjection urogram. AP oblique projection, RPO position.

Urinary System

☒ LATERAL PROJECTION
R or L position

Film: 14 × 17 in (35 × 43 cm) lengthwise.

Position of patient

- Turn the patient to a lateral recumbent position on the right or left side, as indicated.

Position of part

- Flex the patient's knees to a comfortable position and adjust the body so that the median coronal plane is centered to the midline of the grid.
- Place supports between the knees and the ankles.
- Flex the elbows and place the hands under the patient's head (Fig. 18-45).
- Center the cassette at the level of the crests of the ilia.
- *Shield gonads.* (Not shown for illustrative purposes.)
- Ask the patient to suspend respiration at the end of exhalation.

Central ray

- Direct the central ray perpendicular to the film, entering the median coronal plane at the level of the crest of the ilia.

Structures shown

A lateral projection of the abdomen demonstrates the kidneys, ureters, and bladder filled with contrast material. Lateral projections are used to demonstrate such conditions as rotation or pressure displacement of a kidney and to localize calcarous shadows and tumor masses (Fig. 18-46).

☐ Evaluation criteria

The following should be clearly demonstrated:

- Entire urinary system.
- Bladder and symphysis pubis.
- Short scale of contrast clearly demonstrating contrast media in the renal area, ureters, and bladder.
- No rotation of the patient. Check pelvis and lumbar vertebrae.
- Time marker.

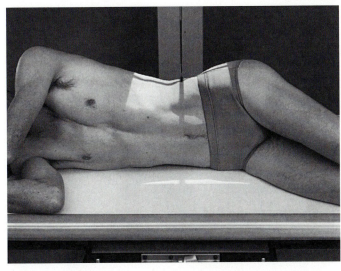

Fig. 18-45. Urogram, lateral projection.

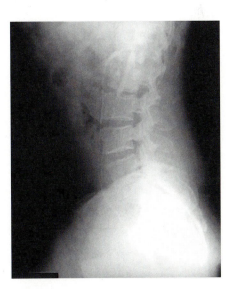

Fig. 18-46. Urogram, lateral projection.

Urinary System

 LATERAL PROJECTION
Dorsal decubitus position

Film: 14 × 17 in (35 × 43 cm).

Position of patient

- Place the patient in the supine position as required on the table with the side in contact with the vertical grid device.
- Place the arms across the upper chest to ensure they are not projected over any abdominal contents, or place them behind the head.
- Flex the patient's knees slightly to relieve strain on the back.

Position of part

- Adjust the height of the vertical grid device so that the long axis of the film is centered to the median coronal plane.
- Position the patient so that a point approximately at the level of the crests of the ilia is centered to the film (Fig. 18-47).
- Adjust the patient to make sure there is no rotation from the supine or prone position.
- *Shield male gonads only.* (Not shown for illustrative purposes.)
- Ask the patient to suspend respiration at the end of exhalation.

Central ray

- Direct the *horizontal* central ray perpendicular to the center of the film, entering the median coronal plane at the level of the crests of the ilia.

Structures shown

Rolleston and Reay[1] recommend the ventral decubitis position for demonstration of the ureteropelvic junction in the presence of hydronephrosis. Cook et al[2] use the position to determine whether an extrarenal mass in the flank is intraperitoneal or extraperitoneal, and they state that the position is an easy way to screen both kidneys and ureters for any abnormal anterior displacement (Fig. 18-48).

---

[1]Rolleston GL and Reay ER: The pelvi-ureteric junction, Br J Radiol 30:617-625, 1957.
[2]Cook IK, Keats TE, and Seale DL: Determination of the normal position of the upper urinary tract in the lateral abdominal urogram, Radiology 99:499-502, 1971.

The following should be clearly demonstrated:

- Entire urinary system.
- Bladder and symphysis pubis.
- Short scale of contrast clearly demonstrating contrast medium in the renal area, ureters, and bladder.
- No rotation of the patient. Check pelvis and lumbar vertebrae.
- Time marker.
- Patient elevated so that entire abdomen is visible.

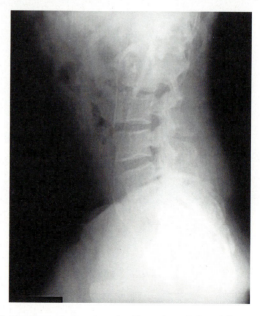

Fig. 18-47. Urogram. Lateral projection, dorsal decubitus position.

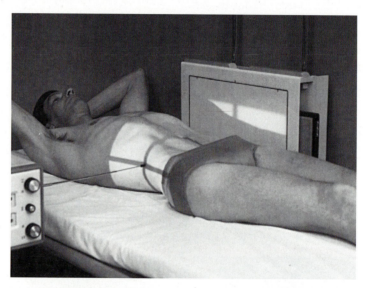

Fig. 18-48. Urogram. Lateral projection, dorsal decubitus position.

(Courtesy Steven J. Bollin, Sr.RT.)

RENAL PARENCHYMA
Nephrotomography and Nephrourography

The renal parenchyma, or the nephrons and collecting tubes, are best visualized by performing tomography immediately after the introduction of contrast medium. Evans et al,[1,2] who introduced nephrotomography, found that, by the use of tomography rather than stationary projections, not only could intestinal-content superimpositions be eliminated, but small intrarenal lesions could be more clearly defined.

Indications and contraindications

Nephrotomography is primarily performed to evaluate renal hypertension. It is also useful in cases of renal cysts and renal tumors.

Contraindications are mainly related to renal failure and contrast media sensitivity as noted for intravenous urography.

Contrast media

Many different contrast agents in various organic iodinated concentrations are available for nephrography. These preparations are packaged in individual bottles with the intravenous tubing included. The actual dose may vary from patient to patient, since contrast medium–induced renal failure appears to be dose related.

[1]Evans JA, Dubilier WJ, and Monteith JC: Nephrotomography, AJR 71:213-223, 1954.
[2]Evans JA: Nephrotomography in the investigation of renal masses, Radiology 69:684-689, 1957.

Contrast medium can be administered rapidly by bolus injection or more slowly by intravenous infusion. Bolus injection nephrotomography was introduced by Weens et al.[1]

This examination is performed by injecting a large bolus of highly concentrated, iodinated contrast medium into the venous bloodstream by way of a large bore needle inserted into an antecubital vein. By this rapid-injection technique, the renal blood vessels and corticomedullary structures are opacified only during the brief passage of the jet of contrast material. This short period requires that the filming procedure be carried out as quickly as possible.

Infusion nephrotomography and nephrourography were introduced by Schencker.[2] This method of administering the contrast medium provides opacification of the renal parenchyma as well as of the renal drainage canals and thus embraces both nephrography and urography. The examination is performed by a procedure

[1]Weens HS et al: Intravenous nephrography: a method of roentgen visualization of the kidney, AJR 65:411-414, 1951.
[2]Schencker B: Drip infusion pyelography; indications and applications in urologic roentgen diagnosis, Radiology 83:12-21, 1964.

somewhat similar to that used for preliminary intravenous urography. The infusion procedure differs from the preliminary procedure in that (1) the contrast medium is introduced into the venous bloodstream by infusion rather than by injection,* and (2) both nephrotomographic and nephrourographic studies are made.

The infusion is made through an 18-gauge needle inserted into an antecubital vein just as for preliminary intravenous urography. The infusion bottle is hung on an IV standard, and the contrast solution is allowed to flow through the needle without restraint; the infusion requires several minutes for completion.

Preparation of patient

When preparation of the intestinal tract is possible, the patient may be placed on a low-residue diet for 1 to 2 days, and a non–gas-forming laxative may be given on the preceding evening.

*An injection is forced into a vessel (or organ), whereas an infusion flows in by gravity.

Examination procedure

The patient is placed in the supine position on a tomographic table. A scout radiograph of the abdomen is made to establish the exposure technique for the nephrourogram, and then a scout radiograph is made to establish the exposure technique and to determine the level for the nephrotomograms.

Before starting the examination, the procedure is explained to the patient so that, knowing what sensations to expect, the patient will be better able to cooperate for the procedure.

The postinjection filming consists of one AP projection of the abdomen during the arterial phase of opacification (Fig. 18-49) and multiple tomograms of the upper abdomen during the nephrographic phase. Immediately after the arterial phase, the renal parenchyma becomes opacified, producing the nephrographic phase, during which tomography is used; hence the term *nephrotomography* (Figs. 18-50 to 18-53). The nephrotic phase normally occurs within 5 minutes after the conclusion of the injection or infusion.

Infusion studies of the urinary canals are usually made at intervals of 10, 20, and 30 minutes. Delayed urograms are taken as required. Studies of the urinary bladder and voiding urethrograms may be made. In addition to the AP projection, tomograms can also be made in the oblique and lateral projections (Fig. 18-54), as these are indicated.

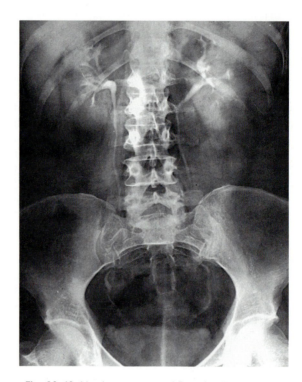

Fig. 18-49. Nephrourogram, AP projection. Arterial phase.

(Courtesy Dr. Marcy L. Sussman.)

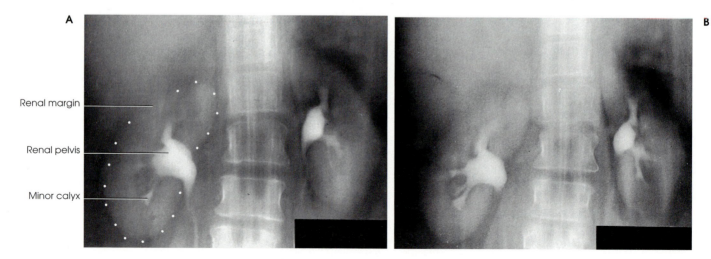

Renal margin

Renal pelvis

Minor calyx

Fig. 18-50. Nephrotomograms, AP projection, at level of 9 cm, **A,** and 10 cm, **B,** on same patient as in Fig. 18-49.

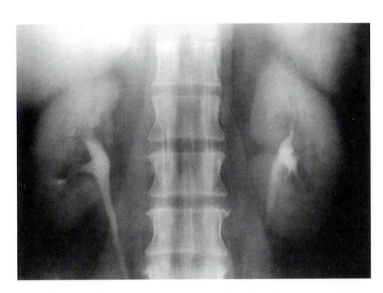

Fig. 18-51. Infusion nephrotomogram, AP projection, at 9 cm level.

(Courtesy of Dr. Joshua A. Becker)

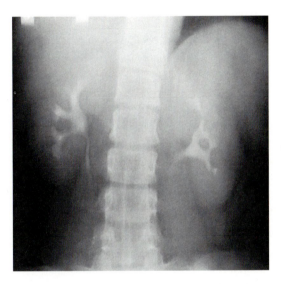

Fig. 18-52. Infusion nephrotomogram, AP projection, at 5 cm level.

(Courtesy Norma Harmon, R.T.)

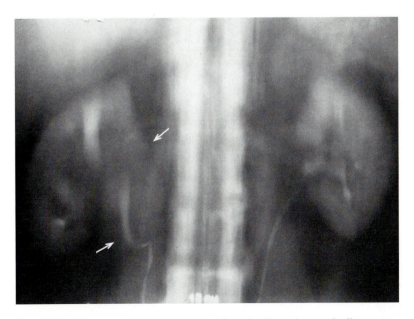

Fig. 18-53. Infusion nephrotomogram, AP projection, demonstrating parapelvic cyst on right kidney *(arrows)*.

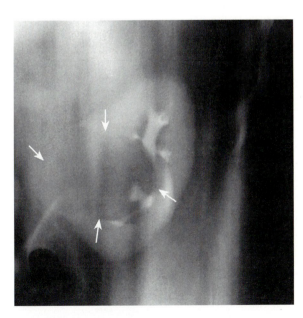

Fig. 18-54. Infusion nephrotomogram, lateral projection, demonstrating parapelvic cyst *(arrows)*.

(Courtesy Dr. Joshua A. Becker.)

Percutaneous renal puncture

Ultrasonic examinations of the kidney have practically eliminated the need for percutaneous renal puncture. When used, percutaneous renal puncture, introduced by Lindblom,[1,2] is a radiologic procedure

[1]Lindblom K: Percutaneous puncture of renal cysts and tumors, Acta Radiol 27:66-72, 1946.
[2]Lindblom K: Diagnostic kidney puncture in cysts and tumors, AJR 68:209-215, 1952.

for the investigation of renal masses. Specifically, it is used to differentiate cysts and tumors of the renal parenchyma. This procedure is performed by the direct injection of contrast medium into the cyst under fluoroscopic control (Figs. 18-55 and 18-56). Ultrasonography now often replaces this procedure as the procedure of choice. In most cases, masses that are clearly diagnosed as cystic by ultrasonic

examination usually are not surgically managed.

By a similar procedure, the renal pelvis is entered percutaneously for direct contrast filling of the pelvicalyceal system in selected patients with hydronephrosis.[1-3] This procedure, called *percutaneous antegrade pyelography*[3] to distinguish it from the retrograde technique of direct pelvicalyceal filling, is usually restricted to the investigation of patients with marked hydronephrosis and of patients with suspected hydronephrosis for which conclusive information could not be gained by either excretory or retrograde urography (Fig. 18-57). Normally, AP abdominal radiographs are obtained for this procedure, although other projections may be requested. See pp. 170-174 in this volume of the atlas for further information on urinary system positioning.

[1]Wickbom I: Pyelography after direct puncture of the renal pelvis, Acta Radiol 41:505-512, 1954.
[2]Weens HS and Florence TJ: The diagnosis of hydronephrosis by percutaneous renal puncture, J Urol 72:589-595, 1954.
[3]Casey WC and Goodwin WE: Percutaneous antegrade pyelography and hydronephrosis, J Urol 74:164-173, 1955.

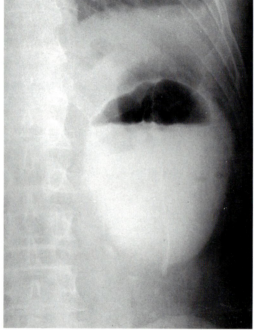

Fig. 18-55. Upright AP left kidney. Percutaneous injection of iodinated contrast material and gas into renal cyst.

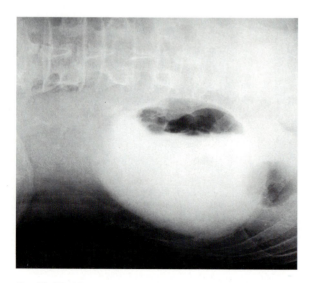

Fig. 18-56. AP projection left kidney, left lateral decubitus position. Same patient as in Fig. 18-55.

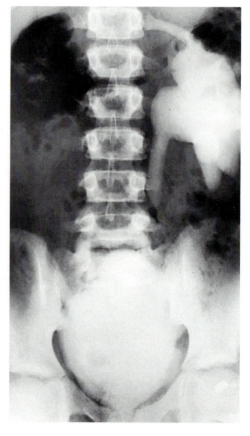

Fig. 18-57. Percutaneous antegrade pyelogram demonstrating hydronephrosis.

(Courtesy Dr. Joshua A. Becker.)

Pelviocalyceal System and Ureters

Retrograde urography requires that the ureters be catheterized so that a contrast agent can be injected directly into the pelvicalyceal system. This technique provides improved opacification of the renal collecting system but little physiologic information about the urinary system.

Indications and contraindications

The retrograde urogram is indicated for evaluation of the collecting system in patients who have renal insufficiency or who are allergic to iodinated contrast media. Because the contrast medium is not introduced into the circulatory system, the incidences of reactions are reduced.

Examination procedure

Retrograde urography is classified, as are all examinations requiring instrumentation, as an operative procedure. This combined urologic-radiologic examination is carried out under careful aseptic conditions by the attending urologist with the assistance of a nurse and radiographer. The examination is performed in a specially equipped cystoscopic-radiographic examining room that, because of the collaborative nature of these examinations, may be located in the urology department or the radiology department. The nurse is responsible for the preparation of the instruments and the care and draping of the patient. One of the responsibilities of the radiographer is to see that the overhead parts of the radiographic equipment are free of dust for the protection of the operative field and the sterile layout. The following steps are then observed:

- Place the patient on the cystoscopic table, and flex the knees over the stirrups of the adjustable leg supports (Fig. 18-58); this is a modified lithotomy position; the true lithotomy position requires acute flexion of the hips and knees.
- If a general anesthetic is not used, explain the breathing procedure to the patient, and check the patient's position on the table. The kidneys and the full extent of the ureters in patients of average height are included on a 14 × 17 in (35 × 43 cm) cassette when the third lumbar vertebra is centered to the grid.

- The elevation of the thighs usually reduces the lumbar curve; if not, readjust the pillow under the head and shoulders so that the back is in contact with the table. Most cystoscopic-radiographic tables are equipped with an adjustable leg rest to permit extension of the patient's legs for certain radiographic studies.
- Catheterization of the ureters is performed through a ureterocystoscope, which is a cystoscope with an arrangement that aids insertion of the catheters into the vesicoureteral orifices. After the endoscopic examination, the urologist passes a ureteral catheter well into one or each ureter (Fig. 18-59) and, leaving the catheters in position, usually withdraws the cystoscope. After taking two catheterized specimens of urine from each kidney for laboratory tests— one specimen for culture and one for microscopic examination—the urologist tests kidney function. For this test, a color dye is injected intravenously, and the function of each kidney is then determined by the time required for the dye substance to appear in the urine as it trickles through the respective catheters.

- Immediately following the kidney function test, the radiographer should recheck the position of the patient and expose the preliminary film, if it has not been done previously, so that it will be ready for inspection by the time the kidney function test has been completed. The urologist will then be ready to inject the contrast medium and to proceed with the urographic examination. When a bilateral examination is to be performed, both sides are filled simultaneously to avoid subjecting the patient to unnecessary radiation exposure. Additional studies in which one side only is refilled may then be made as indicated.
- The most commonly used retrograde urographic series usually consists of three AP projections: the preliminary radiograph showing the ureteral catheters in position (Fig. 18-59), the pyelogram, and the ureterogram. Some urologists recommend that the head of the table be lowered 10 to 15 degrees for the pyelogram to prevent the contrast solution from escaping into the ureters. Other urologists recommend that pressure on the syringe be maintained during the pyelographic exposure to ensure complete filling of the pelvicalyceal system. The head of the table may be elevated 35 to 40 degrees for the ureterogram to demonstrate any tortuosity of the ureters as well as the mobility of the kidneys.

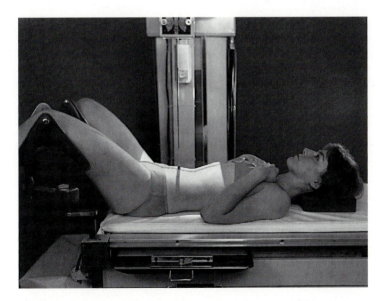

Fig. 18-58. Patient positioned on table for retrograde urography. Modified lithotomy position.

- From 3 to 5 ml of solution will fill the average normal renal pelvis; however, a larger quantity is required when the structure is dilated. The best index of complete filling, and the one most frequently employed, is an indication from the patient as soon as a sense of fullness is felt in the back.
- When both sides are to be filled, the urologist injects the contrast solution through the catheters in an amount sufficient to fill the renal pelves and calyces. When signaled by the physician, the patient is instructed to suspend respiration at the end of exhalation, and the exposure for the pyelogram is then made (Fig. 18-60).

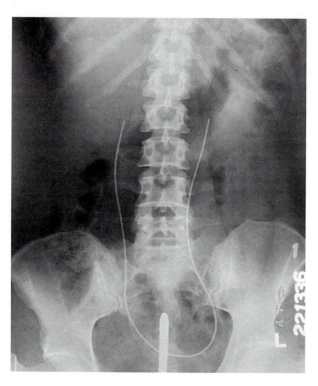

Fig. 18-59. Retrograde urogram with catheters in proximal ureters, AP projection.

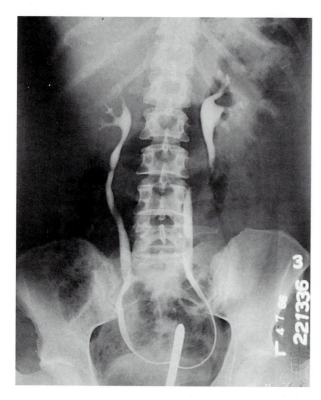

Fig. 18-60. Retrograde urogram with renal pelves filled, AP projection.

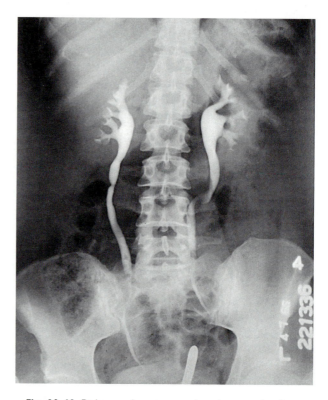

Fig. 18-61. Retrograde urogram showing renal pelves and contrast-filled ureters, AP projection.

(Courtesy Dr. Robert L. Pinck.)

- Following the pyelographic exposure, the cassette is quickly changed, and the head of the table may be elevated in preparation for the ureterogram. For this exposure, the patient is instructed to inhale deeply and then to suspend respiration at the end of full exhalation. Simultaneously with the breathing procedure, the catheters are slowly withdrawn to the lower ends of the ureters as the contrast solution is being injected into the canals. At a signal from the urologist, the ureterographic exposure is made (Fig. 18-61).
- Additional projections are sometimes necessary. RPO or LPO (AP oblique) projections (LPO or RPO) are frequently necessary. Occasionally a lateral projection, with the patient turned onto the affected side, is taken to demonstrate anterior displacement of a kidney or ureter and to delineate a perinephritic abscess. Also, lateral projections with the patient in the ventral or dorsal decubitus positions (as required), are useful to demonstrate the ureteropelvic region in patients with hydronephrosis. For further information on positioning of the urinary system, please see pp. 170-174 in this volume of the atlas.

Urinary bladder, lower ureters, urethra, and prostate

With few exceptions, radiologic examinations of the lower urinary tract are performed with the retrograde technique of introducing the contrast material. These examinations are identified, according to the specific purpose of the investigation, by the terms *cystography, cystoureterography, cystourethrography,* and *prostatography.* Most often they are denoted by the general term *cystography.* Cystoscopy is not required before retrograde contrast filling of the lower urinary canals, but, when both examinations are indicated, they are usually performed in a single-stage procedure to spare the patient preparation and instrumentation for separate examinations. When cystoscopy is not indicated, these examinations are best carried out on an all-purpose radiographic table unless the combination table is equipped with an extensible leg rest.

Indications and contraindications

Retrograde studies of the lower urinary tract are indicated for vesicoureteral reflux, recurrent lower urinary tract infection, neurogenic bladder, bladder trauma, lower urinary tract fistulae, urethral stricture, and posterior urethral valves. Contraindications to lower urinary tract studies are related to catheterization of the urethra.

Contrast media

The contrast agents employed for contrast studies of the lower urinary tracts are ionic solutions of either sodium or meglumine diatrizoates or the newer nonionic contrast media mentioned under the discussion of contrast media earlier in this chapter. These are the same organic compounds used for intravenous urography, but the concentration is reduced for retrograde urography.

Injection equipment

These examinations are performed under careful aseptic conditions. Infants, children, and usually adults may be catheterized before they are brought to the radiology department. When the patient is to be catheterized in the radiology department, a sterile catheterization tray, set up to specifications, must be available. Because of the danger of contamination in transferring a sterile liquid from one container to another, ready-to-use contrast solutions are commercially available and are recommended.

Preliminary preparations

The following guidelines are observed in preparing the patient for the examination:
- Protect the examining table from urine soilage with radioparent plastic sheeting and with disposable underpadding. In addition to a suitable receptacle, correctly arranged, disposable padding does much to reduce soilage during voiding studies and consequently eliminates the need for extensive cleaning between patients.
- Conduct the outpatient, just a few minutes before time for the examination, to a lavatory.
- Give the patient supplies for perineal care and instruct him or her to empty the bladder.
- Place the patient on the examination table for the catheterization procedure.

Patients are usually tense, primarily because of embarrassment. It is important that they be given as much privacy as possible. Only the required personnel should be present during the examination, and the patient should be properly draped and should be covered according to room temperature.

Contrast injection technique

For retrograde cystography (Figs. 18-62 and 18-63), cystoureterography, and voiding cystourethrography, the contrast material is introduced into the bladder by injection or infusion through a catheter passed into position by way of the urethral canal. A small, disposable Foley catheter is used to occlude the vesicourethral orifice in the examination of infants and children and may be used in the examination of adults when interval studies are to be made for the detection of delayed ureteral reflux. Studies are made during voiding for the delineation of the urethral canal and for the detection of ureteral reflux, which may occur only during urination (Fig. 18-64). When urethral studies are to be made during the injection of contrast material, a soft-rubber urethral-orifice acorn is fitted directly onto a contrast-loaded syringe for female patients and, usually, onto a cannula that is attached to a clamp device for male patients.

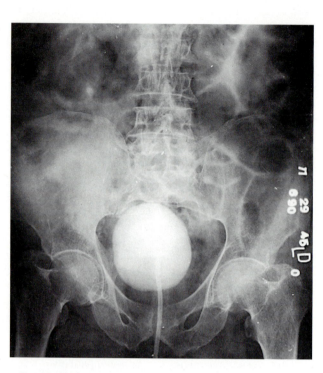

Fig. 18-62. Retrograde cystogram, after introduction of contrast media. AP projection.

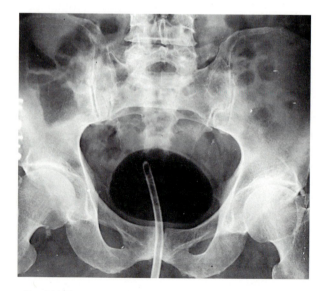

Fig. 18-63. Retrograde cystogram after introduction of air. AP projection.

(Courtesy Dr. Marcy L. Sussman.)

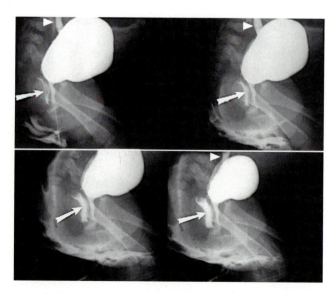

Fig. 18-64. Serial (polygraphic) voiding cystourethrograms of infant girl with bilateral ureteral reflux (*arrowheads*). Urethra is normal. Vaginal reflux (*arrows*) is normal finding.

(Courtesy Dr. Walter E. Berdon and Dr. David H. Baker.)

RETROGRADE CYSTOGRAPHY
Contrast injection technique

In preparing for this examination, the following steps are observed:

- With the urethral catheter in place, adjust the patient in the supine position for a preliminary radiograph and for the first cystogram.
- Usually, take cystograms of adult patients on 10 × 12 in (24 × 30 cm) films that are placed lengthwise.
- Center this size of cassette at the level of the soft tissue depression just above the most prominent point of the greater trochanters. This centering coincides with the middle area of the filled bladder of average size. Therefore a 12-inch (30 cm) film will include the region of the distal end of the ureters for the demonstration of any evidence of ureteral reflux, and it will include the prostate and proximal part of the male urethra.
- Have large films nearby for use when ureteral reflux is shown. Some radiologists have radiographs taken during the filling of the bladder as well as during voiding.

- After inspecting the preliminary radiograph, the catheter is clamped and the bladder drained in preparation for the introduction of the contrast material. Following the introduction of the contrast agent, the physician clamps the catheter and tapes it to the thigh to prevent its displacement during position changes.
- The initial cystographic filming generally consists of four projections: AP, AP obliques, and lateral. Additional studies, including voiding cystourethrograms, are made as indicated.
- The Chassard-Lapiné method (Volume 1, Chapter 7), often called the "squat shot," is sometimes used to obtain an axial projection of the posterior surface of the bladder and of the lower end of the ureters when they are opacified.

These projections of the bladder are also made when it is opacified by the excretory technique of urography.

Pelviocalyceal system and ureters

Urinary Bladder

AP AND PA PROJECTIONS

Film: 10 × 12 in (24 × 30 cm) lengthwise.

Position of patient

- Place the patient supine on the radiographic table for the AP projection of the urinary system. Preliminary (scout) and postinjection radiographs are most commonly obtained with the patient supine. The prone position is sometimes used to image areas of the bladder not clearly seen on the AP projection. An AP projection with the head of the table lowered 15 to 20 degrees and with the central ray directed vertically is sometimes employed to demonstrate the lower ends of the ureters. In this angled position, the weight of the contained fluid stretches the bladder fundus superiorly, giving an unobstructed projection of the lower ureters and the vesicoureteral orifice areas.

Position of part

- Center the median sagittal plane of the body to the midline of the grid device.
- Adjust the shoulders and hips so that they are equidistant from the film.
- Place the arms where they will not cast shadows on the film.
- If the patient is positioned for a supine radiograph, have the patient's legs extended so that the lumbosacral area of the spine is arched enough to tilt the anterior pelvic bones inferiorly. In this position, the pubic bones can more easily be projected below the bladder neck and proximal urethra (Fig. 18-65).
- Center the cassette 2 to 3 inches (5 to 7.5 cm) above the upper border of the symphysis pubis (or at the symphysis pubis for voiding studies).
- Ask the patient to suspend respiration at the end of exhalation.

Central ray

- Direct the central ray perpendicular to the film 2 to 3 inches (5 to 7.5 cm) above the upper border of the symphysis pubis. When the bladder neck and proximal urethra are the main areas of interest, a 5-degree caudal angulation of the central ray is usually sufficient to project the pubic bones below them. When loss of the normal lumbar lordosis occurs, the pelvis is tilted anteriorly and superiorly, so a caudal angulation of 15 to 20 degrees is necessary for these patients (Fig. 18-65).
- When performing PA projections of the bladder, direct the central ray through the region of the bladder neck at an angle of 10 to 15 degrees cephalad. It enters about 1 inch (2.5 cm) distal to the tip of the coccyx and exits a little above the superior border of the symphysis pubis. If the prostate is the area of interest, the central ray is directed 20 to 25 degrees cephalad to project it above the pubic bones.
- Direct the central ray perpendicular to the symphysis pubis for voiding studies.

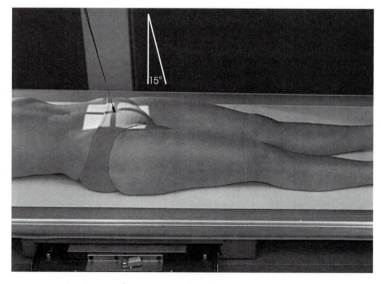

Fig. 18-65. Retrograde cystogram. AP axial bladder with 15-degree caudal angulation of the central ray.

Structures shown

AP or PA projections demonstrate the bladder filled with the contrast medium (Figs. 18-66 and 18-67). If reflux is present, the distal ureters will also be visualized.

□ Evaluation criteria

The following should be clearly demonstrated:

- The regions of the distal end of the ureters, the bladder, and the proximal portion of the urethra.
- Pubic bones projected below the bladder neck and proximal urethra.
- Short scale of contrast clearly demonstrating contrast media in the bladder, distal ureters, and proximal urethra.

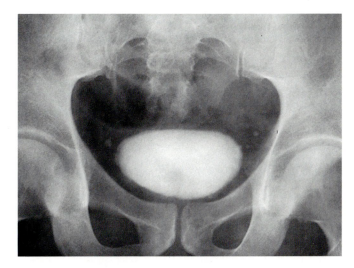

Fig. 18-66. Excretory cystogram, AP projection.

(Courtesy Dr. Joshua A. Becker.)

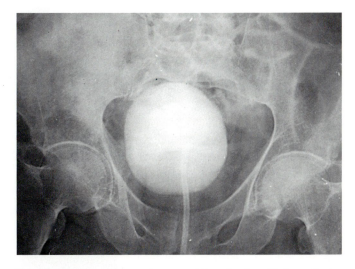

Fig. 18-67. Retrograde cystogram, AP projection. Note catheter in bladder.

Urinary Bladder

 ## AP OBLIQUE PROJECTION
RPO or LPO position

Film: 10 × 12 in (24 × 30 cm) lengthwise.

Position of patient

- Place the patient semi-supine on the radiographic table for AP oblique projections of the urinary system.

Position of part

- Rotate the patient 40 to 60 degrees RPO or LPO, according to the preference of the examining physician (Fig. 18-68).
- Adjust the patient so that the pubic arch closest to the table is aligned over the midline of the grid.
- Extend and abduct the uppermost thigh enough to prevent its superimposition on the bladder area.
- Center the cassette 2 to 3 inches (5 to 7.5 cm) above the upper border of the symphysis pubis approximately 1 inch lateral to the midline on the elevated side (or at the symphysis pubis for voiding studies).
- Ask the patient to suspend respiration at the end of exhalation.

Central ray

- Direct the central ray perpendicular to the film 2 to 3 inches (5 to 7.5 cm) above the upper border of the symphysis pubis. When the bladder neck and proximal urethra are the main areas of interest, a 10-degree caudal angulation of the central ray is usually sufficient to project the pubic bones below them.
- Direct the central ray perpendicular at the level of the symphysis pubis for voiding studies.

Structures shown

Oblique projections demonstrate the bladder filled with the contrast medium. If reflux is present, the distal ureters will also be visualized (Figs. 18-69 and 18-70).

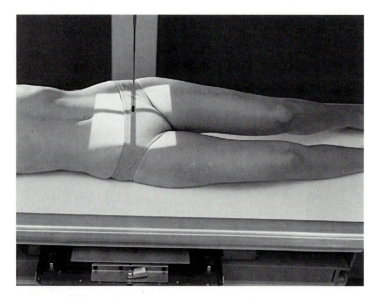

Fig. 18-68. Retrograde cystogram. AP oblique bladder, RPO position.

☐ Evaluation criteria

The following should be clearly demonstrated:

- The regions of the distal end of the ureters, the bladder, and the proximal portion of the urethra.
- Pubic bones projected below the bladder neck and proximal urethra.
- Short scale of contrast clearly demonstrating contrast media in the bladder, distal ureters, and proximal urethra.
- No superimposition of the bladder by the uppermost thigh.

Voiding studies

- Entire urethra visible and filled with contrast media.
- Urethra overlapping the thigh on oblique projections for improved visibility.
- Urethra lying posterior to the superimposed pubic and ischial rami of the side down in oblique projections.

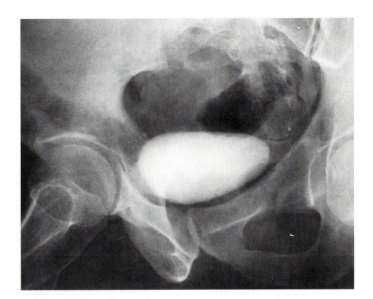

Fig. 18-69. Retrograde cystogram. AP oblique bladder, RPO position.

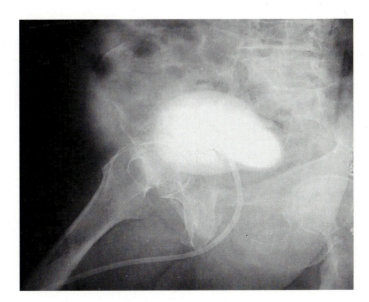

Fig. 18-70. Retrograde cystogram with catheter in bladder.

(Courtesy Dr. Marcy L. Sussman.)

Urinary Bladder

 ## LATERAL PROJECTION
R or L position

Film: 10 × 12 in (24 × 30 cm) lengthwise.

Position of patient

- Place the patient in the lateral recumbent position on the radiographic table on either the right or left side as indicated.

Position of part

- Slightly flex the patient's knees to a comfortable position, and adjust the body so that the median coronal plane is centered to the midline of the grid.
- Flex the elbows and place the hands under the patient's head (Fig. 18-71).
- Center the cassette 2 to 3 inches (5 to 7.5 cm) above the upper border of the symphysis pubis at the median coronal plane.
- Ask the patient to suspend respiration at the end of exhalation.

Central ray

- Direct the central ray perpendicularly to the film 2 to 3 inches (5 to 7.5 cm) above the upper border of the symphysis pubis at the median coronal plane.

Structures shown

A lateral image demonstrates the bladder filled with the contrast medium. If reflux is present, the distal ureters will also be visualized. Lateral projections demonstrate the anterior and posterior bladder walls and the base of the bladder (Fig. 18-72).

□ Evaluation criteria

The following should be clearly demonstrated:

- The regions of the distal end of the ureters, the bladder, and the proximal portion of the urethra.
- Short scale of contrast clearly demonstrating contrast media in the bladder, distal ureters, and proximal urethra.
- The bladder and distal ureters visible through the pelvis.
- Superimposed hips and femora.

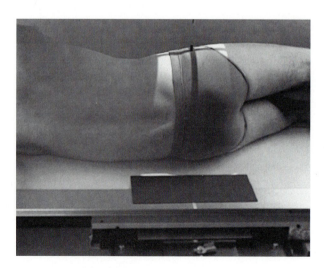

Fig. 18-71. Cystogram, lateral projection.

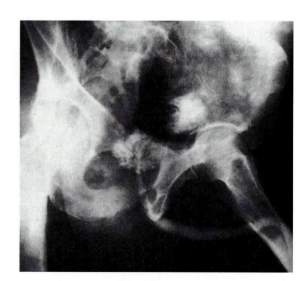

Fig. 18-72. Cystogram, lateral projection.

Male Cystourethrography

AP OBLIQUE PROJECTION
RPO or LPO position

Male cystourethrography may be preceded by an endoscopic examination, following which the bladder is catheterized so that it can be drained just before the injection of the contrast material.

The following steps are observed:

- Use 10 × 12 in (24 × 30 cm) cassettes, placed lengthwise, for cystourethrograms of adult male patients.
- Adjust the patient on the combination table so that the cassette can be centered at the level of the superior border of the symphysis pubis. This centering coincides with the root of the penis, and a 12-in (30 cm) film will include both the bladder and the external urethral orifice.
- After inspecting the preliminary radiograph, the physician drains the bladder and withdraws the catheter.
- Adjust the patient in an oblique position so that the bladder neck and the entire urethra are delineated as free of bony superimposition as possible. Rotate the body 35 to 40 degrees and adjust it so the elevated pubis is centered to the midline of the grid. The superimposed pubic and ischial rami of the down side and the body of the elevated pubis usually are projected anterior to the bladder neck, the proximal part of the urethra, and the prostate (Fig. 18-73).

- Flex the dependent knee only slightly to keep the soft tissues on the medial side of the thigh as near to the center as possible.
- Extend and retract the elevated thigh enough to prevent overlapping.
- With the patient correctly placed, the physician inserts the contrast-loaded urethral syringe or the nozzle of a device such as the Brodney clamp into the urethral orifice. The physician then extends the penis along the soft tissues of the medial side of the dependent thigh to obtain a uniform density of both the deep and the cavernous portions of the urethral canal.

- At a signal from the physician, instruct the patient to hold still, and, while the injection of the contrast material is continued to ensure filling of the entire urethra, make the exposure (Fig. 18-74).
- The bladder may then be filled with a contrast material so that a voiding study can be made (Fig. 18-75). This is usually done without changing the patient's position. When a standing-upright voiding study is required, the patient is adjusted before a vertical grid device and is supplied with a urinal. For further information on positioning, see pp. 170-174 of this volume of the atlas.

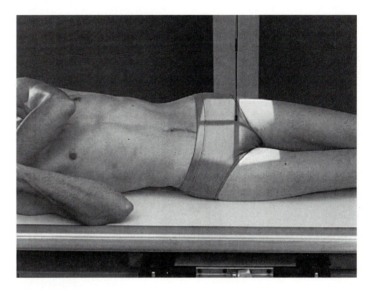

Fig. 18-73. Cystourethrogram. AP oblique projection, RPO position.

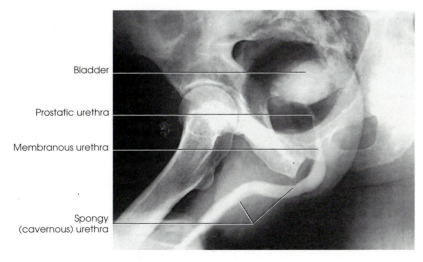

Bladder

Prostatic urethra

Membranous urethra

Spongy
(cavernous) urethra

Fig. 18-74. Injection cystourethrogram. AP oblique urethra, RPO position.

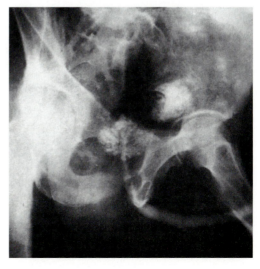

Fig. 18-75. Voiding cystourethrogram. AP oblique urethra, RPO position.

(Courtesy Dr. Oswald S. Lowsley.)

Female Cystourethrography

AP PROJECTION
Contrast injection method

The female urethra averages 3.5 cm in length. Its opening into the bladder is situated at the level of the superior border of the symphysis pubis, from whence the vessel slants obliquely inferiorly and anteriorly to its termination in the vestibule of the vulva, about 1 inch anterior to the vaginal orifice. The female urethra is subject to such conditions as tumors, abscesses, diverticula, dilation, and strictures and to urinary incontinence during the stress of increased intra-abdominal pressure such as occurs during sneezing or coughing. In the investigation of abnormalities other than stress incontinence, contrast studies are made during the injection of the contrast medium or during voiding.

Usually, cystourethrography is preceded by an endoscopic examination. For this reason, it may be performed by the attending urologist or gynecologist with the assistance of a nurse and a radiographer.

The following steps are observed:
- Following the physical examination, the cystoscope is removed and a catheter inserted into the bladder so that the bladder can be drained just before the injection of the contrast solution. Adjust the patient in the supine position on the table. An 8 × 10 in (18 × 24 cm) or 10 × 12 in (24 × 30 cm) cassette is placed lengthwise and centered at the level of the superior border of the symphysis pubis. A 5-degree caudal angulation of the central ray is usually sufficient to free the bladder neck of superimposition.
- After inspecting the preliminary radiograph, the physician drains the bladder and withdraws the catheter. The physician uses a syringe fitted with a blunt-nosed, soft-rubber acorn, which is held firmly against the urethral orifice to prevent reflux as the contrast solution is injected during exposure of the film or films. AP projections are made.

- In addition to the AP projection, obliques may also be required.
- For the latter, rotate the patient 35 to 40 degrees so that the urethra is posterior to the symphysis pubis.
- Extend and abduct the uppermost thigh enough to prevent overlapping.
- For further information on positioning, see pp. 184-188 of this volume of the atlas.
- The physician fills the bladder for each voiding study to be made.
- For an AP projection (Figs. 18-76 and 18-77) maintain the patient in the supine position, or elevate the head of the table enough to place the patient in a semiseated position.
- Perform a lateral voiding study of the female vesicourethral canal with the patient recumbent or upright.
- In either case, center the cassette at the level of the superior border of the symphysis pubis.

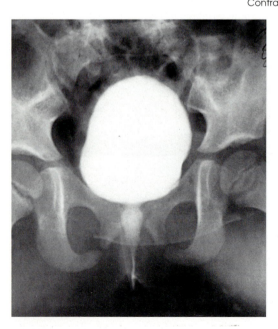

Fig. 18-76. Voiding cystourethrogram, AP projection.

(Courtesy Dr. William B. Seaman.)

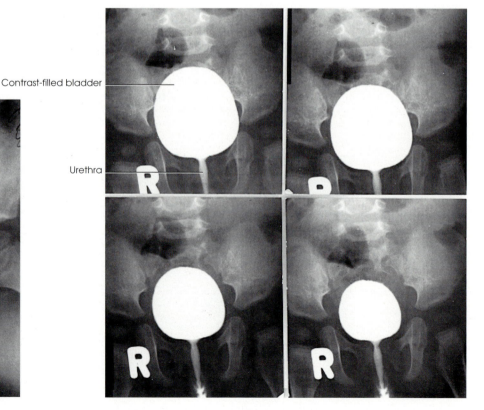

Contrast-filled bladder

Urethra

Fig. 18-77. Serial voiding images showing four stages of bladder emptying.

(Courtesy Dr. Walter E. Berdon and Dr. David H. Baker.)

Metallic bead chain cystourethrography

The metallic bead chain technique of investigating anatomic abnormalities responsible for stress incontinence in women was described by Stevens and Smith[1] in 1937 and by Barnes[2] in 1940. This technique is employed to delineate anatomic changes that occur in the shape and position of the bladder floor, in the posterior urethrovesical angle, in the position of the proximal urethral orifice, and in the angle of inclination of the urethral axis under the stress of increased intra-abdominal pressure as exerted by the Valsalva maneuver. Comparison AP and lateral projections are made with the patient standing at rest (Figs. 18-78 and 18-79) and during straining (Figs. 18-80 and 18-81).

[1]Stevens WE and Smith SP: Roentgenological examination of the female urethra, J Urol 37:194-201, 1937.
[2]Barnes AC: A method for evaluating the stress of urinary incontinence, Am J Obstet Gynecol 40:381-390, 1940.

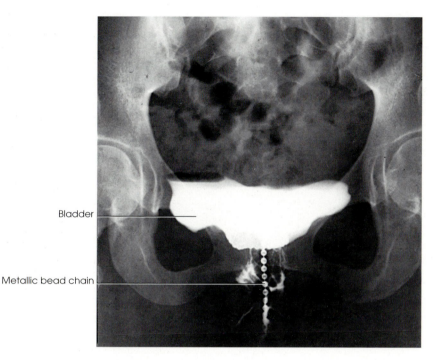

Bladder

Metallic bead chain

Fig. 18-78. Upright cystourethrogram, resting AP projection.

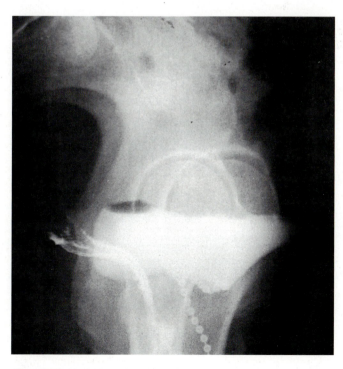

Fig. 18-79. Upright cystourethrogram, resting lateral projection.

Female cystourethrography

For this examination, the physician extends a flexible metallic bead chain through the urethral canal. The proximal portion of the chain rests within the bladder, and the distal end is taped to the thigh. To demonstrate the length of the urethra, a small metal marker is attached with a piece of tape to the vaginal mucosa just lateral to the urethral orifice. After instillation of the metallic chain, a catheter is passed into the bladder, its contents drained, and an opaque contrast solution injected. The catheter is removed for the filming procedure.

Hodgkinson et al[1] recommend the upright position to employ gravity and thus to simulate normal body activity. These physicians obtain two sets of films, AP and lateral projections, and they specify that the rest studies *must* be exposed before the stress studies because the bladder does not immediately return to its normal resting position after straining.

---

[1]Hodgkinson CP, Doub HP, and Kelly WT: Urethrocystograms: metallic bead chain technique, Clin Obstet Gynecol 1:668-677, 1958.

After instillation of the metallic chain and the contrast solution, the patient usually is prepared for upright radiographs. The examining room should be readied in advance so that these patients who will be uncomfortable can be given immediate attention. They must be given kind reassurance and must be examined in privacy. Klawon[2] found that these patients can be relieved of the fear of involuntary voiding, and thus willingly apply full pressure during the stress studies, by the simple act of placing a folded towel or a disposable pad between the thighs before the stress radiographs are taken.

The cassette size and centering point are the same as for other female cystourethrograms. For further information on radiographic positioning of the lower urinary tract, please see pp. 184-188 in this volume of the atlas.

---

[2]Klawon Sister MM: Urethrocystography and urinary stress incontinence in women, Radiol Techn 39:353-358, 1968.

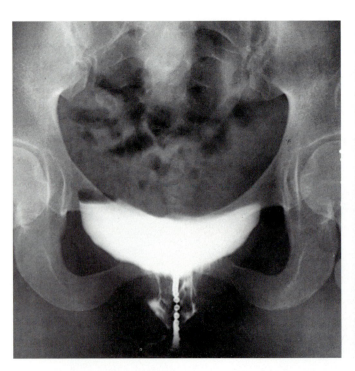

Fig. 18-80. Upright cystourethrogram, stress AP projection. Same patient as in Fig. 18-78.

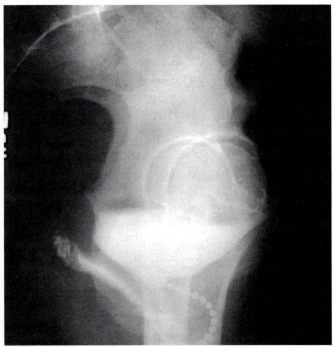

Fig. 18-81. Upright cystourethrogram, stress lateral projection. Same patient as in Fig. 18-79.

(Courtesy Dr. Howard P. Daub.)

Chapter 19

REPRODUCTIVE SYSTEM

Patient positioned against a vertical Potter-Bucky device for lateral pelvimetry examination; 1940s.

Female Reproductive System

The female reproductive system consists of an internal and an external group of organs, the two groups being connected by the vaginal canal. The anatomy of the external genitalia will not be considered, since these structures do not require radiographic demonstration. The internal genital organs consist of the *gonads,* or *ovaries,* which are two glandular bodies homologous to the testes in the male, and of a system of canals made up of the *uterine tubes,* the *uterus,* and the *vagina.* The structures that are near, or adjacent to, the uterus (e.g., ovaries and uterine tubes) are sometimes referred to as the *adnexa uteri.*

The ovaries are small, glandular organs with an internal secretion that controls the menstrual cycle and an external secretion containing the *ova,* or female reproductive cells (Fig. 19-1). The ovaries are shaped approximately like an almond and measure about 1 inch (2.5 cm) in width, ½

inch (1.2 cm) in thickness, and 1½ inches (4 cm) in length. The ovaries lie, one on each side, inferior and posterior to the uterine tube and near the lateral wall of the pelvis, being attached to the posterior surface of the broad ligament of the uterus by the mesovarium.

The ovary is composed of a core of vascular tissue, the medulla, by which it is attached at the hilum to the mesovarium, and of an outer, or cortical, portion of glandular tissue. The cortex contains *ovarian vesicular follicles* (ovisacs), in all stages of development, and each vesicle contains one ovum. A fully developed ovarian vesicular follicle (ovisac) is about ½ inch (1.3 cm) in diameter and is referred to as a *graafian follicle.* As the minute ovum matures, the size of the follicle and its fluid content increase, so that the wall of the follicle sac approaches the surface of the ovary and in time ruptures, liberating the ovum and the follicular fluid into the peritoneal cavity. The extrusion of an ovum by the rupture of a follicle is called *ovulation,* and the process usually

occurs once during the menstrual cycle. Once in the pelvic cavity, the ovum is drawn toward the tubal canal by the current set up by the fimbriae on the end of the uterine tube.

The two *uterine tubes* (fallopian tubes) serve to collect ova liberated by the ovaries and to convey the cells to the uterine cavity. Each tube is 3 to 5 inches (7 to 13 cm) in length (Fig. 19-2) and arises from the lateral angle of the uterus, passes laterally through the superior margin of the broad ligament, forms an arch above the ovary, and opens into the peritoneal cavity. The tube is of small diameter at its uterine end, which opens into the cavity of the uterus by a minute orifice. The uterine tube is divided into three parts: the isthmus, the ampulla, and the infundibulum. The *isthmus* is a short segment near the uterus. The *ampulla* comprises most of the tube and is wider than the isthmus. The terminal and lateral portion of the tube is the *infundibulum* and is flared in appearance. The infundibulum ends in a series of irregular, prolonged processes called *fimbriae.* One of the fimbriae, termed the *ovarian fimbria,* is longer than the other processes and is attached either to or near the ovary.

The mucosal lining of the oviduct is ciliated and is arranged in folds that increase in number and complexity as they approach the fimbriated extremity of the tube. The cilia of the fimbriae draw the liberated ovum into the tube, which then conveys it to the uterine cavity by peristaltic movements. The passage of the ovum through the tube is believed to require several days. Fertilization of the cell occurs in the outer part of the tube with the fertilized ovum next migrating to the uterus for implantation.

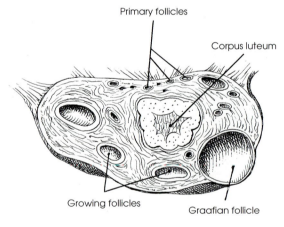

Fig. 19-1. Section of ovary.

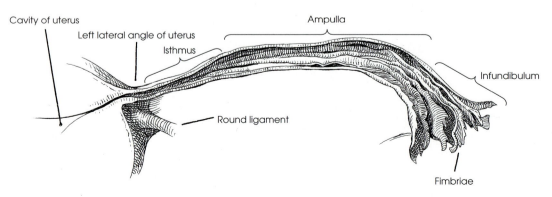

Fig. 19-2. Section of left uterine (fallopian) tube.

The *uterus* is a pear-shaped, muscular organ (Figs. 19-3 and 19-4). The primary functions of the uterus are to receive and retain the fertilized ovum until development of the fetus is complete and, when the fetus is mature, to expel it during parturition.

The uterus consists of four parts: the fundus, the body, the isthmus (internal os), and the cervix. The *fundus* is the bluntly rounded superiormost portion of the uterus and is separated from the body of the uterus by an imaginary line joining the points of entrance of the two uterine tubes. These points of entrance are referred to as the *lateral angles* (cornua). The *body* narrows from the fundus to the isthmus and is the point of attachment for the ligaments that secure the uterus within the pelvis. The *isthmus* (superior part of the cervix) is an approximately ½ inch (1 cm)–long constricted area between the body and the cervix. The *cervix* (neck) is the cylindric vaginal end of the uterus and is approximately 1 inch (2.5 cm) long. The vagina is attached around the circumference of the cervix.

The nulliparous uterus is approximately 3 inches (7.5 cm) in length, almost half of which represents the length of the cervix. The body is about 1 inch (2.5 cm) in thickness and 2 inches (5 cm) in width between the lateral angles of the cornua, its widest part. The cervix is approximately ¾ inch (2 cm) in diameter. During pregnancy the body of the uterus gradually expands into the abdominal cavity, reaching the epigastric region in the eighth month. Following parturition, the organ shrinks to almost its original size but undergoes characteristic changes in shape.

The uterus is situated in the central part of the pelvic cavity, lying posterior and superior to the urinary bladder and anterior to the rectal ampulla. The long axis, which is slightly concave anteriorly, is directed inferiorly and posteriorly at a near right angle to the axis of the vaginal canal, into which the lower end of the cervix projects. The free, vesical surface (undersurface) of the organ rests on the urinary bladder, and its intestinal (upper) surface is in apposition with the small intestine.

It was previously thought that the uterus was supported in position by the ligaments attached to the surrounding structures and to the lateral walls of the pelvis, the most important being the broad and the round ligaments. Anatomists now believe that the ligaments of the uterus maintain the orientation of the organ but are incapable of supporting it. Instead, the uterus is supported in position by the pelvic diaphragm of the pelvic floor, the viscera surrounding the uterus, and the perineal body. The perineal body is a node formed by the converging of fibers from several muscles of the pelvic floor. The round ligament of the uterus holds the fundus anteriorly. The broad ligaments, one on each side, pass laterally from the uterus to the pelvic wall and floor and thus divide the pelvic cavity into anterior and posterior compartments. The body of the uterus moves freely, bending posteriorly or anteriorly on the less movable cervix when the urinary bladder or the rectum becomes distended.

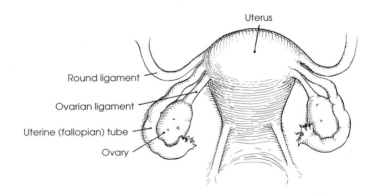

Fig. 19-3. Superoposterior view of uterus, ovaries, and uterine tubes.

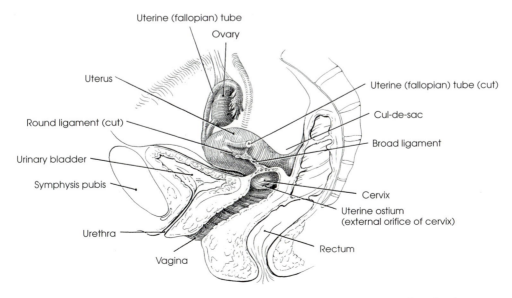

Fig. 19-4. Sagittal section showing relation of internal genitalia to surrounding structures.

The cavity of the body of the uterus, the uterine cavity proper, is triangular in shape when viewed in a frontal plane. In the nongravid state, the anterior and posterior walls of the cavity are in contact, so that the space is more potential than real. The canal of the cervix is dilated in the center and constricted at each extremity. The proximal end of the canal is continuous with the canal of the isthmus (internal os). The distal orifice is called the *uterine ostium* (external os). The latter orifice is bounded by two thick, prominent lips that are normally in contact with the posterior wall of the proximal end of the vaginal canal.

The mucosal lining of the uterine cavity is called the *endometrium*. This lining undergoes cyclic changes, called the menstrual cycle, at about 4-week intervals from puberty to menopause. The endometrium is prepared during each premenstrual period for the implantation and nutrition of the fertilized ovum. If fertilization has not occurred, the menstrual flow of blood and of necrosed particles of uterine mucosa ensues. If fertilization has taken place, the premenstrual histologic changes continue, and the thickened endometrium is then called the *decidua*.

The *vagina* is a muscular structure with walls and a canal lying posterior to the urinary bladder and the urethra and ante-rior to the rectum. Averaging about 3 inches (7.5 cm) in length, the vagina extends inferiorly and anteriorly from the uterus to the vulva, where it opens to the exterior. The proximal portion of the vagina encircles and attaches to the uterine cervix; here, its canal lumen or cavity is known as the *vaginal fornices*. The fornices are shallow anteriorly but gradually deepen to form a pouch, or cul-de-sac, posteriorly, where they are in close proximity to the peritoneal cavity. The space between the labia minora is known as the *vaginal vestibule,* and in it are situated the vaginal orifice and the urethral orifice.

FETAL DEVELOPMENT

The fertilized ovum is passed from the uterine tube into the uterine cavity, where it adheres to and becomes embedded in the decidua; this process is called *implantation*. About 2 weeks after the fertilization of the ovum, the embryo begins to appear. The fertilized ovum is referred to as a *zygote* during the process of implantation (2 weeks), as an *embryo* for the succeeding 5 weeks while the different organs are being formed, and as a *fetus* from approximately the beginning of the third month (week 8), when it assumes a human appearance, until the birth of the baby (Fig. 19-5).

During the first 2 weeks of fetal development, the growing fertilized ovum (zygote) is primarily concerned with the establishment of its nutritive and protective covering, the *chorion* and the *amnion*. As the chorion develops, it forms (1) the outer layer of the protective membranes enclosing the embryo and (2) the embryonic portion of the placenta, by which the umbilical cord is attached to the mother's uterus and through which food is supplied to and waste is removed from the fetus. The amnion, often referred to as the "bag of water" by the laity, forms the inner layer of the fetal membranes and contains amniotic fluid in which the fetus floats. The decidua is expelled with the fetal membranes and the placenta at parturition; these structures constitute the afterbirth. A new endometrium is then regenerated.

The fertilized ovum usually becomes embedded near the fundic end of the uterine cavity, most frequently on the anterior or posterior wall. Implantation occasionally occurs so low, however, that the fully developed placenta encroaches on or obstructs the cervical canal. This condition results in a premature separation of the placenta, which is termed *placenta previa* (Fig. 19-6).

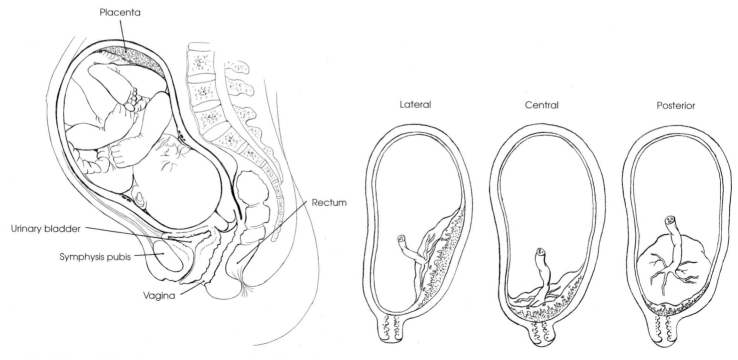

Fig. 19-5. Sagittal section showing fetus of about 7 months.

Fig. 19-6. Schematic drawings of several placental sites in low implantation.

Male Reproductive System

The male genital system consists of (1) a pair of *gonads*, the *testes*, that produce the germ cells or spermatozoa; (2) two excretory channels, the *ductus deferentes,* one leading from each testis and through which the spermatozoa pass from the gonad to the prostatic portion of the urethral canal; and (3) the *prostate*, a *seminal vesicle*, and a pair of *bulbourethral glands* that produce secretions that are added to the secretions of the testes and the ductal mucosa to constitute the final product, the seminal fluid.

The *genital seminal ducts* have anatomic variations along their course that necessitate individual description. The several portions of each duct are called the epididymis, the ductus deferens (vas deferens), the system of prostatic ducts, and the ejaculatory duct. The penis, the scrotum, and the structures enclosed by the scrotal sac (the testes, the epididymides, part of the ductus deferens, and the spermatic cords) are the external genital organs.

The *testes* (or testicles) are ovoid bodies averaging 1½ inches (3.7 cm) in length and about 1 inch (2.5 cm) in both width and depth (Fig. 19-7). Each testis is divided into 200 to 300 partial compartments, each compartment housing one or more of the convoluted, germ cell–producing tubules, which constitute the glandular substance of the testis. These seminiferous tubules converge toward the dorsum of the testis where they empty into a network of tubules, the *rete testis*. These tubules in turn converge and unite to form 15 to 20 tubules that emerge from the testis to enter the head of the epididymis.

The *epididymis* is an oblong structure; its larger proximal part is called the *head* and its distal part the *tail*. The epididymis is attached to the superior and lateroposterior aspects of the testis. The ductules leading out of the testis enter the head of the epididymis to become continuous with the coiled and convoluted ductules that make up this structure. As they pass inferiorly, the ductules progressively unite to form the main duct, which is continuous with the ductus deferens.

The *ductus deferens* is 16 to 18 inches (40 to 46 cm) in length, and only its first part is tortuous, or convoluted. It extends from the tail of the epididymis to the posteroinferior surface of the urinary bladder. From its beginning, the ductus deferens ascends along the medial side of the epididymis on the posterior surface of the testis to join the other constituents of the spermatic cord, with which it emerges from the scrotal sac, to pass into the pelvic cavity through the inguinal canal. The ductus deferens then separates from the other spermatic cord structures and passes inferiorly through the pelvis, over the bladder just medial to the ureter, and then moves medially to the duct of the seminal vesicle (Fig. 19-8). Near its termination, the duct expands into an ampulla for the storage of seminal fluid and then ends by uniting with the duct of the seminal vesicle.

The *seminal vesicle,* a sacculated structure about 2 inches (5 cm) in length (Fig. 19-8), is situated obliquely on the lateroposterior surface of the bladder, where, from the level of the ureterocystic junction, it slants inferiorly and medially to the base of the prostate. The ampulla of the ductus deferens lies along the medial border of the seminal vesicle to form the ejaculatory duct.

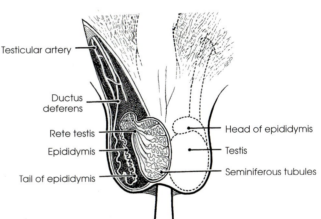

Fig. 19-7. Frontal section of testes and ductus deferens.

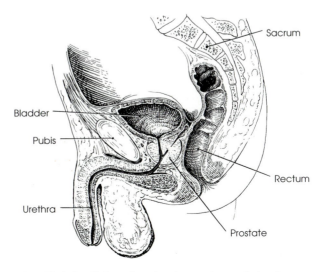

Fig. 19-8. Sagital section showing male genital system.

The *ejaculatory duct* is formed by the union of the ductus deferens and the duct of the seminal vesicle. It averages about ½ inch (1.3 cm) in length and originates behind the neck of the bladder. The two ejaculatory ducts enter the base of the prostate and, passing obliquely inferiorly through the substance of the gland, open into the prostatic urethra at the lateral margins of the prostatic utricle.

The *prostate,* an accessory genital organ, is a somewhat cone-shaped body, the superior part of which is known as the *base* and the inferior part as the *apex.* The prostate averages 1¼ inches (3 cm) from base to apex and somewhat more across its base. The prostate encircles the proximal portion of the male urethra and, extending from the bladder neck to the pelvic floor, lies about 1 inch (2.5 cm) posterior to the lower two thirds of the symphysis pubis and in front of the rectal ampulla (Fig. 19-9). The prostate is composed of both muscular and glandular tissue. The ducts of the prostate open into the prostatic portion of the urethra.

The frequency of performing the radiographic examinations of the male reproductive system described in this chapter has continued to decrease in recent years primarily because of advances in diagnostic ultrasound imaging. The prostate can be ultrasonically imaged either through the urine-filled bladder or by using a special rectal transducer. The seminal ducts can be imaged when the rectum is filled with an ultrasound gel and a special rectal transducer is used. Additionally, testicular ultrasonic scans are performed when the patient has a palpable mass or an enlarged testis or to check for metastasis. The vast majority of the testicular scans are performed because of a palpable mass or an enlarged testis.

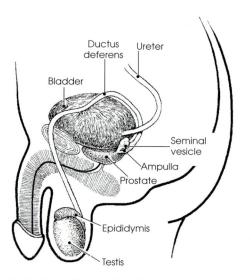

Fig. 19-9. Sagittal section through male pelvis.

Female Radiography
NONGRAVID PATIENT

Radiologic investigation of the nongravid uterus, the adnexa uteri, and vagina are denoted by the terms hysterosalpingography, pelvic pneumography, and vaginography. Each procedure requires the use of a contrast medium, and each is carried out under aseptic conditions.

Hysterosalpingography involves the introduction of a radiopaque contrast agent through a uterine cannula. Hysterosalpingography is performed to determine the size, shape, and position of the uterus and uterine tubes (fallopian tubes); to delineate lesions such as polyps, submucous tumor masses, or fistulous tracts; and to investigate the patency of the uterine tubes in cases of sterility (Fig. 19-10). *Pelvic pneumography* requires the introduction of a gaseous contrast medium directly into the peritoneal cavity, but it is rarely performed today since the development of ultrasonic evaluation techniques of the pelvic cavity. *Vaginography* is performed in the investigation of congenital abnormalities and of vaginal fistulae and other pathologic conditions involving the vagina.

Contrast media

Various opaque media are employed in examinations of the female genital passages. The water-soluble contrast media employed for intravenous urography are widely used for both hysterosalpingography and vaginography as well.

Preparation of intestinal tract

Preparation of the intestinal tract for any of these examinations usually consists of the following: (1) administering a non-gas-forming laxative on the preceding evening if the bowel action is costive, (2) instructing the patient to take cleansing enemas until the return flow is clear before reporting for the examination, and (3) withholding the preceding meal.

Appointment date and care of patient

Gynecologic examinations should be scheduled approximately 10 days following the onset of menstruation. This is the interval during which the endometrium is least congested, and, more importantly, it is a few days before ovulation normally occurs, so there is little danger of irradiating a recently fertilized ovum.

The relatively minor instrumentation required for the introduction of the contrast medium in these examinations normally necessitates neither hospitalization nor premedication. Some patients experience unpleasant but transitory aftereffects; therefore the radiology department should have facilities for outpatients to rest in the recumbent position before returning home.

The patient is requested to completely empty her bladder immediately before the examination. This procedure prevents pressure displacement of and superimposition on the pelvic genitalia. In addition, a vaginal irrigation is administered just before the examination. At this time the patient should be given the necessary supplies and instructed to cleanse the perineal region.

Radiation protection

To deliver the least possible amount of radiation to the gonads, the physician restricts fluoroscopy and filming to the minimum required for a satisfactory examination.

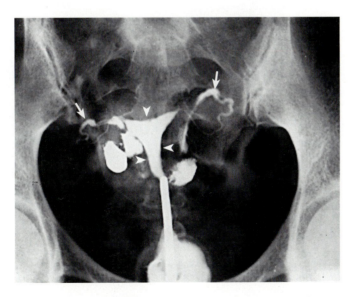

Fig. 19-10. Hysterosalpingography reveals bilateral hydrosalpinx of uterine tubes *(arrows).* Contrast-filled uterine cavity is normal *(arrowheads).*

Hysterosalpingography

Hysterosalpingography is performed by a physician with spot radiographs made with the patient in the supine position on a fluoroscopic table. The examination may also be performed by the physician, and conventional radiographs made with an overhead tube. When fluoroscopy is used, spot radiographs may be the only images obtained. In preparing the patient for the examination, the following steps are observed:

- After irrigation of the vaginal canal, complete emptying of the bladder, and perineal cleansing, place the patient on the examining table.
- Adjust her in the lithotomy position, with knees flexed over leg rests.
- When a combination table is used, adjust the patient's position to permit the films to be centered to a point 2 inches (5 cm) proximal to the symphysis pubis; 10 × 12 in (24 × 30 cm) films are used for all studies and are placed lengthwise.

After inspection of the preliminary radiograph and with a vaginal speculum in position, the physician inserts a uterine cannula through the cervical canal; fits the attached rubber plug, or acorn, firmly against the external cervical os; applies counterpressure with a tenaculum to prevent reflux of the contrast medium; and then withdraws the speculum unless it is radiolucent. An opaque or a gaseous contrast medium may now be injected via the cannula into the uterine cavity. The contrast will flow through the patent uterine tubes and "spill" into the peritoneal cavity (Figs. 19-11 to 19-13). Patency of the uterine tubes can be determined by transuterine gas insufflation (Rubin test), but the length, position, and course of the ducts can be demonstrated only by opacifying the lumina.

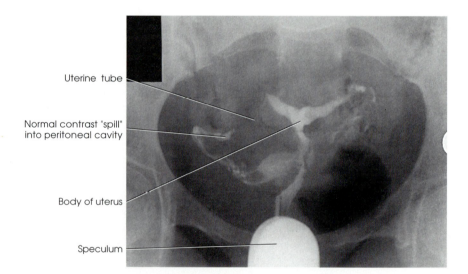

Fig. 19-11. Hysterosalpingogram, AP projection, showing normal uterus and uterine tubes.

(Courtesy Ann Kay, R.T.)

The free-flowing, iodinated organic contrast agents are usually injected at room temperature. These agents pass through patent uterine tubes quickly, and the resultant peritoneal spill is absorbed and eliminated by way of the urinary system, usually within 2 hours or less.

The contrast medium may be injected with a pressometer or a syringe. Intrauterine pressure is maintained for the radiographic studies by closing the cannular valve. To prevent excessive peritoneal spillage, the contrast medium, in the absence of fluoroscopy, is introduced in two to four fractional doses, each of which is followed by a radiographic study to determine whether the filling is adequate as shown by the peritoneal spill.

The filming may consist of no more than a single AP projection taken at the end of each fractional injection. Other projections (oblique, axial, and lateral) are taken as indicated.

□ Evaluation criteria

The following should be clearly demonstrated:
- The pelvic region 2 inches (5 cm) above the symphysis pubis centered on the radiograph.
- All contrast media visible, including any "spill" areas.
- A short scale of contrast on radiographs.

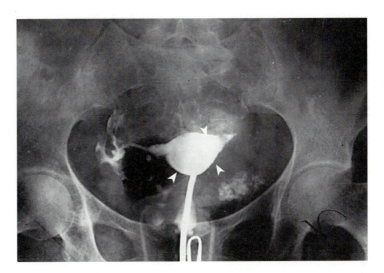

Fig. 19-12. Hysterosalpingogram, AP projection, showing submucous fibroid occupying entire uterine cavity (arrowheads).

(Courtesy Dr. Richard H. Marshak.)

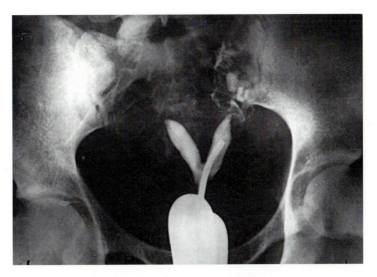

Fig. 19-13. Hysterosalpingogram, AP projection, revealing uterine cavity to be bicornate in outline.

Pelvic pneumography

Pelvic pneumography, gynecography, and *pangynecography* are terms used to denote radiologic examination of the female pelvic organs by means of intraperitoneal gas insufflation (Fig. 19-14). This procedure has essentially been replaced by ultrasonic and other diagnostic techniques. For a description of pelvic pneumography, see the fourth edition of this atlas, Volume 3, p. 840.

Vaginography

Vaginography is used in the investigation of congenital malformations and such pathologic conditions as vesicovaginal and enterovaginal fistulas. The examination is performed by introducing a contrast medium into the vaginal canal. Lambie et al.[1] recommend the use of a thin barium sulfate mixture for the investigation of fistulous communications with the intestine. At the end of the examination, the patient is instructed to expel as much of the barium mixture as possible, and the canal is then cleaned by vaginal irrigation. For the investigation of other conditions, Coe[2] advocates the use of an iodinated organic compound.

---

[1]Lambie RW, Rubin S, and Dann DS: Demonstration of fistulas by vaginography, AJR 90:717-720, 1963.
[2]Coe FO: Vaginography, AJR 90:721-722, 1963.

A rectal retention tube is employed for the introduction of the contrast medium, so that the moderately inflated balloon can be used to prevent reflux. By one technique, the physician inserts only the tip of the tube into the vaginal orifice. The patient is then requested to extend the thighs and to hold them in close approximation to keep the inflated balloon pressed firmly against the vaginal entrance. By another technique, the tube is inserted far enough to place the deflated balloon within the distal end of the vagina, and the balloon is then inflated under fluoroscopic observation. The barium mixture is introduced with the usual enema equipment. The water-soluble medium is injected with a syringe.

Vaginography is performed on a combination fluoroscopic-radiographic table. The contrast medium is injected under fluoroscopic control, and spot radiographs are exposed as indicated during the filling (Fig. 19-15).

The radiographs seen in Figs. 19-16 to 19-18 were taken with the central ray directed perpendicular to the midpoint of the cassette; for localized studies, centering is at the level of the superior border of the symphysis pubis.

In each examination the radiographic projections required are determined by the radiologist according to the fluoroscopic findings. Low rectovaginal fistulas are best shown in the lateral projection, and fistulous communications with the sigmoid and/or ileum are shown to best advantage in oblique projections.

☐ Evaluation criteria

The following should be clearly demonstrated:
- Superior border of the symphysis pubis centered on the radiograph.
- Any fistulas in their entirety.
- Optimal density and contrast to visualize the vagina and any fistula.
- The pelvis on oblique projections not superimposed by the proximal thigh.
- Superimposed hips and femora in the lateral image.

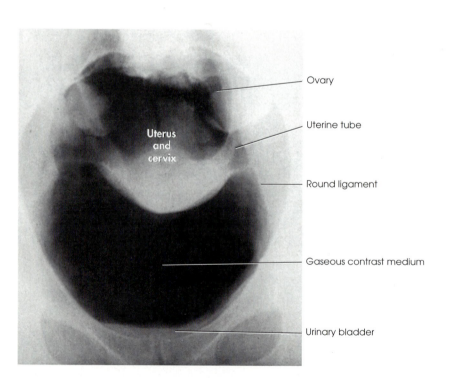

Ovary

Uterine tube

Uterus and cervix

Round ligament

Gaseous contrast medium

Urinary bladder

Fig. 19-14. Normal pelvic pneumogram. See Fig. 19-3 for correlation with radiograph.

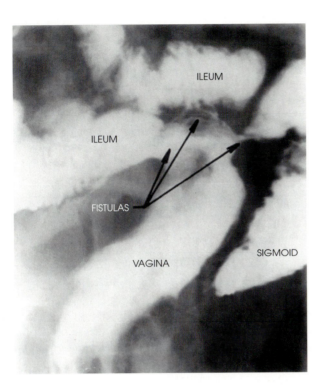

Fig. 19-15. Vaginogram, spot radiograph, PA oblique projection, LAO position. Sigmoid fistula and two ileum fistulas shown.

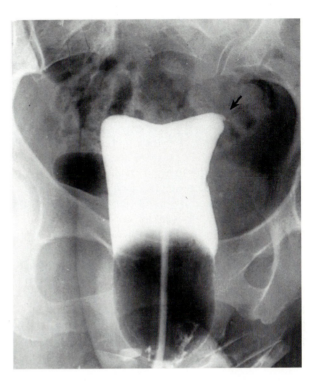

Fig. 19-16. Vaginogram, AP projection, showing small fistulous tract *(arrow)* projecting laterally from apex of vagina and ending in abscess.

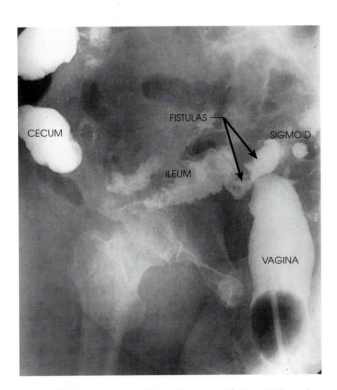

Fig. 19-17. Vaginogram, AP oblique projection, RPO position. Fistulas to ileum and sigmoid shown.

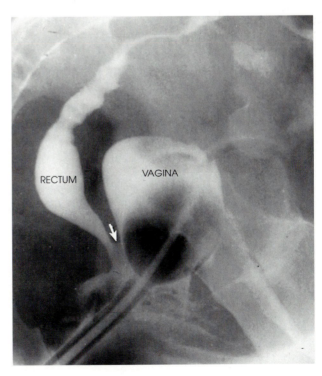

Fig. 19-18. Vaginogram, AP projection, showing low rectovaginal fistula.

(Courtesy Dr. Roger W. Lambie.)

GRAVID PATIENT

Because ultrasound examinations provide visualization of the fetus and placenta with no apparent risk to the patient or fetus, ultrasonography has become the preferred diagnostic tool for examination of the gravid female. In some cases, however, the following radiologic examinations are still indicated:

1. *Fetography* is the demonstration of the fetus in utero. Because of the danger of radiation-induced fetal malformations, this technique of examination is avoided if possible until after the eighteenth week of gestation. Fetography is employed to detect suspected abnormalities of development, to confirm suspected fetal death, to determine the presentation and position of the fetus, and to determine whether the pregnancy is single or multiple.

2. Radiographic *pelvimetry* and *fetal cephalometry* are performed for the purpose of demonstrating the architecture of the maternal pelvis and of comparing the size of the fetal head with the size of the maternal bony pelvic outlet. This procedure is performed to determine whether the pelvic diameters are adequate for normal parturition or whether cesarean section will be used for the delivery.

   Many techniques and combinations of techniques are employed in radiographic pelvimetry, but space permits inclusion in this text of the body positions and pertinent technical factors for only a few. (See the Bibliography for a list of detailed studies of the various measurement techniques.)

3. *Placentography* is the radiographic examination in which the walls of the uterus are investigated to locate the placenta in cases of suspected placenta previa. At one time radiographs were the only means available to detect such conditions. With advances in technology and the concern over the dose of radiation received by the fetus, diagnostic ultrasound (see Volume 3, Chapter 37) has become a valuable diagnostic tool for placenta localization.

Radiation protection

Radiologic examinations of pregnant patients are performed only when information is required that cannot otherwise be obtained. In addition to the danger of genetic changes that may result from reproductive cell irradiation, there is also the danger of radiation-induced malformations of the developing individual. Radiation for any purpose, especially during the first trimester of gestation, is avoided whenever possible, and any examination involving the abdominopelvic region is restricted to the absolute minimum number of radiographs. The radiographer's responsibility, as always, is to carry out the work carefully and thoughtfully to obviate repeat exposures.

Preparation of patient

Although it is desirable to clear the large bowel of gas and fecal material with a cleansing enema shortly before any of these examinations, preliminary preparation of the patient depends entirely on her condition, and under no circumstances is a cleansing enema administered without the express permission of the attending physician. Request that the patient completely empty the bladder immediately before the examination. This is particularly important when the upright position is being used because the filled bladder prevents the fetus from descending to the most dependent portion of the uterine cavity.

Care of patient

Patients who are in labor and those who are bleeding from a placental separation must be treated as emergencies and must be under the constant observation of qualified personnel.

Respiration

A change in the oxygen content of the maternal blood causes the fetus to react quickly by movement. It is recommended that, just before the suspension of respiration for the exposure, the mother's blood be hyperaerated by having her inhale deeply several times and then suspend respiration during the inhalation phase.

Fetography

Fetography has generally been replaced by sonography and therefore is not fully described in this edition. For a more complete description, please see Volume 2 of the seventh or earlier editions of this atlas.

AP or PA and lateral projections are obtained to demonstrate the maternal pelvis and developing fetus (Figs. 19-19 to 19-21). The following steps are observed:

- Whenever possible, place the patient prone to place the fetus closer to the film.
- To accomplish this, place supports under the chest, upper abdomen, and femora (Fig. 19-22).
- If the prone position is not possible, place the patient supine on the radiographic table with a support under the knees to relieve back strain.
- For the lateral projection, with the patient lying on the side, support the abdomen to be parallel to the table if needed.
- Center the perpendicular central ray to the abdomen.

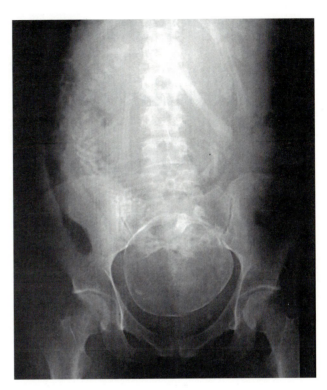

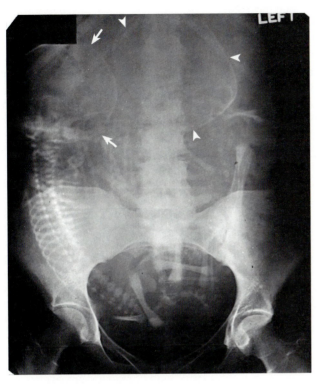

Fig. 19-19. Fetography, PA projection. Twin pregnancy showing two fetal heads (*arrows* and *arrowheads*).

Fig. 19-20. Fetography, AP projection showing one fetus.

(Courtesy Susan M. Orlando, R.T.)

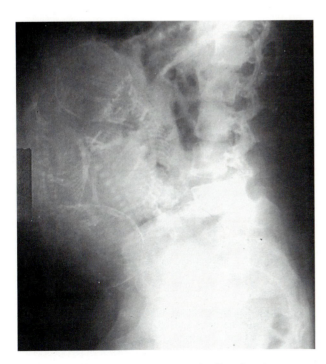

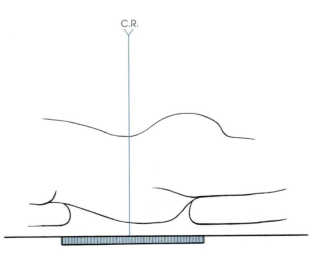

Fig. 19-21. Fetography, lateral projection showing triplet pregnancy.

Fig. 19-22. Fetography, prone position showing support under patient's legs and thorax.

Radiographic pelvimetry and cephalometry

Many different techniques of performing pelvimetry are available, but most have been replaced by sonography. Previous editions of this atlas describe the Ball and Thoms methods, which have been deleted from this edition. For descriptions of the Ball and Thoms methods, see Volume 2 of the seventh or earlier editions of this atlas. The Colcher-Sussman method of pelvimetry is described in this edition following a description of the obtainable pelvic measurements.

External landmarks for plane of pelvic inlet

The entrance to the true pelvis is called the *superior strait* or *pelvic inlet;* it is bounded by the sacral promontory, the linea terminalis, and the crests of the pubic bones and the symphysis. The internal anteroposterior diameter of the inlet is measured from the center of the sacral promontory to the superoposterior margin of the symphysis pubis and is called the *internal conjugate diameter* or the *conjugata vera* (Figs. 19-23 and 19-24). Other internal diameters of the pelvic cavity are shown in the accompanying illustrations.

The *external conjugate diameter* extends from the space between the spinous process of the fourth and fifth lumbar vertebrae to the top of the symphysis pubis. The posterior landmark, the interspinous space, can be palpated at the superior angle of the Michaelis rhomboid, which is the diamond-shaped depression overlying the lumbosacral region. It is bounded laterally by the dimples overlying the posterior superior iliac spines, superior to the fifth lumbar spinous process by the lines formed by the gluteus muscles, and inferior to the groove at the end of the vertebral column.

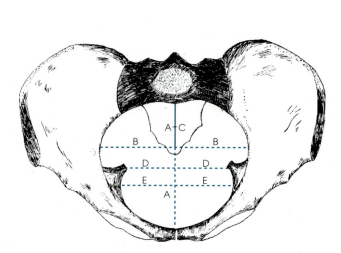

Fig. 19-23. Pelvis seen from above. *A,* Anteroposterior diameter of the inlet; *B,* transverse diameter of inlet; *C,* posterior sagittal diameter of inlet; *D,* interspinous or transverse diameter of midplane; *E,* widest transverse diameter of outlet.

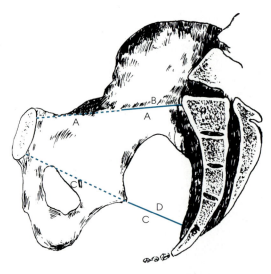

Fig. 19-24. Lateral aspect of pelvis. *A,* Anteroposterior diameter of inlet; *B,* posterior sagittal diameter of inlet; *C,* anteroposterior diameter of midplane; *D,* posterior sagittal diameter of midplane.

Pelvimetry

AP PROJECTION
COLCHER-SUSSMAN METHOD

Each of the two projections (AP and lateral) employed in this method of pelvimetry requires the use of the Colcher-Sussman pelvimeter. This device consists of a metal ruler perforated at centimeter intervals and mounted on a small stand in such a way that it is always parallel with the plane of the film. The ruler can be rotated in a complete circle and adjusted for height (Fig. 19-25).

Film: 14 × 17 in (35 × 43 cm) for each exposure.

Position of patient

- Place the patient in the supine position and center the median sagittal plane of the body to the midline of the grid.
- Flex the knees to elevate the forepelvis, and separate the thighs enough to permit correct placement of the pelvimeter.
- Center the horizontal ruler to the gluteal fold at the level of the ischial tuberosities. The tuberosities are easily palpated through the median part of the buttocks;

if preferred, localize the tuberosities by placing the ruler 10 cm below the superior border of the symphysis pubis (Fig. 19-26).
- Center the film 1½ inches (3.7 cm) superior to the symphysis pubis (Fig. 19-27).
- After determining that the fetus is quiet, instruct the patient to suspend *respiration* at the end of inhalation for the exposure.

Central ray

- Direct the central ray perpendicular to the midpoint of the film 1½ inches (3.7 cm) superior to the symphysis pubis.

□Evaluation criteria

The following should be clearly demonstrated:
- Entire pelvis.
- Metal ruler with centimeter markings visible.
- Density permitting visualization of all pelvic landmarks and intersecting diameters.
- No rotation of the pelvis.
- Entire fetal head.

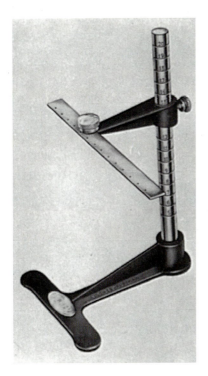

Fig. 19-25. Colcher-Sussman ruler.

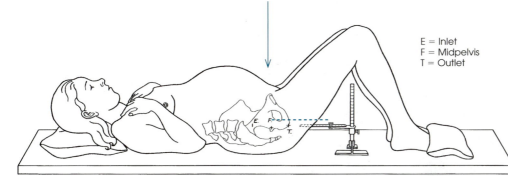

E = Inlet
F = Midpelvis
T = Outlet

Fig. 19-26. Pelvimetry, AP projection with ruler in place.

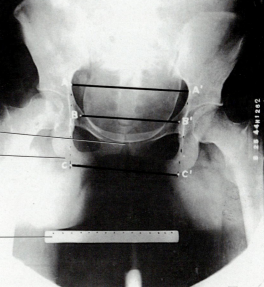

Fig. 19-27. Pelvimetry, AP projection.

Symphysis pubis

Ischial tuberosity

Metal ruler

Pelvimetry

LATERAL PROJECTION
R or L position
COLCHER-SUSSMAN METHOD

Position of patient

- Ask the patient to turn to a lateral position, and center the median coronal plane of the patient's body to the midline of the table.
- Partially extend the thighs so that they will not obscure the pubic bones.
- Place sandbags under and between the knees and ankles to immobilize the legs.
- Place a folded sheet or other suitable support under the lower thorax, and adjust the support so that the long axis of the lumbar vertebrae is parallel with the tabletop.

- Adjust the body in a true lateral position.
- Turn the ruler lengthwise and adjust its height to coincide with the median sagittal plane of the patient's body.
- Place the pelvimeter so that the metal ruler lies within the upper part of the gluteal fold and against the midsacrum (Fig. 19-28).
- Center the cassette at the level of the most prominent point of the greater trochanter (Fig. 19-29).
- Ask the patient to suspend respiration at the end of inhalation.

Central ray

- Direct the central ray perpendicular to the most prominent point of the greater trochanter.

□ Evaluation criteria

The following should be clearly demonstrated:

- Superimposed hips and femora.
- No superimposition of the symphysis pubis by the femurs.
- Entire pelvis, sacrum, and coccyx.
- Metal ruler with centimeter markings visible.
- Density permitting visualization of all pelvic landmarks and intersecting diameters.
- Entire fetal head.

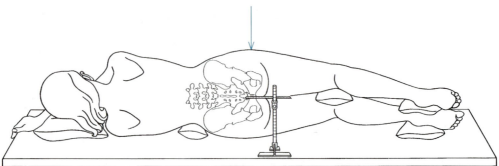

Fig. 19-28. Pelvimetry. Lateral projection with ruler in place.

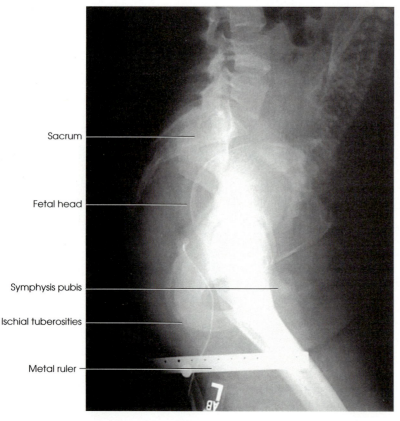
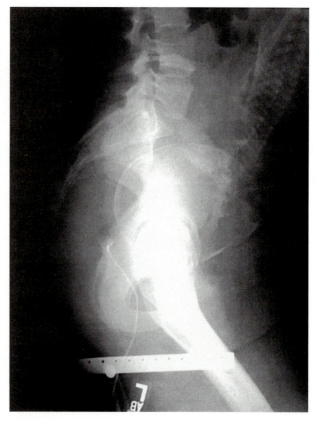

Sacrum

Fetal head

Symphysis pubis

Ischial tuberosities

Metal ruler

Fig. 19-29. Pelvimetry. Lateral projection.

(Courtesy Annette Baldwin, R.T.)

LOCALIZATION OF INTRAUTERINE DEVICES

Intrauterine devices (IUDs) remain a contraceptive option. On occasion, these devices may become dislocated from the uterine cavity. If this occurs, exact location of the IUD must be determined, and in some cases radiography is indicated. Therefore it is necessary to become acquainted with the radiographic appearance of IUDs.

The initial approach in determining the location of an IUD is by physician pelvic examination. If the IUD is not located, a sterile probe may be passed into the uterine cavity and radiographs taken at that time.

AP and lateral projections of the abdomen are suggested for localization, and occasionally oblique projections are indicated. Most IUDs are radiopaque because of their inherent metallic density or because of barium impregnated in the plastic during their manufacture. It should be emphasized that radiography alone is *not* a reliable way to diagnose extrauterine localization of an IUD.

In the early 1980s, five IUDs were available for use. In the late 1980s, three IUDs were removed from the American market by the manufacturers. In the mid-1990s, only two IUDs are available for use in the United States: the Paragard and the Progestasert (Fig. 19-30).

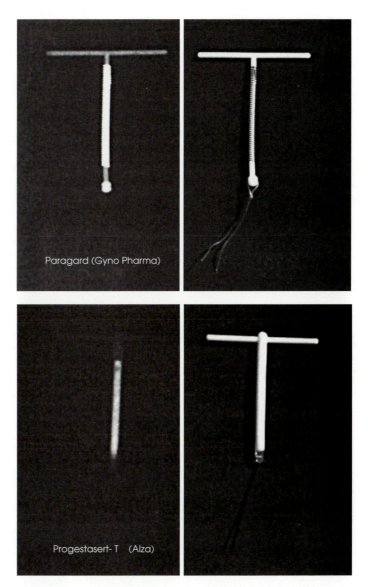

Fig. 19-30. Comparison of IUDs by radiography *(left images)* and photography *(right images)*. Actual size shown.

Male Radiography

SEMINAL DUCTS

Radiologic examinations of the seminal ducts[1-3] are performed in the investigation of selected genitourinary abnormalities such as cysts, abscesses, tumors, inflammation, and sterility. The regional terms applied to these examinations are *vesiculography, epididymography,* and, when combined, *epididymovesiculography.*

The contrast medium employed for these procedures is one of the water-soluble, iodinated compounds used for intravenous urography. Gaseous contrast medium can be injected into each scrotal sac to improve contrast when examining the extrapelvic structures.

The seminal vesicles are sometimes opacified directly by urethroscopic catheterization of the ejaculatory ducts. More frequently, the entire duct system is inspected by introducing the contrast solution into the canals by way of the ductus deferens. This requires that small bilateral incisions be made in the upper part of the scrotum for the exposure and identification of these ducts. The needle that is used for the injection of the contrast medium is

---

[1]Boreau J et al: Epididymography, Med Radiogr Photogr 29:63-66, 1953.
[2]Boreau J: L'étude radiologique des voies séminales normales et pathologiques, Paris, 1953, Masson & Cie.
[3]Vasselle B: Etude radiologique des voies séminales de l'homme, Paris, 1953 (thesis).

inserted into the duct in the direction of the portion of the tract under investigation—distally for the study of the extrapelvic ducts and then proximally for the study of the intrapelvic ducts.

A nongrid exposure technique is used for the delineation of extrapelvic structures (Figs. 19-31 to 19-33). The examining urologist places the film and adjusts the position of the testes for the desired projections of the ducts. A grid technique is used to demonstrate the intrapelvic ducts (Figs. 19-34 to 19-36). AP and oblique projections are made on 8 × 10 in (18 × 24 cm) or 10 × 12 in (24 × 30 cm) cassettes that are placed lengthwise and centered at the level of the superior border of the symphysis pubis.

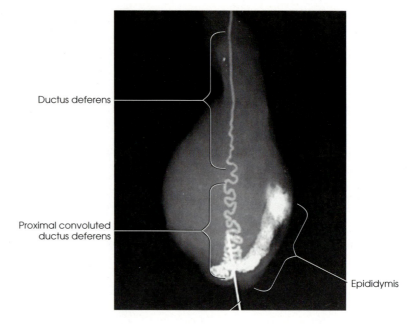

Ductus deferens

Proximal convoluted ductus deferens

Epididymis

Fig. 19-31. Epididymogram. Normal epididymis showing origin of ductus deferens. Needle is at epididymovasal kink, which can be palpated.

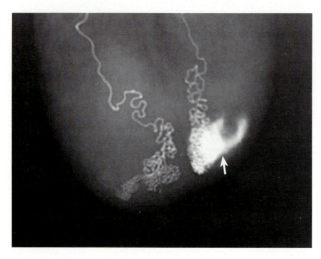

Fig. 19-32. Epididymogram. Tuberculosis (cold abscess) of epididymis *(arrow).*

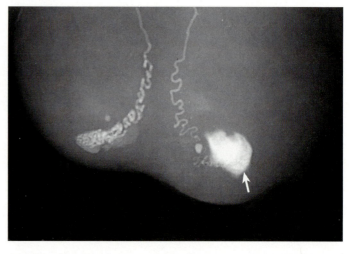

Fig. 19-33. Epididymogram. Epididymal abscess *(arrow)* observed during acute orchitis (third relapse). Epididymovasal kink is atrophic.

(Courtesy Dr. Jacques Boreau.)

□Evaluation criteria

The following should be clearly demonstrated:

AP

- Film centered at the level of the superior border of the symphysis pubis.
- No rotation of the patient.
- A short scale of contrast on radiograph to optimally demonstrate the seminal ducts.

Oblique

- Film centered at the level of the superior border of the symphysis pubis.
- No superimposition of the seminal ducts by the ilia.
- No overlap of the region of the prostate or urethra by the uppermost thigh.

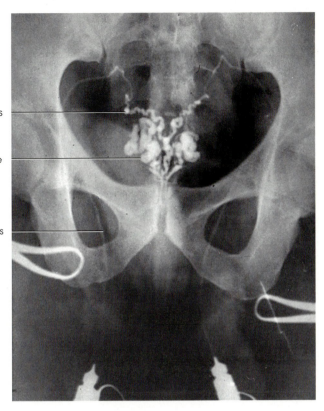

Distal ductus deferens

Seminal vesicle

Proximal ductus deferens

Fig. 19-34. Normal vesiculogram.

(Courtesy Dr. David Benninghoff.)

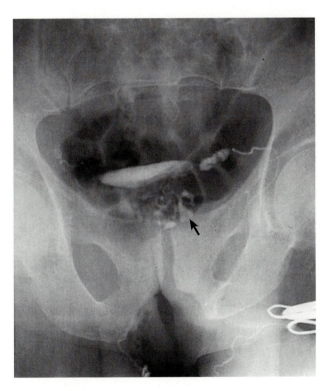

Fig. 19-35. Vesiculogram. Tuberculous seminal vesicle associated with deferentitis demonstrating small abscesses, ampulitis, and considerable vesiculitis on left (*arrow*).

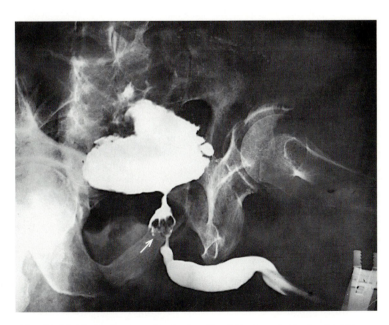

Fig. 19-36. Vesiculogram. Beginning (budding) metastasis of crista urethralis (*arrow*) discovered 2 years after prostatectomy for cancer of prostate.

PROSTATE

Prostatography is a term applied to the investigation of the prostate by either radiographic, cystographic, or vesiculographic procedures. It is seldom performed today because of advancements in the diagnostic value of ultrasound.

The normal prostate cannot be demonstrated radiographically. Radiographic studies are made for the detection of calcareous deposits and, as shown by urinary retention, of prostatic enlargement. Other known or suspected abnormalities of the gland are investigated by cystourethrographic or vesiculographic procedures. Sugiura and Hasegawa[1] reported a method of contrast prostatography wherein a water-soluble contrast medium is injected directly into the prostate by way of the rectal wall. Since ultrasonography is widely being used as a technique to evaluate the prostate, the following procedure therefore may be used only on special patients.

Preparation of the patient for radiographic studies usually consists of evacuating the lower bowel with a cleansing enema and requesting the patient to empty his bladder immediately before the examination.

---

[1]Sugiura H and Hasegawa S: Clinical evaluation of transrectal prostatography, AJR 111:157-164, 1971.

The following steps are then observed:
- Place the patient in the supine position, with the central ray directed to a point about 1 inch (2.5 cm) above the symphysis pubis at a caudal angulation of 15 degrees. The prone position is preferred because it places the prostate closer to, and the sacrococcygeal vertebrae farther from, the film, where their shadows can be projected above the region of the prostate (Fig. 19-37).
- With the patient in the prone position, center the median sagittal plane of the body to the midline of the grid.
- Place an 8 × 10 in (18 × 24 cm) cassette lengthwise in the Bucky tray and center it approximately 2 inches (5 cm) above the symphysis pubis.
- Direct the central ray through the region of the anus at an angle of 20 to 25 degrees cephalad to project the prostate above the pubic arch (Figs. 19-38 to 19-39).

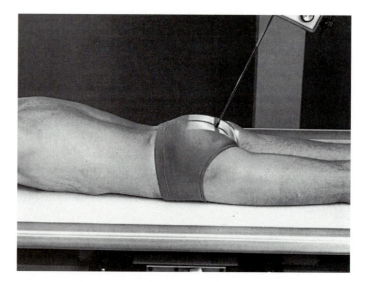

Fig. 19-37. Prostatography. PA axial projection.

Tom McMahon

□ Evaluation criteria

The following should be clearly demonstrated:

- Film centered slightly above the symphysis pubis.
- Prostate projected between the symphysis pubis and the coccyx.

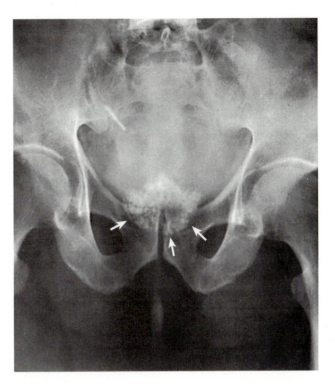

Fig. 19-38. Prostatography. PA projection showing prostatic enlargement with extensive glandular calcification (*arrows*).

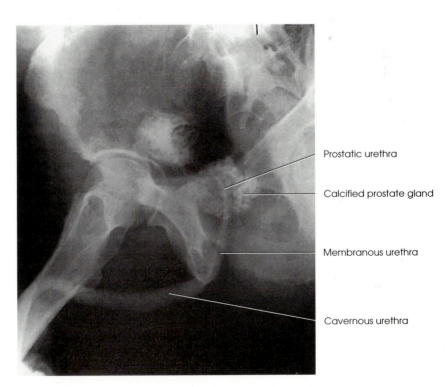

Prostatic urethra

Calcified prostate gland

Membranous urethra

Cavernous urethra

Fig. 19-39. Retrograde urethrogram of same patient as in Fig. 19-38. Note relationship of proximal urethra to prostate gland.

(Courtesy Dr. Oswald S. Lowsley.)

Chapter 20

SKULL

Patient positioned for a PA skull radiograph. The head is immobilized with head clamps.

Skull

The skull, or bony framework of the head, is divided into two parts: (1) the *cranium*, which is composed of eight bones (Figs. 20-1 to 20-4), and (2) the *face*, which is composed of 14 bones (Figs. 20-24 and 20-25). The cranial bones are rigidly jointed together by articulations called *sutures*, and they form the protective housing for the brain. These bones are as follows: one *frontal*, one *ethmoid*, two *parietal*, one *sphenoid*, two *temporal* (that contain the organs of hearing and balance), and one *occipital*. The facial bones, with the exception of the mandible, are also rigidly jointed together by sutures. These bones form the protective housing for the upper ends of the respiratory and digestive tracts and, with several of the cranial bones, form the orbital sockets for the protection of the organs of sight. The facial bones are as follows: two *nasal bones*, two *lacrimal bones*, two *maxillae*, two *zygomatic bones* or *malars*, two *palatine bones* (Fig. 20-4), two *inferior nasal con-chae* or *turbinates*, one *vomer*, and one *mandible*. The *hyoid bone* is commonly included with this group of bones; it will be considered later.

The bones of the cranial vault are composed of two plates of compact tissue separated by an inner layer of spongy tissue called *diploe*. The outer plate, or table, is thicker than the inner table over most of the vault, and the thickness of the layer of spongy tissue varies considerably. The internal surfaces of the bones forming the vault of the cranium are marked with narrow, branchlike grooves (the *meningeal grooves*) and with relatively larger channels (called *sulci*), which lodge blood vessels of various sizes.

The bones of the cranium and face, except for the mandible, are joined by synarthrodial joints called *sutures*. The most commonly referred to sutures are the coronal, sagittal, squamosal, and lambdoidal (Figs. 20-1 and 20-2). The *coronal suture* is found between the frontal and parietal bones. The *sagittal suture* is located between the two parietal bones and just behind the coronal suture line. Thus, it is the only suture discussed here which is not visible in these two figures. The junction of the coronal and sagittal sutures is the *bregma*. Between the temporal bones and the parietal bones are the *squamosal sutures*. Between the occipital bone and the parietal bones is the *lambdoidal suture*. The *lambda* is the junction of the lambdoidal and sagittal sutures. On the lateral aspect of the skull, the junction of the parietal bone, the squamosal suture, and the greater wing of the sphenoid is the *pterion*, which overlies the middle meningeal artery. At the junction of the occipital bone, the parietal bone, and the mastoid portion of the temporal bone is the *asterion*.

In the newborn infant the bones are thin and incompletely developed. They contain a small amount of calcium, are indistinctly marked, and present six areas of in-

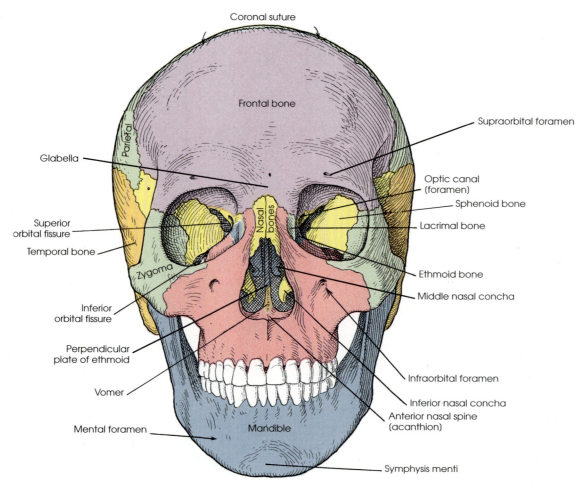

Fig. 20-1. Anterior aspect of cranium. For anatomy of the facial bones, see Figs. 20-24 and 20-25.

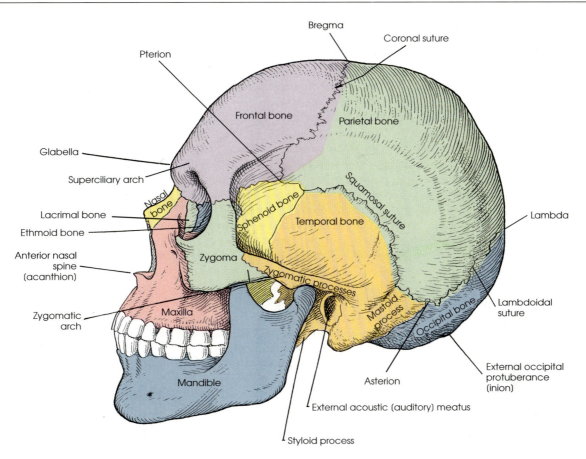

Fig. 20-2. Lateral aspect of cranium. For anatomy of the facial bones, see Fig. 20-24 and 20-25.

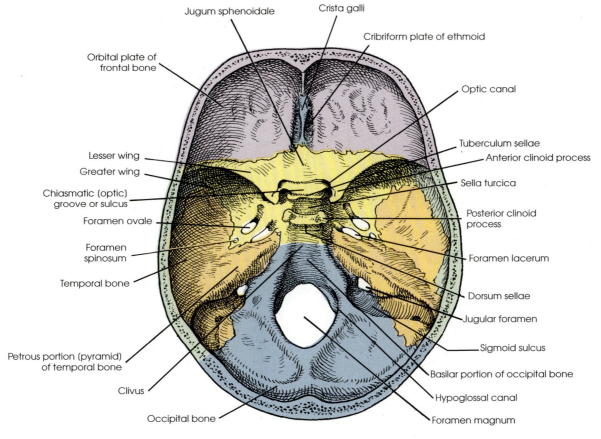

Fig. 20-3. Superior aspect of cranial base.

complete ossification called *fontanels.* Two of the fontanels are situated in the median sagittal plane at the superior and posterior angles of the parietal bones. The anterior fontanel is located at the junction of the two parietal and the one frontal bone at the bregma. Posteriorly and also in the median sagittal plane is the posterior fontanel, located at the point labeled *lambda* on Fig. 20-2. Two fontanels are also on each side at the inferior angles of the parietal bones. Each sphenoidal (anterolateral) fontanel is found at the site of the pterion; the mastoid (posterolateral) fontanels are found at the asterions. The posterior and sphenoidal (anterolateral) fontanels normally close at the first and third months, respectively, and the anterior and mastoid (posterolateral) fontanels close during the second year. The cranium develops rapidly in size and density during the first 5 or 6 years, after which time there is a gradual increase to adult size and density, usually reached by the age of 12 years. The thickness and degree of mineralization in normal adult crania show comparatively little difference in radiopacity from subject to subject, and the

atrophy of old age is less marked than in other regions of the body.

Internally, the cranium appears to be divided into three regions: the anterior, middle, and posterior cranial fossae (Fig. 20-3). The *anterior cranial fossa* extends from the anterior frontal bone to the lesser wings of the sphenoid. It is mainly associated with the frontal lobes of the cerebrum. The *middle cranial fossa* accommodates the temporal lobes and associated neurovascular structures and extends from the lesser wings of the sphenoid bone to the apices of the petrous portions of the temporal bones. The deep depression posterior to the petrous ridges is the *posterior cranial fossa,* which protects the cerebellum, pons, and medulla oblongata.

The average, or so-called normal, cranium is more or less oval in shape, being wider behind than in front. The average cranium measures approximately 6 inches (15 cm) at its widest point from side to side, 7 inches (18 cm) at its longest point from front to back, and 9 inches (22 cm) at its deepest point from the vertex to the submental region. Crania vary in size and shape, resulting in a variation in the position and relationship of internal parts.

Internal deviations from the normal are usually indicated by the external deviations and thus can be estimated with a reasonable degree of accuracy. There is a 1-inch (2.5 cm) difference between the width and length of the normally shaped head. Any deviation from this relationship indicates a comparable change in relationship of the internal structures. If the deviation involves more than a 5-degree change, it must be compensated for either by a change in part rotation or by the central ray angulation. This rule applies to all images except direct laterals. A ½-inch (1 cm) change in the 1-inch (2.5 cm) width-to-length measurement indicates an approximate 5-degree change in the direction of the internal parts with reference to the median sagittal plane.

It is not necessary for the radiographer to know the minute details of the complex structure of the cranium. However, it is necessary to understand cranial anatomy from the standpoint of size and shape and the position and relationship of the cranium's component parts, so that estimations and compensations can be made for deviations from the normal.

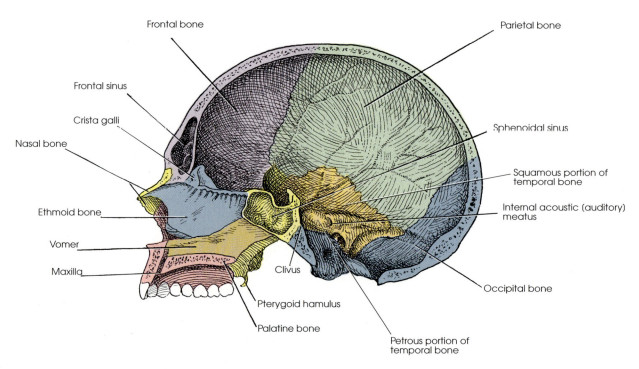

Fig. 20-4. Lateral aspect of interior of cranium.

Cranial Bones

FRONTAL BONE

The frontal bone consists of a vertical portion, called the *squama,* which forms the forehead and the anterior part of the vault, and horizontal portions, which form the orbital plates (roofs of the orbits), part of the roof of the nasal cavity, and the greater part of the anterior cranial fossa (Figs. 20-5 to 20-7).

On each side of the median sagittal plane of the superior portion of the squama is a rounded elevation called the *frontal eminence* (frontal tuberosity). Below the frontal eminences, just above the supraorbital margins, are two arched ridges that correspond in position to the eyebrows. These ridges are called the *superciliary arches* (ridges). The smooth elevation between the superciliary arches (ridges) is termed the *glabella.*

The *frontal air sinuses* are situated between the two tables of the squama on each side of the median sagittal plane, and from the lower margin of the squama they extend superiorly, laterally, and posteriorly. These sinuses are separated by a bony wall, the intersinus septum, which may be incomplete and usually deviates from the midline. The frontal sinuses vary greatly in size, and they are frequently divided into a number of loculi by the presence of other septa.

The squama articulates with the parietal bones at the coronal suture, with the greater wing of the sphenoid bone at the frontosphenoidal suture and with the nasal bones at the frontonasal suture. The midpoint of the frontonasal suture is termed the *nasion.*

The orbital plates of the horizontal portion of the frontal bone are separated by a notch, called the *ethmoidal notch,* that receives the cribriform plate of the ethmoid bone. At the anterior edge of the ethmoidal notch is a small inferior projection of bone, the *nasal (frontal) spine,* which is the most superior component of the bony nasal septum. The posterior margins of the orbital plates articulate with the lesser wings of the sphenoid bone.

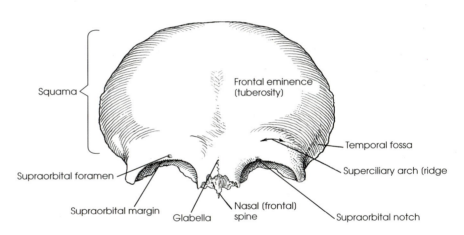

Fig. 20-5. Anterior aspect of frontal bone.

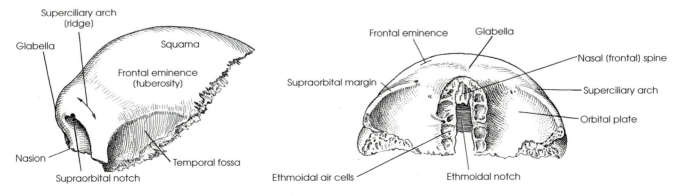

Fig. 20-6. Lateral aspect of frontal bone.

Fig. 20-7. Inferior aspect of frontal bone.

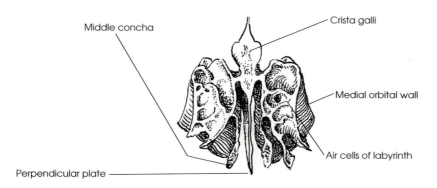

Fig. 20-8. Anterior aspect of ethmoid bone.

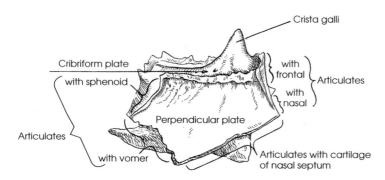

Fig. 20-9. Lateral aspect of ethmoid bone with labyrinth removed.

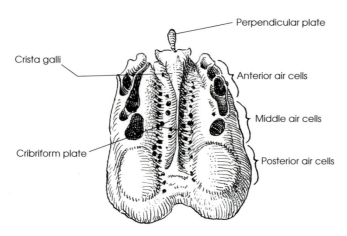

Fig. 20-10. Superior aspect of ethmoid bone.

ETHMOID BONE

The ethmoid bone is a small, cube-shaped bone (Figs. 20-8 to 20-10) that consists of a horizontal plate, a vertical plate, and two light, spongy lateral labyrinths (masses). Situated between the orbits, the ethmoid bone forms part of the anterior cranial fossa and part of the nasal and orbital walls and nasal septum.

The horizontal portion, called the *cribriform plate,* is received into the ethmoidal notch of the frontal bone. Perforated by many foramina for the transmission of the olfactory nerves, the cribriform plate has a thick, conical process, called the *crista galli,* projecting superiorly from its anterior midline which serves as the anterior attachment for the falx cerebri.

The vertical portion is called the *perpendicular plate.* This plate is a thin, flat bone that projects inferiorly from the inferior surface of the cribriform plate and, with the nasal (frontal) spine, forms the superior portion of the bony septum of the nose.

The *labyrinths* (lateral masses) contain the ethmoidal air cells. The cells of each side are arbitrarily divided into three groups, called the anterior, the middle, and posterior ethmoidal air cells. The walls of the labyrinths (lateral masses) form a part of the medial walls of the orbits and a part of the lateral walls of the nasal cavity. Projecting inferiorly from each medial wall of the labyrinths are two thin, scroll-shaped processes called the *superior* and *middle nasal conchae* (turbinates).

Skull

PARIETAL BONES

The two parietal bones are square in shape and have a convex external surface and a concave internal surface (Figs. 20-11 and 20-12). The parietal bones form a large portion of the sides of the cranium, and by their articulation with each other at the sagittal suture in the median sagittal plane, they form the posterior portion of its roof.

Each parietal bone presents a prominent bulge, called the *parietal eminence* (tuberosity), near the central portion of its external surface. In radiography the width of the head should be measured at this point, the widest point of the head.

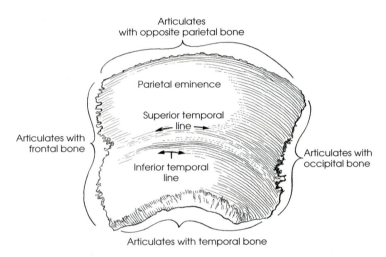

Fig. 20-11. External surface of parietal bone.

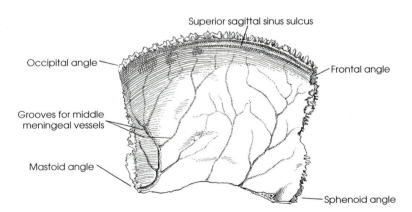

Fig. 20-12. Internal surface of parietal bone.

SPHENOID BONE

The sphenoid bone is an irregularly wedge-shaped bone situated in the base of the cranium between the horizontal portion of the frontal bone, the basilar portion of the occipital bone, and the petrous and squamous portions of the temporal bone (Figs. 20-13 to 20-15). The sphenoid bone consists of a body, two lesser wings and two greater wings, which project laterally from the sides of the body, and two pterygoid processes, which project inferiorly from each side of the inferior surface of the body.

The *body* of the sphenoid bone contains the two sphenoidal air sinuses, which are incompletely separated by a median septum. The anterior surface of the body forms the posterior bony wall of the nasal cavity. The superior surface presents a deep depression that is called the *hypophyseal fossa* and lodges a gland known as the *hypophysis* (pituitary body). The bone surrounding the hypophyseal fossa is termed the *sella turcica* because of its resemblance to a turkish saddle. The sella turcica lies in the median sagittal plane of the cranium at a point ¾ inch (2 cm) anterior to and ¾ inch (2 cm) superior to the level of the external acoustic (auditory) meatus. The sella turcica is bounded anteriorly by the *tuberculum sellae* and posteriorly by the *dorsum sellae*, which bears the *posterior clinoid processes*. The slanted area of bone posterior and inferior to the dorsum sellae is continuous with the basilar portion of the occipital bone and is called the *clivus*. The clivus supports the pons. On either side of the sella turcica is a groove, the *carotid sulcus*, in which lies the internal carotid artery and the cavernous sinus.

The *chiasmatic* (optic) *groove* or *sulcus* extends across the anterior portion of the superior surface of the body of the sphenoid bone. This groove accommodates the *optic chiasma*, which is the structure formed by the approach and crossing of the two optic nerves. The groove is bounded anteriorly by the jugum sphenoidale and posteriorly by the tuberculum sellae. The groove ends on each side at the optic canal, the passage opening into the apex of the orbit for the transmission of the optic nerve and ophthalmic artery.

The *lesser wings* are triangular in shape and nearly horizontal in position. They arise, one on each side, from the anterosuperior portion of the body of the sphenoid bone and project laterally, where they end in sharp points. The lesser wings form the posteromedial portion of the roofs of the orbits (the ridge between the lesser wings is known as the *jugum sphenoidale* [Fig. 20-13]), the posterior portion of the anterior cranial fossa, the upper margin of the *superior orbital fissures*, and the *optic canals*. The medial ends of their posterior borders form the *anterior clinoid processes*. Each arises from two roots. The anterior (superior) root is thin and flat, and the posterior (inferior) root, referred to as the *sphenoid strut*, is thick and rounded. The circular opening between the two roots is known as the optic foramen or, because of its length, as the *optic canal*. The canals measure from 4 to 9 mm in length and about 5.5 mm in diameter.

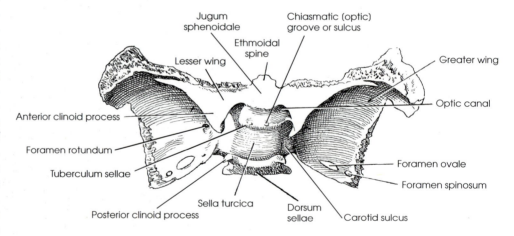

Fig. 20-13. Superior aspect of sphenoid bone.

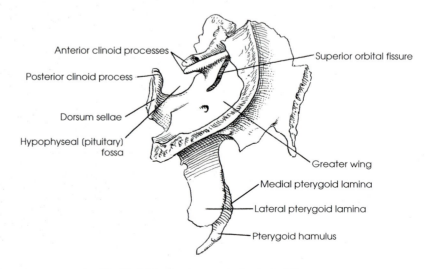

Fig. 20-14. Lateral aspect of sphenoid bone.

The *greater wings* arise from the sides of the body and curve laterally, posteriorly, anteriorly, and superiorly. The greater wings form a part of the middle cranial fossa, the posterolateral walls of the orbits, the lower margin of the superior orbital fissures, and the greater part of the posterior margin of the inferior orbital fissures. The foramina rotundum, ovale, and spinosum are paired and are situated in the greater wings. These foramina transmit nerves and blood vessels, so they are subject to radiologic investigation for the detection of erosive lesions of neurogenic or vascular origin. The *foramen rotundum* is a round aperture and is horizontally placed in the anteromedial portion of the greater wing adjacent to the lateral wall of the sphenoidal sinus. The *foramen ovale,* the largest of these foramina, is usually oval in shape and is situated laterally and posteriorly to the foramen rotundum. The *foramen spinosum,* the smallest of these foramina, is situated near the posterior angle of the greater wing, just lateral and posterior to the foramen ovale.

The *pterygoid processes* arise from the lateral portions of the inferior surface of the body and the medial portions of the inferior surfaces of the greater wings and project inferiorly and curve laterally. Each pterygoid process consists of two plates of bone, the *medial* and *lateral pterygoid laminae,* that are fused at their superoanterior parts. The inferior extremity of the medial lamina possesses an elongated, hook-shaped process, the *pterygoid hamulus,* which makes it longer and narrower than the lateral lamina. The pterygoid processes articulate with the palatine bones anteriorly and with the alae of the vomer where they enter into the formation of the nasal cavity.

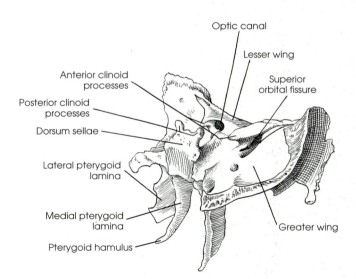

Fig. 20-15. Oblique aspect of upper and lateroposterior aspects of sphenoid bone (right lateral pterygoid lamina removed).

OCCIPITAL BONE

The *occipital bone* is situated at the posteroinferior part of the cranium. It forms the posterior and almost half of the base of the cranium and the greater part of the posterior cranial fossa (Figs. 20-16 to 20-18). The occipital bone consists of four parts and has a large aperture, the *foramen magnum*, that contains the inferior portion of the medulla oblongata as it passes into the cranial cavity. The four parts of the occipital bone are (1) the squama, which is saucer-shaped, being convex externally; and (2 and 3) two lateral condylar portions that extend anteriorly, one on each side of the foramen magnum, from the squama to their junction with (4) the *basilar part*.

The *squama* curves posteriorly and superiorly from the foramen magnum and is also curved from side to side. It articulates with the parietal bones at the lambdoidal suture and with the mastoid portions of the temporal bones at the occipitomastoid sutures. On the external surface of the squama, midway between its summit and the foramen magnum, there is a prominent process termed the *external occipital protuberance* (inion), which corresponds in position to the internal occipital protuberance. Extending laterally and inferiorly from the external occipital protuberance (inion) are the *superior, median, and inferior nuchal lines*. The internal surface of the squama is divided into four fossae, which are separated by sulci for the transverse, occipital, and sagittal venous sinuses. The two upper fossae accommodate the occipital lobes of the cerebrum, and the two lower fossae accommodate the hemispheres of the cerebellum.

The *lateral condylar portions* project anteriorly, one from each side of the squama. Part of each lateral portion curves medially to fuse with the basilar portion and thus to complete the foramen magnum, and part of it projects laterally to form the jugular process. On the inferior surface of the curved parts, extending from the level of the middle of the foramen magnum anteriorly to the level of its anterior margin, there are reciprocally shaped condyles for articulation with the superior facets of the atlas. These articulations are known as the *occipitoatlantal joints,* and they are the only bony articulations between the skull and the neck. The *hypoglossal canals* are found at the anterior ends of the condyles and transmit the hypoglossal nerves. At the posterior end of the condyles are the condylar canals.

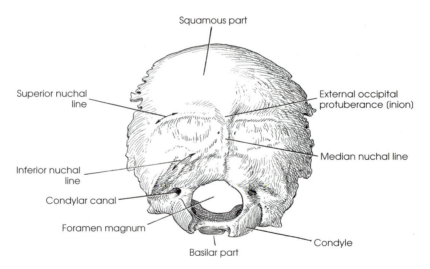

Fig. 20-16. External surface of occipital bone.

Squamous part

Superior nuchal line

External occipital protuberance (inion)

Inferior nuchal line

Median nuchal line

Condylar canal

Foramen magnum

Condyle

Basilar part

Skull

The *jugular process* presents, on its anterior border, a deep notch that forms the posterior and medial boundary of a venous passage known as the *jugular foramen*. The extremity of the process articulates with a reciprocally shaped process on the inferior surface of the temporal petrosa beside a deep depression, the jugular fossa, that forms the anterior and lateral boundary of the jugular foramen. The right jugular foramen is normally somewhat larger than the left, and each opening is partially divided by bony projections into medial and lateral parts. The jugular foramen is situated directly below the internal acoustic (auditory) meatus, with its floor at the level of, and just lateral to, the anterior third of the occipital condyles.

The *basilar portion* curves anteriorly and superiorly to its junction with the body of the sphenoid. In the adult the basilar part of the occipital bone fuses with the body of the sphenoid bone, resulting in formation of a continuous bone. The sloping surface of this junction between the dorsum sellae of the sphenoid bone and the basilar portion of the occipital bone is called the *clivus*.

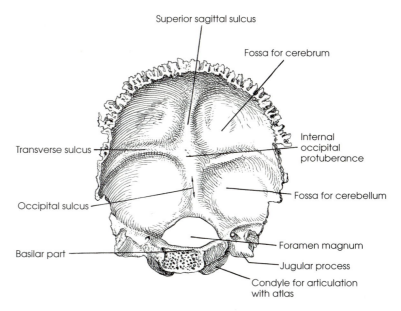

Fig. 20-17. Internal surface of occipital bone.

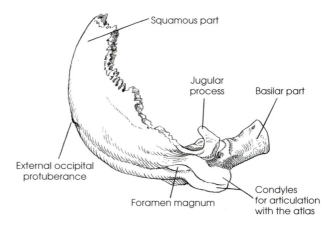

Fig. 20-18. Lateroinferior aspect of occipital bone.

TEMPORAL BONES

The temporal bones are irregular in shape (Figs. 20-19 to 20-22) and are situated on each side of the base of the cranium between the greater wings of the sphenoid bone and the occipital bone. The temporal bones form a large part of the middle fossa of the cranium and part of the posterior fossa. Each temporal bone consists of a squamous portion, a tympanic portion, a styloid process, a zygomatic process, and a petromastoid portion (a mastoid portion and a petrous portion) that contains the auditory organs and organs of balance.

The *squama* is the thin, upper portion of the temporal bone. This portion of the bone forms a part of the side wall of the cranium and has a prominent arched process, the *zygomatic process,* that projects anteriorly to articulate with the zygomatic bone of the face and thus complete the zygomatic arch. The superior border of the zygomatic process extends posteriorly above the external acoustic (auditory) meatus, where it merges with the *temporal line,* a smooth ridge that extends posteriorly and superiorly across the posterior part of the squama. The articular part of the mandibular fossa is formed by the inferior surfaces of the anterior portion of the squama and the posterior portion of the zygomatic process.

The *tympanic portion,* situated below the squama and in front of the mastoid and petrous portions of the temporal bone, forms the posterior part of the mandibular fossa. The tympanic portion also forms the anterior, the inferior, and part of the posterior walls of the *external acoustic meatus* (auditory canal); the superior part of the posterior wall and the superior wall, or roof, of the canal are formed by the squama. The external acoustic (auditory) meatus is approximately ½ inch (1.25 cm) in length and projects medially, slightly posteriorly, and slightly superiorly.

The *styloid process,* a slender, pointed bone of variable length, projects inferiorly, anteriorly, and slightly medially from the posteroinferior portion of the tympanic part of the temporal bone.

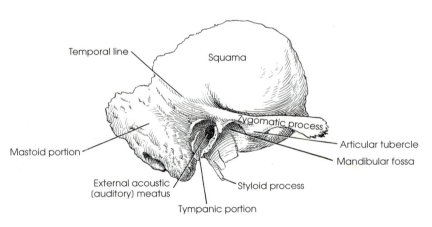

Fig. 20-19. Lateral aspect of temporal bone.

Temporal line — Squama — Zygomatic process — Articular tubercle — Mandibular fossa — Styloid process — Tympanic portion — External acoustic (auditory) meatus — Mastoid portion

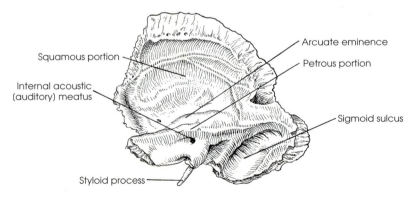

Fig. 20-20. Internal surface of temporal bone.

Squamous portion — Internal acoustic (auditory) meatus — Styloid process — Arcuate eminence — Petrous portion — Sigmoid sulcus

THE PETROMASTOID PORTIONS

The *petromastoid portion,* which is prolonged into the conical *mastoid process,* forms the inferior, posterior part of the temporal bone (Figs. 20-21 and 20-22). The mastoid portion articulates with the parietal bone at its superior border through the parietomastoid suture and with the occipital bone at its posterior border through the occipitomastoid suture, which is continuous with the lambdoidal suture. The mastoid process varies considerably in size, depending on its pneumatization, and is larger in the male than in the female. The first of the air cells to develop is situated at the upper anterior part of the process. The first air cell communicates with the tympanic cavity, is large in size, and is termed the *mastoid antrum* (tympanic antrum) to distinguish it from the other mastoid air cells. The mastoid antrum and the tympanic cavity are covered by a thin plate of bone called the *tegmen tympani.* Shortly before or after birth, smaller air cells begin to develop around the mastoid antrum and continue to increase in number and size until full development of the process is reached around puberty. However, the air cells vary considerably in both size and number; they sometimes extend well superiorly, posteriorly, and medially into the petrosa, and inferiorly to the tip of the process, ranging in size from large to very small cells. Occasionally they are absent altogether, in which case the mastoid process is solid bone and is usually small in size.

The *petrous portion* (also called the pars petrosa and the petrous pyramid) is conical or pyramidal in form and is the thickest, densest bone in the cranium. From its base at the squamous and mastoid portions, the petrous portion projects medially and anteriorly between the greater wing of the sphenoid bone and the occipital bone to the posterolateral angle of the body of the sphenoid bone, with which its apex articulates. The carotid artery, in the carotid canal, enters the inferior aspect of the petrous portion, passes superior to the cochlea, then passes medially to exit the petrous apex. At the center of the posterior aspect of the petrous portion is the *internal acoustic* (auditory) *meatus,* which transmits the vestibulocochlear and facial nerves. In the normally shaped head, the upper border of the pyramid lies at the infraorbitomeatal line, and its long axis forms an angle of 47 degrees, open posteriorly, with the median sagittal plane of the head. The petrous portion contains the organs of hearing and balance.

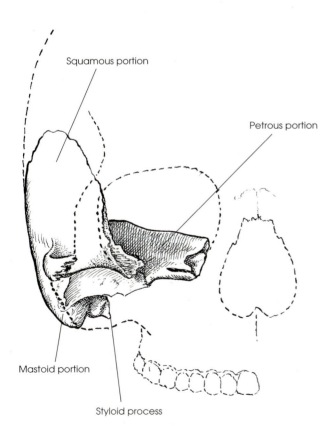

Fig. 20-21. Anterior aspect of temporal bone in relation to surrounding structures. (Chin slightly tucked for illustration.)

Squamous portion

Petrous portion

Mastoid portion

Styloid process

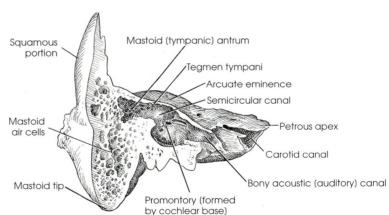

Fig. 20-22. Coronal section through mastoid and petrous portions of the temporal bone.

Squamous portion

Mastoid air cells

Mastoid tip

Mastoid (tympanic) antrum

Tegmen tympani

Arcuate eminence

Semicircular canal

Petrous apex

Carotid canal

Bony acoustic (auditory) canal

Promontory (formed by cochlear base)

Cranial bones

Vestibulocochlear Organ (Organ of Hearing and Balance)

The ear is the organ of hearing and balance and is therefore called the *vestibulocochlear* organ. The *ear* is a compound organ comprising the peripheral sensory apparatus of equilibrium as well as the acoustic (auditory) apparatus (Fig. 20-23). The essential parts of the ear are housed in the petrous portion of the temporal bone. The organ of hearing consists of three main divisions: the external ear, the middle ear, and the cochlea of the internal ear.

The *external ear* consists of two parts: (1) the oval-shaped, fibrocartilaginous, sound-collecting organ situated on the side of the head and known as the *auricle*, or *pinna*, and (2) a sound-conducting canal called the *external acoustic* (auditory) *meatus*. The auricle presents a deep central depression, the *concha*, the lower part of which leads into the external acoustic (auditory) meatus. At its anterior margin the auricle presents a prominent lip, the *tragus*, that projects posteriorly over the entrance of the meatus. The outer rim of the ear is the *helix*. The external acoustic (auditory) meatus is about 1 inch (2.5 cm) in length. The outer third of the canal wall is cartilaginous, and the inner two thirds are osseous. From the meatal orifice, the canal forms a slight curve as it passes medially and anteriorly in line with the axis of the internal acoustic (auditory) meatus. The external acoustic (auditory) meatus ends at the tympanic membrane of the middle ear.

The *middle ear* is situated between the external and the internal ear. The middle ear proper, called the *tympanum*, consists of (1) the *tympanic membrane* (or eardrum), (2) an irregularly shaped, air-containing compartment called the *tympanic cavity*, and (3) three small bones called the *auditory ossicles*. The middle ear communicates with the *mastoid* (tympanic) *antrum* and the *auditory* (eustachian or pharyngotympanic) *tube*, which are air-containing parts with which the tympanic cavity shares a continuous mucosal lining.

The tympanic membrane is a thin, concavoconvex membranous disk that has an elliptical shape. The disk, the convex surface of which is directed medially, is situated obliquely over the medial end of the external acoustic (auditory) meatus and serves as a partition between the external and the middle ear. The function of the tympanic membrane is the transmission of sound vibrations.

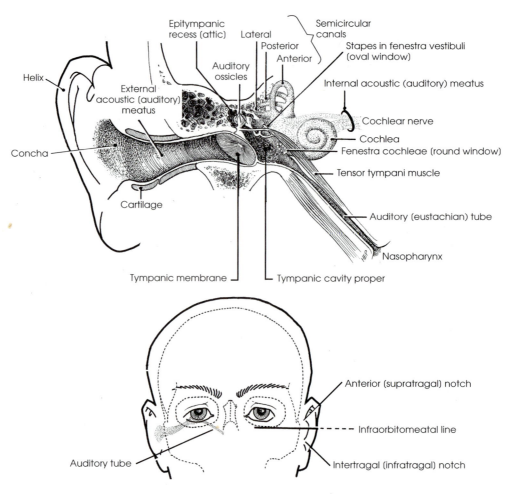

Fig. 20-23. Frontal section through right ear showing internal structures.

The tympanic cavity is a narrow, irregularly shaped chamber that lies just posteriorly and medially to the mandibular fossa. The cavity is separated from the external ear by the tympanic membrane and from the internal ear by the structures that occupy the fenestra vestibuli and fenestra cochleae (oval and round windows) on the intervening medial, or labyrinthine, wall; this wall presents a bulge called the *promontory,* the concave opposite side of which accommodates the first turn of the cochlea. The *fenestra vestibuli* (oval window) is situated above and posterior to the promontory, and the *fenestra cochlea* (round window) is located below and behind the promontory. The tympanic cavity communicates with the nasopharynx through the auditory (eustachian or pharyngotympanic) tube, a passage by which air pressure in the middle ear is equalized with the outside air passages. The auditory (eustachian or pharyngotympanic) tube is about 1¼ inches (3 cm) in length. The comparatively wide lateral ½ inch (1 cm) of the wall of the tube is osseous, and the gradually tapering medial portion is cartilaginous. From its entrance into the tympanic cavity, the auditory (eustachian or pharyngotympanic) tube passes medially and inferiorly to its orifice on the lateral wall of the nasopharynx.

The portion of the tympanic cavity lying below the level of the superior margin of the external acoustic auditory meatus is called the *tympanic cavity proper,* and the part lying above this level is called the *epitympanic recess* (tympanic attic). Through a large opening known as the *aditis ad antrum,* the epitympanic recess (tympanic attic) communicates posterosuperiorly with the mastoid antrum and mastoid air cells. The *mastoid antrum* is a large air cavity situated in the temporal bone above the mastoid air cells and immediately behind the epitympanic recess (tympanic attic). This area—the mastoid antrum, the epitympanic recess, and the intercommunicating aditus—is frequently referred to as the *key area.*

The auditory ossicles, named for their shape, are the *malleus* (hammer), the *incus* (anvil), and the *stapes* (stirrup). These three delicate bones are articulated to permit vibratory motion and are situated partly in the epitympanic recess (attic) and partly in the tympanic cavity proper. They bridge the middle ear cavity for the transmission of sound vibrations from the tympanic membrane to the internal ear. The handle of the malleus, the outermost of the ossicles, is attached to the tympanic membrane, and its head articulates with the central ossicle, the incus. The head of the stapes, the innermost of the ossicles, articulates with the incus, and its base, or footplate, is fitted into the fenestra vestibuli (oval window) of the inner ear.

The *internal ear* contains the essential sensory apparatus of hearing and equilibrium and lies on the densest portion of the petrous pyramid immediately below the arcuate eminence. Composed of an irregularly shaped bony chamber, called the *bony labyrinth,* the internal ear is housed within the bony chamber and is an intercommunicating system of ducts and sacs known as the *membranous labyrinth.* The bony labyrinth consists of three distinctly shaped parts: (1) a spirally coiled, tubular part called the *cochlea* (snail shell), which communicates with the middle ear through the membranous covering of the fenestra cochleae (round window); (2) a small, ovoid central compartment that is behind the cochlea and is known as the *vestibule,* which communicates with the middle ear by way of the fenestra vestibuli (base of the stapes); and (3) three unequally sized semicircular canals that form right angles to one another and are called, according to their positions, the *anterior* (superior), *posterior,* and *lateral semicircular canals.* The basal, or first turn of the cochlea is in close relationship with the labyrinthine wall, on which it produces the bulging promontory on the middle ear side and from whence its long axis is directed posteriorly and medially toward the internal acoustic (auditory)

meatus. From its cranial orifice the internal acoustic (auditory) meatus passes inferiorly and laterally for a distance of about ½ inch (1 cm). It is this canal through which the cochlear and vestibular nerves pass from their fibers in the respective parts of the membranous labyrinth to the brain. The membranous labyrinth corresponds in general form to the bony labyrinth but does not fill it, being partially suspended in fluid (the perilymph). The portions of the membranous labyrinth occupying the cochlea and the semicircular canals are ducts correspondingly named for the region each occupies. The vestibular portion of the membranous labyrinth consists of two sacs, the *utriculus* (utricle) and the *sacculus* (saccule), that are centrally connected by a narrow duct and that communicate with the cochlear and the semicircular ducts. In addition to the sensory apparatus, the ducts contain fluid called endolymph. The cochlea is concerned with hearing, and the vestibule and semicircular canals are concerned with equilibrium.

Facial Bones

NASAL BONES

The nasal bones are small and thin and vary in size and shape in different subjects (Figs. 20-24 and 20-25). They form the superior bony wall (called the "bridge" of the nose) of the nasal cavity. The nasal bones articulate with each other in the median sagittal plane, where at their posterosuperior surface they also articulate with the perpendicular plate of the ethmoid bone. They articulate with the frontal bone above and with the maxillae at the sides.

LACRIMAL BONES

The lacrimal bones, which are small and quite thin, are situated at the anterior part of the medial wall of the orbits between the labyrinth (lateral mass) of the ethmoid bone and the maxilla (Figs. 20-24 and 20-25). The lacrimal bones, together with the maxillae, form the lacrimal fossae, which accommodate the lacrimal sacs.

MAXILLAE

The maxillary bones are the largest of the immovable bones of the face (Figs. 20-24 and 20-25). They form part of the lateral walls and most of the floor of the nasal cavity, part of the floor of the orbital cavities, and three-fourths of the roof of the mouth. Their zygomatic processes articulate with the zygomatic bones and assist in the formation of the prominence of the cheeks. The body of each maxilla contains a large, pyramidal cavity called the *maxillary sinus* (antrum of Highmore).

At their inferior border, the maxillae present a thick, spongy ridge, called the *alveolar process,* that is excavated for the reception of the roots of the teeth. There is a depression on each side directly above the premolar teeth, at the level of the anterior nasal spine, which is termed the *canine fossa.* In the anterior median sagittal plane at their junction with each other and with the vomer, the maxillae form a pointed, forward-projecting process called the *anterior nasal spine.* The midpoint of this projection is called the *acanthion.*

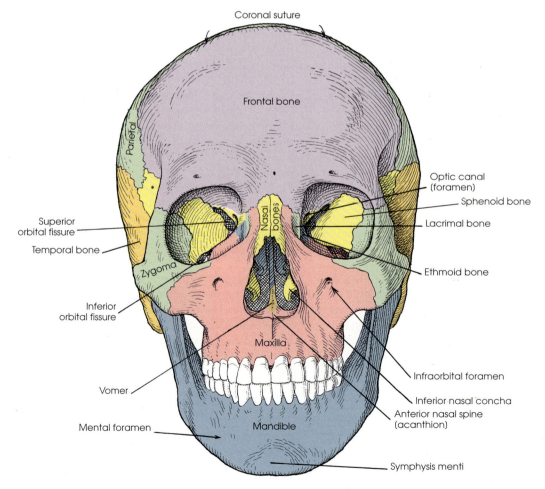

Fig. 20-24. Anterior aspect of skull demonstrating facial bones. For anatomy of the cranium, see Figs. 20-1 to 20-4.

ZYGOMATIC BONES

The zygomatic (malar) bones form the prominence of the cheeks and a part of the side wall and floor of the orbital cavities (Figs. 20-24 and 20-25). They articulate with the frontal bone superiorly, with the zygomatic process of the temporal bone at the side, with the maxilla anteriorly, and with the sphenoid bone posteriorly.

PALATINE BONES

The two palatine bones are L-shaped bones composed of vertical and horizontal plates. The horizontal plates articulate with the maxillae to complete the posterior fourth of the bony palate. The vertical portions of the palatine bones extend upward between the maxillae and the pterygoid processes of the sphenoid bone in the posterior nasal cavity. The superior tips of the vertical portions of the palatine bones assist in forming the posteromedial bony orbit.

INFERIOR NASAL CONCHAE

The inferior nasal conchae extend diagonally and inferiorly from the lateral walls of the nasal cavity at approximately its lower third (Fig. 20-24). They are long, narrow, and extremely thin and curl laterally, which gives them a scroll-like appearance. Each inferior concha presents two extremities, or processes of bone, that project superiorly from the attached superior border. One of these, the *ethmoid process,* articulates with the ethmoid bone. The other, called the *lacrimal process,* projects anteriorly and superiorly, articulates with the lacrimal bone, and enters into the formation of the bony lacrimal canal.

The three nasal conchae, the upper two of which are processes of the ethmoid bone, project into and divide the lateral portion of the respective side of the nasal cavity into superior, middle, and inferior meatuses. The space between the conchae and the nasal septum is called the *common nasal meatus.*

VOMER

The vomer is a thin plate of bone situated in the median sagittal plane of the floor of the nasal cavity, where it forms the inferior part of the bony septum of the nose (Fig. 20-24). The anterior border of the vomer slants superiorly and posteriorly from the anterior nasal spine to the body of the sphenoid bone, with which its superior border articulates. The superior part of its anterior border articulates with the perpendicular plate of the ethmoid bone; its posterior border is free.

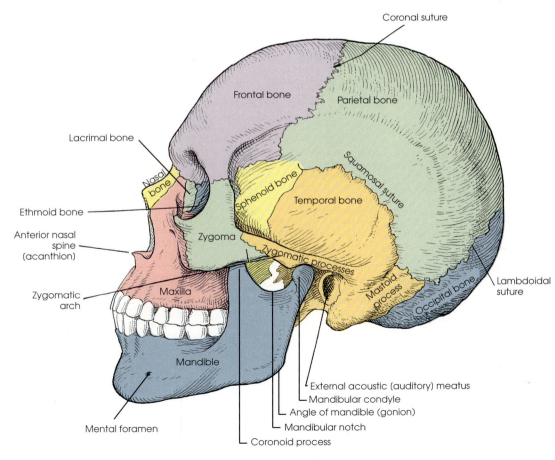

Fig. 20-25. Lateral aspect of skull demonstrating facial bones. For anatomy of the cranium, see Figs. 20-1 to 20-4.

MANDIBLE

The mandible is the largest and densest bone of the face (Figs. 20-26 and 20-27) and consists of a curved horizontal portion, called the *body,* and two vertical portions, called the *rami.* At birth the mandible consists of bilateral pieces held together by a fibrous symphysis that ossifies during the first year. At the site of ossification there is a slight ridge that ends below in a triangular prominence, the *mental protuberance,* the midpoint of which is called the *mental point.*

The superior border of the body of the mandible consists of spongy bone, called the *alveolar portion,* that presents excavations for the reception of the roots of the teeth. Below the second premolar tooth, approximately halfway between the superior and inferior borders of the bone, there is a small opening on each side for the transmission of nerves and blood vessels. These openings are called the *mental foramina.*

The rami project superiorly at an obtuse angle to the body of the mandible, and their broad surface forms an angle of approximately 110-120 degrees. Each ramus presents two processes at its upper extremity, one coronoid and one condylar, that are separated by a concave area called the *mandibular notch.* The anterior process, the *coronoid,* is thin and tapered and projects to a higher level than the posterior process. The *condylar* (condyloid) *process* consists of a constricted area, the neck, above which is a broad, thick, almost transversely placed *condyle* (head) that articulates with the mandibular fossa of the temporal bone. This articulation, called the *temporomandibular joint,* slants posteriorly approximately 15 degrees and inferiorly and medially approximately 15 degrees. Radiographic projections, being made from the opposite side, must reverse these directions; that is, the central ray angulation must be superior and anterior in order to coincide with the long axis of the joint. The temporomandibular joint is situated immediately in front of the external acoustic (auditory) meatus.

HYOID BONE

The hyoid bone is a small, U-shaped structure situated at the base of the tongue, where it is held in position in part by the stylohyoid ligaments extending from the styloid processes of the temporal bones (Fig. 20-28). The hyoid bone is divided into a *body,* two *greater cornua* (horns), and two *lesser cornua* (horns). The bone serves as an attachment for certain muscles of the throat and tongue.

Articulations of the Skull

The sutures of the skull are connected by teethlike projections of bone interlocked with a thin layer of fibrous tissue. These articulations allow for no movement and are classified as fibrous (synarthrotic) joints. The articulations of the facial bones, including the joints between the roots of the teeth and the jawbones, are fibrous (synarthrotic). The exception is the point at which the rounded condyle (head) of the mandible articulates with the mandibular fossa of the temporal bone to form the temporomandibular joint (TMJ). The TMJ articulation is a synovial (diarthrotic) ellipsoidal (condyloid) joint.

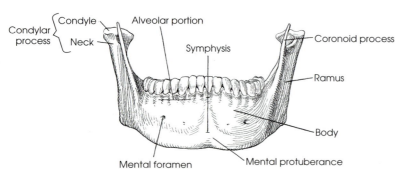

Fig. 20-26. Anterior aspect of mandible.

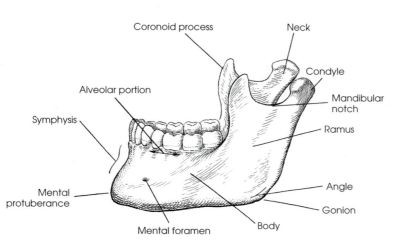

Fig. 20-27. Lateral aspect of mandible.

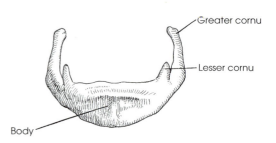

Fig. 20-28. Anterior aspect of hyoid.

Skull Topography

The basic localization points and planes (all of which can be either seen or palpated) used in radiographic positioning are illustrated in Figs. 20-29 and 20-30.

The *orbitomeatal line* is sometimes referred to as the radiographic base line. In the past some authors have referred to a less specific anatomic line simply as base line, a term that is usually reserved for the base line of the cranium. To eliminate doubt, the term *base line* is not used in this text, and the base line of the cranium is referred to as the *infraorbitomeatal line*.

In the adult, there exists an average 7-degree angle difference between the orbitomeatal line and the infraorbitomeatal line. An average 8-degree angle difference exists between the orbitomeatal line and the glabellomeatal line. The degree difference between the cranial positioning lines must be realized. Often the relationship of the patient, film, and central ray is the same, but the angle described may vary depending on the cranial line of reference.

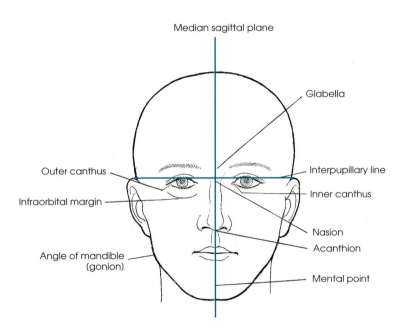

Median sagittal plane

Glabella

Outer canthus

Interpupillary line

Inner canthus

Infraorbital margin

Nasion

Acanthion

Angle of mandible (gonion)

Mental point

Fig. 20-29. Anterior landmarks.

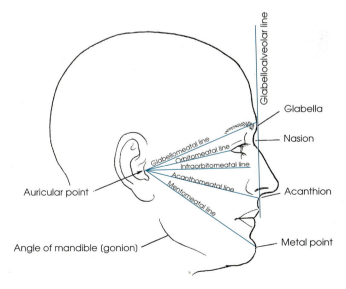

Glabelloalveolar line

Glabellomeatal line

Orbitomeatal line

Infraorbitomeatal line

Acanthomeatal line

Mentomeatal line

Glabella

Nasion

Acanthion

Auricular point

Metal point

Angle of mandible (gonion)

Fig. 20-30. Lateral landmarks.

Skull topography

Skull Morphology

Radiographic images of the skull are all based on the normal size and shape of the cranium. The rules for centering and adjustment of the localization points and planes and for the exact degree of angulation of the central ray have been established for each position. Although a majority of heads fall within the limits of normality and can be radiographed satisfactorily by using the established positions, a considerable number vary in shape enough to require an adjustment of the standard procedure in order to obtain an undistorted image.

In the typically shaped head (Fig. 20-31), the petrous pyramids project anteriorly and medially at an angle of 47 degrees and open posteriorly to the median sagittal plane of the skull; their superior borders are situated in the base of the cranium. The optic foramina lie at an angle of approximately 37 degrees, open anteriorly to the median sagittal plane.

The atypical cranium will, depending on its shape, require more or less rotation of the head or an increase or decrease in the angulation of the central ray compared with the typical, or *mesocephalic,* skull (Fig. 20-31). In the *brachycephalic* skull (Fig. 20-32), which is short from front to back, broad from side to side, and shallow from vertex to base, the internal structures are higher with reference to the infraorbitomeatal line and their long axes are more frontal in position; that is, they form a wider angle with the median sagittal plane. The petrous pyramids lie at an average angle of 54 degrees, open posteriorly. In the *dolichocephalic* skull (Fig. 20-33), which is long from front to back, narrow from side to side, and deep from vertex to base, the internal structures are lower with reference to the infraorbitomeatal line and their long axes are less frontal in position; that is, they form a narrower angle with the median sagittal plane. The petrous pyramids form an average angle of 40 degrees in the dolichocephalic skull.

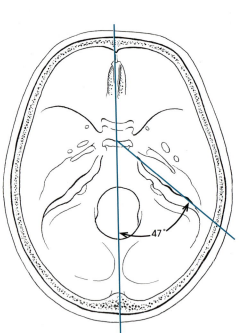

Fig. 20-31. Mesocephalic skull.

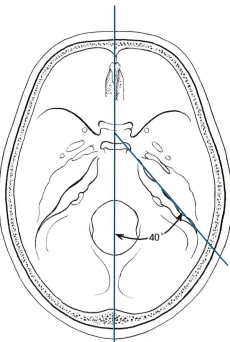

Fig. 20-33. Dolichocephalic skull.

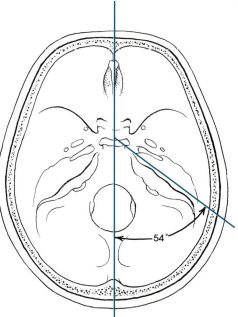

Fig. 20-32. Brachycephalic skull.

Asymmetry must also be considered. To name a few anomalies, the orbits are not always symmetric in size and shape, the lower jaw is often asymmetric, and the nasal bones and cartilage are frequently deviated from the median sagittal plane. There are many deviations that are not as obvious as these, but if the radiographer adheres to the fundamental rules of positioning, there will be comparatively little trouble. Varying the position of the part or the degree of angulation of the central ray to compensate for structural variations becomes a simple procedure if care and precision are used initially.

It is advisable to obtain a dry skull specimen, if possible, and radiograph it in the standard positions. This affords the best technique of studying the anatomy of the different parts of the cranium from both actual and radiographic standpoints. Compare the actual structure, its position in the head, its relationship to each of the adjacent structures in each position, and its relationship to the film and the angulation of the central ray with the resultant shadow on the radiograph. In this way the radiographer can develop the ability to look at a head as if it were transparent—to visualize the location and direction of the internal parts according to the shape of the cranium. By studying the shadow cast by the part being examined with reference to its relationship to the shadows of the adjacent structures, the radiographer learns to detect quickly and accurately any error in the image and any deviation from the normal cranium that requires compensation.

It is also advisable to keep a complete set of radiographs of a normally shaped skull. These radiographs can be used for comparison with atypical patients in determining the deviation and in deciding the correct adjustment to make in the degree and direction of part rotation or central ray angulation. Radiographic examples of correct and incorrect rotation of the skull are shown in Figs. 20-34 and 20-35.

The radiographic positions depicted in this volume show the patient either seated at a head unit or lying on a radiographic table. Whether the radiographer elects to perform the examination with the patient in the recumbent or upright position depends on three variables: (1) the equipment available, (2) the age and condition of the patient, and (3) the preference of the radiographer and/or radiologist.

With the exception of paranasal sinuses, which should be radiographed upright, the remaining radiographic positions are shown with the patient *either* upright or recumbent. To show all patient positions in *both* the upright and recumbent positions is indeed duplicative and not possible with the space available.

The reader is advised that comparable radiographs can usually be obtained with the patient either upright or recumbent. (For example, a recumbent skull radiograph can also be obtained with the patient upright as long as the radiographic base line and central ray angulation remain constant.) *Unless specifically noted in the text, the photographic illustration does not constitute a recommendation for performing the examination with the patient in either the upright or recumbent position.* To assist the reader, however, line drawings illustrating both table and upright radiography are included for most radiographic positions in this volume.

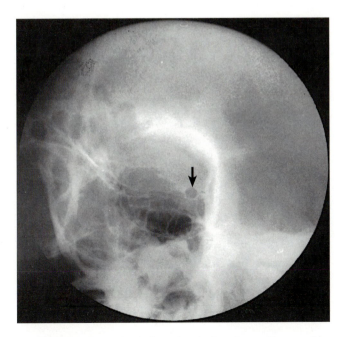

Fig. 20-34. Correct rotation clearly showing optic canal (*arrow*).

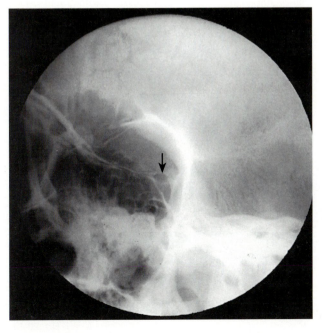

Fig. 20-35. Incorrect rotation for optic canal (*arrow*).

General Body Position

The position of the body is important in radiography of the skull. A majority of repeat examinations caused by rotation and by motion are the result of an uncomfortable body position. We often become so engrossed in adjusting the head that we forget it is attached to a body, which, if not correctly adjusted, will place so great a strain on the muscles that they cannot support the position.

- Place the body so that (1) its long axis will, depending on the image, either coincide with or be parallel to the midline of the table in order to prevent lateral rotation of the head and (2) the long axis of the cervical vertebrae will coincide with the level of the midpoint of the foramen magnum in order to prevent superior or inferior pull on the head, resulting in longitudinal angulation or tilt.
- Support any elevated part, such as the shoulder or hip, on a pillow or sandbags to relieve strain.
- In examinations of a hyposthenic or asthenic patient, elevate the chest on a small pillow to raise the cervical vertebrae to the correct level for the lateral, PA, and oblique projections when the patient is recumbent.
- An obese or hypersthenic patient presents problems that are not as easily overcome as those of a thin patient. In table radiography of such a patient, elevate the head on a radioparent pad in order to obtain the correct part-film relationship if needed. An advantage of a head unit is that it simplifies the handling of these patients.

- While adjusting the body position, stand in a position that will facilitate estimation of the approximate part position. That is, stand so that the longitudinal axis of the table is visible while centering the median sagittal plane of the body. This allows a view of the anterior surface of the forehead when the degree of body rotation for a lateral projection of the skull is adjusted. Thus, the body can be adjusted in such a way that it will not interfere with the final adjustment of the head, and it will be comfortable for the patient.

When the body is correctly placed and adjusted so that the long axis of the cervical vertebrae is supported at the level of the foramen magnum, the final position of the head requires only minor adjustments. The average patient will be able to maintain this relatively comfortable position without the aid of elaborate immobilization devices, although the following techniques may be helpful:

- Apply a head clamp with equal pressure on the two sides of the head, if needed.
- If such a clamp is not available, use a suitably backed strip of adhesive tape where it will not be projected onto the film. Do not place adhesive tape directly on patient's skin. When the film area to be exposed is small, immobolize the head with sandbags placed against the sides or vertex.

The correct basic body positions and adjustments made to compensate are illustrated in Figs. 20-36 to 20-43.

RADIATION PROTECTION

Protection of the patient from unnecessary radiation is a professional responsibility of the radiographer. (See Chapter 1, Volume 1, for specific guidelines.) In this chapter, radiation shielding of the patient is not specified or illustrated, since the professional community and the federal government have reported that placing a lead shield over the patient's pelvis does not significantly reduce the gonadal exposure during imagining of the skull.

The pediatric patient, however, should receive radiation shielding of the thyroid and thymus glands and gonads. The protective lead shielding used to cover the thyroid and thymus glands can also assist in immobilizing the pediatric patient while providing improved radiation protection.

The most effective way to protect the patient from unnecessary radiation is to restrict the radiation beam by using proper collimation. Taking care to ensure that the patient is properly instructed and immobilized also reduces the chance of having to repeat the procedure, thus further limiting the radiation exposure received by the patient.

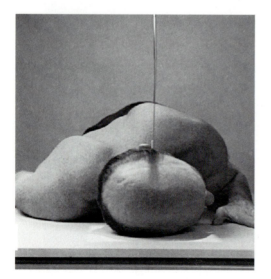

Fig. 20-36. Horizontal sagittal plane.

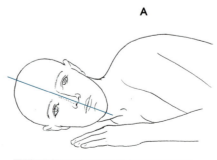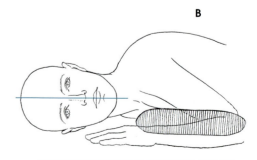

Fig. 20-37. Adjusting the sagittal planes to horizontal position. **A,** Asthenic or hyposthenic patient. **B,** Angulation corrected.

Skull

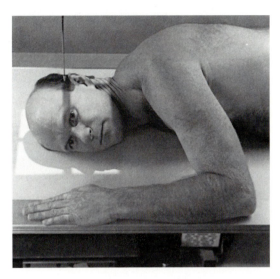

Fig. 20-38. Horizontal sagittal plane.

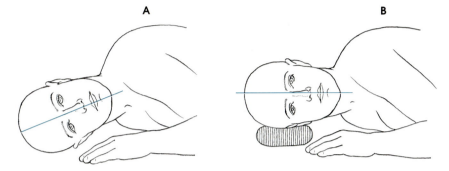

Fig. 20-39. Adjusting the sagittal plane to horizontal position. **A,** Hypersthenic patient. **B,** Angulation corrected.

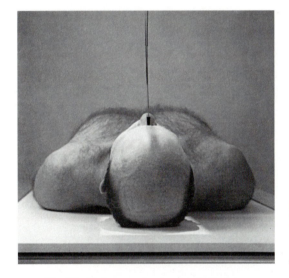

Fig. 20-40. Perpendicular sagittal plane.

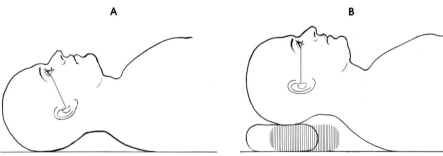

Fig. 20-41. Adjusting the orbitomeatal line to vertical position. **A,** Hypersthenic or round-shouldered patient. **B,** Angulation corrected.

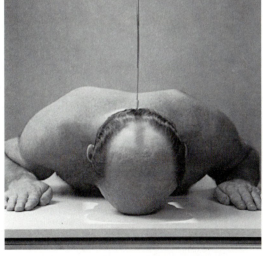

Fig. 20-42. Perpendicular sagittal plane.

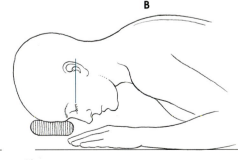

Fig. 20-43. Adjusting the orbitomeatal line to vertical position. **A,** Correction for hyposthenic patient. **B,** Correction for hypersthenic patient.

Cranium

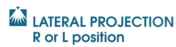

LATERAL PROJECTION
R or L position

Film: 10 × 12 in (24 × 30 cm) crosswise.

Position of patient

- Place the patient in the seated-upright or semiprone position.
- With the patient in a semiprone position, have him or her rest on the forearm and flexed knee of the elevated side.
- Adjust the position of the body so that the region of the external acoustic (auditory) meatus is centered to the midline of the grid, and adjust the rotation of the body so that the median sagittal plane of the head is parallel to the plane of the film.
- If possible, examine in the seated-upright position the patient whose breathing is somewhat labored and who is difficult to hold in the recumbent position.

Position of part

- While standing with the eyes directly focused above the midline of the table at the level of the sella turcica, place one hand under the mandibular region of the patient's head and ask him or her to relax the muscles of the neck.
- With the opposite hand on the upper parietal region of the patient's head to aid in guiding it into position, center the external acoustic (auditory) meatus to the midline of the grid.
- Adjust the head so that the median sagittal plane is horizontal.
- Adjust the flexion of the neck so that the infraorbitomeatal line is parallel with the horizontal axis of the film.

- Place a support under the side of the mandible to prevent it from sagging.
- Check the head position so that the interpupillary line is perpendicular to the film (Figs. 20-44 to 20-47).
- With the cassette in the Bucky tray, center it at a level 2 inches (5 cm) above the external acoustic (auditory) meatus.
- When the head is too large or too long for the entire cranium to be included on the film, use a larger cassette.
- Immobilize the head.
- Ask the patient to suspend respiration for the exposure.

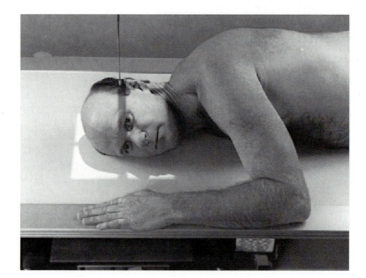

Fig. 20-44. Lateral skull.

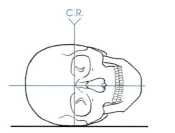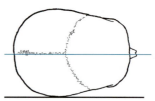

Fig. 20-45. Table radiography.

Central ray

- Direct the central ray perpendicular to the midpoint of the film.
- For a general survey examination, have the central ray enter 2 inches (5 cm) superior to the external acoustic (auditory) meatus.
- When the sella turcica is of primary interest, have the central ray enter ¾ inch (1.8 cm) superior and ¾ inch (1.8 cm) anterior to the external acoustic (auditory) meatus.
- Center the cassette to the central ray.

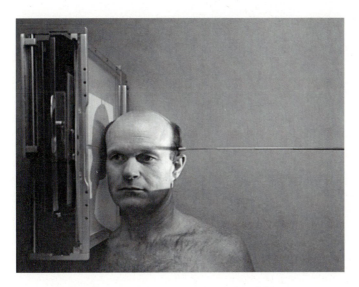

Fig. 20-46. Lateral skull centered over sella turcica.

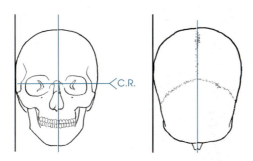

Fig. 20-47. Upright radiography.

Cranium

LATERAL PROJECTIONS
R or L postion
CROSS TABLE TECHNIQUE

Cross-table lateral

- With the patient supine, adjust the shoulders to lie in the same horizontal plane.
- After ruling out cervical injury, place the side of interest closest to the cassette, then elevate the head enough to center it to the vertically placed cassette and support it on a radiolucent sponge.
- Adjust the head so that the median sagittal plane is vertical and the interpupillary line is perpendicular to the film (Fig. 20-48).
- Direct the central ray perpendicular to the plane of the film and center it 2 inches (5 cm) above the external acoustic (auditory) meatus.

Robinson et al.[1] recommend use of the cross-table lateral projection for the demonstration of traumatic sphenoid sinus effusion (Fig. 20-49). They state that this finding may be the only clue to the presence of a basal skull fracture.

---

[1]Robinson AE, Meares BM, and Goree JA: Traumatic sphenoid sinus effusion, AJR 101:795-801, 1967.

Supine lateral

- With the patient supine, turn the head toward the side being examined.
- Elevate and support the opposite shoulder and hip enough so that the median sagittal plane of the head is parallel and the interpupillary line is perpendicular to the film.
- Adjust the position of the body so that a point 2 inches (5 cm) above the external acoustic (auditory) meatus is centered to the midline of the grid (Fig. 20-50).

Structures shown

A lateral image of the superimposed halves of the cranium, showing the detail of the side adjacent to the film, is seen. The sella turcica, the anterior clinoid processes, the dorsum sellae, and the posterior clinoid processes are well demonstrated in the lateral projection (Fig. 20-51).

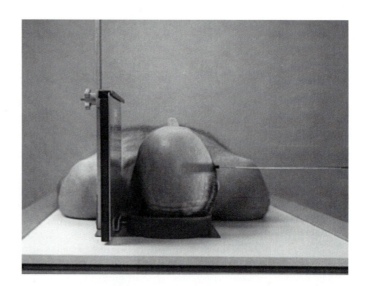

Fig. 20-48. Cross-table lateral skull.

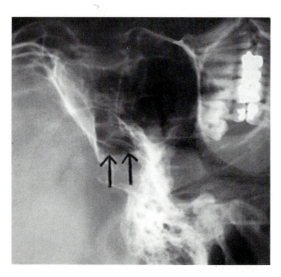

Fig. 20-49. Cross table lateral skull showing sphenoid sinus effusion *(arrows)*.

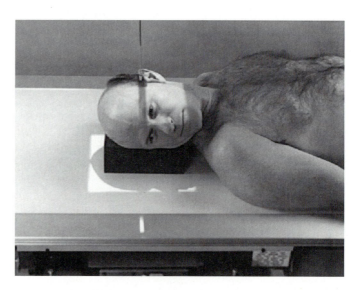

Fig. 20-50. Lateral skull with patient supine.

□ Evaluation criteria

The following should be clearly demonstrated:
- Entire cranium without rotation or tilt.
- Superimposed mandibular rami.
- Superimposed orbital roofs.
- Superimposed mastoid regions.
- Superimposed external acoustic (auditory) meati.
- Superimposed temporomandibular joints.
- No rotation of sella turcica.
- Penetration of parietal region.
- No overlap of the cervical spine by the mandible.

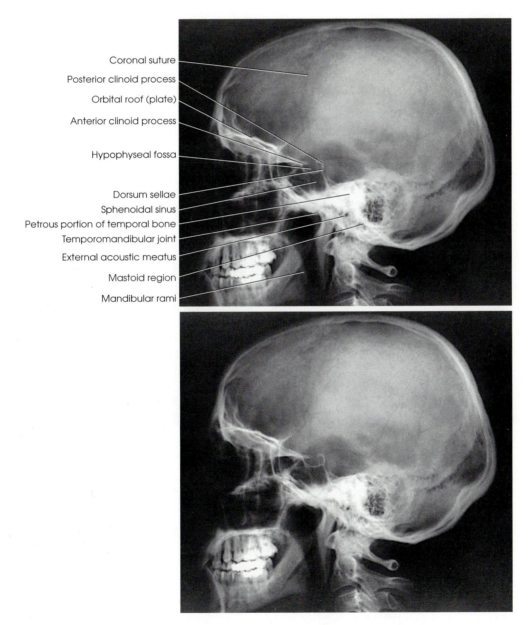

Coronal suture
Posterior clinoid process
Orbital roof (plate)
Anterior clinoid process
Hypophyseal fossa
Dorsum sellae
Sphenoidal sinus
Petrous portion of temporal bone
Temporomandibular joint
External acoustic meatus
Mastoid region
Mandibular rami

Fig. 20-51. Lateral skull.

241

Cranium

 PA AND PA AXIAL PROJECTION
CALDWELL METHOD

Film: 10 × 12 in (24 × 30 cm) lengthwise.

Position of patient

- Place the patient in either the prone or the seated-upright position.
- Center the median sagittal plane of the body to the midline of the grid.
- Flex the patient's elbows, place the arms in a comfortable position, and adjust the shoulders to lie in the same horizontal plane.

Position of part

- Rest the patient's forehead and nose on the table with the median sagittal plane perpendicular to the midline of the grid.
- Adjust the flexion of the neck so that the orbitomeatal line is perpendicular to the plane of the film.
- If the patient is recumbent, support the chin on a radiolucent sponge if needed.
- Immobilize the head and center the cassette to the nasion (Figs. 20-52 to 20-55).
- Ask the patient to suspend respiration for the exposure.

Central ray

- For the *PA projection,* when the frontal bone is of primary interest, direct the central ray perpendicular to the nasion.
- For the *Caldwell method,* direct the central ray to the nasion at an angle of 15 degrees caudad.

- For the demonstration of the superior orbital fissures, direct the central ray through the midorbits at an angle of 20 to 25 degrees caudad.
- For the demonstration of the rotundum foramina, direct the central ray to the nasion at an angle of 25 to 30 degrees caudad. The Waters method is also used for the demonstration of the rotundum foramina (see Chapter 22, pp. 382 and 383).

NOTE: For the demonstration of the superior and lateral portions of the frontal bone, rest the patient's head on the chin and adjust it so that the vertically directed central ray will pass through the frontal bone alone; it will enter near the coronal suture and exit through the supraorbital ridges.

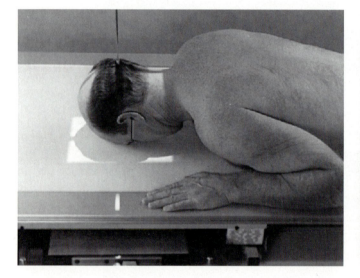

Fig. 20-52. PA skull: central ray angulation of 0 degrees for frontal bone.

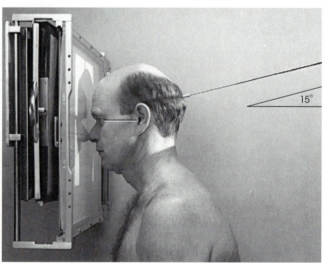

Fig. 20-53. PA axial skull, Caldwell method: central ray angulation of 15 degrees.

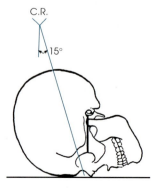

Fig. 20-54. Table radiography.

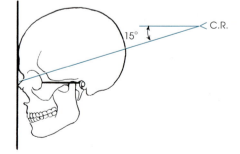

Fig. 20-55. Upright radiography.

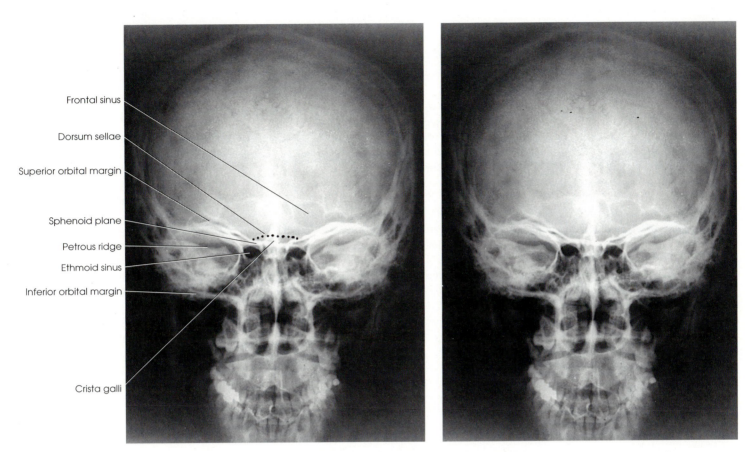

Frontal sinus

Dorsum sellae

Superior orbital margin

Sphenoid plane

Petrous ridge

Ethmoid sinus

Inferior orbital margin

Crista galli

Fig. 20-56. PA skull with 0-degree central ray angulation.

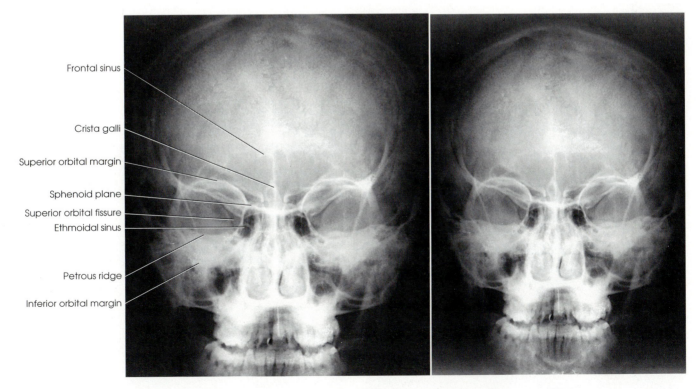

Frontal sinus

Crista galli

Superior orbital margin

Sphenoid plane

Superior orbital fissure

Ethmoidal sinus

Petrous ridge

Inferior orbital margin

Fig. 20-57. PA axial skull. Caldwell method: central ray angulation of 15 degrees.

(Courtesy Rinette Tavitri, R.T.)

243

Cranium—cont'd

Structures shown

For the PA projection with a perpendicular central ray (Fig. 20-57), the orbits are filled by the shadows of the petrous pyramids. Other structures demonstrated include the posterior ethmoidal air cells, the crista galli, the frontal bone, and the frontal sinuses. The dorsum sellae is seen as a curved line extending between the orbits just above the ethmoidal air cells. When the central ray is angled 15 degrees caudad to the nasion for the Caldwell method, many of the same structures that appear in the direct PA projection are seen (Fig. 20-58). The petrous ridges, however, are projected into the lower third of the orbits. The Caldwell method also demonstrates the anterior ethmoidal air cells.

Schüller[1] who first described this positioning for the skull, recommended a caudal angle of 25 degrees.

---

[1]Schüller A: Die Schädelbasis im Rontgenbild, Fortschr Roentgenstr 11:215, 1905.

□ Evaluation criteria

The following should be clearly demonstrated:
- Distance from the lateral border of the skull to the lateral border of the orbit equal on both sides.
- Symmetric petrous ridges.
- Petrous bones lying in the lower third of the orbit with a caudal central ray angulation of 15 degrees and filling the orbits with no central ray angulation.
- Penetration of frontal bone without excessive density at the lateral borders of the skull.
- Entire cranial vertex.

AP PROJECTION AND AP AXIAL PROJECTIONS

Film: 10 × 12 in (24 × 30 cm) lengthwise.

Position of patient/position of part

- When the patient cannot be rotated from the supine position, obtain a similar, although somewhat magnified, projection by adjusting the head for an AP projection with the orbitomeatal line perpendicular.

Central ray

- Use a perpendicular central ray (Fig. 20-58) or direct the central ray to the nasion at an angle of 10 to 15 degrees cephalad (Fig. 20-59).
- For the demonstration of the frontal bone only, direct the central ray midway between the frontal tuberosity (eminences) at a caudal angulation that is parallel to the supraorbitomeatal line.

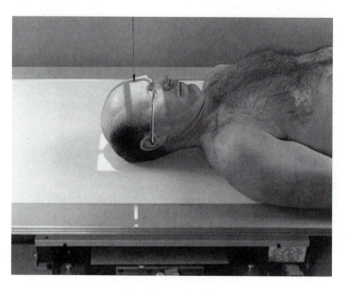

Fig. 20-58. AP skull.

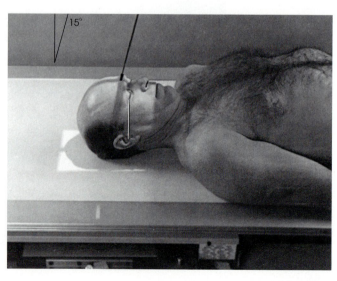

Fig. 20-59. AP axial skull with 15-degree cephalad central ray.

Structures shown

The structures shown on the AP projection are the same as those demonstrated on the PA projection described on the previous page. On the AP projection (Fig. 20-60), the orbits are considerably magnified due to the increased orbit-to-image receptor distance. Similarly, the distance from the lateral margin of the orbit to the lateral margin of the temporal bone measures less on the AP than on the PA due to the magnification.

☐ Evaluation criteria

The following should be clearly demonstrated:

- Distance from the lateral border of the skull to the lateral border of the orbit equal on both sides.
- Symmetric petrous ridges.
- Petrous bones lying in the lower third of the orbit with a cephalad central ray angulation of 15 degrees and filling the orbits with no central ray angulation.
- Penetration of frontal bone without excessive density at the lateral borders of the skull.
- Entire cranial vertex.

Stretcher and bedside examinations

- When the patient cannot be turned to the prone position, and after ruling out cervical spine injury, elevate one side enough to place the head in a lateral position and support the shoulder and hip on pillows or sandbags if needed.
- Elevate the head on a suitable support and adjust its height to center the median sagittal plane of the head to a vertically positioned grid.
- Adjust the head so that the orbitomeatal line is perpendicular to the plane of the film (Fig. 20-61).
- Direct the horizontal central ray 15 degrees caudad to exit the nasion.

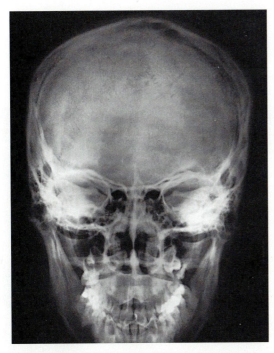

Fig. 20-60. AP skull: central ray angulation of 0 degrees.

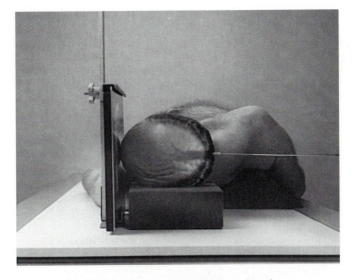

Fig. 20-61. PA skull with patient semi-supine.

Cranium

Cranium

AP AXIAL PROJECTION
TOWNE METHOD

Film: 10 × 12 in (24 × 30 cm) lengthwise.

NOTE: Although it is most commonly referred to as the Towne[1] method, numerous authors have described slightly different variations. In 1912, Grashey[2] presented the first description of the AP axial projection of the cranium. In 1926 Altschul[3] and Towne[1] described the position. Altschul recommended strong depression of the chin and that the central ray be directed through the foramen magnum at a caudal angle of 40 degrees. Towne (citing Chamberlain) recommended that, with the chin depressed, the central ray be directed through the median sagittal plane from a point about 3 inches (7.5 cm) above the eyebrows to the foramen magnum. Towne gave no specific central ray angulation, but this would, of course, depend on the flexion of the neck.

---

[1]Towne EB: Erosion of the petrous bone by acoustic nerve tumor, Arch Otolaryngol 4:515-519, 1926.
[2]Grashey R: Atlas typischer Röntgenbilder vom normalen Menschen. In Lehmann's medizinische Atlanten, ed 2, vol 5, Munich, 1912, JF Lehmann.
[3]Altschul W: Beiträg zur Röntgenologie des Gehörorganes, Z Hals Nas Ohr 14:335-340, 1926.

Position of patient

- With the patient either supine or seated upright, center the median sagittal plane of the body to the midline of the grid.
- Place the arms in a comfortable position and adjust the shoulders to lie in the same horizontal plane.
- For the purpose of obtaining the correct image receptor relationship without increasing the image receptor distance, as well as for the patient's comfort, examine hypersthenic patients in the seated-upright position if possible.
- When this is not possible, obtain the desired projection of the occipitobasal region by angling the central ray caudad with the head elevated and adjusted in the horizontal position. The total angulation can be divided between tube tilt and image receptor tilt. Stewart,[4] who recommended a total angulation of 40 degrees, suggested adjusting the head on a 25-degree caudally inclined plane and directing the central ray at a caudal angle of 15 degrees. The occipitofrontal projection devised by Haas[5] (p. 251) can be used in place of the AP axial projection on hypersthenic patients. The Haas method is the reverse of the AP axial projection and produces a comparable result.

---

[4]Stewart WH and Lucket WH: Skull fractures, Ann Roentgenol 6:14-28, 1925.
[5]Haas L: Über die nuchofrontale Aufnahme des Schädels, Fortschr Roentgenstr 45:532-557, 1932.

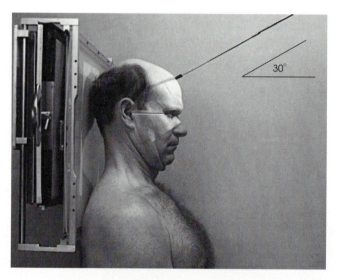

Fig. 20-62. AP axial skull, Towne Method.

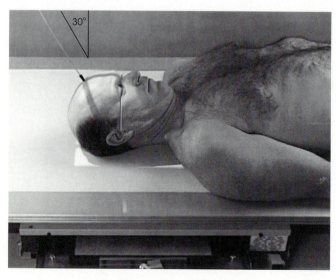

Fig. 20-63. AP axial skull, Towne Method.

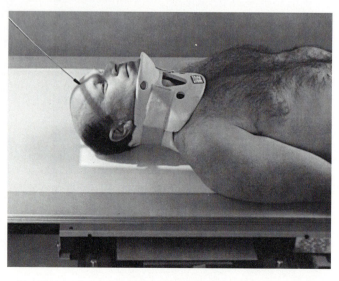

Fig. 20-64. AP axial skull, Towne Method on trauma patient.

Position of part

- Adjust the patient's head so that the median sagittal plane is perpendicular to the midline of the cassette.
- Flex the neck enough to place the orbitomeatal line perpendicular to the plane of the film.
- When the patient cannot flex the neck to this extent, adjust it so that the infraorbitomeatal line is perpendicular and then increase the central ray angulation 7 degrees (Figs. 20-62 to 20-66).
- For the demonstration of the entire occipitobasal region, adjust the position of the film so that its upper margin is at the level of the highest point of the cranial vertex. The cassette will be centered at or near the level of the foramen magnum.
- For a localized image of the dorsum sellae and petrous pyramids, adjust the cassette so that its midpoint will coincide with the central ray; it will be centered at or slightly below the level of the occlusal plane.
- Recheck the position and immobilize the head.
- Ask the patient to suspend respiration for the exposure.

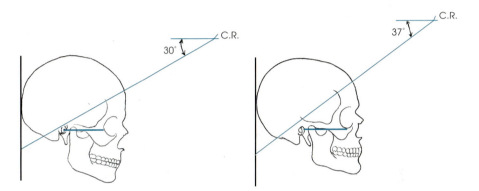

Fig. 20-65. Upright radiography. Same result with central ray directed 30 degrees to orbitomeatal line or 37 degrees to infraorbitomeatal line.

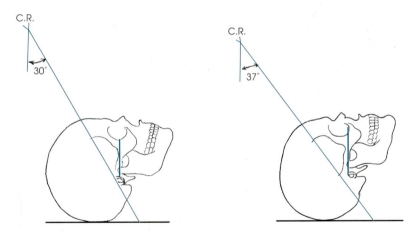

Fig. 20-66. Table radiography.

Central ray

- For general survey examinations, direct the central ray through the foramen magnum at a caudal angle of (1) 30 degrees to the orbitomeatal line or (2) 37 degrees to the infraorbitomeatal line. The central ray enters approximately 2 to 2½ inches above the glabella.

Structures shown

The AP axial projection shows a symmetric image of the petrous pyramids, the posterior portion of the foramen magnum, the dorsum sellae and posterior clinoid processes projected within the foramen magnum, the occipital bone, and the posterior portion of the parietal bones (Fig. 20-67).

This projection is also used for tomographic studies of the ears, the facial canal, the jugular foramina, and the rotundum foramina.

☐ Evaluation criteria

The following should be clearly demonstrated:

- Distance from the lateral border of the skull to the lateral margin of the foramen magnum equal on both sides.
- Symmetric petrous pyramids.
- Dorsum sellae and the posterior clinoid processes visible within the foramen magnum.
- Penetration of occipital bone without excessive density at the lateral borders of the skull.

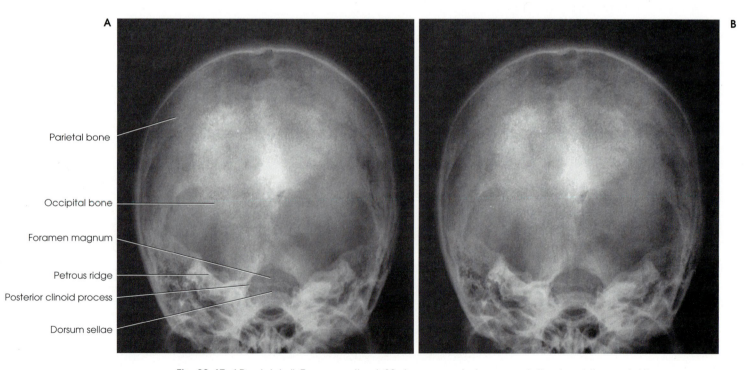

Parietal bone
Occipital bone
Foramen magnum
Petrous ridge
Posterior clinoid process
Dorsum sellae

Fig. 20-67. AP axial skull, Towne method: 30-degree central ray angulation to orbitomeatal line.

(Courtesy Kimberly Edgar, RT.)

Skull

Pathology or trauma patients

For the demonstration of the entire foramen magnum and the jugular foramina,
increase the caudal angulation of the central ray to anywhere from 40 to 60 degrees, according to the flexion of the head
(Figs. 20-68 to 20-71).

If, because of trauma, pathologic conditions, or deformity such as a strongly ac-
centuated dorsal kyphosis, the patient cannot be examined in a direct supine or
prone position, the following steps should
be observed:

- Adjust and support the body in a recumbent position, which will allow
  the head to be placed in an exact lateral position.
- Immobilize the cassette and grid in a
  vertical position behind the occiput.
- Direct the central ray 30 degrees caudally to the orbitomeatal line (Fig.
  20-72).

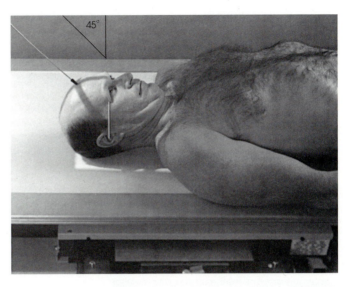

Fig. 20-68. AP axial skull: central ray angulation of 40 to 45 degrees.

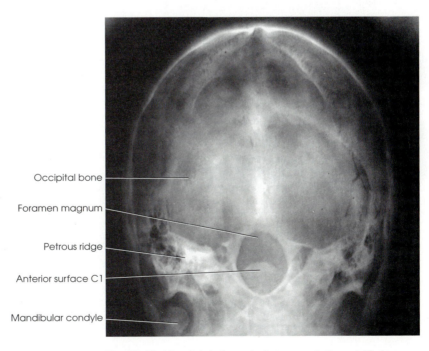

Occipital bone

Foramen magnum

Petrous ridge

Anterior surface C1

Mandibular condyle

Fig. 20-69. AP axial skull: central ray angulation of 45 degrees.

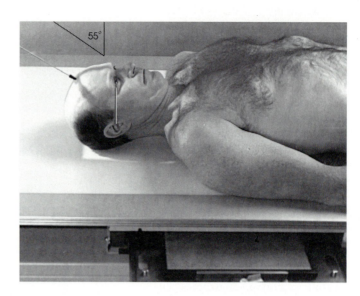

Fig. 20-70. AP axial foramen magnum and jugular foramina.

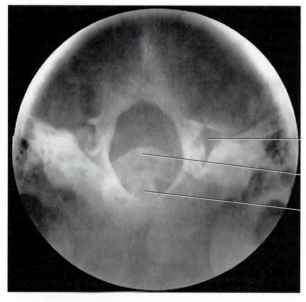

Jugular foramen

Anterior surface of C1

Dens

Fig. 20-71. AP axial foramen magnum and jugular foramina: central ray angulation of 55 degrees.

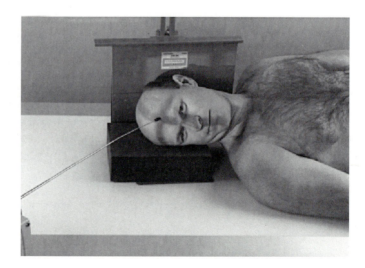

Fig. 20-72. AP axial skull. Head in lateral position, cassette and grid vertical.

Cranium

PA AXIAL PROJECTION
HAAS METHOD

Haas[1] devised this projection for obtaining an image of the sellar structures projected within the foramen magnum of hypersthenic or other patients who cannot be adjusted correctly for the reverse (AP) axial projection. He recommended that the head be rested on the forehead and nose and the central ray be angled cephalad to enter 1½ inches (3.7 cm) below the external occipital protuberance (inion) and emerge approximately 1½ inches (3.7 cm) above the nasion. When the head of average shape (mesocephalic) is adjusted so that the orbitomeatal line is perpendicular to the plane of the film, a central ray angulation of 25 degrees meets the Haas recommendation and produces the desired result. For demonstration of the sella in patients with atypically shaped heads, the entrance and exit points remain as above and the degree of central ray angulation should be determined by means of a protractor.

Film: 10 × 12 in (24 × 30 cm) lengthwise.

Position of patient

- Adjust the patient in the prone position and center the median sagittal plane of the body to the midline of the grid.
- Flex the patient's elbows, place the arms in a comfortable position, and adjust the shoulders to lie in the same horizontal plane.

Position of part

- Rest the patient's forehead and nose on the table with the median sagittal plane perpendicular to the midline of the grid.
- Adjust the flexion of the neck so that the orbitomeatal line is perpendicular (Figs. 20-73 to 20-75).
- Immobilize the head.
- Ask the patient to suspend respiration for the exposure.
- For a localized image of the sellar region and/or the petrous pyramids, adjust the position of the film so that the midpoint will coincide with the central ray; shift the cassette cephalad approximately 3 inches (7.5 cm) to include the vertex of the skull.

[1]Haas L: Verfahren zur sagittalen Aufnahme der Sellagegend, Fortschr Roentgenstr 36:1198-1203, 1927.

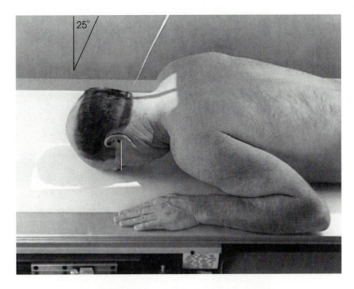

Fig. 20-73. PA axial skull, Haas method.

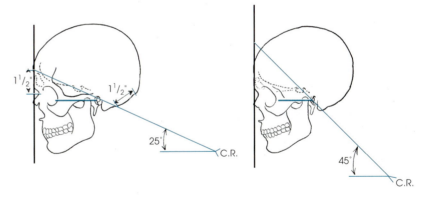

Fig. 20-74. Upright radiography.

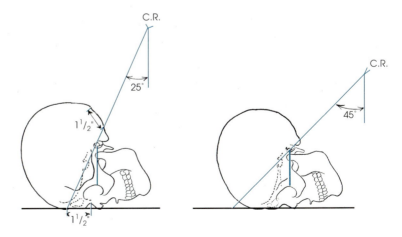

Fig. 20-75. Table radiography.

Central ray

- Direct the central ray at a cephalad angle of 25 degrees, to exit a point 1½ inches (3.7 cm) above the nasion. The central ray enters a point 1½ inches (3.7 cm) below the external occipital protuberance (inion). The central ray can be varied to demonstrate other cranial anatomy as shown (Figs. 20-74 and 20-75).

Structures shown

A PA axial projection demonstrates the occipital region of the cranium, showing a symmetric image of the petrous pyramids and showing the dorsum sellae and other structures within the foramen magnum (Figs. 20-76 and 20-77).

□ Evaluation criteria

The following should be clearly demonstrated:

- Projection of dorsum sellae within the foramen magnum.
- Distance from the lateral border of the skull to the lateral margin of the foramen magnum equal on both sides.
- Symmetric petrous pyramids.
- Entire cranium.

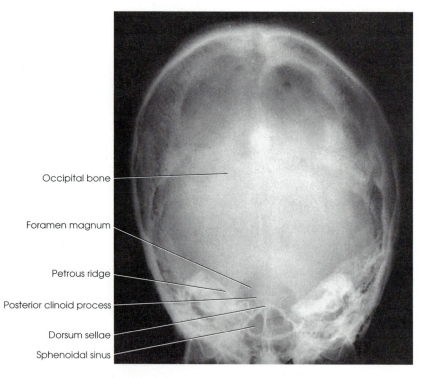

Occipital bone

Foramen magnum

Petrous ridge

Posterior clinoid process

Dorsum sellae

Sphenoidal sinus

Fig. 20-76. PA axial skull, Haas method: central ray angulation of 25 degrees.

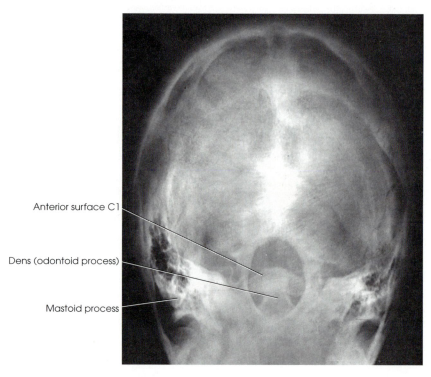

Anterior surface C1

Dens (odontoid process)

Mastoid process

Fig. 20-77. PA axial skull: central ray angulation of 45 degrees.

Cranial Base

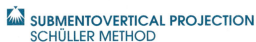

SUBMENTOVERTICAL PROJECTION
SCHÜLLER METHOD

Film: 10 × 12 in (24 × 30 cm) lengthwise.

Position of patient

The success of the submentovertical (SMV) projection of the cranial base depends on (1) placing the infraorbitomeatal line as nearly as possible parallel with the plane of the film and (2) directing the central ray perpendicular to the infraorbitomeatal line.

- Place the patient in either the supine or the upright position, although the latter is more comfortable. If a chair that supports the back is used, the upright position also allows greater freedom in positioning the body to place the infraorbitomeatal line parallel with the film. If the patient is seated far enough away from the vertical grid device, the head can usually be adjusted.
- Place patients with short necks and hypersthenic patients in the upright position if possible. An advantage of a head unit is that it can be angled from the vertical position.

- When the patient is placed in the supine position, elevate the torso on firm pillows or a suitable pad to allow the head to rest on the vertex, with the neck in complete extension.
- Flex the patient's knees to relax the abdominal muscles.
- Center the median sagittal plane of the body to the midline of the grid.
- Place the arms in a comfortable position and adjust the shoulders to lie in the same horizontal plane.
- The supine position places considerable strain on the neck; do not keep the patient in the final adjustment longer than is absolutely necessary.

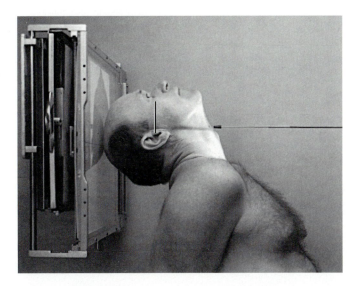

Fig. 20-78. Submentovertical cranial base.

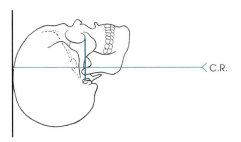

Fig. 20-79. Upright radiography.

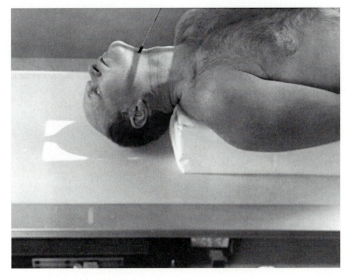

Fig. 20-80. Submentovertical cranial base.

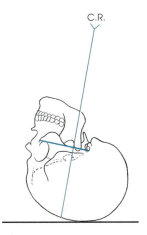

Fig. 20-81. Table radiography.

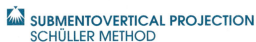

253

Position of part

- With the median sagittal plane of the body centered to the midline of the grid, extend the patient's neck as far as possible and rest the head on the vertex.
- Adjust the head so that the median sagittal plane is perpendicular to the midline of the film.
- Adjust the tube so that the central ray is perpendicular to the infraorbitomeatal line and center to the sella turcica (Figs. 20-78 to 20-81).
- In the absence of a head clamp, place a suitably backed strip of adhesive tape across the tip of the chin and anchor it to the sides of the radiographic unit if needed.
- Ask the patient to suspend respiration for the exposure.

Central ray

- Direct the central ray through the sella turcica perpendicular to the infraorbitomeatal line. It enters the median sagittal plane of the throat between the angles of the mandible and passes through a point ¾ inch (1.8 cm) anterior to the level of the external acoustic (auditory) meatuses.

Structures shown

An SMV projection of the cranial base demonstrates symmetric images of the petrosae, the mastoid processes, the bony part of the auditory (eustachian) tubes, the foramina ovale and spinosum (which are best shown in this projection), the carotid canals, the sphenoidal sinuses, the mandible, the the nasal septum, the dens of the axis, and the entire atlas. The maxillary sinuses are superimposed over the mandible (Fig. 20-82).

The SMV projection is also used for axial tomography of the orbits, optic canals, the ethmoid bones and maxillary sinuses, and the mastoid processes.

With a decrease in the exposure factors the zygomatic arches are well demonstrated in this position. (See Facial Bones, Chapter 22.)

□Evaluation criteria

The following should be clearly demonstrated:

- Distance from the lateral border of the skull to the mandibular condyles equal on both sides.
- Superimposition of mandibular symphysis over anterior frontal bone.
- Mandibular condyles anterior to the petrous pyramids.
- Symmetric petrosae.
- Clearly visible structures of the cranial base, indicated by adequate penetration.

NOTE: Schüller described and illustrated the basal projections, submentovertical and verticosubmental, in 1905, but it was Pfeiffer[1] who gave specific directions for the central ray angulation.

[1]Pfeiffer W: Beitrag zum Wert des axialen Schädelskiagrammes, Arch Laryngol Rhinol 30:1-14, 1916.

A

B

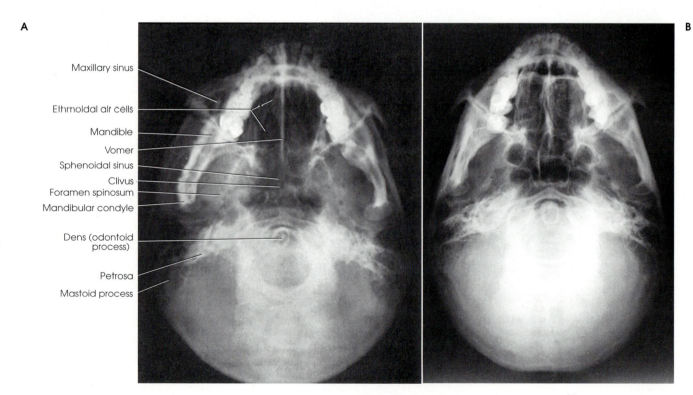

Maxillary sinus
Ethmoidal air cells
Mandible
Vomer
Sphenoidal sinus
Clivus
Foramen spinosum
Mandibular condyle
Dens (odontoid process)
Petrosa
Mastoid process

Fig. 20-82. Submentovertical cranial base.

Cranial Base

VERTICOSUBMENTAL PROJECTION
SCHÜLLER METHOD

Film: 10 × 12 in (24 × 30 cm) lengthwise.

Position of patient

The *verticosubmental* (VSM) projection is used to demonstrate the base of the cranium when the submentovertical projection is contraindicated by the patient's condition.

- Place the patient in the prone position and center the median sagittal plane of the body to the midline of the grid.
- Flex the elbows, place the arms in a comfortable position, and adjust the shoulders to lie in the same horizontal plane.

Position of part

- Rest the patient's fully extended chin on the table and adjust it so that the median sagittal plane is vertical (Fig. 20-83).
- Immobilize the head.
- Ask the patient to suspend respiration for the exposure.

Central ray

- Direct the central ray through the sella turcica perpendicular to the infraorbitomeatal line. The central ray passes through a point ¾ inch (1.8 cm) anterior to the level of the external acoustic (auditory) meatuses.

Structures shown

The VSM projection (Fig. 20-84) of the cranial base is somewhat similar to the SMV projection demonstrated previously. Because of the increase in object-to-image receptor distance and the increase in angle between the cranial base and the plane of the film, the basal structures, particularly those in the midbase region, are somewhat distorted and magnified. However, this projection is useful in studies of the anterior cranial base and sphenoidal sinuses, where magnification and distortion can be reduced by placing the cassette in contact with the throat.

☐ **Evaluation criteria**

The following should be clearly demonstrated:

- Distance from the lateral border of the skull to the mandibular condyles equal on both sides.
- Mandibular condyles anterior to the petrous pyramids.
- Symmetric petrosae.
- Structures of the cranial base.
- Superimposition of mandibular symphysis over anterior frontal bone.

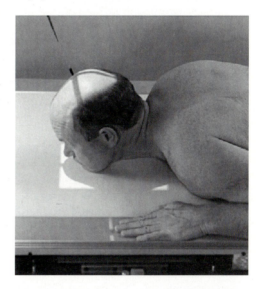

Fig. 20-83. Verticosubmental cranial base.

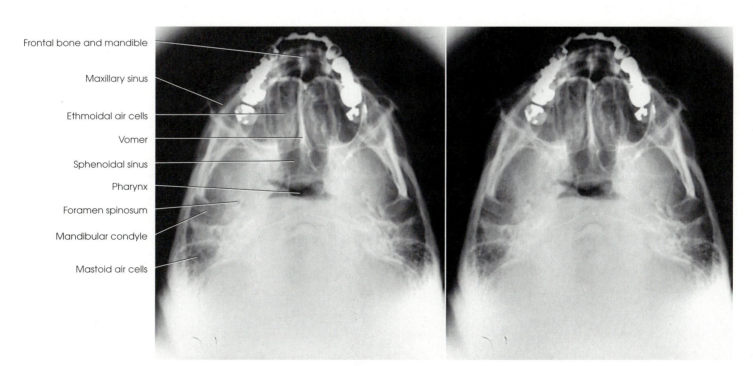

Frontal bone and mandible

Maxillary sinus

Ethmoidal air cells

Vomer

Sphenoidal sinus

Pharynx

Foramen spinosum

Mandibular condyle

Mastoid air cells

Fig. 20-84. Verticosubmental cranial base.

(Courtesy Nina Kowalczyk, R.T.)

Cranial Base
AXIOLATERAL PROJECTION
R and L positions
LYSHOLM METHOD

Film: 10 × 12 in (24 × 30 cm) crosswise.

Position of patient

- Place the patient in the seated-upright or semiprone position.
- Align the body so that the external acoustic (auditory) meatus is centered to the midline of the grid.
- Adjust the rotation of the body so that the median sagittal plane of the head is approximately horizontal.
- Have the patient rest on the forearm and flexed knee of the elevated side.
- Adjust the shoulders to lie in the same horizontal plane.

Position of part

- Place a hand under the patient's neck and mandibular region and the other hand on the upper parietal region to aid in the adjustment of the position.
- Center the external acoustic (auditory) meatus of the side being examined to the midline of the grid and adjust the head in a true lateral position.
- Extend the neck enough to place the infraorbitomeatal line parallel with the transverse axis of the cassette.
- Support the mandible to prevent rotation.
- Using a suitable protractor, check the head position so that the interpupillary line is perpendicular to the film (Figs. 20-85 to 20-87).
- Immobilize the head.
- Ask the patient to suspend respiration for the exposure.

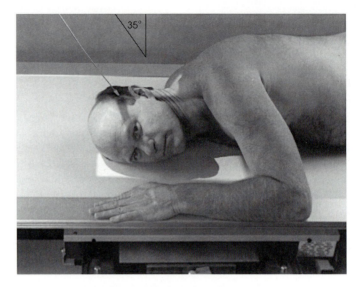

Fig. 20-85. Axiolateral cranial base.

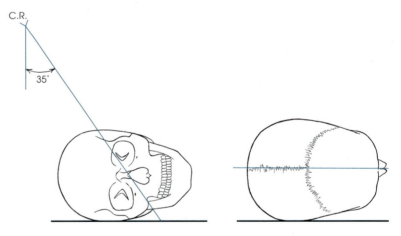

Fig. 20-86. Table radiography.

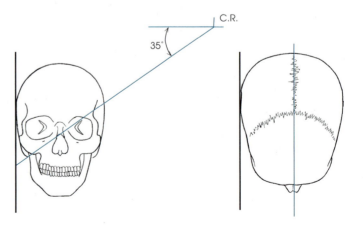

Fig. 20-87. Upright radiography.

Skull

Central ray

- Direct the central ray to the midline of the grid so that it exits a point 1 inch (2.5 cm) distal to the lower external acoustic (auditory) meatus at an angle of 30 to 35 degrees caudad.
- Adjust the cassette to coincide with the central ray. The central ray enters approximately 3 inches (7.5 cm) superior and ¾ inch (2 cm) anterior to the external acoustic meatus on the side up.

Structures shown

An axiolateral projection of the lateral aspect of the base of the cranium closest to the film is demonstrated in Fig. 20-88. Both sides are usually examined for comparison.

Lysholm[1] recommends this projection for use with patients who cannot extend their head enough for a satisfactory submentovertical projection.

---

[1]Lysholm E: Apparatus and technique for the roentgen examination of the skull, Acta Radiol 12 (suppl):53-55, 1931.

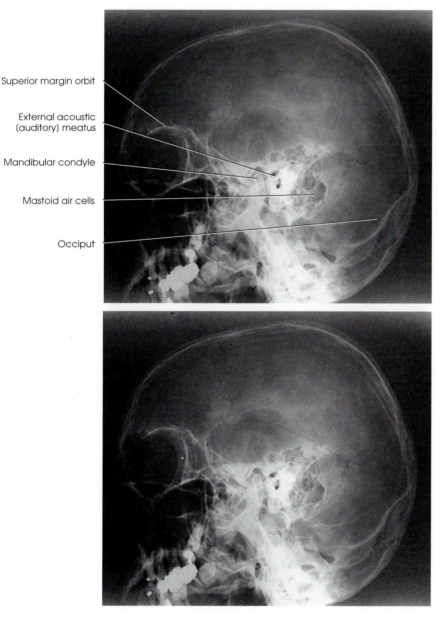

Superior margin orbit

External acoustic (auditory) meatus

Mandibular condyle

Mastoid air cells

Occiput

Fig. 20-88. Axiolateral cranial base.

□Evaluation criteria

The following should be clearly demonstrated:

- Entire cranium.
- Some distortion of structures of the cranial base.

Cranium, Sella Turcica, and Ear
PA AXIAL PROJECTION
VALDINI METHOD

This PA axial projection is used to demonstrate the cranium, sella-turcica, and the ear. It requires accurate adjustment of the head on patients who cannot, because of basal deformity (platybasia) or other reasons, assume the Grashey or Haas position.

Valdini[1] devised this method using a perpendicular central ray to project the dorsum sellae in the foramen magnum without angular distortion. This method requires that the head be rested on the upper frontal region and adjusted so that an imaginary line extends from the external occipital protuberance (inion) to a point directly anterior and 0.5 cm distal to the nasion at an angle of 28 degrees, open posteroinferiorly, to the perpendicular central ray. When the head of average shape (mesocephalic) is so adjusted, the infraorbitomeatal line forms an angle of 50 degrees to the plane of the film.

An excellent projection of the organs of hearing is obtained by this method.

Film: 8 × 10 in (18 × 24 cm) lengthwise.

---

[1]Valdini L: La sella turcica in proiezione occipitofrontale, Radiol Med 15:881-886, 1928.

Position of patient

- Place the patient in either the recumbent or seated-upright position. The upright position is more comfortable; however, accurate adjustment of the head requires that it be acutely flexed. When the prone position is used, elevate the thorax on several firm pillows to enable the patient to achieve adequate flexion of the neck without strain.
- Center the median sagittal plane of the body to the midline of the grid.
- Place the arms in a comfortable position and adjust the shoulders to lie in the same horizontal plane.

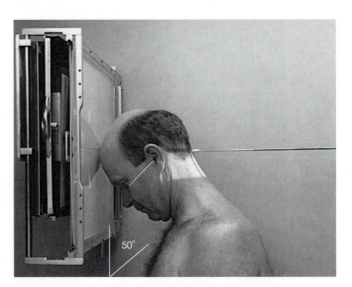

Fig. 20-89. PA axial cranium, sella turcica, and inner ear: Valdini method.

Position of part

- Rest the upper frontal region of the patient's skull on the table and adjust it so that the median sagittal plane is perpendicular to the midline of the grid.
- Using a protractor, flex the neck so that the following requirements are met:
  1. The *infraorbitomeatal* line forms a 50-degree angle with the plane of the film for the demonstration of the dorsum sellae or of the internal acoustic (auditory) canals and the labyrinths of the ears (Figs. 20-89 to 20-91).
  2. The *orbitomeatal* line forms a 50-degree angle with the plane of the film for the demonstration of the external acoustic (auditory) canals, the tympanic cavities, and the bony part of the eustachian tubes (Fig. 20-92).

- Center the film approximately 1 inch (2.5 cm) superior to the level of the external acoustic (auditory) meatus for the inclusion of the vertex.
- Use a head clamp for immobilization as needed.
- Ask the patient to suspend respiration for the exposure.

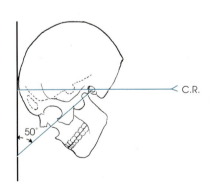

Fig. 20-90. Upright radiography.

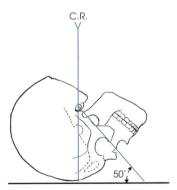

Fig. 20-91. Table radiography.

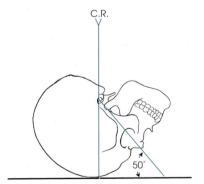

Fig. 20-92. Table radiography.

Cranium, sella turcica, and ear

259

Central ray

With the central ray perpendicular to the plane of the film:

- Center to a point 0.5 cm distal to the nasion for the demonstration of the dorsum sellae (Figs. 20-93 and 20-94).
- Center to the foramen magnum at or slightly above the level of the external acoustic (auditory) meatus to demonstrate the petrosae (Figs. 20-95 and 20-96).

Structures shown

The Valdini method, using the infraorbitomeatal line, shows the dorsum sellae and posterior clinoid processes within or slightly above the foramen magnum and the tuberculum sellae and anterior clinoid processes just below this point; the anterior processes are usually superimposed by the petrous apices. This projection, because of the absence of angular distortion, clearly demonstrates the entire labyrinth and the internal acoustic canal. When the orbitomeatal line is positioned and the central ray is centered at the level of the

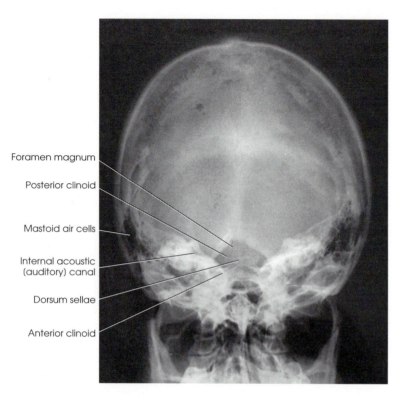

Foramen magnum

Posterior clinoid

Mastoid air cells

Internal acoustic (auditory) canal

Dorsum sellae

Anterior clinoid

Fig. 20-93. PA axial projection, Valdini method: infraorbitomeatal line, 50 degrees to film.

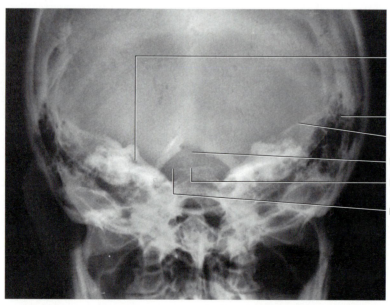

Internal acoustic canal

Mastoid air cells

Petrous ridge

Foramen magnum

Dorsum sellae

Posterior clinoid process

Fig. 20-94. PA axial projection, Valdini method: infraorbitomeatal line, 50 degrees to film.

external acoustic (auditory) canals, the sella is most frequently projected below the foramen magnum. The external acoustic canal, the tympanic cavity, and the bony part of the auditory (eustachian) tube are more clearly shown when the head is adjusted by the orbitomeatal line. The mastoid pneumatization is shown in all images.

☐ Evaluation criteria

The following should be clearly demonstrated:
- Distance from the lateral border of the skull to the lateral margin of the foramen magnum equal on both sides.
- Symmetric petrous pyramids.
- Dorsum sellae and the posterior clinoid processes visible within the foramen magnum when the infraorbitomeatal line is used.
- Anterior surface of the cervical atlas visible within the foramen magnum when the orbitomeatal is the positioning line of reference.

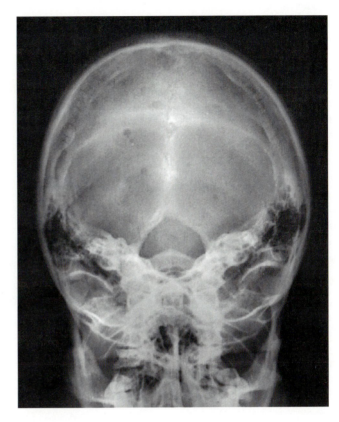

Fig. 20-95. PA axial projection, Valdini method: orbitomeatal line, 50 degrees to film.

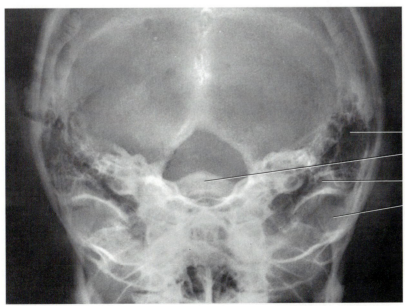

Mastoid air cells

Anterior surface C1

External acoustic (auditory) canal

Mandibular condyle

Fig. 20-96. PA axial projection, Valdini method: orbitomeatal line, 50 degrees to film.

Sella Turcica

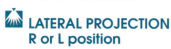

LATERAL PROJECTION
R or L position

Film: 8 × 10 in (18 × 24 cm).

Position of patient

- A closely collimated projection of the sella turcica is often requested in addition to the lateral projection of the entire cranium.
- Place the patient in the seated-upright or semiprone position.
- Adjust the rotation of the body so that the median sagittal plane of the head is parallel to the plane of the film.
- Adjust the shoulders to lie in the same horizontal plane.

Position of part

- If the patient is hypersthenic, elevate the head enough to place the median sagittal plane parallel to the film and support it on a radiolucent sponge.
- Center the cassette to the region of the sella turcica, a point ¾ inch (1.8 cm) anterior to, and ¾ inch (1.8 cm) superior to the external acoustic (auditory) meatus.
- Adjust the head in a true lateral position so that the median sagittal plane is parallel with, and the interpupillary line is perpendicular to, the plane of the film.
- Adjust the head so that the infraorbitomeatal line is parallel with the horizontal axis of the film (Figs. 20-97 to 20-99).
- Immobilize the head as necessary.
- Ask the patient to suspend respiration for the exposure.

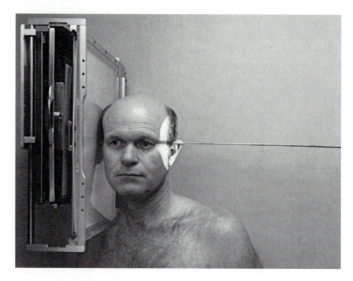

Fig. 20-97. Lateral skull for sella turcica.

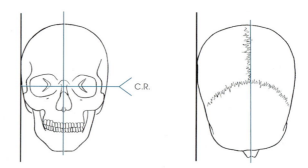

Fig. 20-98. Upright radiography.

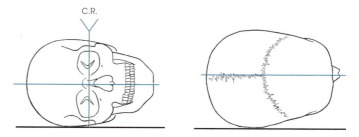

Fig. 20-99. Table radiography.

Central ray

- Direct the central ray perpendicular to a point ¾ inch (1.8 cm) anterior to, and ¾ inch (1.8 cm) superior to, the external acoustic (auditory) meatus.
- Collimate to the sphenoid bone.

Structures shown

A lateral projection of the sellar region of the cranium is seen (Fig. 20-100).

□Evaluation criteria

The following should be clearly demonstrated:
- No rotation of sella turcica.
- Superimposed anterior clinoid processes.
- Superimposed posterior clinoid processes.
- Sella turcica centered on the radiograph.
- Close beam restriction of sellar region.

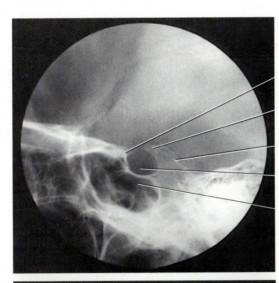

Anterior clinoid

Posterior clinoid

Dorsum sellae

Hypophyseal fossa

Sphenoidal sinus

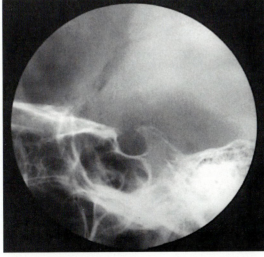

Fig. 20-100. Lateral sella turcica.

Sella Turcica (Dorsum Sellae and Posterior Clinoid Processes)

AP AXIAL PROJECTION

Film: 8 × 10 in (18 × 24 cm) lengthwise.

Position of patient

• With the patient seated upright or supine, center the median sagittal plane of the body to the midline of the grid.
• Place the patient's arms along the sides of the body and adjust the shoulders to lie in the same horizontal plane.

Position of part

• With the median sagittal plane centered and perpendicular to the midline of the grid, adjust the flexion of the neck so that the infraorbitomeatal line is perpendicular to the plane of the film (Figs. 20-101 to 20-103).
• Adjust the film so that its midpoint will coincide with the central ray.
• Immobilize the head.
• Ask the patient to suspend respiration for the exposure.

Central ray

• Direct the central ray to the midline of the film to a point that will exit the foramen magnum. (1) A 37-degree caudal angulation will project the dorsum sellae and posterior clinoid processes within the foramen magnum (Fig. 20-104) or (2) a 30-degree caudal angulation of the central ray to the infraorbitmeatal line will project the dorsum and tuberculum sellae and the anterior clinoid processes through the occipital bone above the level of the foramen magnum (Fig. 20-105).

Structures shown

AP axial images of the sellar region and the petrous pyramids are demonstrated.

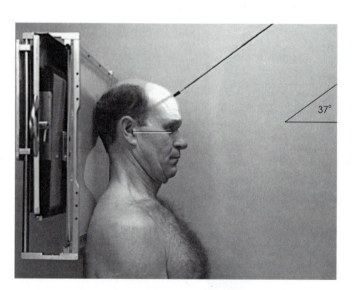

Fig. 20-101. AP axial sella turcica.

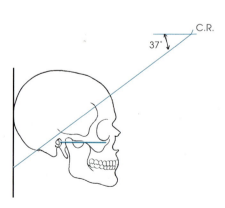

Fig. 20-102. Upright radiography.

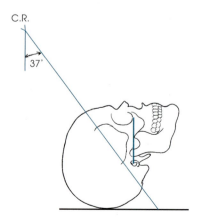

Fig. 20-103. Table radiography.

□ Evaluation criteria

The following should be clearly demonstrated:

- Sellar structures within the foramen magnum with a 37-degree angulation and through the occipital bone with a 30-degree angulation.
- No rotation of cranium.
- Symmetric petrous pyramids.
- Close beam restriction of sellar region.

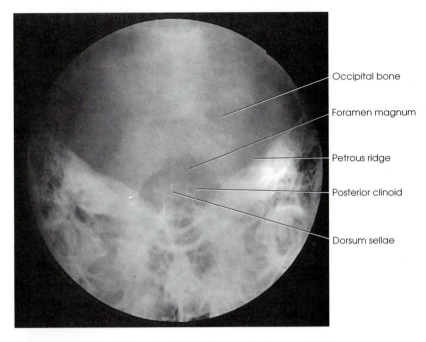

Occipital bone
Foramen magnum
Petrous ridge
Posterior clinoid
Dorsum sellae

Fig. 20-104. AP axial sella turcica: 37-degree central ray angulation.

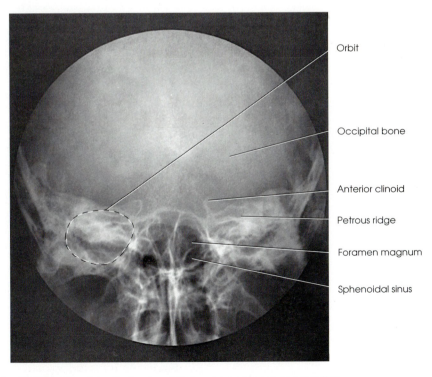

Orbit
Occipital bone
Anterior clinoid
Petrous ridge
Foramen magnum
Sphenoidal sinus

Fig. 20-105. AP axial sella turcica: 30-degree central ray angulation.

Sella Turcica

PA AXIAL PROJECTION
HAAS METHOD

Film: 8 × 10 in (18 × 24 cm) lengthwise.

Position of patient

- With the patient in the prone or seated position, center the median sagittal plane of the body to the midline of the grid.
- Flex the patient's elbows, place the arms in a comfortable position, and adjust the shoulders to lie in the same horizontal plane.

Position of part

- Adjust the median sagittal plane to be perpendicular and centered to the midline of the grid.
- Rest the forehead and nose on the table and center the film to a point 2 inches (5 cm) above the nasion.
- Adjust the flexion of the neck so that the orbitomeatal line is perpendicular to the plane of the film (Fig. 20-106).
- Place a support under the chin if needed.
- Immobilize the head.
- Ask the patient to suspend respiration for the exposure.

Central ray

- Direct the central ray to exit a point 1½ inches (3.7 cm) above the nasion at an angle of 25 degrees cephalad (Figs. 20-107 to 20-108). The central ray enters a point 1½ inches (3.7 cm) below the external occipital protuberance (inion).
- When examining heads of atypical shape, adjust the central ray angulation to coincide with the above points of entrance and exit.
- Use close collimation.

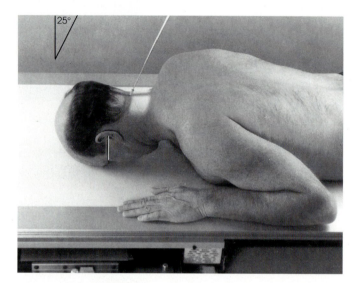

Fig. 20-106. PA axial sella turcica.

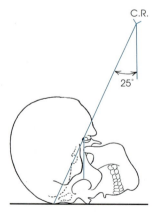

Fig. 20-107. Table radiography.

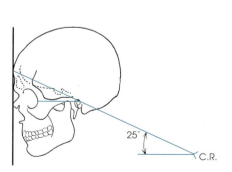

Fig. 20-108. Upright radiography.

Structures shown

An axial projection of the dorsum sellae and posterior clinoid processes projected within the foramen magnum and a symmetric image of the petrosae are shown (Fig. 20-109).

□ Evaluation criteria

The following should be clearly demonstrated:
- Dorsum sellae and the posterior clinoid processes within the foramen magnum.
- No rotation of the cranium.
- Symmetric petrous pyramids.
- Close collimation of the sellar region.

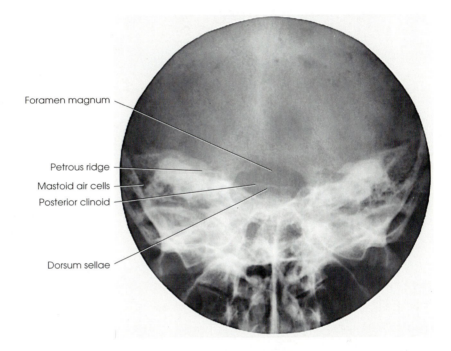

Foramen magnum

Petrous ridge
Mastoid air cells
Posterior clinoid

Dorsum sellae

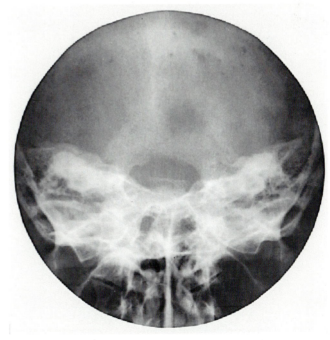

Fig. 20-109. PA axial sella turcica.

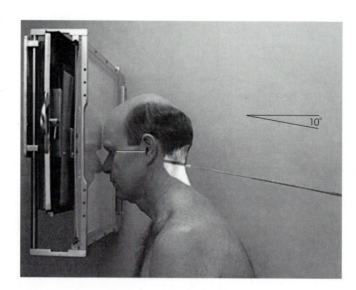

Fig. 20-110. PA sella turcica.

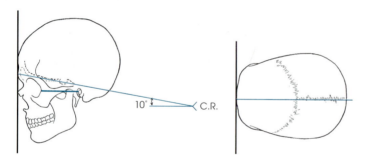

Fig. 20-111. Upright radiography.

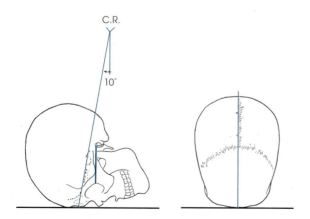

Fig. 20-112. Table radiography.

Sella Turcica
PA PROJECTION

Film: 8×10 in (18×24 cm) lengthwise.

Position of patient

- With the patient in the prone or seated position, center the median sagittal plane of the body to the midline of the grid.
- Flex the patient's elbows, place the arms in a comfortable position, and adjust the shoulders to lie in the same horizontal plane.

Position of part

- With the median sagittal plane of the patient's head perpendicular and centered to the midline of the grid, rest the forehead and nose on the table.
- Adjust the head so that the orbitomeatal line is perpendicular to the film (Fig. 20-110).
- Support the chin to prevent angulation if needed.
- Immobilize the head.
- Ask the patient to suspend respiration for the exposure.

Central ray

- Direct the central ray to exit the glabella at an angle of 10 degrees cephalad.
- Adjust the position of the cassette so that the midpoint will coincide with the central ray (Figs. 20-111 and 20-112).
- Use close collimation.

Structures shown

The dorsum and tuberculum sellae and the posterior and anterior clinoid processes are projected through the frontal bone just above the ethmoidal sinuses (Fig. 20-113).

□Evaluation criteria

The following should be clearly demon-strated:

- Adequate penetration of sellar struc-tures visible through the frontal bone.
- No rotation of the cranium.
- Symmetric petrous pyramids.
- Close beam restriction of sellar region.

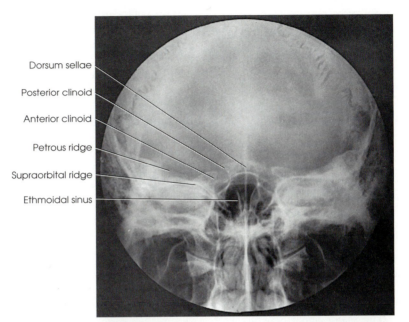

Dorsum sellae
Posterior clinoid
Anterior clinoid
Petrous ridge
Supraorbital ridge
Ethmoidal sinus

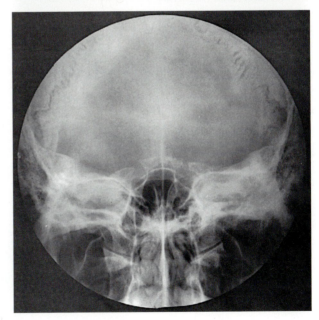

Fig. 20-113. PA sella turcica.

Orbit

The orbits are cone-shaped, bony-walled cavities, one situated on each side of the median sagittal plane of the head (Fig. 20-114). They are formed by the seven previously described and illustrated frontal, ethmoid, and sphenoid bones of the cranium, and the lacrimal, palatine, maxillary, and zygomatic bones of the face. Each orbit presents a roof, a medial and a lateral wall, and a floor. The easily palpable, quadrilateral-shaped anterior circumference of the orbit is called its *base*. Its *apex* corresponds to the optic canal (foramen). The long axis of each orbit is directed obliquely, posteriorly, and medially at an average angle of 37 degrees to the median sagittal plane of the head and also superiorly at an angle of about 30 degrees from the orbitomeatal line (Fig. 20-115).

The orbits serve primarily as bony sockets for the eyeballs and the structures associated with them, but they also contain blood vessels and nerves that pass through openings in their walls to other regions. The major and frequently radiographed openings are the previously described optic canal (foramina) and the superior and inferior orbital fissures.

The *superior orbital,* or sphenoid, fissure is the cleft between the greater and lesser wings of the sphenoid bone. It extends from the body of the sphenoid, from a point near the orbital apex, superiorly and laterally between the roof and the lateral wall of the orbit. The *inferior orbital,* or sphenomaxillary, fissure is the narrow cleft extending from the lower anterolateral aspect of the body of the sphenoid bone anteriorly and laterally between the floor and the lateral wall of the orbit. The anterior margin of the cleft is formed by the orbital plate of the maxilla, and its posterior margin is formed by the greater wing of the sphenoid bone and the zygomatic bone (zygoma).

The walls of the orbits are thin, so they are subject to fracture. For example, when a victim is forcibly struck squarely on the eyeball (by a fist, sporting equipment, etc.), the resulting pressure directed to the eyeball forces the eyeball into the cone-shaped orbit and "blows out" the thin and delicate bony floor of the orbit (Figs. 20-116 and 20-117). Accurate diagnosis and treatment must occur so that the vision of the victim is not jeopardized. For radiographic demonstration of blow-out fractures, images are obtained using any combination of radiographs with the patient positioned for the parietoacanthial projection (Waters method), radiographic tomography, and/or computed tomography.

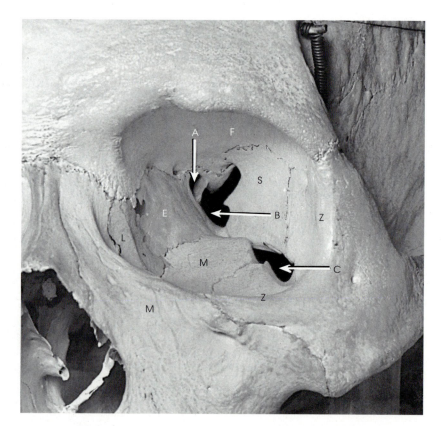

Fig. 20-114. Bones of left orbit of dry specimen; *E*, ethmoid; *F*, frontal; *L*, lacrimal; *M*, maxilla; *S*, sphenoid; *Z*, zygomatic (palatine not shown). *A*, Optic canal (foramen); *B*, superior orbital fissure; *C*, inferior orbital fissure.

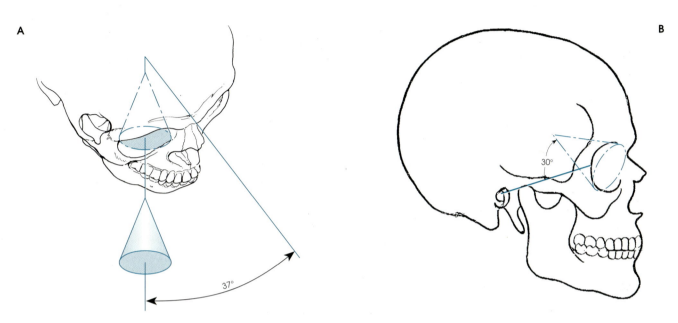

Fig. 20-115. Cone-shaped orbit. **A,** Average angles of 37 degrees from the median sagittal plane, and **B,** 30 degrees superior to the median orbitomeatal line.

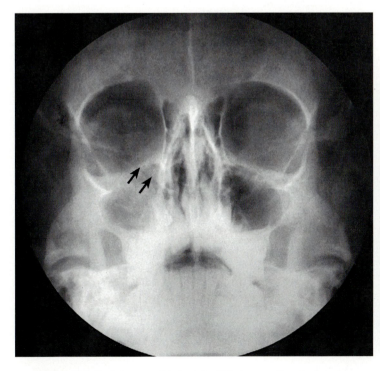

Fig. 20-116. Parietoacanthial orbits, (Waters method): showing blowout fracture of orbit *(arrows).*

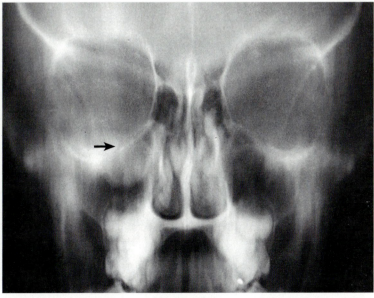

Fig. 20-117. Tomogram, AP projection showing fracture *(arrow)* on same patient as Fig. 20-116.

(Courtesy Dr. Judah Zizmor.)

Orbit

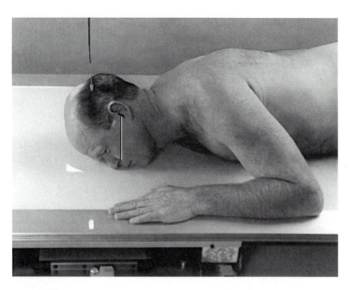

Fig. 20-118. Parieto-orbital oblique projection, Rhese method, for optic canal.

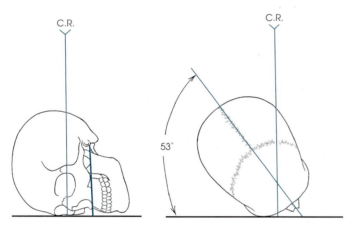

Fig. 20-119. Table radiography.

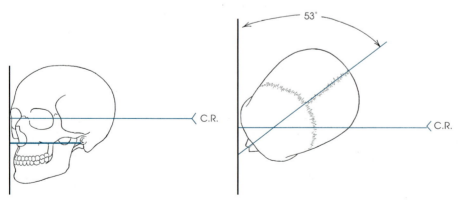

Fig. 20-120. Upright radiography.

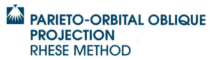

Optic Canal (Foramen)

◢ PARIETO-ORBITAL OBLIQUE PROJECTION
RHESE METHOD

Film: 8 × 10 in (18 × 24 cm).

Position of patient

- Place the patient in the prone or seated-upright position.
- Place the arms in a comfortable position and adjust the shoulders to lie in the same horizontal plane.

Position of part

- Center the affected orbit to the unmasked half of the cassette and rest the zygomatic bone (zygoma), the nose, and the chin on the table.
- Adjust the flexion of the neck to place the acanthomeatal line perpendicular to the plane of the film.
- Adjust the rotation of the head so that the median sagittal plane forms an angle of 53 degrees from the plane of the film (Figs. 20-118 to 20-120).
- When placed opposite the vertex, a protractor set to 53 degrees will parallel the median sagittal plane of the head if the rotation is correct. Check the position of the acanthomeatal line with one of the right-angle sides of the triangle.
- Immobilize the head.
- Ask the patient to suspend respiration for the exposure.

Central ray

- Direct the central ray perpendicular entering approximately 1 in (2.5 cm) superior and posterior to the top of ear attachment. The central ray exits through the affected orbit closest to the film.
- Use close collimation to orbit resting on table.

Structures shown

This projection demonstrates the optic canal in cross section, lying in the inferior and lateral quadrant of the projected orbit (Fig. 20-121). Any lateral deviation of this location indicates incorrect rotation of the head. Any longitudinal deviation indicates incorrect angulation of the acanthomeatal line. The supraorbital margins should lie in the same horizontal line. Both sides are examined for comparison.

☐ Evaluation criteria

The following should be clearly demonstrated:

- Optic canal (foramen) lying in the inferior and lateral quadrant of the orbit.
- Optic canal (foramen) visible enface at the end of the sphenoid ridge.
- Entire orbital rim.
- Close beam restriction of the orbital region.

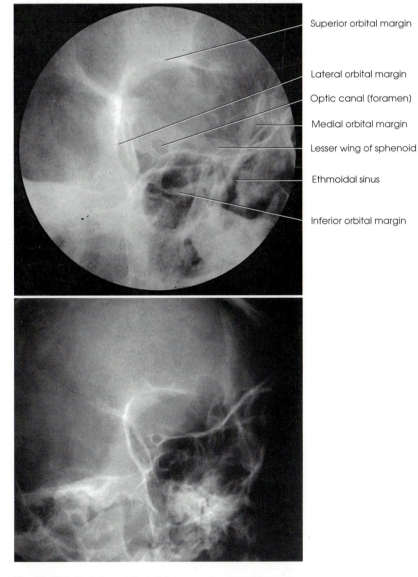

Superior orbital margin

Lateral orbital margin

Optic canal (foramen)

Medial orbital margin

Lesser wing of sphenoid

Ethmoidal sinus

Inferior orbital margin

Fig. 20-121. Parieto-orbital oblique projection, Rhese method, for optic canal.

(**B,** courtesy Deborah Meeker, RT.)

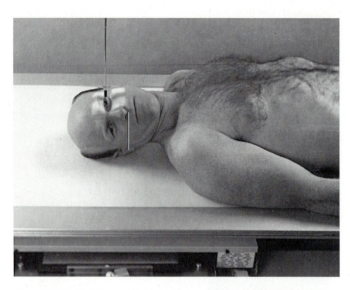

Fig. 20-122. Orbitoparietal oblique projection, Rhese method, for optic canal.

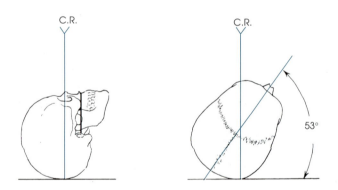

Fig. 20-123. Table radiography.

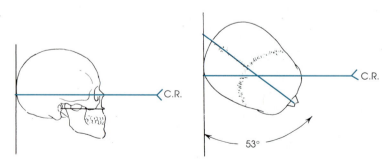

Fig. 20-124. Upright radiography.

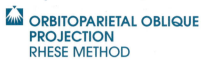

Optic Canal (Foramen)

ORBITOPARIETAL OBLIQUE PROJECTION
RHESE METHOD

Film: 8 × 10 in (18 × 24 cm).

Position of patient

- With the patient in the seated-upright or supine position, center the median sagittal plane of the body to the midline of the grid.
- Place the arms along the sides of the body and adjust the shoulders to lie in the same horizontal plane.

Position of part

- Rotate the head so that the median sagittal plane forms an angle of 53 degrees from the plane of the film.
- With the acanthomeatal line perpendicular, center the cassette to the orbit farthest from the film (Figs. 20-122 to 20-124).
- Immobilize the head.
- Ask the patient to suspend respiration for the exposure.

Central ray

- Direct the central ray perpendicular to the midpoint of the film entering the uppermost orbit at its inferior and lateral quadrant.

Structures shown

A cross-sectional image of the optic canal is seen in the inferior and lateral quadrant of the orbit (Fig. 20-125). This projection, the exact reverse of the parieto-orbital projection described previously, produces a comparable image.

NOTE: This projection should be used with patients who cannot be turned to the prone position. The radiographer should note that placing the patient supine will result in a certain degree of magnification on the radiograph because of the increased OID. Additionally, the orbitoparietal projection results in a greater amount of radiation exposure to the lens of the eye than does the parieto-orbital projection.

□ Evaluation criteria

The following should be clearly demonstrated:
- Optic canal (foramen) lying in the inferior and lateral quadrant of the orbit.
- Optic canal (foramen) visible enface at the end of the sphenoid ridge.
- Entire orbital rim.
- Close beam restriction of the orbital region.

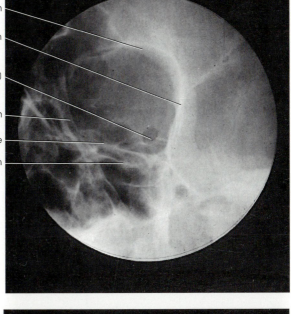

Superior orbital margin
Lateral orbital margin
Optic canal (foramen)
Medial orbital margin
Sphenoid ridge
Inferior orbital margin

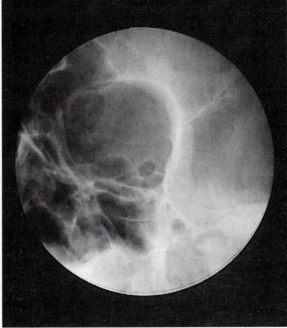

Fig. 20-125. Orbitoparietal oblique projection, Rhese method, for optic canal.

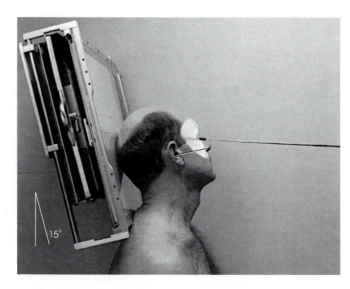

Fig. 20-126. Orbitoparietal oblique projection, Alexander method, for optic canal.

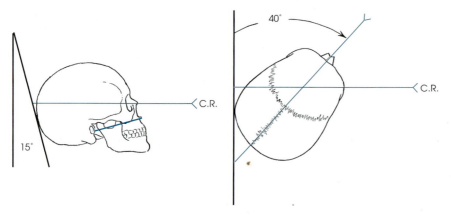

Fig. 20-127. Upright radiography.

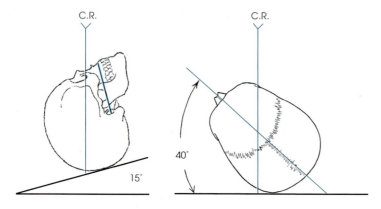

Fig. 20-128. Table radiography.

Optic Canal (Foramen)

ORBITOPARIETAL OBLIQUE PROJECTION
ALEXANDER METHOD

Film: 8 × 10 in (18 × 24 cm).

Position of patient

- Place the patient in the upright or supine position.
- With the patient in the supine position, elevate the shoulders several inches on a firm pillow or on sandbags so that the head can be adjusted on a 15-degree inclined angle sponge.
- Place the arms along the sides of the body and adjust the shoulders to lie in the same horizontal plane.

Position of part

- Place the cassette horizontally under the occiput on a 15-degree inclined angle sponge.
- If the patient is seated at a head unit, angle the film and grid device so that it forms a 15-degree angle from the vertical position (Figs. 20-126 to 20-128).
- Rotate the head with the side of interest farthest from the film, and adjust the head so that the median sagittal plane forms an angle of 40 degrees to the plane of the film.
- Extend the neck to place the acanthomeatal line perpendicular to the plane of the film.
- Immobilize the head.
- Ask the patient to suspend respiration for the exposure.

Central ray

- The central ray will be horizontal or vertical, depending on the patient position. This results in a 75-degree angle between the central ray and the film. It enters at the inferior and lateral margin of the outermost orbit.

Structures shown

This projection shows the optic canal in cross section, lying in the inferior and lateral quadrant of the orbital rim (Fig. 20-129). Both sides are examined for comparison.

□Evaluation criteria

The following should be clearly demonstrated:
- Optic canal (foramen) lying in the inferior and lateral quadrant of the orbit.
- Optic canal (foramen) visible enface at the end of the sphenoid ridge.
- Entire orbital rim.
- Close beam restriction of the orbital region.

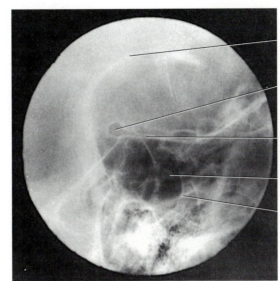

Superior orbital margin

Optic canal (foramen)

Sphenoid ridge

Ethmoidal sinus

Inferior orbital margin

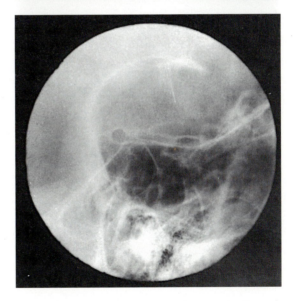

Fig. 20-129. Orbitoparietal oblique projection, Alexander method, for optic canal.

(Courtesy Sidney Alexander.)

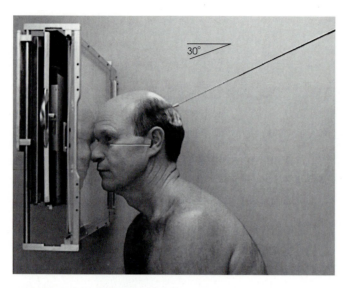

Fig. 20-130. Parieto-orbital axial oblique projection, modified Lysholm method: 30-degree central ray angulation.

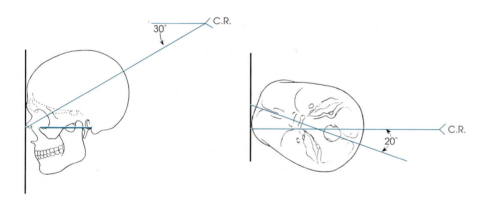

Fig. 20-131. Upright radiography.

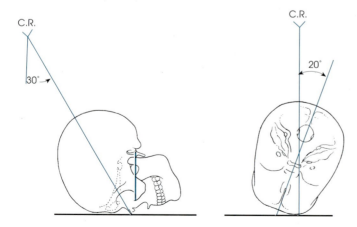

Fig. 20-132. Table radiography.

Optic Canal (Foramen), Superior Orbital Fissure, and Anterior Clinoid Process

PARIETO-ORBITAL AXIAL OBLIQUE PROJECTION
MODIFIED LYSHOLM METHOD

Film: 8 × 10 in (18 × 24 cm).

Position of patient

- Place the patient in the seated-upright or prone position.
- Center the median sagittal plane to the midline of the cassette.
- Place the arms in a comfortable position and adjust the shoulders to lie in the same plane.

Position of part

- Center the orbit of interest to the midline of the cassette.
- Rest the forehead and nose on the film holder.
- Adjust the head so that the median sagittal plane forms a 20-degree angle from the vertical.
- Rest the nose and zygomatic bone (zygoma) firmly on the grid device so that the infraorbitomeatal line is perpendicular to the plane of the film (Figs. 20-130 to 20-132).
- Immobilize the head.
- Ask the patient to suspend respiration for the exposure.

Central ray

- Direct the central ray to exit the affected orbit at the following angles:
  1. 20 degrees caudad for the demonstration of the optic canal (foramen) and the anterior clinoid process.
  2. 30 degrees caudad for the demonstration of the superior orbital fissure.
- Use close collimation.

Structures shown

The 20-degree angulation projection shows the anterior clinoid process and a slightly oblique image of the optic canal (foramen) projected into the center of the orbital shadow (Fig. 20-133).

The 30-degree angulation projection shows the superior orbital fissure to better advantage (Fig. 20-134).

The following should be clearly demonstrated:
- Optic canal (foramen) lying in the center of the orbit with a 20-degree angulation.
- Superior orbital fissure lateral to the optic canal (foramen) with a 30-degree angulation.
- Entire orbital rim.
- Close beam restriction of the orbital region.

NOTE: This method, originally described by Lysholm, used a double-tube angulation. The method presented has been modified by rotating the median sagittal plane 20 degrees. However, the basic geometry of the positioning has remained unchanged.

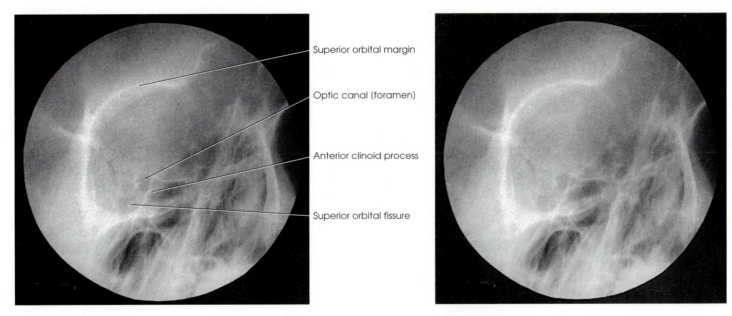

Superior orbital margin

Optic canal (foramen)

Anterior clinoid process

Superior orbital fissure

Fig. 20-133. Parieto-orbital axial oblique projection, modified Lysholm method. 20-degree central ray angulation.

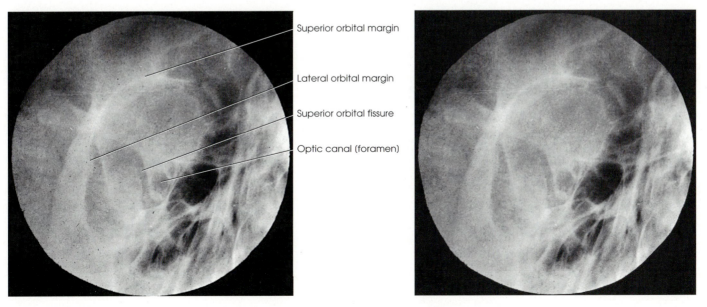

Superior orbital margin

Lateral orbital margin

Superior orbital fissure

Optic canal (foramen)

Fig. 20-134. Parieto-orbital axial oblique projection, modified Lysholm method. 30-degree central ray angulation.

Optic canal, superior orbital fissure, & anterior clinoid process

279

Sphenoid Strut

PARIETO-ORBITAL OBLIQUE PROJECTION
HOUGH METHOD[1]

Sphenoid strut is the term often used to describe the inferior root of the lesser wing of the sphenoid bone (Fig. 20-135). This root, or strut, of bone forms the floor and part of the lateral wall of the optic canal, the opening through which the optic nerve and the ophthalmic artery pass from the brain to the eye. The Hough method presents a nondistorted projection of the strut and is of particular value for the demonstration of erosion of the bone caused by a lesion involving the adjacent cavernous sinus.

Film: 8 × 10 in (18 × 24 cm).

[1]Hough JE: Sphenoid strut: parieto-orbital projection, Radiol Technol 39:197-209, 1968.

Position of patient

- Place the patient in the prone position or seated before a vertical grid device.
- Place the arms in a comfortable position and adjust the shoulders to lie in the same horizontal plane to prevent rotation.

Position of part

- Center the affected orbit to the cassette and rest the superciliary arch (ridge) and the side of the nose on the film holder.
- Adjust the extension of the neck so that the infraorbitomeatal line is perpendicular to the plane of the film.
- Adjust the rotation of the head so that the median sagittal plane is rotated 20 degrees toward the side being examined (Figs. 20-136 to 20-138).
- Immobilize the head.
- Ask the patient to suspend respiration for the exposure.

Central ray

- Direct the central ray 7 degrees caudad to exit the affected orbit to the center of the film.
- Use close collimation.

Structures shown

An unobstructed and undistorted image of the sphenoid strut is visible in the center of the orbital rim, where it separates the optic canal from the superior orbital fissure (Fig. 20-139). The sphenoid strut is seen lying between the sphenoidal sinus and the combined shadows of the adjacent anterior clinoid process and the lesser wing of the sphenoid bone. The superior root of the lesser wing of the sphenoid bone, forming the roof of the optic canal, can be traced medially to the jugum sphenoidale and laterally to the sphenoid ridge.

□Evaluation criteria

The following should be clearly demonstrated:

- Sphenoid strut visible in the center of the orbit between the optic canal (foramen) and superior orbital fissure.
- Entire orbital shadow.
- Close beam restriction of the orbital region.

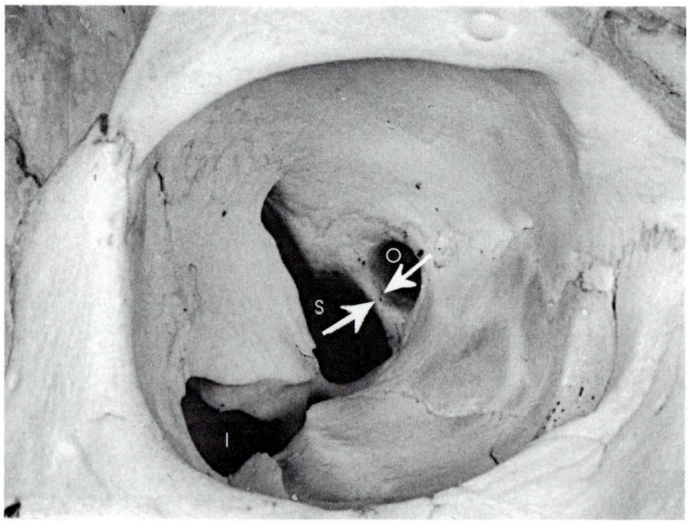

Fig. 20-135. Oblique image of right orbit *(dry specimen);* sphenoid strut indicated by arrows. *O,* Optic foramen; *S,* superior orbital fissure; *I,* inferior orbital fissure.

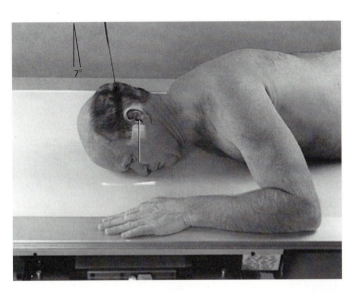

Fig. 20-136. Parieto-orbital oblique projection, Hough method, for sphenoid strut.

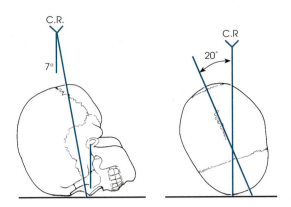

Fig. 20-137. Table radiography.

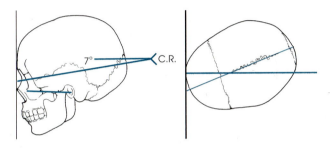

Fig. 20-138. Upright radiography.

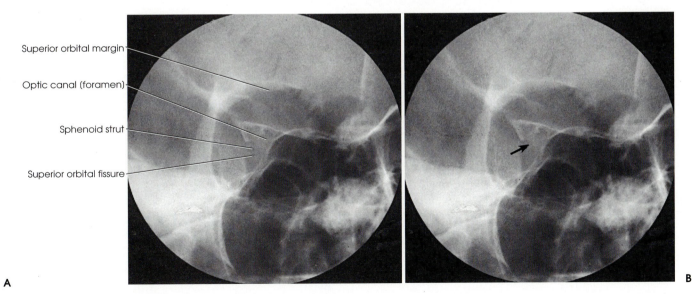

Superior orbital margin

Optic canal (foramen)

Sphenoid strut

Superior orbital fissure

A

B

Fig. 20-139. A, Normal right sphenoid strut. **B,** Abnormal *(eroded)* left sphenoid strut on patient with spontaneous carotid-cavernous fistula.

(Courtesy Dr. John A. Goree.)

Superior Orbital Fissures

PA AXIAL PROJECTION

Film: 8 × 10 in (18 × 24 cm) lengthwise.

Position of patient

- Place the patient in the prone or seated-upright body position.
- Adjust to center the median sagittal plane of the body to the midline of the grid.

Position of part

- Rest the forehead and nose on the grid device with the median sagittal plane centered and perpendicular to the midline of the film.
- Adjust the flexion of the neck so that the orbitomeatal line is perpendicular to the plane of the film (Figs. 20-140 to 20-142).
- Center the film at the level of the inferior margin of the orbits.
- Ask the patient to suspend respiration for the exposure.

Central ray

- Direct the central ray at an angle of 20 to 25 degrees caudad, exiting the midline at the level of the inferior margin of the orbit.
- Use close collimation.

Structures shown

The superior margin of the petrous portions of the temporal bones should be projected at or just below the inferior margin of the orbits (Fig. 20-143). The superior orbital (sphenoid) fissures are seen as elongated dark areas lying on the medial side of the orbits between the greater and lesser wings of the sphenoid bones.

The margins of the superior orbital (sphenoid) fissures, although somewhat narrowed, are frequently well shown on the 15-degree caudad angle PA skull (Fig. 20-144).

□ Evaluation criteria

The following should be clearly demonstrated:

- No rotation of the cranium.
- Projection of petrous ridges below the superior orbital fissures.
- Close beam restriction of both orbital regions.

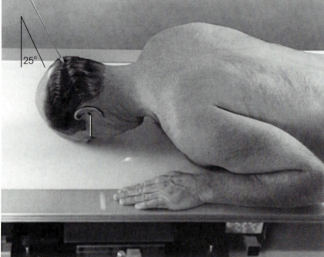

Fig. 20-140. PA axial superior orbital fissure. Central ray angled 25 degrees.

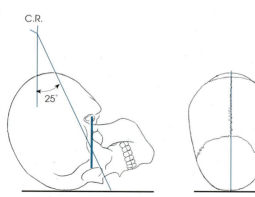

Fig. 20-141. Table radiography.

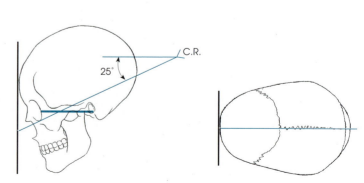

Fig. 20-142. Upright radiography.

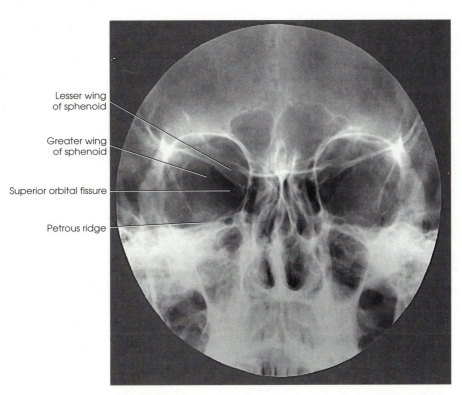

Lesser wing
of sphenoid

Greater wing
of sphenoid

Superior orbital fissure

Petrous ridge

Fig. 20-143. PA axial superior orbital fissures: central ray angulation 25 degrees.

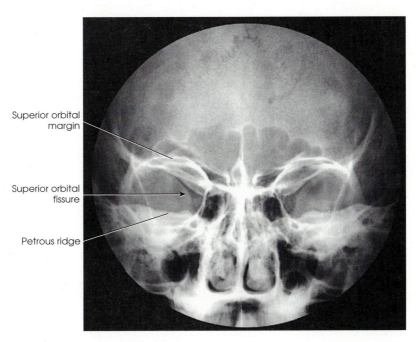

Superior orbital
margin

Superior orbital
fissure

Petrous ridge

Fig. 20-144. PA axial skull, Caldwell method: central ray angulation 15 degrees.

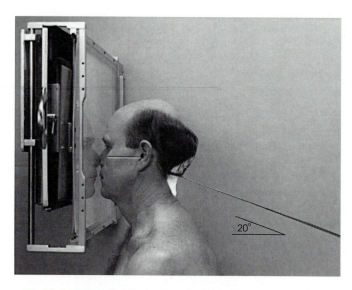

Fig. 20-145. PA axial projection, Bertel method, for inferior orbital fissures.

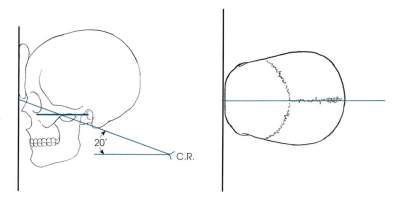

Fig. 20-146. Upright radiography.

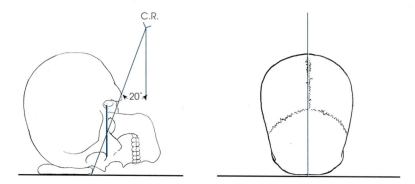

Fig. 20-147. Table radiography.

Inferior Orbital Fissures

PA AXIAL PROJECTION
BERTEL METHOD

Film: 8 × 10 in (18 × 24 cm) lengthwise.

Position of patient

- Place the patient in the seated-upright or prone position.
- Center the median sagittal plane of the body to the midline of the grid device.
- Place the arms in a comfortable position and adjust the shoulders to lie in the same horizontal plane.

Position of part

- Rest the forehead and nose on the grid device with the median sagittal plane perpendicular to the midline of the grid.
- Adjust the flexion of the neck so that the infraorbitomeatal line is perpendicular to the plane of the film; elevate the forehead somewhat on a radiolucent pad if needed (Figs. 20-145 to 20-147).
- With the cassette in the Bucky tray, adjust it so that the midpoint of the film will coincide with the central ray.
- Immobilize the head.
- Ask the patient to suspend respiration for the exposure.

Central ray

- Direct the central ray to exit the nasion at an angle of 20 to 25 degrees cephalad. The central ray enters the midline approximately 3 in (7.5 cm) below the external occipital protuberance.

NOTE: Lower exposure factors are typically used because the orbital area in this projection requires less penetration.

Structures shown

A PA axial projection of each orbital floor and inferior orbital fissure is demonstrated between the shadows of the pterygoid process of the sphenoid bone and the mandibular ramus (Fig. 20-148).

□ Evaluation criteria

The following should be clearly demonstrated:
- No rotation of the cranium.
- Inferior orbital fissures visible within the orbits.
- Close beam restriction of both orbital regions.

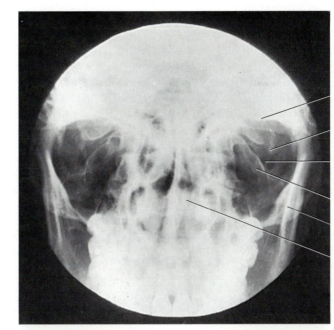

Superior orbital margin

Styloid process

Inferior orbital fissure

Lateral pterygoid lamina

Mandibular ramus

Nasal cavity

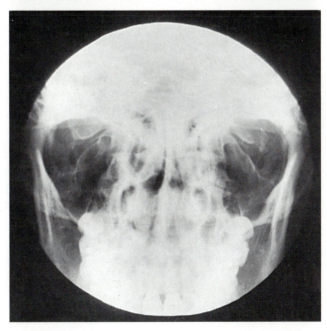

Fig. 20-148. PA axial projection, Bertel method, for inferior orbital fissures. Note exposure factors for orbital area different than skull.

Eye

The organ of vision, or eye (L. *oculus;* Gr. *ophthalmos),* consists of the eyeball; the optic nerve, which connects the eyeball to the brain; the blood vessels; and such accessory organs as the extrinsic muscles, the lacrimal apparatus, and the eyelids (Figs. 20-149 and 20-150).

The *eyeball,* or optic bulb, is situated in the anterior part of the orbital cavity, where its posterior segment, about two thirds of the bulb, is in relation to the soft parts that occupy the remainder of the orbital cavity—chiefly muscles, fat, and connective tissue. The anterior portion of the eyeball is exposed, and it projects somewhat beyond the base of the orbit, so that bone-free radiographic images can be obtained of the anterior segment of the eye. The exposed part of the eyeball is covered by a thin mucous membrane known as the *conjunctiva,* reflections of which line the eyelids. The conjunctival

membrane is kept moist by tear secretions from the lacrimal gland, which prevent drying and friction irritation during movements of the eyeball and eyelids.

The eyeball consists of (1) a thin but firm-walled capsule composed of three concentric membranous coats and (2) the enclosed fluid-to-gelatinous refracting media of the eye. The eyeball is nearly spherical in shape. It is slightly flattened from above inferiorly, and it presents an anterior bulge in its outer coat, so that the front-to-back diameter is slightly greater than the vertical and transverse diameters. Killian and Elstrom[1] state that while the average AP diameter of the eyeball is 24 mm, this measurement varies from 20 to 26 mm. They further state that the average horizontal diameter is 23.7 mm, and the

---

[1]Killian CH and Elstrom ER: Localization of intraorbital and intraocular foreign bodies, Med Radiogr Photogr 28:78-94, 1952.

average vertical diameter is 23.5 mm. The female eyeball is said to measure 0.5 mm less in all diameters than the male eyeball.

The outer, supporting coat of the eyeball is a firm, fibrous membrane consisting of a posterior segment called the *sclera* and an anterior segment called the *cornea.* The opaque, white sclera is commonly referred to as the white of the eye. The cornea is situated in front of the iris, with its center point corresponding to the pupil. The corneal part of the membrane is modified to transparence for the passage of light, and it serves as one of the four refractive media of the eye. A shallow groove, the scleral sulcus, encircles the edge, or *limbus,* of the cornea at its junction with the sclera. The cornea is bulged anteriorly for the accommodation of the fluid-containing anterior chamber of the eyeball, the space situated between the cornea and the iris and pupil.

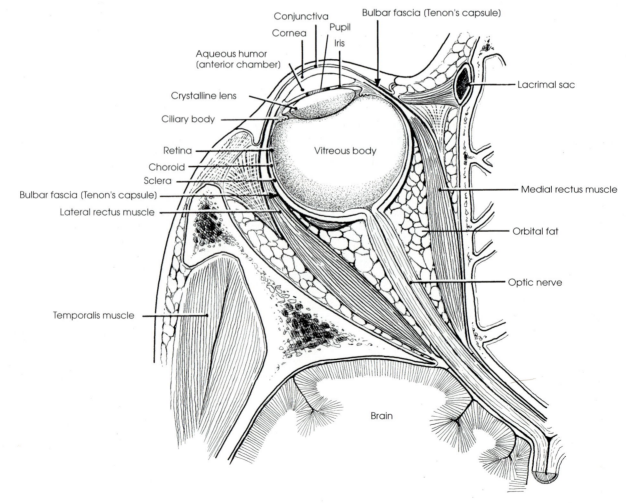

Conjunctiva
Cornea
Pupil
Iris
Bulbar fascia (Tenon's capsule)
Aqueous humor (anterior chamber)
Crystalline lens
Ciliary body
Retina
Choroid
Sclera
Bulbar fascia (Tenon's capsule)
Lateral rectus muscle
Temporalis muscle
Vitreous body
Lacrimal sac
Medial rectus muscle
Orbital fat
Optic nerve
Brain

Fig. 20-149. Diagrammatic horizontal section of right orbital region.

The middle coat of the eyeball is vascular and pigmented. It consists of three continuous segments: (1) the *choroid,* which covers the posterior two thirds of the eyeball, (2) the *ciliary body,* which is a wedge-shaped muscular ring surrounding the iris and associated with the focusing power of the eye, and (3) the *iris,* which is the colored muscular diaphragm. The iris, by controlling the size of the pupillary opening, regulates the amount of light admitted to the eye.

The inner coat of the eyeball is called the *retina.* This delicate membrane is continuous with the optic nerve. The retina is chiefly composed of nervous tissue and the several million minute receptor organs, called rods and cones, that transmit light impulses to the brain.

The refractive media contained within the eyeball are (1) the *crystalline lens,* which is a transparent viscous fluid contained within a transparent membranous capsule that is held in place behind the iris by a system of ligamentous fibers extending from the circumference of the capsule to the ciliary body; (2) the *aqueous hu-mor,* which is a watery fluid filling the space between the cornea and the iris and crystalline lens and which produces the forward bulge in the cornea; and (3) the *vitreous body,* which is a clear, jellylike substance filling the space behind the crystalline lens.

Movements of the eyeball in directing the pupillary aperture are controlled by six extrinsic muscles arranged in opposing pairs. These muscles are the superior and inferior and the medial and lateral *rectus* (straight) *muscles* and the superior and inferior *oblique muscles.* The four rectus muscles and the superior oblique muscle arise from a fibrous ring attached around the circumference of the optic canal (foramen), and the inferior oblique muscle arises from the anteromedial margin of the floor of the orbit. Each muscle has its other attachment on the sclerotic coat of the eyeball. The retrobulbar space situated central to the divergent straight muscles is called the *muscle cone.* The muscles stretch or contract and turn with the eyeball, so that a foreign body lodged in a muscle, as well as one located within the optic bulb, will show a shift in position with movements of the eye.

A fibrous tunic known as the *bulbar fascia,* or *Tenon's capsule,* ensheathes the posterior portion of the eyeball, the part corresponding to the sclera, and by tubelike prolongations joins the somewhat thinner fascial sheaths enclosing the extrinsic muscles. Tenon's capsule serves to separate the eyeball from the surrounding orbital contents. The space between the sclera and capsule, called the *interfascial space of Tenon,* provides a synovial-like sac in which friction-free movement of the eyeball is possible.

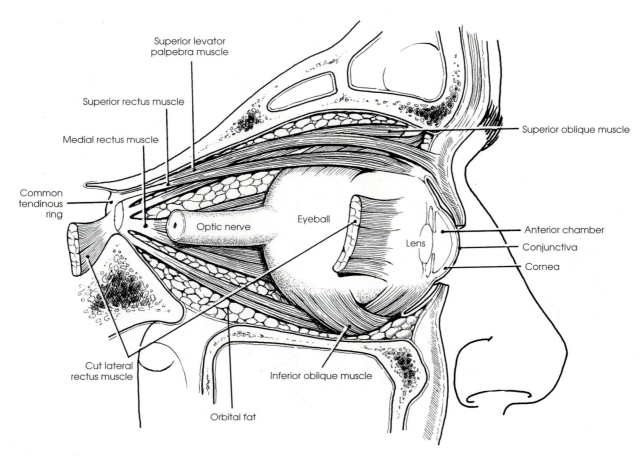

Fig. 20-150. Diagrammatic sagittal section of right orbital region.

Superior levator palpebra muscle

Superior rectus muscle

Medial rectus muscle

Common tendinous ring

Cut lateral rectus muscle

Orbital fat

Optic nerve

Eyeball

Inferior oblique muscle

Lens

Superior oblique muscle

Anterior chamber

Conjunctiva

Cornea

LOCALIZATION OF FOREIGN BODIES WITHIN ORBIT OR EYE

Ultrasound and computed tomography (Fig. 20-151) have been increasingly used in locating foreign bodies in the eye. (The use of magnetic resonance imaging in foreign body localization is contraindicated since movement of a metallic foreign body by the magnetic field could lead to hemorrhage or other serious complications.) Whether ultrasound or a radiographic approach is used, accurate localization of foreign particles lodged within the orbit or eye necessitates using a precision localization technique. Each of the numerous precision methods and modifications of these methods, approximately 30 in all, requires the use of a specially designed accessory device. For a detailed study of the different methods, the reader is referred to the works listed in the bibliography. The method or methods selected for radiographic use by the individual radiologist and radiographer varies, but the Sweet method[1] and the Pfeiffer modification[2,3] of the Comberg method[4] are the two procedures most widely employed in the United States.

Technical precision is essential in these examinations. Full information on the use of each method of localization can be obtained from the literature (see bibliography in this volume), but skill in the application of any precision technique can be gained only through instruction and supervised practice until proficiency is attained.

Film quality

Ultra fine recorded detail is essential to the detection and localization of minute foreign particles located within the orbit or eyeball. First, the geometric unsharpness must be reduced as much as possible by a close OID and by the use of a small, undamaged focal spot at a source–to–im-

[1]Sweet WH: Improved apparatus for localizing foreign bodies in the eyeball by the roentgen rays, Trans Am Ophthalmol Soc 12:320-329, 1909.
[2]Pfeiffer RL: Localization of intraocular foreign bodies with the contact lens, AJR 44:558-563, 1940.
[3]Pfeiffer RL: Localization of intraocular foreign bodies by means of contact lens, Arch Ophthalmol 32:261-266, 1944.
[4]Comberg W: Ein neues Verfahren zur Röntgenlokalisation am Augapfel, Arch Ophthalmol 118: 175-194, 1927.

age receptor distance (SID)—that is, as long as is consistent with the exposure factors required. Second, secondary radiation must be minimized by close collimation. Third, motion must be eliminated by firm immobilization of the patient's head and by securing cooperation in immobilizing the eyeballs with a steady gaze at a fixed object.

An artifact can cast an image that simulates the appearance of a foreign body located within the orbit or eye. Therefore cassettes and screens must be impeccably cleaned before each examination. Where these examinations are often performed, an adequate number of film holders are held in reserve for eye studies only, thus protecting them from the wear of routine use in less critical procedures.

PRELIMINARY EXAMINATION

The scout radiographs consist of lateral and PA projections, and bone-free studies, which are taken to determine whether a radiographically demonstrable foreign body is present. For these radiographs, the patient may be placed in the recumbent position or seated upright before a vertical grid device.

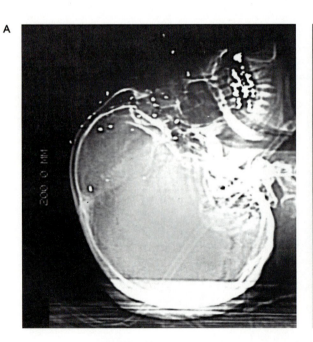
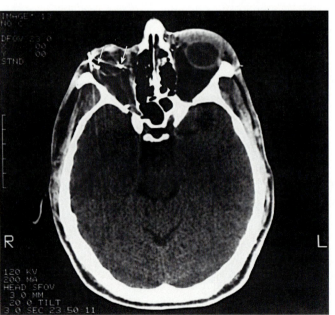

Fig. 20-151. A, Lateral localizer computed tomography image of narcotics agent shot in face with shotgun, demonstrating multiple buckshot. **B,** Axial computed tomography image on same patient showing shotgun pellets within the eye *(arrow).*

LATERAL PROJECTION
R or L position

A non-grid technique is recommended to reduce magnification and eliminate possible artifacts in, or on, the table and grid; the following steps are observed:

- With the patient either semiprone or seated upright, place the outer canthus of the affected eye adjacent to and centered over the midpoint of the film.
- Adjust the head to place the median sagittal plane parallel with and the interpupillary line perpendicular to the plane of the film.
- Ask the patient to suspend respiration for the exposure.

Central ray

- Direct the central ray perpendicular through the outer canthi.
- Instruct the patient to look straight ahead for the exposure (Figs. 20-152 and 20-153).

□ Evaluation criteria

The following should be clearly demonstrated:

- Density and contrast permitting optimal visibility of the orbit and eye for foreign bodies.
- Superimposed orbital roofs.
- No rotation of sella turcica.
- Close beam restriction centered to the orbital region.

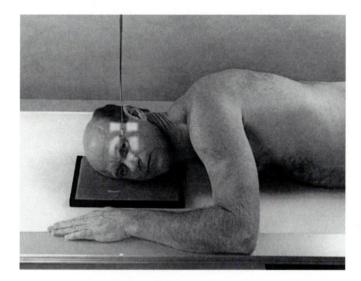

Fig. 20-152. Lateral projection, orbital foreign body localization.

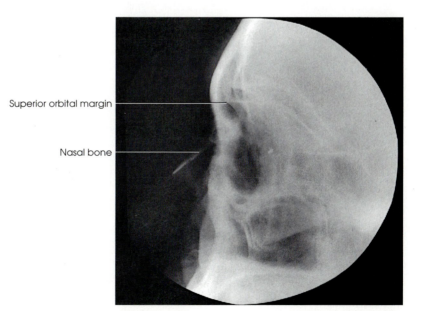

Superior orbital margin

Nasal bone

Fig. 20-153. Lateral projection with foreign body (*white speck*).

(Courtesy Dr. Judah Zizmor.)

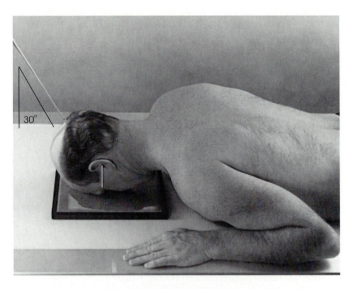

Fig. 20-154. PA axial projection orbital foreign body localization.

PA AXIAL PROJECTION

A non-grid technique is recommended to reduce magnification and eliminate possible artifacts in, or on, the table and grid, and the following steps are observed:

- Rest the forehead and nose on the film holder, and center the film holder ¾ inch (1.9 cm) distal to the nasion.
- Adjust the head so that the median sagittal plane and the orbitomeatal line are perpendicular to the plane of the film.
- Ask the patient to suspend respiration for the exposure.

Central ray

- Direct the central ray through the center of the orbits at a caudal angulation of 30 degrees. This angulation is used to project the petrous portions of the temporal bones below the inferior margin of the orbits (Figs. 20-154 and 20-155).
- Instruct the patient to close the eyes and to concentrate on holding them still for the exposure.

☐ Evaluation criteria

The following should be clearly demonstrated:

- ■ Petrous pyramids lying below the orbital shadows.
- ■ No rotation of the cranium.
- ■ Close beam restriction centered to the orbital region.

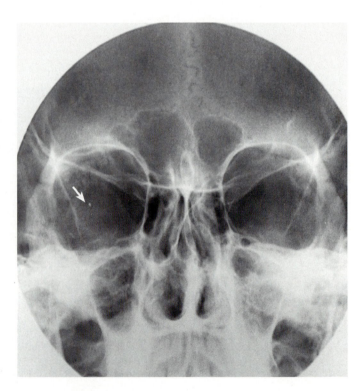

Fig. 20-155. PA axial projection demonstrating foreign body *(arrow)* in right eye.

(Courtesy Dr. Raymond Pfeiffer.)

PARIETOACANTHIAL PROJECTION
MODIFIED WATERS METHOD

Some physicians prefer to have the PA projection done with the head adjusted in a modified Waters method so that the petrous margins are displaced by part adjustment rather than by central ray angulation.

- With the film centered at the level of the center of the orbits, rest the patient's chin on the film holder.
- Adjust the head so that the median sagittal plane is perpendicular to the plane of the film.
- Adjust the flexion of the neck so that the orbitomeatal line forms an angle of 37 to 50 degrees with the plane of the film.
- Ask the patient to suspend respiration for the exposure.

Central ray

- Direct the central ray perpendicular through the midorbits (Figs. 20-156 and 20-157).
- Instruct the patient to close the eyes and to concentrate on holding them still for the exposure.

□ Evaluation criteria

The following should be clearly demonstrated:
- Petrous pyramids lying well below the orbital shadows.
- No rotation of the cranium.
- Close beam restriction centered to the orbital region.

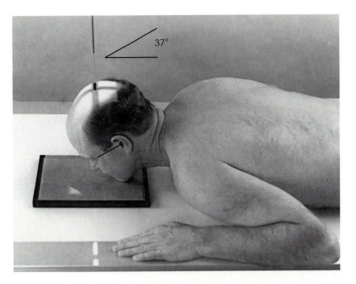

Fig. 20-156. Parietoacanthial projection, modified Waters method, for orbital foreign body localization.

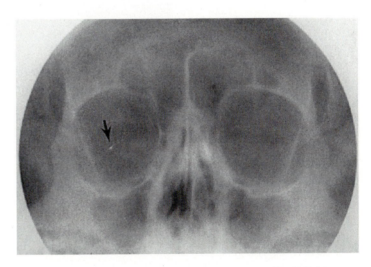

Fig. 20-157. Parietoacanthial projection, modified Waters method, demonstrating foreign body *(arrow)*.

Eye

291

VOGT BONE-FREE PROJECTIONS

Vogt[1] bone-free projections are taken to detect small or low-density foreign particles located in the anterior segment of the eyeball or in the eyelids. Lateromedial and, when the eye is not too deeply set, superoinferior images are taken. These projections are produced on standard periapical (1¼ × 1⅝ in) or occlusal size (2 × 2¾ in) dental films (Figs. 20-158 and 20-159).

---

[1]Vogt A: Skelettfreie Röntgenaufnahmen des vorderen Bulbusabechnittes, Schweiz Med Wochenschr 2:145-146, 1921.

In bone-free studies the eyes may be directed straight forward and/or the eyeball may be in different positions.

- For vertical movement images, make one exposure in which the patient looks up as far as possible, and make a second exposure in which the patient looks down as far as possible.
- For horizontal movement images, make one exposure while the patient is looking to the extreme right and the other exposure while the patient is looking to the extreme left.
- Make the latter studies from the superoinferior direction when the eyes are not too deeply set.
- For detailed information on performing the Vogt bone-free projections, please see pp. 278 and 279 of the seventh edition of this atlas, or earlier editions.

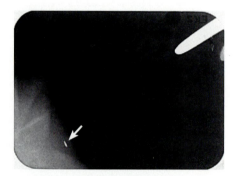

Fig. 20-158. Lateral eye, bone free, demonstrating foreign body *(arrow).*

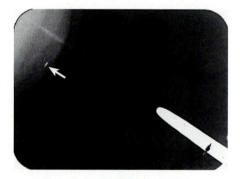

Fig. 20-159. Superoinferior eye, bone free, demonstrating foreign body *(arrow).*

PARALLAX MOTION METHOD

The parallax motion method of determining whether a foreign body is located within the eyeball requires no special apparatus. This procedure, first described by Richards,[1] consists of producing two lateral and two PA projections with the eyeball in different positions. Each pair of projections may be made on one film or on separate films, as preferred.

---

[1]Richards GE: Localization of foreign bodies in the eye: an additional safeguard, AJR 18:387-389, 1927.

Anteriorly and posteriorly placed intraocular foreign bodies move with the eyeball, whereas centrally placed intraocular foreign bodies (Fig. 20-160) do not change position. Foreign bodies lodged in the extrinsic muscles or attached to the fascial sheaths outside the bulb also move with the eyeball. For this reason it is not considered a precision localization procedure, but it is widely used as a preliminary evaluation. Parallax movement of the eyeball is, as described previously, also used in bone-free studies of the anterior segment of the eye.

For more complete information on positioning for the parallax motion method, please see pp. 280 and 281 of the seventh edition of this atlas, or earlier editions.

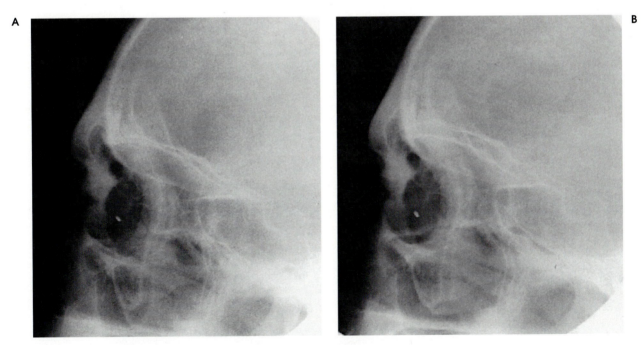

Fig. 20-160. Lateral eye on patient with foreign body. **A,** Patient looking superiorly. **B,** Same patient looking inferiorly. Note slight movement of foreign body.

SWEET METHOD

The Sweet method of orbital foreign body localization determines the exact location of a foreign body by the use of a geometric calculation. This method requires a device that contains two markers of known position and relationship, from which measurements can be made.

The apparatus designed for this method comprises the localizer device and an 8 × 10 in (18 × 24 cm) film tunnel of the pedestal type (Fig. 20-161). The legs can be removed if the user prefers. The localizer consists of a small, heavy-based metal stand on which is mounted a vertically adjustable arm bearing the essential parts of the device. These parts are (1) a *metal ball* and a *metal cone*, each attached to the end of a slender metallic rod so mounted that the ball is held 15 mm directly above the cone and each at right angles to the stand; (2) a recoil spring and trigger release arrangement that permits an exact 10 mm forward-backward movement of the ball and cone support; and (3) two sighting notches for use in aligning the indicator ball and rod.

The pedestal tunnel is equipped with a sliding film tray, a head clamp, and a small pneumatic cushion on which the patient's head rests. Except for the central exposure area, the bakelite top of the tunnel is backed with radiopaque metal to mask one half of the film for each exposure, so that the two lateral projections required for this examination can be made on one film. The outline of the exposure area and longitudinal and horizontal centering lines are etched on the top of the tunnel.

A

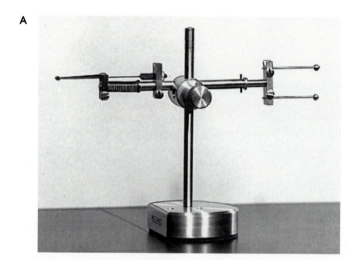

B

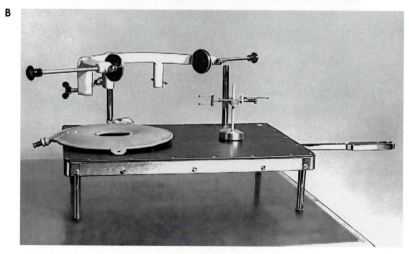

Fig. 20-161. A, Sweet localizing device. **B,** Sweet film pedestal device (legs attached).

Examination procedure

The procedure is conducted in the following manner:

- Immobilize the patient's head in the true lateral position, and center the localizer device to the center of the affected pupil.
- Instruct the patient to hold the eye still by focusing on an object.
- Make two exposures, one with a perpendicular central ray and another with the central ray directed 15 to 25 degrees cephalad (Fig. 20-162). The location of the foreign body is geometrically mapped using a special Sweet Localizing Graph paper using measurements from the two lateral radiographic images (Fig. 20-163).
- For more detailed information on performing this procedure, please refer to pp. 282 to 284 of the seventh edition of this atlas, or earlier editions.

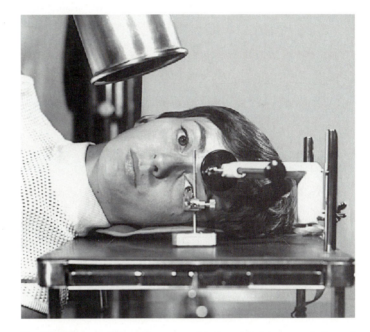

Fig. 20-162. Lateral eye, Sweet method, central ray angulation of 15 degrees.

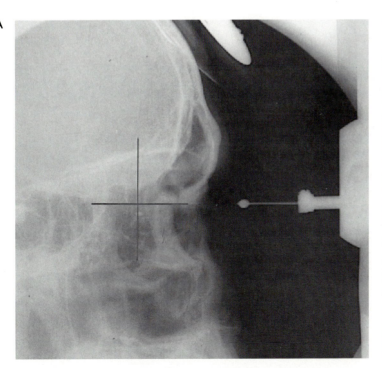

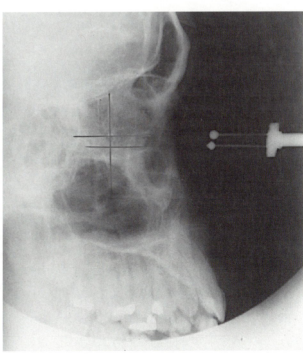

Fig. 20-163. Lateral eye, Sweet method. **A,** Central ray angulation of 0 degrees and, **B,** angulation of 15 degrees cephalad.

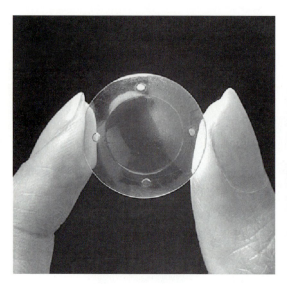
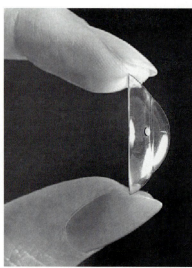

Fig. 20-164. Pfeiffer-Comberg contact lens localization device.

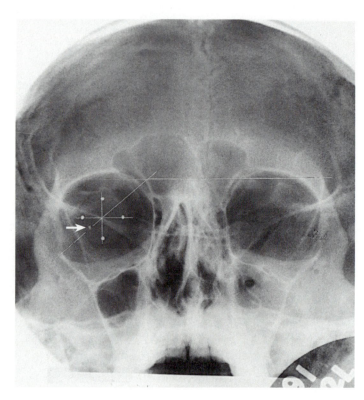

Fig. 20-165. PA projection, Pfeiffer-Comberg localization image demonstrating foreign body *(arrow)*. Lateral projection not shown.

PFEIFFER-COMBERG METHOD

In the Pfeiffer-Comberg method, a sterilized leaded contact lens is placed directly over the patient's locally anesthetized cornea, and intraorbital and intraocular foreign bodies are then localized in relation to the limbus and the corneoscleral junction, instead of to the visual axis of the eye, as in the Sweet method.

The apparatus designed for this procedure comprises the contact lens localization device and a pedestal type of film holder. The contact lens (Fig. 20-164) has embedded around its periphery four lead markers spaced at 90-degree intervals. When in position on the cornea, the lead markers indicate the horizontal and vertical meridians of the eyeball.

Examination procedure

The procedure is conducted in the following manner:

- With the patient positioned using the special Pfeiffer-Comberg film holder device, have the patient bite a special "bite bar" to ensure the patient does not move between the PA and lateral projections. Make the exposure for the PA projection (Fig. 20-165). Without moving the patient, move the x-ray tube around the patient and make the exposure for the lateral projection.
- Using special localizing graph paper, calculate the location of the foreign body.
- For more complete information on performing the Pfeiffer-Comberg procedure, please refer to pp. 285 to 287 of the seventh edition of this atlas, or earlier editions.

Nasolacrimal Drainage System

Dacryocystography (Gr. *dakryon,* tear) is the term used to denote radiologic examinations of the nasolacrimal drainage system by filling the lumina of the canals with a radiopaque medium. This examination is performed in the investigation of such abnormalities of these passages as defective development, stenosis, and chronic mucosal thickening.

The *lacrimal gland* (L. *lacrima,* tear) is a small, almond-shaped, bipartite body situated anteriorly on the lateral side of the roof of the orbit, where it is lodged in the lacrimal fossa of the frontal bone (Fig. 20-166). The function of the gland is to secrete watery fluid. The tear secretion serves to lubricate and wet the delicate membrane that lines the eyelids and covers the front of the eyeball. This membrane is called the *conjunctiva,* and the space between the lids and the surface of the eyeball is called the *conjunctival sac.* Six to twelve minute ducts convey the tear secretion from the gland to the conjunctival sac, and the blinking movements of the lids spread the fluid over the surface of the eyeball. Part of the fluid evaporates, and part of it flows into the *lacrimal lake.* The lacrimal lake is the shallow, triangular pouch, or cul-de-sac, formed by the conjunctiva at the inner angle, or canthus, of the eye. The lake is in large part occupied by the *lacrimal caruncle,* which is the fleshy, reddish eminence situated in the inner angle of the eye.

The tear secretion that collects in the lacrimal lake is drained into the inferior nasal meatus through the *nasolacrimal* system of ducts. This system of channels is the part of the lacrimal apparatus often subjected to radiologic investigation. The nasolacrimal system of channels consists of (1) two small canals called *lacrimal canaliculi,* one canaliculus leading from the free margin of the inner angle of each eyelid, and (2) the *lacrimal sac,* which is the upper, rounded, and slightly dilated part of (3) the *nasolacrimal duct.*

Each canaliculus begins at a minute orifice called the *punctum lacrimale.* The punctum lacrimale is so situated on a small elevation, the *lacrimal papilla,* that it is directed into the lacrimal lake for the drainage of accumulating fluid. From its orifice, or punctum, the canaliculus passes within the margin of the respective eyelid, first vertically and then medially, to its junction with the lacrimal sac, for a distance of about 10 mm. The canaliculi sometimes unite into a single passage as they converge toward their entrance into the lacrimal sac.

The lacrimal sac is 12 mm in length, is rounded above, and is slightly constricted at its junction with the nasolacrimal duct proper. The sac is situated anteroinferiorly on the medial wall of the orbit, where it is lodged in the fossa formed for it by the lacrimal and maxillary bones, and on the other side of which are the anterior ethmoidal air cells. The lacrimal fossa is the beginning of the osseous lacrimal canal, through which the nasolacrimal duct passes. The bony canal is formed by the lacrimal bone, the maxilla, and the lacrimal process of the inferior nasal concha. It passes inferiorly, posteriorly, and laterally between the medial wall of the maxillary sinus and the lateral wall of the nasal cavity.

The nasolacrimal duct proper varies in length but is believed to average approximately 17 mm. The duct narrows somewhat as it approaches the nasal cavity, where it opens under the inferior concha approximately in line with the first molar tooth.

CONTRAST MEDIUM

Because oil is immiscible with the watery tear secretion, an oil-based, iodinated contrast medium is employed in examinations of the nasolacrimal duct system. A compound having low viscosity or ethiodized oil may be used after warming it to body temperature to further reduce its viscosity.

INJECTION SUPPLIES

The items required for the injection are (1) sterile cotton balls, gauze sponges, and cotton-tipped applicators; (2) sterile sponge forceps; (3) a sterile pack containing punctum dilators, lacrimal needles, and 2 ml Luer-Lok syringes; (4) local anesthetic solution; (5) sterile normal saline solution; (6) the contrast medium; and (7) a waste basin.

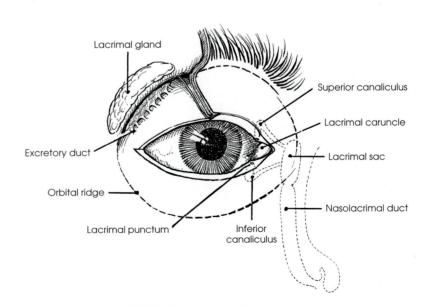

Fig. 20-166. Nasolacrimal drainage system.

DACRYOCYSTOGRAPHY
Examination procedure

Preliminary in Caldwell, Waters, and lateral radiographs are usually taken for evaluation of the paranasal sinuses, and the following steps are observed:

- To expedite filming after the introduction of the contrast medium, perform the injection procedure with the patient seated before a vertical grid device.
- If preferred, place the patient in the supine position for the introduction of the medium and then turn the patient to the prone position for filming.

- After anesthetizing the conjunctiva and puncta, the radiologist dilates the punctum of the canaliculus to be injected (the upper when the lower is blocked) and then inserts the round-tipped lacrimal needle into the canaliculus. The patency of the canals is tested by irrigating them with normal saline solution, and, if they are found to be patent, the examination may be terminated.
- Immediately following the introduction of the contrast medium and the withdrawal of the needle, take the Caldwell or Waters and lateral projections in rapid succession.
- Repeat the same images at specified intervals to follow the progress of the medium through the channels.

- Usually, take the follow-up radiographs at a postinjection interval of 7 to 10 minutes and again at a 15 to 20-minute interval, at which time the medium will have passed through patent ducts and be seen on the floor of the nasal cavity and on the pharyngeal mucosa.
- Inject the contralateral side after the initial filming of the first side if needed.
- When this is done, rotate the head slightly (10 to 15 degrees) away from the film to separate the bilaterally opacified ducts in the lateral projection.
- The exposure factors that are used for routine paranasal sinus studies are satisfactory for contrast studies of the nasolacrimal duct system (Figs. 20-167 and 20-168).

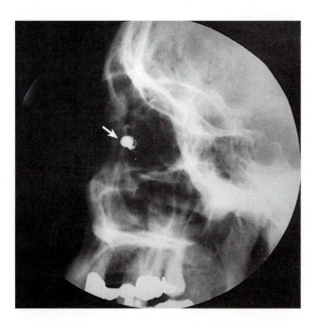

Fig. 20-167. Right lateral nasolacrimal drainage system showing complete blockage between dilated lacrimal sac and nasolacrimal duct *(arrow).*

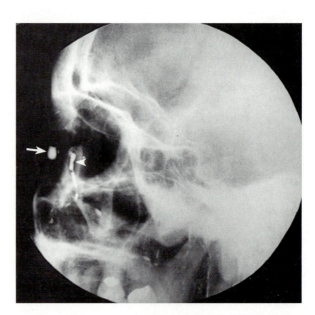

Fig. 20-168. Right lateral nasolacrimal drainage system demonstrating nasolacrimal ducts and patent communication with contrast in nasal cavity on left side *(arrowhead).* Patient's head rotated slightly so right nasolacrimal duct *(arrow)* is not superimposed on left duct.

Chapter 21

FACIAL BONES*

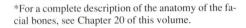

*For a complete description of the anatomy of the facial bones, see Chapter 20 of this volume.

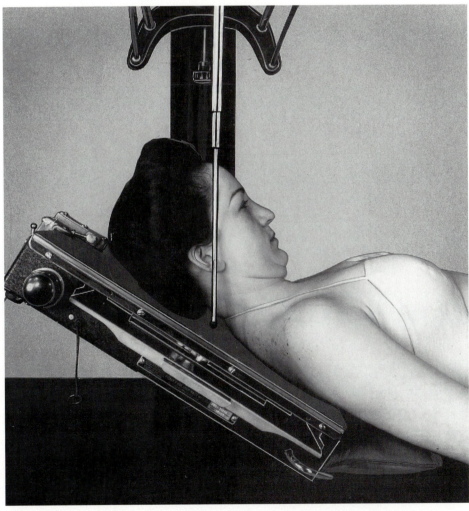

Patient positioned for temporomandibular joint radiography. The head is resting on a portable Potter-Bucky diaphragm. The Potter-Bucky device had a string hanging down, and the operator had to "cock" the single stroke (non-reciprocating) Bucky. The operator adjusted the length of the exposure time by turning a timer knob. The timer knob is shown on the left border (upper middle) of the illustration.

Radiation Protection

Protection of the patient from unnecessary radiation is a professional responsibility of the radiographer. (See Chapter 1, Volume 1 for specific guidelines.) In this chapter *with a few exceptions* (due to central ray angulations), radiation shielding of the patient is not specified or illustrated because the professional community and the federal government have reported that a lead shield over the patient's pelvis does not significantly reduce the gonadal exposure during radiography of the facial bones.

The pediatric patient, however, should be protected from radiation by shielding the thyroid and thymus glands and gonads. The protective lead shielding used to cover the thyroid and thymus glands can also assist in immobilizing the pediatric patient.

The most effective way to protect the patient from unnecessary radiation is to restrict the radiation beam by using proper collimation. Taking care to ensure that the patient is properly instructed and immobilized also reduces the chance of having to repeat the procedure, further limiting the radiation exposure received by the patient.

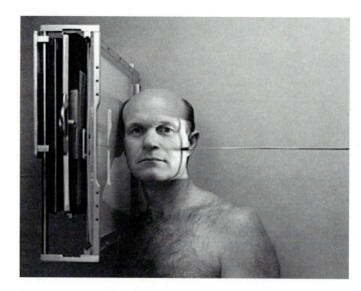

Fig. 21-1. Lateral facial bones.

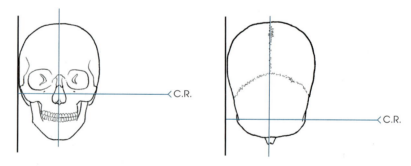

Fig. 21-2. Upright radiography.

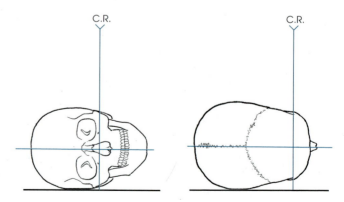

Fig. 21-3. Table radiography.

Facial Bones

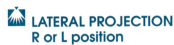

LATERAL PROJECTION
R or L position

Film: 8 × 10 in (18 × 24 cm) lengthwise.

Position of patient

- Place the patient in a semiprone position or seated obliquely before a vertical grid device.
- Place the arms in a comfortable position and adjust the shoulders to lie in the same transverse plane.

Position of part

- Adjust the head so that the median sagittal plane is parallel with, and the interpupillary line is perpendicular to, the film.
- Adjust the flexion of the patient's neck so that the infraorbitomeatal line is parallel with the transverse axis of the film.
- Place a radiolucent pad under the side of the mandible to prevent rotation.
- With the cassette in the Bucky tray, center the cassette to the zygomatic bone (zygoma) (Figs. 21-1 to 21-3).
- Immobilize the head.
- Ask the patient to suspend respiration for the exposure.

Central ray

- Direct the central ray perpendicular to the midpoint of the film entering the lateral surface of the zygomatic bone.

Structures shown

A lateral image of the bones of the face is demonstrated, with the right and left sides superimposed (Fig. 21-4).

□ Evaluation criteria

The following should be clearly demonstrated:
- ■ All facial bones in their entirety with the zygomatic bone (zygoma) in the center.
- ■ Almost perfectly superimposed mandibular rami.
- ■ Superimposed orbital roofs.
- ■ No rotation of sella turcica.

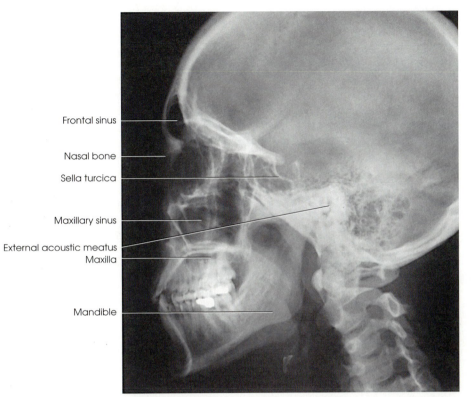

Frontal sinus

Nasal bone

Sella turcica

Maxillary sinus

External acoustic meatus
Maxilla

Mandible

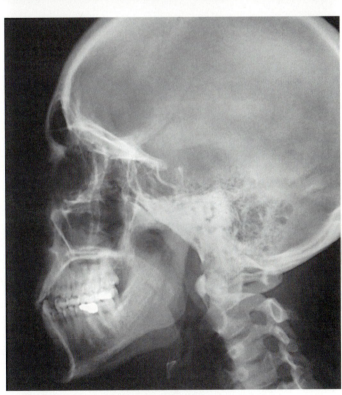

Fig. 21-4. Lateral facial bones.

(Courtesy John Syring, R.T.)

Facial bones

Facial Profile
LATERAL PROJECTION
R or L position
RELATIONSHIP OF BONY AND SOFT TISSUE CONTOURS

One film is placed in the cassette in the usual manner, and a second film is placed in a light-tight, nonscreened film holder and placed on top of the cassette; the two films are exposed simultaneously with the factors called for in lateral facial bone technique.

Film: 8 × 10 in (18 × 24 cm) placed lengthwise.

Position of patient

- Place the patient in a semiprone position or seated before a vertical grid device.

Position of part

- Rest the patient's head in a lateral position, with the region of the zygomatic bone (zygoma) centered to the film.
- Adjust the flexion of the neck so that the infraorbitomeatal line is parallel with the transverse axis of the film.
- Adjust the head so that the median sagittal plane is parallel with, and the interpupillary line is perpendicular to, the plane of the film.
- Support the mandible on a radiolucent pad to prevent rotation.
- Immobilize the head.
- Ask the patient to suspend respiration for the exposure.

Central ray

- Direct the central ray perpendicular to the lateral surface of the zygomatic bone.

Structures shown

The film placed between the intensifying screens shows a bone-negative lateral image of the bony structures of the face (Fig. 21-5). The film packet placed on top of the cassette (soft tissue-negative image, Fig. 21-6), lacking the effect of the intensifying screens, shows the soft tissue structures. The bone-negative image of Fig. 21-5 can be contact-printed in the darkroom to obtain a tone-reversed image (bone-positive image, Fig. 21-7). This bone-positive image can be superimposed on the soft tissue-negative projection (Fig. 21-6) to demonstrate the relationship between the bony and the soft tissue structures as shown in Fig. 21-8.

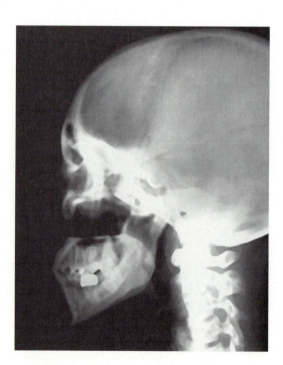

Fig. 21-5. Lateral facial profile: normal bony demonstration.

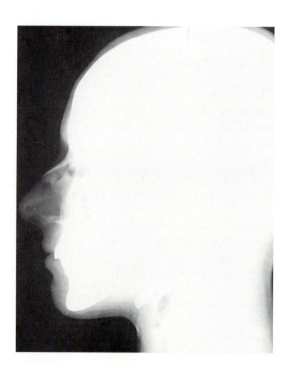

Fig. 21-6. Lateral facial profile: non-screen exposure for soft tissue.

□ Evaluation criteria

The following should be clearly demonstrated:
- Soft tissue of the face.
- No rotation of the face.
- Relation between bony and soft tissue structures visible if the bone-positive and soft tissue-negative images are superimposed.

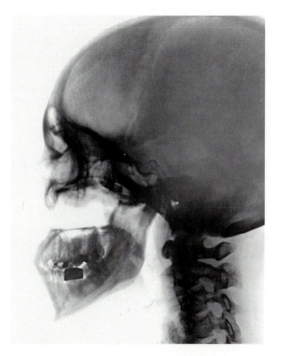

Fig. 21-7. Lateral facial profile: bone-positive reversal image.

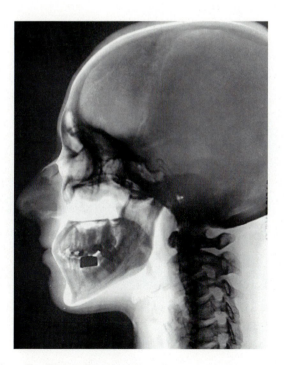

Fig. 21-8. Lateral facial profile: superimposed bone. Positive reversal image.

Facial Bones

 PARIETOACANTHIAL PROJECTION
WATERS METHOD[1]

Film: 8 × 10 in (18 × 24 cm) lengthwise.

Position of patient

- Place the patient in the prone or seated-upright position.
- Center the median sagittal plane of the body to the midline of the grid device.
- Place the arms in a comfortable position and adjust the shoulders to lie in the same transverse plane.

---

[1]Waters CA: Modification of the occipito-frontal position in roentgenography of the accessory nasal sinuses, Arch of Radiol and Electrotherapy 20:15-17, 1915.

Position of part

- Center the median sagittal plane of the patient's head to the midline of the grid and rest it on the tip of the extended chin. The average patient's nose will be ¾ inch (2 cm) away from the grid device.
- Extend the neck so that the orbitomeatal line forms a 37-degree angle with the *plane of the film*. The mentomeatal line will be approximately perpendicular to the film plane.
- Adjust the head so that the median sagittal plane is perpendicular to the plane of the film (Figs. 21-9 to 21-11).
- Center the cassette at the level of the acanthion.
- Immobilize the head.
- Ask the patient to suspend respiration for the exposure.

Central ray

- Direct the central ray perpendicular to exit the acanthion.

Structures shown

The Waters method demonstrates the orbits, the maxillae, and the zygomatic arches (Fig. 21-12).

□ Evaluation criteria

The following should be clearly demonstrated:

- Distance between the lateral border of the skull and orbit equal on each side.
- Petrous ridges projected immediately below the maxillae.

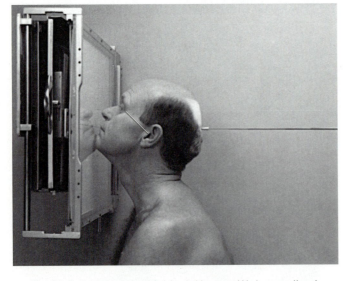

Fig. 21-9. Parietoacanthial facial bones, Waters method.

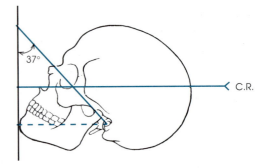

Fig. 21-10. Upright radiography.

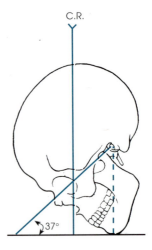

Fig. 21-11. Table radiography.

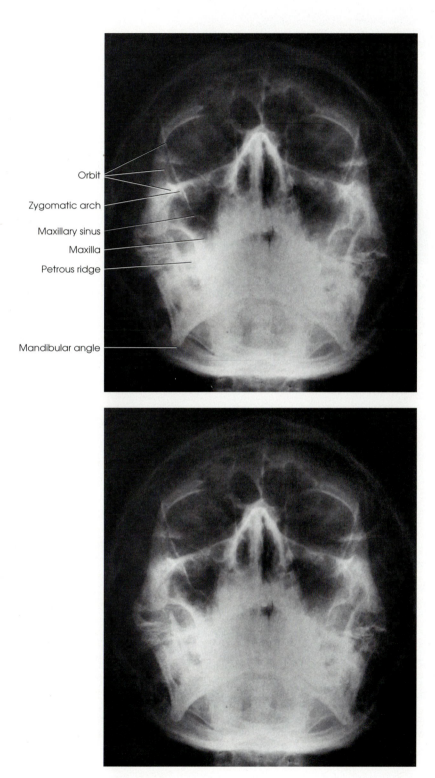

Orbit

Zygomatic arch

Maxillary sinus

Maxilla

Petrous ridge

Mandibular angle

Fig. 21-12. Parietoacanthial facial bones, Waters method.

(Courtesy Jane Kober, R.T.)

PARIETOACANTHIAL MODIFICATION

Although the parietoacanthial projection (Waters method) is widely used, many institutions modify the projection by radiographing the patient using less extension of the neck. This modification, while sometimes called a "shallow" Waters, actually increases the angulation of the orbitomeatal line by placing it more perpendicular with the film plane. The patient's head is positioned as described using the Waters method but the neck is extended a lesser amount. In the modification the orbitomeatal line is adjusted to be approximately 55 degrees with the plane of the film (Figs. 21-13 to 21-15). The resulting radiograph demonstrates the facial bones with less axial angulation than using the Waters method seen in Fig. 21-12. With the modification, the petrous ridges are projected immediately below the inferior border of the orbits as seen in Fig. 21-16.

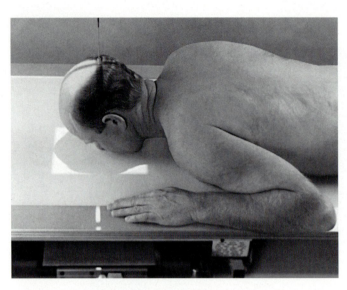

Fig. 21-13. Modified parietoacanthial facial bones, Waters method.

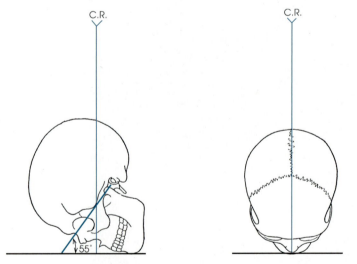

Fig. 21-14. Table radiography, modified parietoacanthial facial bones, Waters method, with orbitomeatal line adjusted to 55 degrees.

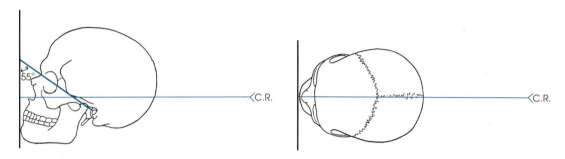

Fig. 21-15. Upright radiography, modified parietoacanthial facial bones, Waters methods, with orbitomeatal line adjusted to 55°.

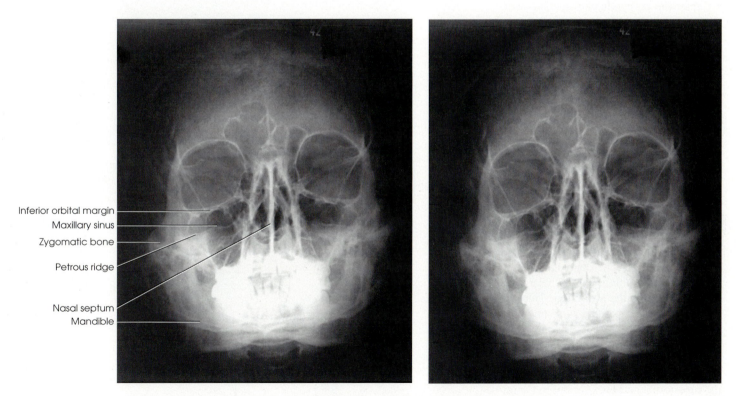

Inferior orbital margin
Maxillary sinus
Zygomatic bone

Petrous ridge

Nasal septum
Mandible

Fig. 21-16. Modified parietoacanthial facial bones, Waters method.

Facial Bones

ACANTHOPARIETAL PROJECTION
REVERSE WATERS METHOD

Film: 10 × 12 in (24 × 30 cm) lengthwise.

The reverse Waters method is used to demonstrate the facial bones when the patient cannot be placed in the prone position.

Position of patient

- With the patient in the supine position, center the median sagittal plane of the body to the midline of the grid.
- Place the arms along the sides of the body and adjust the shoulders to lie in the same transverse plane.

Position of part

- Adjust the cassette so that the midpoint will coincide with the central ray. It will lie approximately 3 inches (7.5 cm) above the external occipital protuberance.
- Center the perpendicular median sagittal plane of the head to the midline of the cassette.
- Adjust the flexion of the neck so that the infraorbitomeatal line is perpendicular to the plane of the film (Figs. 21-17 to 21-19).
- Immobilize the head.
- Ask the patient to suspend respiration for the exposure.

Central ray

- Direct the central ray to exit from a point approximately 2 inches (5 cm) above the external occipital protuberance at an angle of 30 degrees cephalad to the infraorbitomeatal line (this is the same as angling it 37 degrees to the orbitomeatal line). It enters the face at, or slightly below, the acanthion. The central ray will be parallel with the mentomeatal line.

Structures shown

The *reverse* Waters method demonstrates the superior facial bones similar to the image obtained with the Waters method, although the structures are considerably magnified (Fig. 21-20).

□ Evaluation criteria

The following should be clearly demonstrated:
- Distance between the lateral border of the skull and orbit equal on each side.
- Petrous ridges projected in the maxillary sinuses.

AP AXIAL PROJECTION FOR TRAUMA

For the trauma patient who is unable to assume the prone or supine body position to demonstrate the facial bones, the acanthoparietal projection, or "Reverse Waters," can be achieved in one of several ways.

- When the neck can be safely extended, adjust the orbitomeatal line to an angle of approximately 37 degrees to the plane of the film. This degree of angulation places the mentomeatal line approximately perpendicular to the film plane. The perpendicular central ray enters the patient at the acanthion (Fig. 21-21).

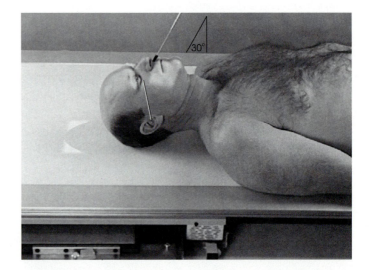

Fig. 21-17. Acanthoparietal facial bones, reverse Waters method.

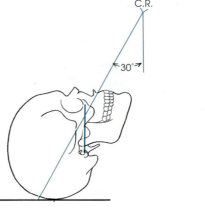

Fig. 21-18. Table radiography.

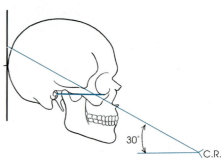

Fig. 21-19. Upright radiography.

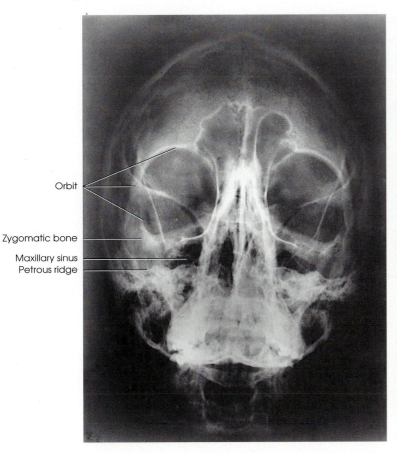
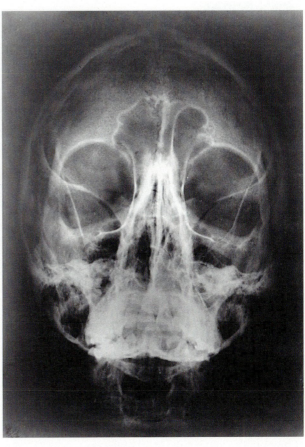

Orbit

Zygomatic bone

Maxillary sinus
Petrous ridge

Fig. 21-20. Acanthoparietal facial bones, reverse Waters method.

• When the patient's neck cannot be moved because of trauma, radiograph the patient in the position in which he or she arrives. Maintain the same angle relationships as above but adjust the central ray to be 37 degrees from the plane of the film. Another way to achieve approximately the same image is to adjust the central ray to enter the acanthion while remaining parallel with the mentomeatal line (Fig. 21-22).

Trauma radiography guidelines

For a detailed description of adapting any body position for the trauma patient, see Trauma Radiography Guidelines, Volume 1, Chapter 13. The example given in that section is the "Reverse Waters" discussed above.

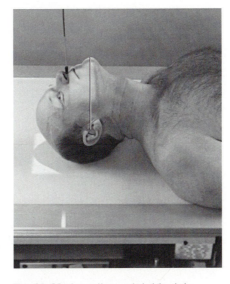

Fig. 21-21. Acanthoparietal facial bones, reverse Waters method. Neck extended. Note mentomeatal line perpendicular to film.

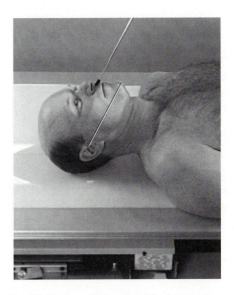

Fig. 21-22. Acanthoparietal facial bones, reverse Waters method. Central ray parallel with mentomeatal line.

Facial Bones

PARIETO-ORBITAL OBLIQUE PROJECTION

NOTE: This projection is identical to the parieto-orbital oblique, Rhese method, described in Chapters 20 and 22. The only difference is the central ray is centered slightly lower.

Film: 8 × 10 in (18 × 24 cm) lengthwise.

Position of patient

• Place the patient in a semiprone position or seated before a vertical grid device.

Position of part

• Rest the patient's head on the affected zygomatic bone (zygoma), the nose, and the chin, with the orbit centered to the midline of the grid.
• Adjust the flexion of the neck so that the acanthomeatal line is parallel with the transverse axis of the film.
• Using a suitable protractor as a guide, adjust the rotation of the head so that the median sagittal plane forms an angle of 53 degrees from the plane of the film (Figs. 21-23 to 21-25).
• Center the cassette at the level of the infraorbital margin.
• Immobilize the head.
• Ask the patient to suspend respiration for the exposure.

Central ray

• Direct the central ray to the infraorbital margin of the orbit closest to the film either (1) perpendicular or (2) at an angle of 10 to 15 degrees cephalad, depending on the region to be demonstrated.

Structures shown

An oblique projection of the facial bones is demonstrated. Both sides are examined for comparison (Fig. 21-26).

☐Evaluation criteria

The following should be clearly demonstrated:
■ All facial bones.
■ Side being demonstrated not superimposed by the opposite side.

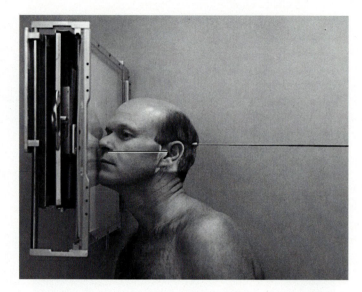

Fig. 21-23. Parietal-orbital oblique facial bones.

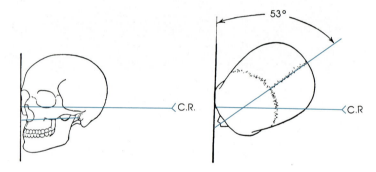

Fig. 21-24. Upright radiography.

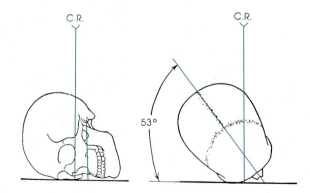

Fig. 21-25. Table radiography.

Frontal sinus

Dependent orbit

Coronoid process

Elevated maxillary sinus
Mandibular ramus

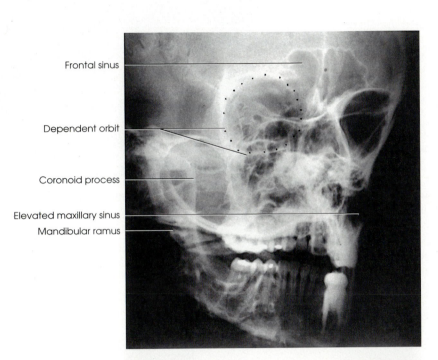

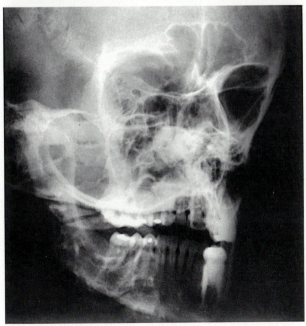

Fig. 21-26. Parieto-orbital oblique facial bones.

Facial Bones

PA AXIAL OBLIQUE PROJECTION
LAW METHOD

Film: 8 × 10 in (18 × 24 cm) lengthwise.

Position of patient

- Adjust the patient in a seated-upright or a semiprone position.
- Place the arms in a comfortable position and adjust the shoulders to lie in the same transverse plane.

Position of part

- With the patient's neck fully extended, center the region of the maxillary sinus closest to the film to the midline of the grid.
- Rest the nose, the zygomatic bone (zygoma), and the chin on the grid device (Figs. 21-27 to 21-29).
- Center the cassette to the orbit closest to the film. This places the midpoint of the film approximately 2 inches (5 cm) above the floor of the maxillary sinuses.
- Immobilize the head.
- Ask the patient to suspend respiration for the exposure.

Central ray

- Direct the central ray to the lower maxillary sinus at an angle of 25 to 30 degrees cephalad. It enters the neck just posterior to the angle of the mandible.

Structures shown

Although Law[1] developed this position primarily to demonstrate the floor and posterior wall of the maxillary sinus (antrum) of the side adjacent to the film, he also recommended that it be used to demonstrate the external orbital wall, the zygomatic bone (zygoma), and the anterior wall of the maxillary sinuses of the side farther from the film (Fig. 21-30).

□ Evaluation criteria

The following should be clearly demonstrated:

- All facial bones.
- Side being demonstrated not superimposed by the opposite side.

[1]Law FM: Nasal accessory sinuses, Ann Roentgenol 15:32-51, 53-76, 1933.

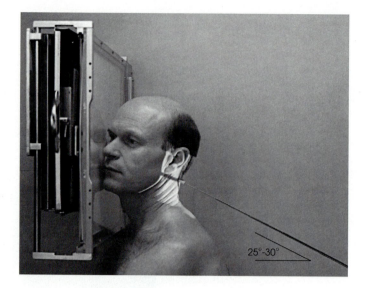

Fig. 21-27. PA axial oblique facial bones.

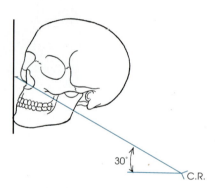

Fig. 21-28. Upright radiography.

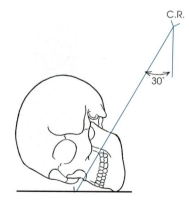

Fig. 21-29. Table radiography.

Facial bones

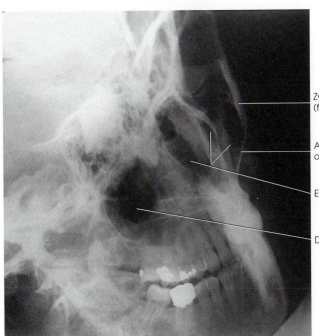

Zygomatic bone
(farthest from film)

Anterior wall
of elevated maxillary sinus

Elevated maxillary sinus

Dependent maxillary sinus

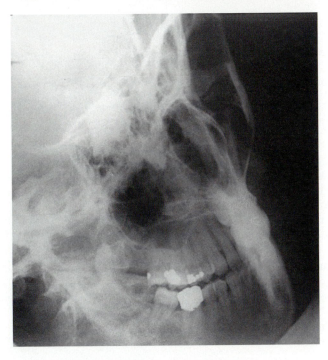

Fig. 21-30. PA axial oblique facial bones.

Nasal Bones

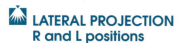
LATERAL PROJECTION
R and L positions

Film: 8 × 10 in (18 × 24 cm) placed crosswise for two exposures on one film or a 2¼ × 3 in (57 × 76 mm) occlusal film for each side.

Position of patient

Although the patient may be seated upright before a vertical grid device, the recumbent position facilitates placement of the small films used in lateral examinations of the nasal bones.

- With the patient in a semiprone position, adjust the rotation of the body so that the median sagittal plane of the head can be placed horizontal.
- Place the arms in a comfortable position and adjust the shoulders to lie in the same transverse plane.

Position of part

- Adjust the head so that the median sagittal plane is parallel with, and the interpupillary line is perpendicular to, the tabletop.
- Adjust the flexion of the neck so that the infraorbitomeatal line is parallel with the transverse axis of the cassette (Figs. 21-31 and 21-32).
- Support the mandible to prevent rotation.
- Ask the patient to suspend respiration for the exposure.

Placement of film

- When using an 8 × 10 in (18 × 24 cm) film, slide the unmasked half of the cassette under the frontonasal region and center it to the nasion (Fig. 21-31). This centering allows space for the identification marker to be projected across the upper part of the film. Tape the side marker (R or L) in position.
- When using occlusal film for the examination, tape the side marker onto the lower, outer corner of the pebbled side of the film packet.
- Place a sandbag under the side of the nose, against the orbit and cheek, for the support of the film packet.
- Adjust the film packet so that the pebbled surface faces, and is parallel with, the median sagittal plane and so that its upper border projects approximately ½ inch (1.2 cm) above the supraorbital ridge.
- Press it firmly against the maxilla and the supraorbital ridge (Fig. 21-33).

314

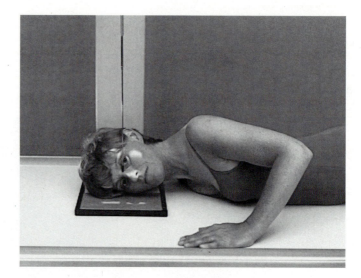

Fig. 21-31. Lateral nasal bones.

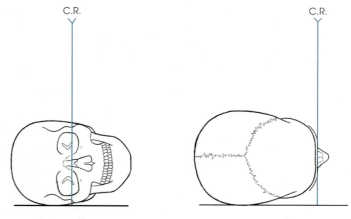

Fig. 21-32. Table radiography.

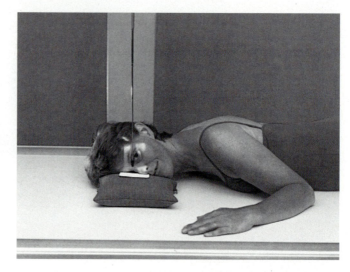

Fig. 21-33. Lateral nasal bones using occlusal film.

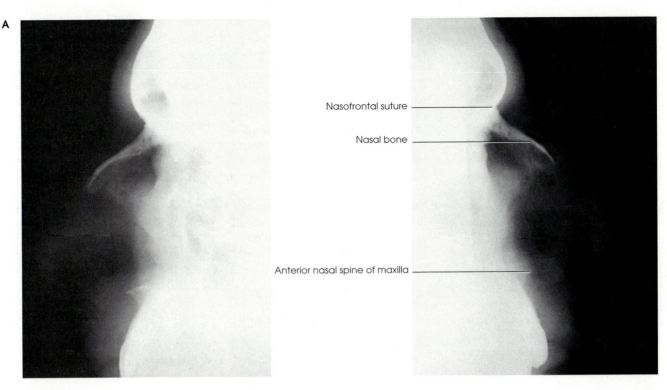

A   B

Nasofrontal suture _____

Nasal bone _____

Anterior nasal spine of maxilla _____

Fig. 21-34. A, Right lateral. **B,** Left lateral, nasal bones.

(Courtesy Jane Kober, R.T.)

If the bridge of the nose is flat or concave, the following steps are observed:
- Place the film packet at an angle under the supraorbital ridge.
- Turn the corner of the packet back enough to ease the sharp edge, so that it can be placed without discomfort to the patient.
- Place the rounded corner just medial to the inner canthus and press the upper border firmly against the inferior surface of the supraorbital ridge.
- Instruct the patient to hold the film packet in position so that its plane is parallel with the median sagittal plane of the head.

Central ray

- Direct the central ray perpendicular to the bridge of the nose at a point ¾ inch (1.9 cm) distal to the nasion.
- Use close collimation.

Structures shown

Lateral images of the nasal bones are demonstrated, showing the detail of the side nearer the film and of the soft structures of the nose (Figs. 21-34 and 21-35). Both sides are examined for comparison.

□ Evaluation criteria

The following should be clearly demonstrated:
- No rotation of the nasal bone and soft tissue.
- Anterior nasal spine and frontonasal suture.

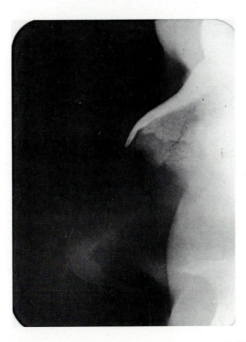

Fig. 21-35. Lateral nasal bones using occlusal film.

Nasal Bones
TANGENTIAL PROJECTION

The success of this projection depends on (1) adjusting and having the patient hold the occlusal film packet between the teeth, or using the larger film placed under the chin, so that the plane of the film is perpendicular to the glabelloalveolar line and (2) directing the central ray along the glabelloalveolar line perpendicular to the plane of the film.

Whether a patient can hold an occlusal film at the correct angle or must be examined with an extraoral film depends largely on the dental occlusion and availability and processing capability of occlusal film. The following guidelines are observed:

- Examine patients who have abnormal occlusion with an extraoral film.
- Have the average patient, by protrusive or retractive movement of the mandible, approximate the anterior teeth to hold an occlusal film at the correct angle.
- When the patient's normal bite does not hold the film packet correctly, instruct the patient to adjust the mandible according to the direction of film displacement.
- That is, if the film is angled upward, instruct the patient to retract the mandible; if the film is angled downward, instruct the patient to protract the mandible anteriorly.

Film: 8 × 10 in (18 × 24 cm) film placed crosswise under the chin or a 2¼ × 3 in (57 × 76 mm) occlusal film held between the anterior teeth. The use of occlusal film is recommended because of the reduced object-to-image receptor distance.

Position of patient

- Place the patient in either a recumbent or a seated position.
- Seat the patient so that the chin can be rested on a sandbag or on an inclined cassette for support.

Position of part
Extraoral film

- Elevate the side of the cassette adjacent to the patient on a small sandbag or a folded towel.
- Rest the head on the fully extended chin and center the film to the median sagittal plane just anterior to the chin.
- Adjust the inclination of the cassette so that its plane is perpendicular to the glabelloalveolar line.
- Adjust the head so that the median sagittal plane is perpendicular to the plane of the film (Fig. 21-36).
- Immobilize the head.
- Ask the patient to suspend respiration for the exposure.

Intraoral film

- Tape a side marker (R or L) onto one side of the pebbled surface of the film packet.
- With the patient supine, rest the head on the table or elevate it on a sponge.
- With the median sagittal plane of the head vertical, adjust it so that the glabelloalveolar line is horizontal if the head is resting on the table or so that it is parallel with the plane of the sponge if the head is elevated.
- Immobilize the head.
- With its long axis directed anteroposteriorly and the pebbled surface facing upward, insert the film packet approximately 1 inch (2.5 cm) into the mouth.
- Center the packet to the median sagittal plane and then instruct the patient to close the lips and teeth so that the film is held in position with its plane perpendicular to the glabelloalveolar line (Figs. 21-37 and 21-38).
- Ask the patient to suspend respiration for the exposure.

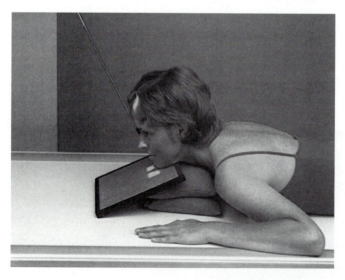

Fig. 21-36. Tangential nasal bones.

Central ray

• Direct the central ray parallel to glabel-loalveolar line perpendicular to the plane of the film.

Structures shown

A tangential projection of only a portion of the nasal bones that extend beyond the glabelloalveolar line is shown (Fig. 21-39). This projection is primarily used to demonstrate any medial or lateral displacement of fragments in fractures.

☐ Evaluation criteria

The following should be clearly demonstrated:

■ Nasal bones with minimal superimposition unless the patient has a prominent forehead, recessed nose, or protruding upper teeth.
■ No rotation of the nose.
■ Soft tissue.

NOTE: Because the nasal bones do not have sufficient body to cast a shadow through the dense superjacent and subjacent structures, the tangential projection cannot be used successfully with children or with adults who have very short nasal bones, a concave face, or protruding upper teeth.

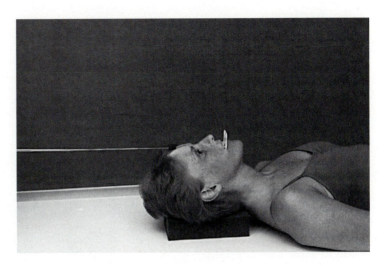

Fig. 21-37. Tangential nasal bones.

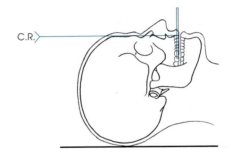

Fig. 21-38. Table radiography.

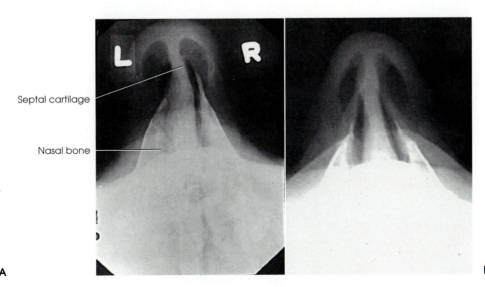

Septal cartilage

Nasal bone

A

B

Fig. 21-39. Tangential nasal bones.

Zygomatic Arches

⬥ TANGENTIAL PROJECTION

This projection is performed similar to the SMV projection described in Chapter 20.

Film: 8 × 10 in (18 × 24 cm) crosswise.

Position of patient

- Place the patient in either the seated-upright or the supine position. A vertical head unit greatly assists the patient unable to hyperextend the neck.
- When the supine position is used, elevate the trunk on several firm pillows or a suitable pad to allow complete extension of the neck and flex the knees to relax the abdominal muscles.
- Center the median sagittal plane of the body to the midline of the grid device.
- Place the arms in a comfortable position and adjust the shoulders to lie in the same transverse plane.

Position of part

- Extend the patient's neck completely so that the infraorbitomeatal line, which passes through the long axis of the zygomatic arches, is as nearly parallel with the plane of the film as possible.
- Rest the head on the vertex and adjust it so that the median sagittal plane is perpendicular to the plane of the film (Figs. 21-40 to 21-42).
- Attach a strip of adhesive tape to the inferior surface of the chin and then anchor it to the edge of the table or stand. This usually provides sufficient support. Do not put adhesive surface directly on patient's skin.
- Adjust the cassette position so that the midpoint of the film will coincide with the central ray.
- Ask the patient to suspend respiration for the exposure.

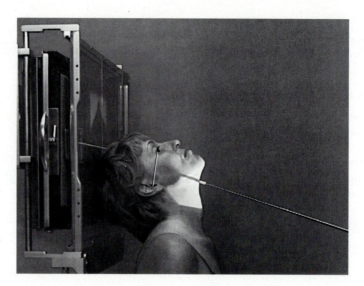

Fig. 21-40. Tangential zygomatic arches.

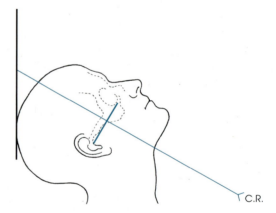

Fig. 21-41. Upright radiography.

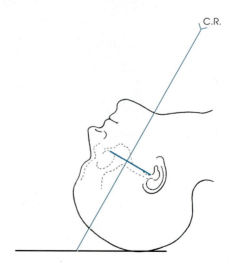

Fig. 21-42. Table radiography.

Central ray

- Direct the central ray perpendicular to the infraorbitomeatal line and centered midway between the zygomatic arches. It passes through a coronal plane lying approximately 1 inch (2.5 cm) posterior to the outer canthi.

Structures shown

Symmetric tangential images of the zygomatic arches are shown, projected free of superimposed structures (Fig. 21-43). Unless they are very flat or are traumatically depressed, the arches, being farther from the film, are projected beyond the prominent parietal eminences by the divergent x-ray beam.

□Evaluation criteria

The following should be clearly demonstrated:
- Zygomatic arches free from overlying structures.
- Zygomatic arches symmetric and without foreshortening.
- No rotation of the head.

NOTE: The zygomatic arches are well demonstrated with a decrease in the exposure factors used for this projection of the cranial base.

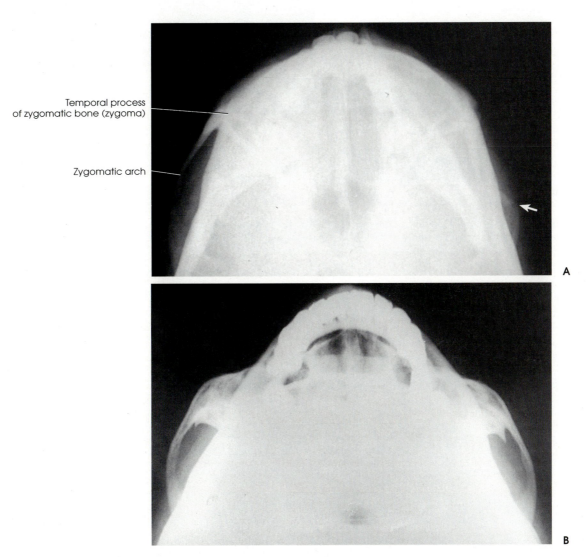

Temporal process of zygomatic bone (zygoma)

Zygomatic arch

A

B

Fig. 21-43. Tangential zygomatic arches. **A,** Intact arch and depressed fracture *(arrow).* **B,** Tangential zygomatic arches.

(**A,** courtesy Jana Hoffman, R.T.; **B,** courtesy Dr. Albert A. Dunn.)

Zygomatic Arch

▲ TANGENTIAL PROJECTION

Film: 8 × 10 in (18 × 24 cm).

Position of patient

- Seat the patient with the back against a vertical grid device, or place the patient in the supine position, with the trunk elevated on several firm pillows and with the knees flexed to permit complete extension of the neck.
- Place the arms in a comfortable position and adjust the shoulders to lie in the same transverse plane.

Position of part

With the patient in the seated position, the following steps are observed:

- Extend the neck and rest the head on the vertex.
- If possible, adjust the position of the body so that the infraorbitomeatal line is parallel with the plane of the film.
- Rotate the median sagittal plane approximately 15 degrees toward the side being examined.
- Tilt the top of the head approximately 15 degrees away from the side examined. This rotation and tilt ensures that the central ray will be tangent to the lateral surface of the skull. The central ray will thus skim across the lateral portion of the mandibular angle and the parietal bone to project the zygomatic arch onto the film.
- Center the zygomatic arch to the cassette (Figs. 21-44 and 21-45).

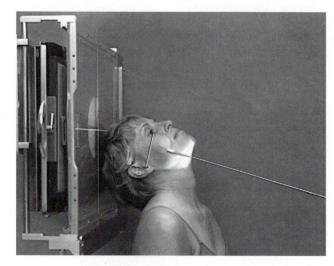

Fig. 21-44. Tangential zygomatic arch.

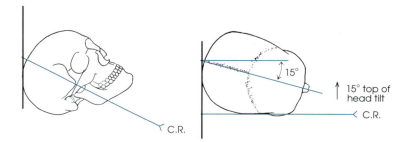

Fig. 21-45. Upright radiography.

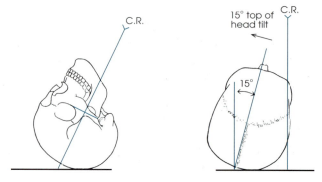

Fig. 21-46. Table radiography.

Facial bones

320

With the patient in the supine position, the following steps are observed:
- Rest the head on the vertex.
- Elevate the upper end of the cassette on sandbags, or place it on an angle sponge of suitable size.
- Adjust the elevation of the cassette and the extension of the neck so that the infraorbitomeatal line is placed as nearly parallel with the plane of the film as possible.
- Rotate and tilt the median sagittal plane approximately 15 degrees toward the side being examined similar to the upright position.
- If the infraorbitomeatal line is parallel with the plane of the film, center the film to the zygomatic arch; if not, displace the cassette so that the midpoint of the film will coincide with the central ray (Fig. 21-46).
- Attach a strip of adhesive tape to the inferior surface of the chin and then draw it upward and anchor it to the edge of the table or cassette stand. This usually affords sufficient support. Do not put adhesive surface directly on patient's skin.
- Ask the patient to suspend respiration for the exposure.

Central ray

- Direct the central ray perpendicular to the infraorbitomeatal line and center it to the zygomatic arch.

Structures shown

A tangential image of one zygomatic arch is seen free of superimposition (Fig. 21-47). This projection is particularly useful with patients who have depressed fractures or "flat" cheekbones.

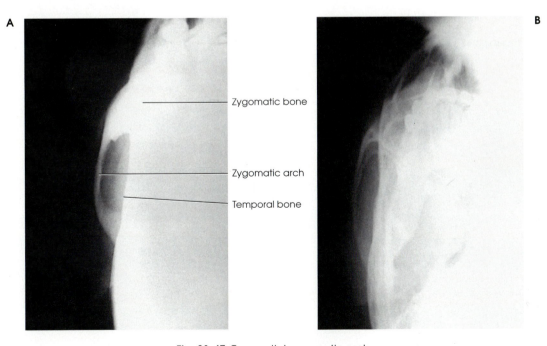

Fig. 21-47. Tangential zygomatic arch.

(Courtesy Deborah Wolfenberger, R.T.)

Zygomatic bone

Zygomatic arch

Temporal bone

Zygomatic Arch
TANGENTIAL PROJECTION
MAY METHOD

Film: 8 × 10 in (18 × 24 cm) crosswise for two exposures.

Position of patient

- Place the patient in the prone position or seated before a vertical grid device.

Position of part

- Fully extend the patient's neck and rest the chin on the grid device.
- Center the cassette 3 inches (7.5 cm) distal to the most prominent point of the zygomatic bone (zygoma).
- Completely extend the patient's neck so that the infraorbitomeatal line is as parallel with the plane of the film as possible.
- Using a protractor as a guide, rotate the median sagittal plane approximately 15 degrees away from the side being examined, then tilt the top of the head away from the side examined approximately 15 degrees. This rotation and tilt ensures that the central ray will be tangent to the lateral surface of the skull. The central ray will thus skim across the lateral portion of the parietal bone and the mandibular angle to project the zygomatic arch onto the film (Figs. 21-48 to 21-50).
- Ask the patient to suspend respiration for the exposures.

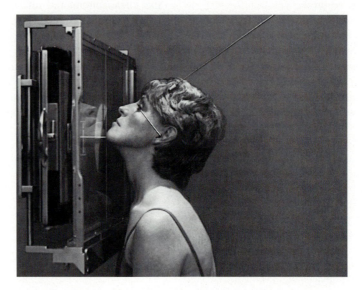

Fig. 21-48. Tangential zygomatic arch, May method.

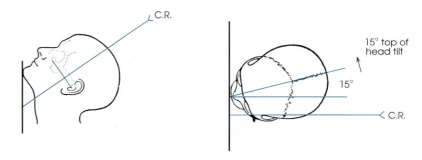

Fig. 21-49. Upright radiography.

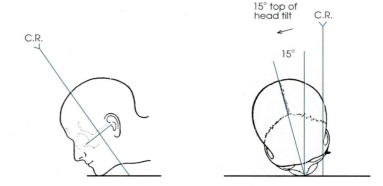

Fig. 21-50. Table radiography.

Central ray

- With the central ray perpendicular to the infraorbitomeatal line, direct it through the zygomatic arch at a point approximately 1½ inches (3.8 cm) posterior to the outer canthus.

Structures shown

The May method demonstrates the zygomatic arch free of superimposition (Fig. 21-51). This projection is particularly useful with patients who have depressed fractures or "flat" cheekbones.

The following should be clearly demonstrated:

- ■ Zygomatic arch in its entirety and free from overlying structures.

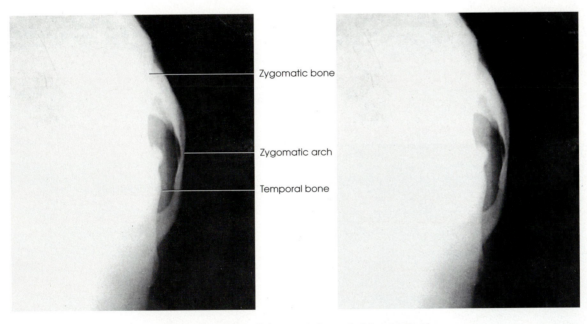

Zygomatic bone

Zygomatic arch

Temporal bone

Fig. 21-51. Tangential zygomatic arch, May method.

Zygomatic Arches

PA AXIAL PROJECTION
MODIFIED TITTERINGTON METHOD

Film: 8 × 10 in (18 × 24 cm).

Position of patient

- Place the patient in the prone or seated position before the grid device.
- Center the median sagittal plane of the head to the midline of the grid.
- Place the arms in a comfortable position and adjust the shoulders to lie in the same transverse plane.

Position of part

- Rest the tip of the nose and chin on the grid device with the chin centered to the midpoint of the grid.
- Adjust the head so that the median sagittal plane is perpendicular to the film (Figs. 21-52 to 21-54).
- Ask the patient to suspend respiration for the exposure.

Central ray

- Direct the central ray at a caudal angle of 23 to 38 degrees. It enters the vertex midway between the zygomatic arches.

Structures shown

The zygomatic arches are well shown in this projection (Figs. 21-55 and 21-56). The image presented is similar in appearance to the parietoacanthial projection (Waters method) previously described.

□ **Evaluation criteria**

The following should be clearly demonstrated:

- Zygomatic arches symmetric.
- Distance from the lateral border of the skull to the arches equal on both sides.

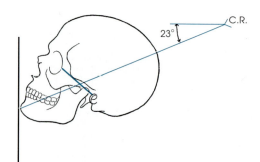

Fig. 21-53. Upright radiography.

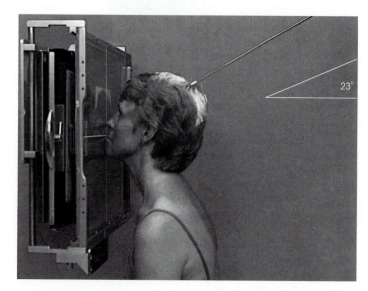

Fig. 21-52. PA axial zygomatic arches, modified Titterington method.

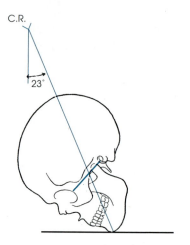

Fig. 21-54. Table radiography.

Facial bones

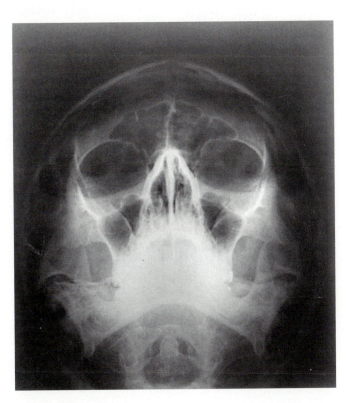

Fig. 21-55. PA axial zygomatic arches, modified Titterington method: caudal central ray angulation of 23 degrees.

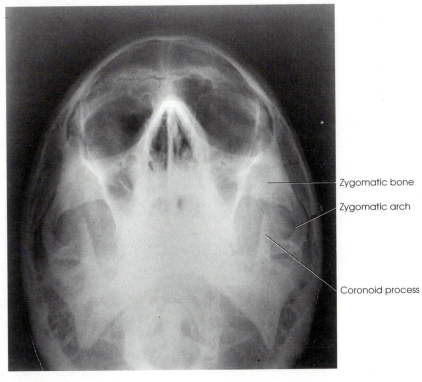

Zygomatic bone

Zygomatic arch

Coronoid process

Fig. 21-56. PA axial zygomatic arches, modified Titterington method: caudal central ray angulation of 38 degrees.

Zygomatic Arches

 AP AXIAL PROJECTION

Film: 8 × 10 in (18 × 24 cm) crosswise.

Position of patient

- Place the patient in the seated-upright or supine position.
- Center the median sagittal plane of the body to the midline of the grid.
- Place the arms in a comfortable position and adjust the shoulders to lie in the same transverse plane.

Position of part

- Adjust the patient's head so that the median sagittal plane is perpendicular to the midline of the grid.
- Adjust the flexion of the neck so that the orbitomeatal line is perpendicular to the plane of the film (Figs. 21-57 to 21-59).
- Center the cassette at the level of the mandibular angles.
- If necessary, immobilize the head with a suitably backed strip of adhesive tape that is applied across the patient's chin and is anchored to the sides of the grid. Do not put adhesive surface directly on patient's skin.
- Ask the patient to suspend respiration for the exposure.

Central ray

- Direct the central ray to enter the glabella, approximately 1 inch above the nasion, at an angle of 30 degrees caudad.
- For the patient unable to sufficiently flex the neck, adjust the infraorbitomeatal line perpendicular with the film and direct the central ray 37 degrees caudad.

Structures shown

A symmetric AP axial projection of both zygomatic arches is demonstrated. The arches should be projected free of superimposition (Fig. 21-60).

□ Evaluation criteria

The following should be clearly demonstrated:

- No overlap of the zygomatic arches by the mandible.
- No rotation evident since the arches are symmetric.
- Zygomatic arches projected lateral to mandibular rami.

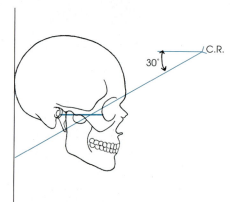

Fig. 21-58. Upright radiography.

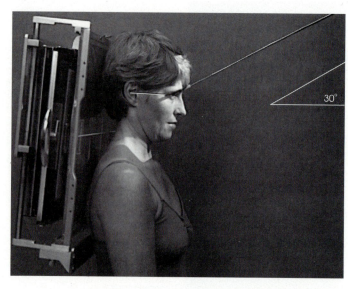

Fig. 21-57. AP axial zygomatic arches.

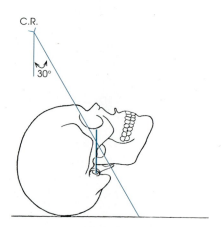

Fig. 21-59. Table radiography.

Occipital bone

Mandible

Zygomatic arch

Mandible

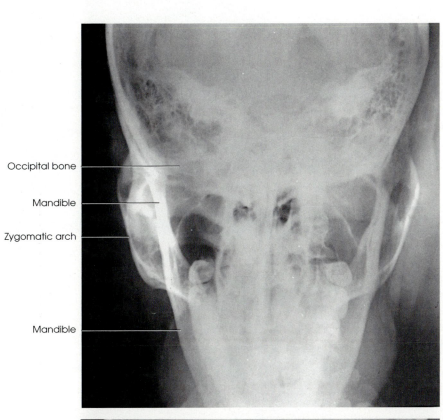

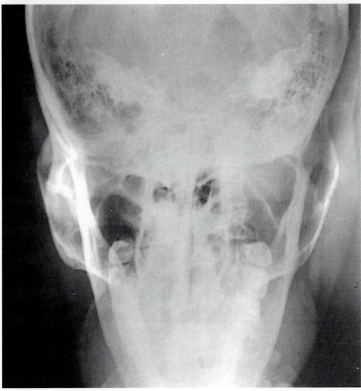

Fig. 21-60. AP axial zygomatic arches.

Zygomatic Arch

PA AXIAL OBLIQUE PROJECTION
MODIFIED FUCHS METHOD

Film: 8 × 10 in (18 × 24 cm) lengthwise.

Position of patient

- Place the patient in the prone position or seated before a vertical grid device.
- Place the arms in a comfortable position and adjust the shoulders to lie in the same transverse plane.

Position of part

- Rest the patient's cheek of the unaffected side on the grid device, with the most lateral point (the zygion) of the uppermost zygomatic bone (zygoma) lying directly above the center point of the film. The lips will be just above the transverse midline of the cassette.
- Adjust the flexion of the patient's neck so that the acanthomeatal line is perpendicular to the plane of the film.
- Using a protractor as a guide, rotate the median sagittal plane approximately 45 degrees, then tilt the top of the head away from the side being examined approximately 15 degrees. This rotation and tilt ensure that the central ray will be tangent to the lateral surface of the skull. The central ray will thus skim across the lateral portion of the parietal bone and the mandibular angle to project the zygomatic arch onto the film (Figs. 21-61 to 21-63).
- Immobilize the head.
- Ask the patient to suspend respiration for the exposure.

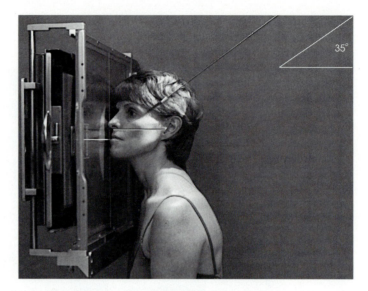

Fig. 21-61. PA axial oblique zygomatic arch, modified Fuchs method.

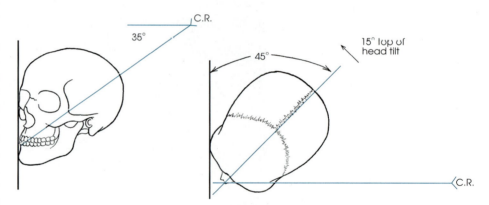

Fig. 21-62. Upright radiography.

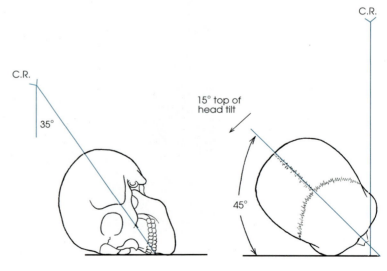

Fig. 21-63. Table radiography.

Central ray

• Direct the central ray 35 degrees caudad to enter the most prominent point of the zygomatic bone (zygoma) farthest from the film.

Structures shown

An oblique image of the uppermost zygomatic arch is shown, projected free of superimposition shadows (Fig. 21-64). The lateral portion of the maxillary sinus is also well demonstrated.

□ Evaluation criteria

The following should be clearly demonstrated:

■ Zygomatic arch projected free from overlying structures.

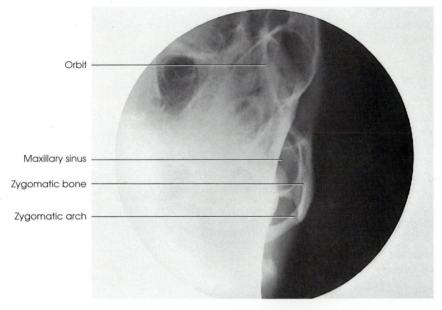

Orbit

Maxillary sinus

Zygomatic bone

Zygomatic arch

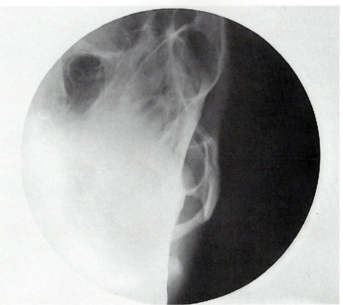

Fig. 21-64. PA axial oblique zygomatic arch, modified Fuchs method.

Maxillae

Hard Palate and Dental Arch

SUPEROINFERIOR PROJECTION (INTRAORAL)

Film: 2¼ × 3 in (57 × 76 mm) occlusal film.

Position of patient

- Place the patient in the supine position.

Position of part

- With the patient in the supine position, rest the head on the table or on a caudally inclined sponge and adjust it so that the median sagittal plane is vertical.
- Extend the head enough so that the occlusal plane is vertical.
- Immobilize the head.

Placement of film

- To spare the patient undue discomfort, do not insert the film packet into the mouth until after the head has been positioned and immobilized and the central ray has been adjusted in its approximate position.
- Tape a side marker (R or L) onto the correct corner of the pebbled surface of the film packet.
- With the pebbled surface of the packet facing the x-ray tube and its long axis directed tranversely, center the packet to the median sagittal plane of the head and then gently insert it far enough into the mouth so that it is in contact with the anterior borders of the mandibular rami.
- Instruct the patient to lightly close the mouth to hold the film in position (Figs. 21-65 and 21-66).
- Recheck the position of the head.
- Ask the patient to suspend respiration for the exposure.

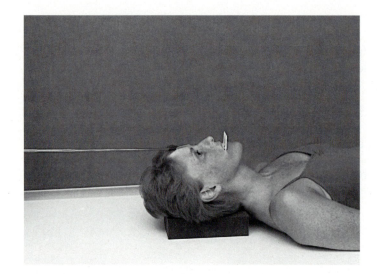

Fig. 21-65. Superoinferior hard palate.

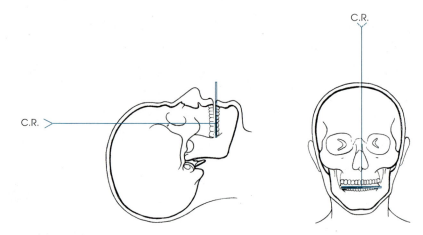

Fig. 21-66. Table radiography.

Central ray

• Direct the central ray perpendicular to the plane of the film and center it to the intersection of the median sagittal plane and a coronal plane that passes anterior to the outer canthi.

Structures shown

A superoinferior projection of the roof of the mouth (the palatine processes of the maxillae and the horizontal plates of the palatine bones) and of the entire dental arch is demonstrated (Fig. 21-67).

The following should be clearly demonstrated:

■ Horizontal plates of the palatine bones in their entirety along with all the teeth and the palatine processes of the maxillae.

■ No elongation or foreshortening of the roof of the mouth.

■ Distance between the teeth and the median palatine suture equal on both sides.

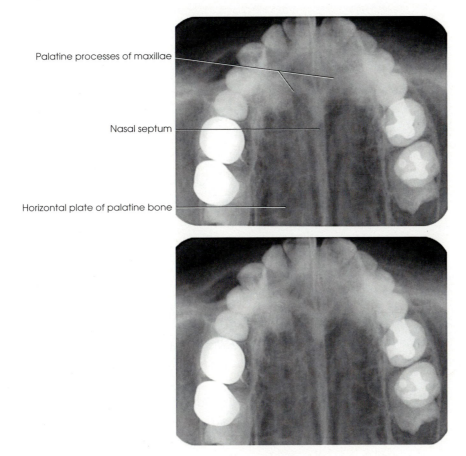

Palatine processes of maxillae

Nasal septum

Horizontal plate of palatine bone

Fig. 21-67. Superoinferior maxillae.

Maxillae

Maxillae

Anterior Hard Palate and Alveolar Process
AP AXIAL PROJECTION (INTRAORAL)

Film: 2¼ × 3 in (57 × 76 mm) occlusal film.

Position of patient

- Place the patient in the supine position.

Position of part

- Adjust the head so that the median sagittal plane is vertical and the occlusal plane is perpendicular to the table.
- Immobilize the head.
- Ask the patient to suspend respiration for the exposure.

Placement of film

- To spare the patient undue discomfort, do not insert the film packet into the mouth until after the head has been positioned and immobilized and the central ray has been adjusted in approximately the correct position (Figs. 21-68 and 21-69).
- Tape a side marker (R or L) onto the correct corner of the pebbled surface of the film packet.
- With the pebbled surface of the packet facing superiorly and its long axis directed anteroposteriorly, center the packet to the median sagittal plane and then gently insert it far enough into the mouth so that it is in contact with the anterior borders of the mandibular rami.
- Have the patient close the mouth to maintain the packet in position.
- Place a lead apron/shield over the patient's neck and pelvis for radiation protection.

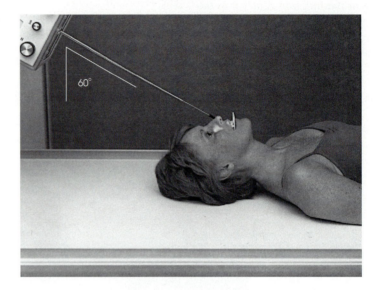

Fig. 21-68. AP axial maxillae.

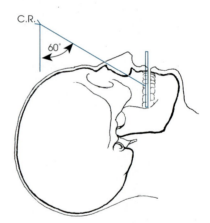

Fig. 21-69. Table radiography.

Central ray

- Direct the central ray to the distal lower third of the nose at an angle of 60 to 65 degrees caudad from the vertical.

Structures shown

The image shows an AP axial projection of the anterior portion of the hard palate, the alveolar process, and the upper incisors (Fig. 21-70).

□ Evaluation criteria

The following should be clearly demonstrated:

- Most of the elongated hard palate.
- Distance between the teeth and the median palatine suture equal on both sides.

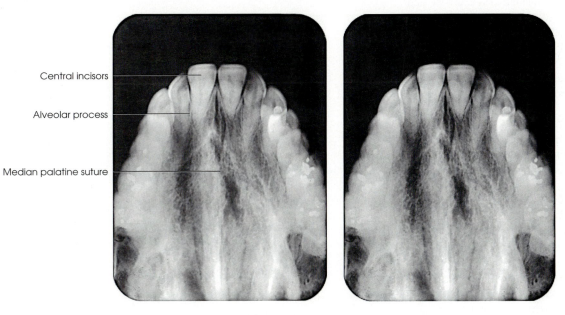

Central incisors

Alveolar process

Median palatine suture

Fig. 21-70. AP axial maxillae.

Maxillae

Posterior Hard Palate and Alveolar Process
AP AXIAL OBLIQUE PROJECTION (INTRAORAL)

Film: 2¼ × 3 in (57 × 76 mm) occlusal film.

Position of patient

- Place the patient in the supine position.

Position of part

- With the patient's head resting on the table, rotate it 30 degrees away from the side being examined.
- Adjust the flexion of the neck so that the occlusal plane is vertical.
- Check the rotation of the head and immobilize it if needed (Figs. 21-71 and 21-72).
- Place a lead apron/shield over the patient's neck and pelvis for radiation protection.
- Ask the patient to suspend respiration for the exposure.

Placement of film

- To spare the patient undue discomfort, position and immobilize the head and adjust the central ray before placing the film packet in the mouth.
- Tape a side marker (R or L) onto one corner of the pebbled surface of the film packet.
- With the pebbled surface facing the x-ray tube and the long axis directed anteroposteriorly, place the film packet into the mouth, adjust it approximately ½ inch (1.2 cm) off center toward the side being examined, and then gently insert it far enough into the mouth so that it is in contact with the anterior border of the mandibular ramus.
- Instruct the patient to hold the film packet lightly between the teeth.

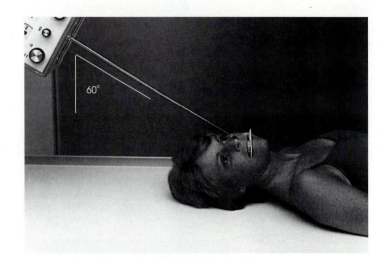

Fig. 21-71. AP axial oblique maxillae.

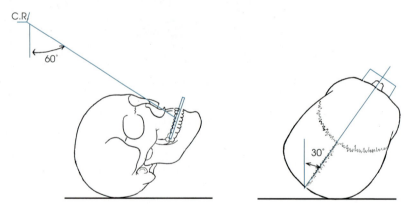

Fig. 21-72. Table radiography.

Central ray

- Direct the central ray to the canine fossa at an angle of 60 degrees caudad from the vertical.

Structures shown

The image shows an AP axial oblique projection of the posterior part of the hard palate, the alveolar process, and the canine, premolars, and molars of one side of the upper maxilla (Fig. 21-73).

□ Evaluation criteria

The following should be clearly demonstrated:

- All of the teeth on the side being demonstrated along with the posterior part of the hard palate.

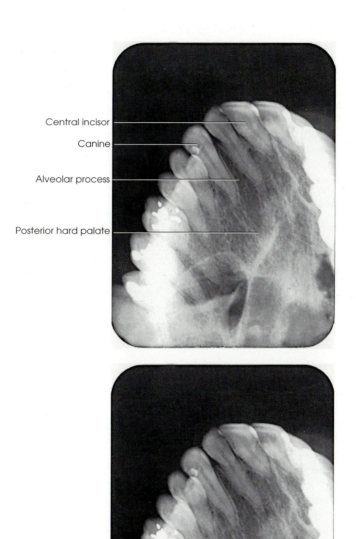

Central incisor

Canine

Alveolar process

Posterior hard palate

Fig. 21-73. AP axial oblique maxillae.

Mandible

Body and Dental Arch
INFEROSUPERIOR PROJECTION
(INTRAORAL)

Film: 2¼ × 3 in (57 × 76 mm) occlusal film.

Position of patient

- Elevate the patient's thorax on firm pillows or sandbags and flex the knees to relax the abdominal muscles, so that the neck can be fully extended.
- Place the arms in a comfortable position and adjust the shoulders to lie in the same transverse plane.

Position of part

- Fully extend the neck, rest the head on the vertex, and adjust it so that the median sagittal plane is vertical.
- Immobilize the head (Figs. 21-74 and 21-75).
- Ask the patient to suspend respiration for the exposure.

Placement of film

- To spare the patient undue discomfort, position and immobilize the head and adjust the central ray before placing the film packet in the mouth.
- Tape a side marker (R or L) onto one corner of the pebbled surface of the packet.
- With the film packet facing the x-ray tube and its long axis directed transversely, center it to the median sagittal plane and then gently insert it far enough into the mouth so that it is in contact with the anterior surfaces of the mandibular rami.
- Instruct the patient to hold the film packet lightly between the teeth.

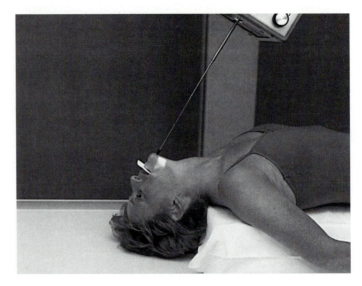

Fig. 21-74. Inferosuperior mandible.

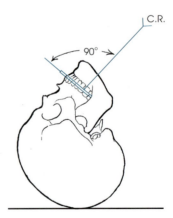

Fig. 21-75. Table radiography.

Central ray

- Direct the central ray perpendicular to the plane of the film packet and center it to the intersection of the median sagittal plane and a coronal plane passing through the second molars.

Structures shown

The projection demonstrates the floor of the mouth, the entire lower dental arch, and that portion of the mandibular body which it supports (Fig. 21-76).

The projection is commonly employed for the demonstration of any medial or lateral displacement of fragments in fractures and, with a lighter exposure, for the examination of the submaxillary and sublingual salivary glands.

□ Evaluation criteria

The following should be clearly demonstrated:

- All of the lower teeth so that the mandibular body will be almost entirely included.
- Distance between the teeth and the outer border of the mandible symmetric on both sides.

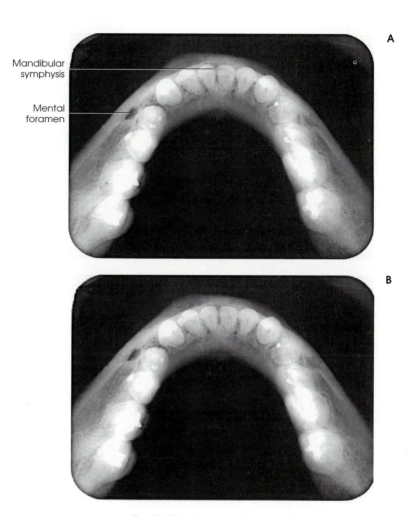

Fig. 21-76. Inferosuperior mandible.

Mandibular symphysis

Mental foramen

Mandible

Mandibular Symphysis

AP AXIAL PROJECTION (INTRAORAL)

Film: 2¼ × 3 in (57 × 76 mm) occlusal film.

Position of patient

- Place the patient in the supine position.
- Place the arms along the sides of the body and adjust the shoulders to lie in the same transverse plane.

Position of part

- Rest the patient's head on the occiput, and, with the median sagittal plane vertical, adjust the flexion of the neck so that the occlusal plane is vertical.
- Immobilize the head if needed (Figs. 21-77 and 21-78).

To modify for the upright patient, observe the following steps:
- Seat the patient in a chair that has an adjustable headrest.
- Tilt the head backward, support it on the headrest, and adjust it so that the median sagittal plane is vertical and the occlusal plane forms an angle of 55 degrees to the horizontal.
- Ask the patient to suspend respiration for the exposure.

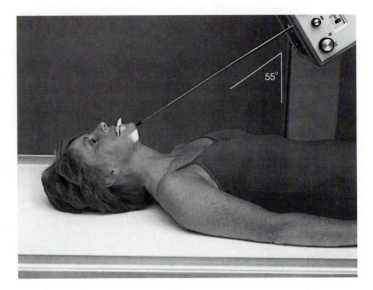

Fig. 21-77. AP axial mandibular symphysis.

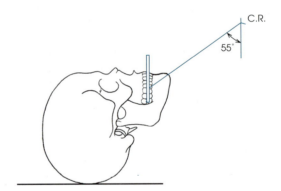

Fig. 21-78. Table radiography.

Placement of film

- To spare the patient undue discomfort, position and immobilize the head and adjust the central ray angulation before placing the film packet in the mouth.
- Tape a side marker (R or L) onto one corner of the pebbled surface of the film packet.
- With the pebbled surface of the film packet facing the x-ray tube and its long axis directed anteroposteriorly, center the packet to the median sagittal plane and then gently insert it far enough into the mouth so that it is in contact with the anterior borders of the mandibular rami.
- Instruct the patient to close the mouth lightly to hold the film packet in position.

Central ray

- Direct the central ray to the tip of the chin at an angle of 55 degrees cephalad for the supine patient.
- Direct the central ray horizontal to the tip of the chin for the upright patient.

Structures shown

This image shows an AP axial projection of the region of the mandibular symphysis, showing the alveolar portion, the incisors, and the canine teeth (Fig. 21-79).

□ Evaluation criteria

The following should be clearly demonstrated:

- No self-superimposition of the symphysis of mandible.
- No rotation of the mandible.

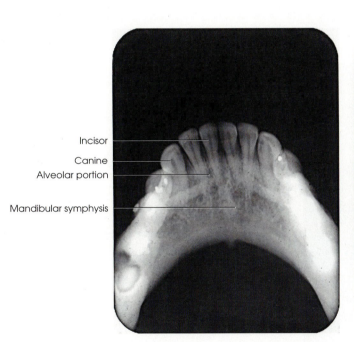
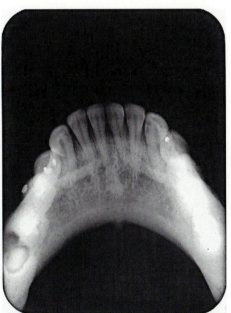

Incisor
Canine
Alveolar portion

Mandibular symphysis

Fig. 21-79. AP axial mandibular symphysis.

Mandibular Symphysis

AP AXIAL PROJECTION (EXTRAORAL)

Film: 2¼ × 3 in (57 × 76 mm) occlusal film or 8 × 10 in (18 × 24 cm) crosswise.

Position of patient: Upright

- Seat the patient at one end of the radiographic table.
- Elevate the film packet on a suitable support so that the patient can extend the neck and maintain the position of the chin in a horizontal plane in order to place it in close contact with the film holder.
- Tape a side marker (R or L) onto one corner of the occlusal film, and place the film in position, with its pebbled surface up and its long axis directed anteroposteriorly.

Position of part

- With the median sagittal plane of the patient's head perpendicular and centered to the midline of the film, adjust the fully extended chin well forward on the film to allow for the angulation of the central ray. The support under the chin is usually sufficient to maintain the head in position (Figs. 21-80 and 21-81).
- *Shield gonads.*
- Ask the patient to suspend respiration for the exposure.

Central ray

- Direct the central ray posteriorly at an angle of 40 to 45 degrees and center it to the mandibular symphysis (midway between the lips and the tip of the chin) for the upright patient.

Position of patient: Supine

If the patient is unable to sit, conduct the examination in the supine position observing the following steps:

- Rest the patient's head on the occiput with the median sagittal plane vertical.
- Adjust the flexion of the neck so that the inferior border of the body of the mandible is vertical (Fig. 21-82).
- Immobilize the head.
- Adjust the film packet in position, with its pebbled surface in contact with the chin and its long axis in the median sagittal plane.
- Either tape the packet to the skin or have the patient hold it in position if possible.
- Ask the patient to suspend respiration for the exposure.
- Direct the central ray to the mandibular symphysis at an angle of 40 or 45 degrees caudad for the supine patient.

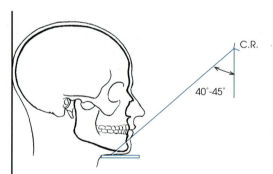

Fig. 21-81. Upright radiography.

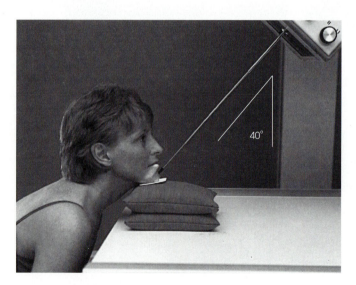

Fig. 21-80. AP axial mandibular symphysis.

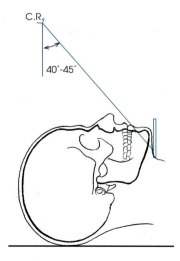

Fig. 21-82. Table radiography.

Structures shown

The AP axial projection shows the mandibular symphysis, the mental foramina, and the roots of the lower incisors and canines (Fig. 21-83).

☐ Evaluation criteria

The following should be clearly demonstrated:
- Mandibular symphysis and the adjacent mentum.
- Roots of the lower anterior teeth.
- No rotation of the mandible.

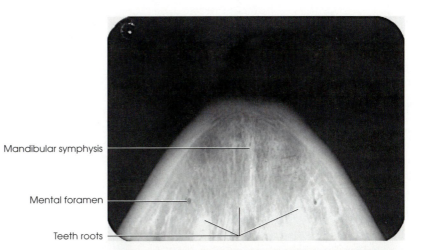

Mandibular symphysis

Mental foramen

Teeth roots

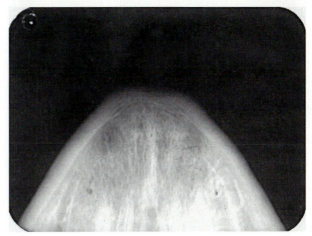

Fig. 21-83. AP axial mandibular symphysis.

Mandibular Rami

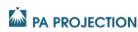 PA PROJECTION

Film: 8 × 10 in (18 × 24 cm) crosswise.

Position of patient

- Place the patient in the prone position or seated before a vertical grid device.
- Place the arms in a comfortable position and adjust the shoulders to lie in the same transverse plane.

Position of part

- Rest the patient's forehead and nose on the film holder. For a general projection of the mandibular rami, center the tip of the nose to the midpoint of the film.
- Adjust the film so that the midpoint will coincide with the central ray.
- Adjust the head so that the median sagittal plane is perpendicular to the plane of the film (Fig. 21-84).
- Immobilize the head.
- Ask the patient to suspend respiration for the exposure.

Central ray

- Direct the perpendicular central ray to exit the acanthion.

Structures shown

The PA projection shows the mandibular body and rami (Fig. 21-85). The central part of the body is not well shown because of the superimposed spine. This radiographic approach is usually employed to demonstrate any medial or lateral displacement of fragments in fractures of the rami.

□ Evaluation criteria

The following should be clearly demonstrated:

- Mandibular body and rami symmetric on each side.
- Entire mandible.

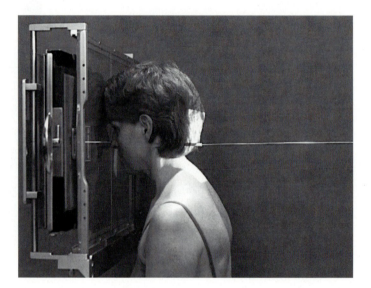

Fig. 21-84. PA mandibular rami.

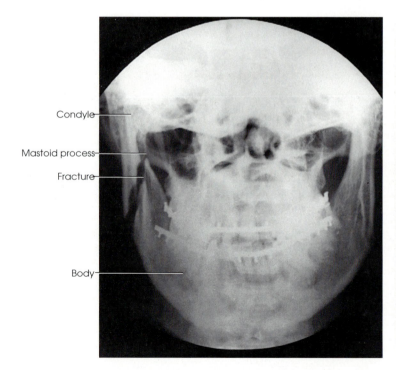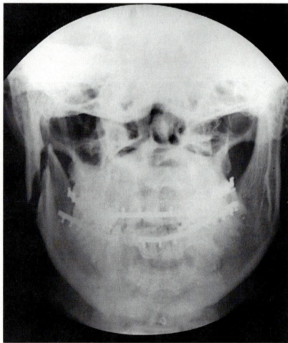

Condyle

Mastoid process

Fracture

Body

Fig. 21-85. PA mandibular rami showing fracture of right superior ramus.

(Courtesy Dr. William H. Shehadi.)

Mandibular Rami

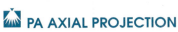 PA AXIAL PROJECTION

Film: 8 × 10 in (18 × 24 cm) crosswise.

Position of patient

- Place the patient in the prone position or seated before a vertical grid device.
- Place the arms in a comfortable position and adjust the shoulders to lie in the same transverse plane.

Position of part

- Rest the patient's forehead and nose on the film holder and (1) for a general projection of the mandibular rami, center the tip of the nose to the midpoint of the film, or (2) for the demonstration of the condylar processes, center the glabella to the midpoint of the film.
- Adjust the film so that the midpoint will coincide with the central ray.
- Adjust the head so that the median sagittal plane is perpendicular to the plane of the film (Fig. 21-86).
- Immobilize the head.
- Ask the patient to suspend respiration for the exposure.

Central ray

- Direct the central ray 20 or 25 degrees cephalad to exit above the tip of the nose.

Structures shown

The PA axial projection shows the mandibular body and rami (Fig. 21-87). The central part of the body is not well shown because of the superimposed spine. This radiographic approach is usually employed to demonstrate any medial or lateral displacement of fragments in fractures of the rami.

☐ Evaluation criteria

The following should be clearly demonstrated:

- Mandibular body and rami symmetric on each side.
- Condylar processes.
- Entire mandible.

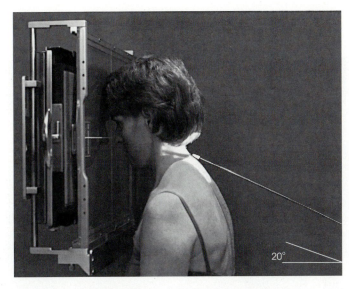

Fig. 21-86. PA axial mandibular rami.

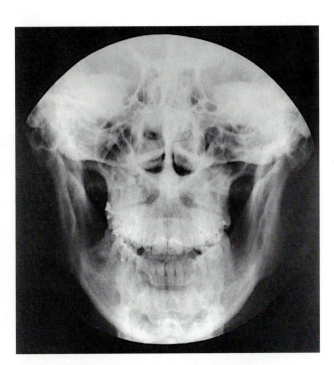

Fig. 21-87. PA axial mandibular rami.

Mandibular Body
PA PROJECTION

Film: 8×10 in $(18 \times 24$ cm$)$ lengthwise.

Position of patient

• Place the patient in the prone position or seated before a vertical grid device.

Position of part

• With the median sagittal plane of the head centered to the midline of the cassette, rest the weight of the skull on the nose and chin so that the anterior surface of the mandibular symphysis is parallel with the plane of the film. This position places the acanthomeatal line nearly perpendicular to the film plane.
• Adjust the head so that the median sagittal plane is perpendicular to the plane of the film.
• Center the film at the level of the lips (Fig. 21-88).
• Ask the patient to suspend respiration for the exposure.

Central ray

• Direct the central ray perpendicular to the level of the lips.

Structures shown

This image demonstrates the mandibular body (Fig. 21-89).

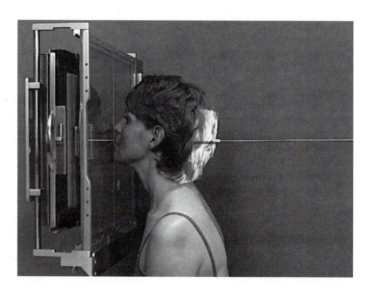

Fig. 21-88. PA mandibular body.

□ Evaluation criterion

The following should be clearly demonstrated:
■ Mandibular body symmetric on each side.

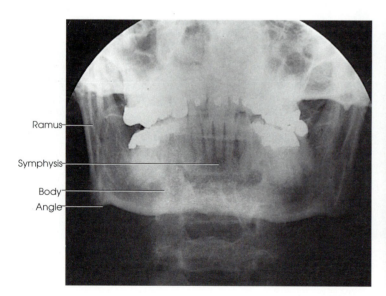
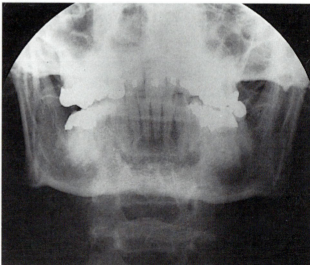

Ramus
Symphysis
Body
Angle

Fig. 21-89. PA mandibular body.

Mandibular Body
PA AXIAL PROJECTION

Film: 8 × 10 in (18 × 24 cm) lengthwise.

Position of patient

- Place the patient in the prone position or seated before a vertical grid device.

Position of part

- With the median sagittal plane of the head centered to the midline of the cassette, rest the weight of the skull on the nose and chin so that the anterior surface of the mandibular symphysis is parallel with the plane of the film. This position places the acanthomeatal line nearly perpendicular to the film plane.
- Adjust the head so that the median sagittal plane is perpendicular to the plane of the film.
- To include the rami and temporomandibular joints (TMJs), center the film to the tip of the nose, approximately 2 inches (5 cm) above the mandibular symphysis (Fig. 21-90).
- Ask the patient to suspend respiration for the exposure.

Central ray

- Direct the central ray midway between the TMJs at an angle of 30 degrees cephalad. Zanelli[1] recommends that the patient be instructed to fill the mouth with air for this projection in order to obtain better contrast around the TMJs.

[1]Zanelli A: Le proiezioni radiografiche dell'articolazione temporomandibolare, Radiol Med 16:495-499, 1929.

Structures shown

This image shows the mandibular body and TMJs (Fig. 21-91).

□ Evaluation criterion

The following should be clearly demonstrated:

- TMJs just inferior to the mastoid process.
- Symmetric rami.

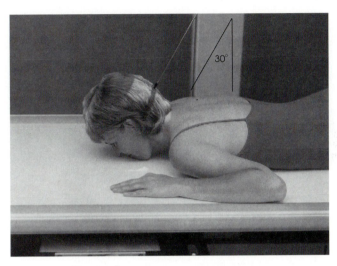

Fig. 21-90. PA axial mandibular body.

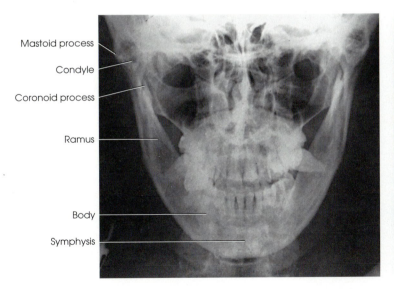
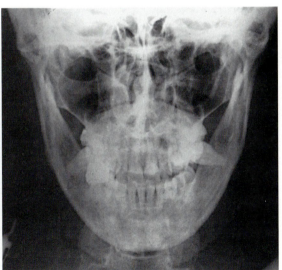

Mastoid process
Condyle
Coronoid process
Ramus
Body
Symphysis

Fig. 21-91. PA axial mandibular body.

Mandibular body

Mandible

AXIOLATERAL OBLIQUE PROJECTION

The goal of this position is to place the desired portion of the mandible parallel with the film.

Film: 8 × 10 in (18 × 24 cm) placed according to region.

Position of patient

- Place the patient in the prone position or seated.
- When the patient is in the prone position, oblique the body slightly and have the patient support the body on the opposite hand and forearm. For the seated position, rotate the body slightly so the side of the face can be placed next to the cassette.

Body of mandible
Position of part

- Adjust the cassette under the cheek with the mouth closed and teeth together.
- Extend the neck enough so that the long axis of the mandibular body is parallel with the transverse axis of the film.
- Center the film to the region of the first molar.
- Adjust the rotation of the head so that the broad surface of the mandibular body is parallel with the plane of the film (Figs. 21-92 and 21-93).
- Ask the patient to suspend respiration for the exposure.

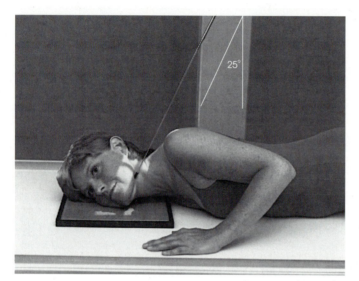

Fig. 21-92. Prone axiolateral oblique mandibular body.

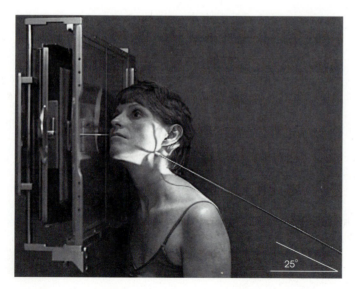

Fig. 21-93. Upright axiolateral oblique mandibular body.

Facial bones

Central ray

- Direct the central ray to enter slightly posteriorly to the mandibular angle on the side farthest from the film at an angle of approximately 25 degrees cephalad.

Structures shown

The axiolateral oblique projection demonstrates the body of the mandible from the angle to the region of the canine (Fig. 21-94).

The following should be clearly demonstrated:

- Mandibular body to the canine tooth.
- No overlap of the mandibular body by the opposite side of the mandible.

NOTE: To reduce the possibility of projecting the shoulder over the mandible when radiographing muscular or hypersthenic patients, the median sagittal plane of the patient's skull can be adjusted with an approximate 15-degree angle, open inferiorly. The cephalad angulation of 10 degrees of the central ray will maintain the optimal 25-degree central ray/part angle relationship.

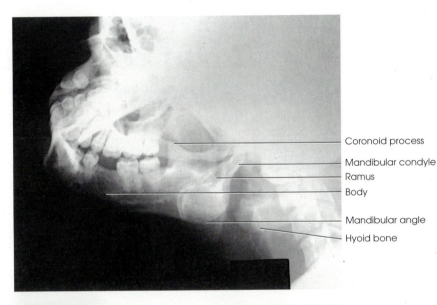

Coronoid process
Mandibular condyle
Ramus
Body
Mandibular angle
Hyoid bone

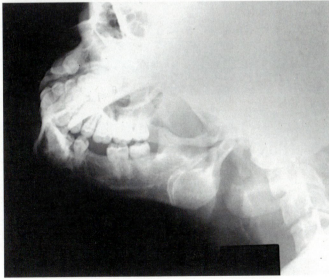

Fig. 21-94. Prone axiolateral oblique mandibular body.

(Courtesy Sharon A. Coffey, R.T.)

Symphysis of mandible
Position of part

- With the cassette placed under the patient's cheek, center the cassette to the occlusal surface of the canine region, extend the neck, and rest the mandible on the film holder (Fig. 21-95).
- Rest the head on the extended chin, the nose, and the zygomatic bone (zygoma).
- Ask the patient to suspend respiration for the exposure.

Central ray

- Direct the central ray to the midpoint of the film at an angle of 20 degrees cephalad. The central ray exits the mandibular symphysis.

Structures shown

This projection shows the region of the symphysis of the mandible and the lower incisor teeth (Fig. 21-96).

☐ Evaluation criteria

The following should be clearly demonstrated:

- No overlap of the symphysis and the adjacent region by the opposite side of the mandible.

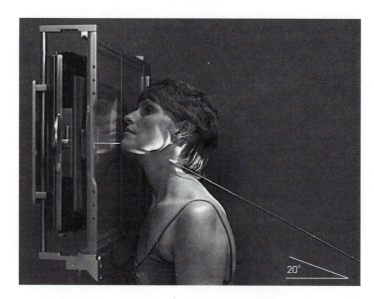

Fig. 21-95. Axiolateral oblique mandibular symphysis.

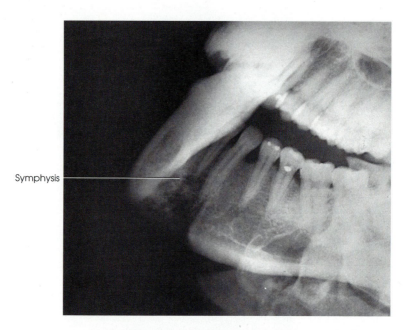

Symphysis

Fig. 21-96. Axiolateral oblique mandibular symphysis.

Ramus of mandible
Position of part

- Place the cassette under the patient's cheek.
- Center the film to a point ½ inch (1.2 cm) anterior and 1 inch (2.5 cm) inferior to the external acoustic (auditory) meatus.
- With the patient's cheek resting on the grid device so that the broad surface of the ramus is parallel with the plane of the film, extend the neck fully to prevent the spine from being superimposed on that of the ramus (Fig. 21-97).
- Ask the patient to suspend respiration for the exposure.

Central ray

- Direct the central ray to enter slightly posterior to the mandibular angle on the side *farthest* from the film at an angle of 25 degrees cephalad.

Structures shown

The mandibular ramus (except the condyle) and the angle and posterior part of the body of the mandible are demonstrated (Fig. 21-98).

□Evaluation criteria

The following should be clearly demonstrated:

- No overlap of the ramus by the opposite side of the mandible.
- No elongation or foreshortening of the ramus.
- No overlap of the ramus by the cervical vertebrae.

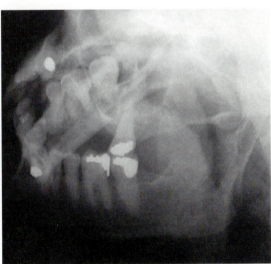

Fig. 21-97. Axiolateral oblique for mandibular ramus.

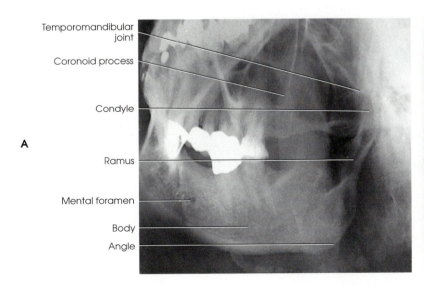

Temporomandibular joint
Coronoid process
Condyle
Ramus
Mental foramen
Body
Angle

A

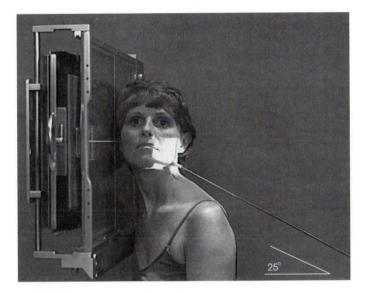

B

Fig. 21-98. Axiolateral oblique for mandibular ramus.

(Courtesy Jeffrey L. Rowe, RT.)

Mandible

AXIOLATERAL OBLIQUE PROJECTION

This position is useful when the patient is unable to sit or lie prone. The position is easily modified to accommodate the trauma patient.

Film: 8 × 10 in (18 × 24 cm) placed according to region.

Position of patient

- Place the patient in a semisupine position, the affected side down.
- Support the elevated hip and shoulder on sandbags or firm pillows.
- Adjust the rotation of the body so that the head can be placed in a lateral position on a cranially inclined cassette.

Body and symphysis of mandible
Position of part

- Place the cassette crosswise under the cheek.
- Using a support or sponge, elevate the side of the cassette adjacent to the shoulder so that it will be in close contact with the mandible.
- Extend the neck so that the long axis of the mandibular body is parallel with the transverse axis of the film and then center the distal half of the film to the body of the mandible.
- Place a small sandbag against the upper edge of the cassette if needed so that it will not slip during the adjustment of the head.
- Rotate the patient's head enough so that the broad surface of the mandibular body is parallel with the plane of the film, and (1) for the posterior two thirds of the body, rest the head on the cheek (Fig. 21-99), or (2) for the anterior third of the body, rest the head on the side of the chin.
- Ask the patient to suspend respiration for the exposure.

Central ray

- Direct the central ray to the midpoint of the film at an angle of 20 degrees cephalad entering approximately 2 inches (5 cm) distal to the mandibular angle on the side farthest from the film.

Structures shown

This projection shows the posterior portion of the mandibular body, the angle, and part of the ramus (Figs. 21-100 and 21-101).

□ Evaluation criteria

The following should be clearly demonstrated:

- Mandibular body including the symphysis.
- The canine tooth.
- No superimposition or overlap of the body by the opposite side of the mandible.

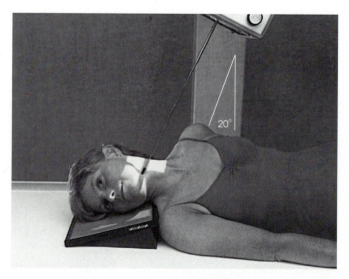

Fig. 21-99. Semisupine axiolateral oblique mandibular body and symphysis.

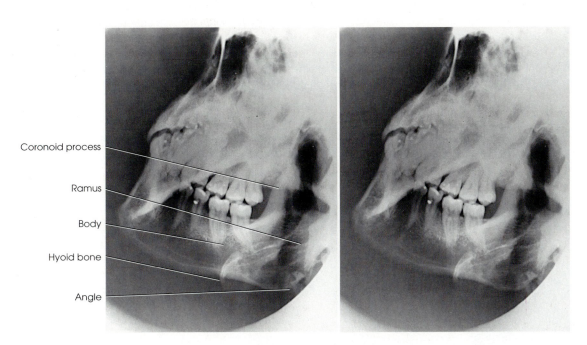

Coronoid process

Ramus

Body

Hyoid bone

Angle

Fig. 21-100. Axiolateral oblique mandibular body and symphysis.

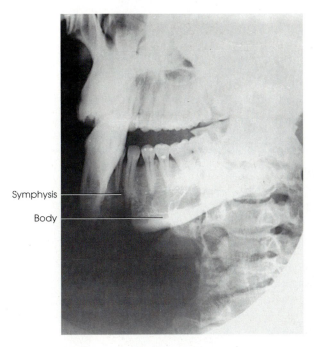

Symphysis

Body

Fig. 21-101. Axiolateral oblique mandibular
symphysis.

Ramus of mandible
Position of part

- Place the cassette lengthwise under the patient's cheek, elevate the end adjacent to the shoulder enough so that the cassette is in close contact with the mandible, and provide support.
- Center the film to a point ½ inch (1.2 cm) anterior to and 1 inch (2.5 cm) inferior to the external acoustic (auditory) meatus and place a small sandbag against the upper end of the cassette to prevent it from slipping during the adjustment of the head.

- Adjust the rotation of the head so that the broad surface of the ramus is parallel with the plane of the film.
- Extend the neck enough so that the acanthomeatal line is parallel with the transverse axis of the film; this moves the ramus forward so it will not be superimposed by the spine (Fig. 21-102).
- Ask the patient to suspend respiration for the exposure.

Central ray

- Direct the central ray to the midpoint of the film at an angle of 25 degrees cephalad, entering approximately 2 inches (5 cm) distal to the mandibular angle on the side farthest from the film.
- When the neck cannot be extended enough for correct placement of the acanthomeatal line, also direct the central ray posteriorly at an angle of 10 degrees.

Structures shown

This projection shows the ramus, the angle, and part of the body of the mandible (Fig. 21-103).

□Evaluation criteria

The following should be clearly demonstrated:
- No overlap of the ramus by the opposite side of the mandible.
- No elongation or foreshortening of the ramus.
- No overlap of the ramus by the cervical vertebrae.

NOTE: Trauma patients sometimes have other injuries that contraindicate rotation of the body or head. The cassette is then placed in the vertical position parallel with the median sagittal plane and is centered to the occlusal plane. The central ray is directed horizontally at an angle of 30 to 35 degrees cephalad, plus a 10-degree angle anteriorly or posteriorly, as indicated.

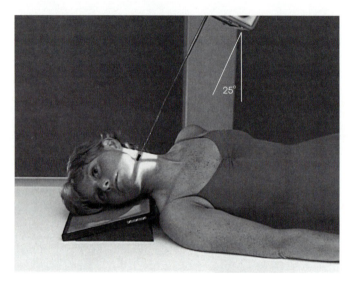

Fig. 21-102. Semisupine axiolateral oblique mandibular ramus.

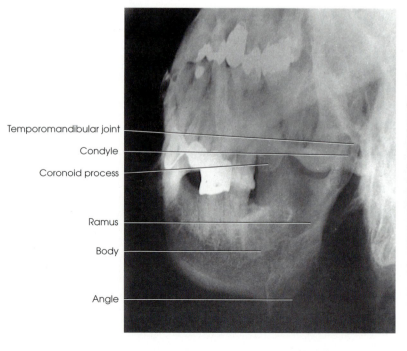
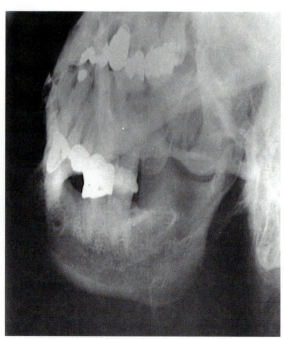

Temporomandibular joint
Condyle
Coronoid process
Ramus
Body
Angle

Fig. 21-103. Axiolateral oblique mandibular ramus.

Mandible
SUBMENTOVERTICAL PROJECTION

Film: 8 × 10 in (18 × 24 cm) lengthwise.

Position of patient

- Place the patient in front of a vertical grid device or in the supine position for the submentovertical (SMV) projection.
- In the latter case, elevate the trunk 7 or 8 inches (17.5 to 20 cm) on firm pillows or on a suitable pad to permit complete extension of the neck.
- Flex the patient's knees to relax the abdominal muscles and thus relieve strain on the neck muscles.
- Center the median sagittal plane of the body to the midline of the grid device.
- Place the arms in a comfortable position and adjust the shoulders to lie in the same transverse plane.

Position of part

- With the neck fully extended, rest the head on the vertex and adjust it so that the median sagittal plane is vertical.
- Adjust the infraorbitomeatal line as parallel as possible with the film plane (Fig. 21-104).
- When the neck cannot be extended enough so that the infraorbitomeatal line is parallel with the film plane, angle the *grid device* and place it parallel to the infraorbitomeatal line.
- Immobilize the head.
- Ask the patient to suspend respiration for the exposure.

Central ray

- Direct the central ray perpendicularly to the infraorbitomeatal line and center it midway between the angles of the mandible.

Structures shown

The SMV projection of the mandibular body is demonstrated, showing the coronoid and condyloid processes of the rami (Fig. 21-105).

The following should be clearly demonstrated:

- Distance between the lateral border of the skull and the mandible equal on both sides.
- Condyles of the mandible anterior to the pars petrosae.
- Symphysis extending almost to the anterior border of the face so that the mandible is not foreshortened.

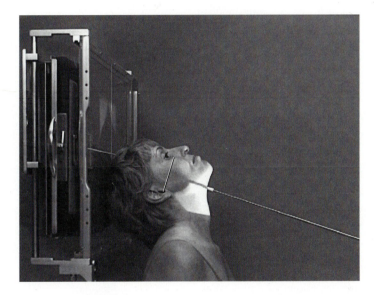

Fig. 21-104. Submentovertical mandible.

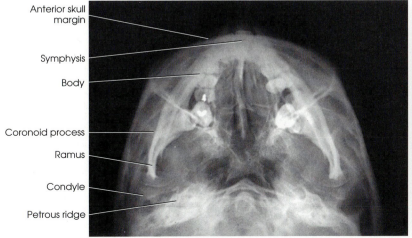
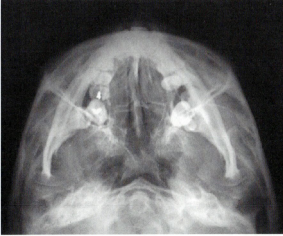

Anterior skull margin

Symphysis

Body

Coronoid process

Ramus

Condyle

Petrous ridge

Fig. 21-105. Submentovertical mandible.

Mandible

VERTICOSUBMENTAL PROJECTION

Film: 8 × 10 in (18 × 24 cm).

Position of patient

- Examine the patient in the prone position, or seated so that the chin can be positioned across the cassette.
- Place the arms in a comfortable position and adjust the shoulders to lie in the same transverse plane.

Position of part

- Place the cassette on a small sandbag and adjust it, either horizontally or at a cranial inclination, so that it is in close contact with the patient's throat.
- Center the median sagittal plane of the patient's head to the midline of the cassette.
- With the transverse midline of the cassette lying directly below the external acoustic (auditory) meatuses, fully extend the neck and rest the chin on the cassette.
- Adjust the head so that the median sagittal plane is vertical.
- Adjust the infraorbitomeatal line to be parallel with the film (Fig. 21-106).
- Immobilize the head. When the mandible is painful, do not employ the compression technique of immobilization.
- *Shield gonads.*
- Ask the patient to suspend respiration for the exposure.

Central ray

- Direct the central ray through the median sagittal plane entering at the level just posterior to the outer canthi, either (1) perpendicular to the infraorbitomeatal line (Fig. 21-106) or (2) perpendicular to the occlusal plane.

Structures shown

The VSM projection demonstrates the mandible as seen from above the patient. The coronoid processes are well shown on either image, but the condyle and neck of the condylar processes are better shown with the greater angle, that is, with the central ray at right angles to the occlusal plane (Figs. 21-107 and 21-108).

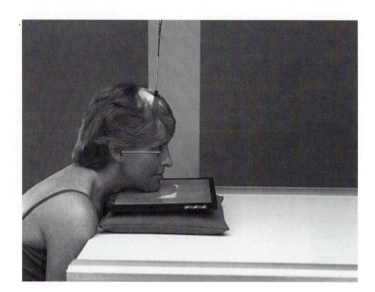

Fig. 21-106. Verticosubmental mandible.

The following should be clearly demonstrated:
- Distance between the lateral border of the skull and the mandible equal on both sides.
- Angles of the mandible anterior to the petrosae.

NOTE: Be sure to provide gonadal shielding for the patient in this projection. The use of a sheet of leaded rubber placed across the lap is sufficient in addition to close collimation.

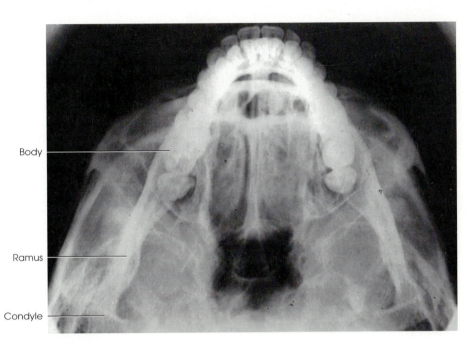

Body

Ramus

Condyle

Fig. 21-107. Verticosubmental mandible with central ray perpendicular to infra-orbitomeatal line.

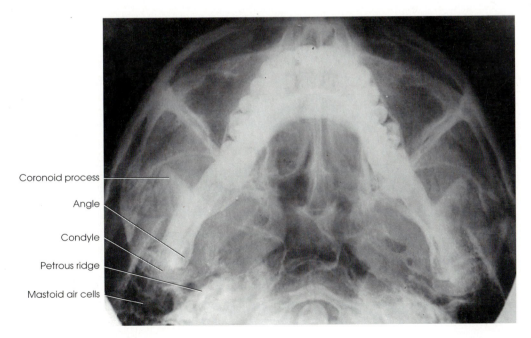

Coronoid process

Angle

Condyle

Petrous ridge

Mastoid air cells

Fig. 21-108. Verticosubmental mandible with central ray perpendicular to occlusal plane.

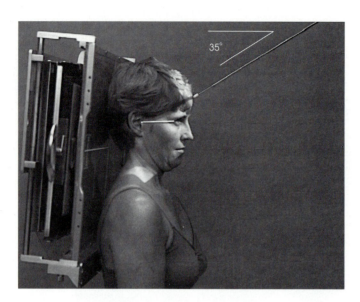

Fig. 21-109. AP axial TMJs.

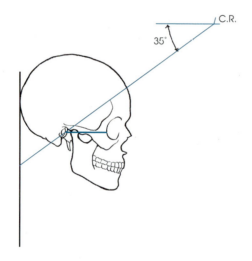

Fig. 21-110. Upright radiography.

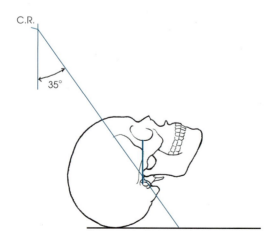

Fig. 21-111. Table radiography.

Temporomandibular Articulations

AP AXIAL PROJECTION

For radiography of the temporomandibular joints (TMJs) in the closed- and open-mouth positions, it must be remembered that in the closed-mouth position the patient must occlude the posterior teeth rather than the incisors. Occlusion of the incisors places the mandible in a position of protrusion, and the condyles are carried out of the mandibular fossae. In the open-mouth position, the mouth should be opened as wide as possible but not with the mandible protruded (jutted forward).

The open-mouth position should not be attempted if there has been recent injury because of the danger of fragment displacement. Trauma patients are examined without any stress movement of the mandible. Tomography is particularly useful when a fracture or dislocation is suspected.

Film: 8 × 10 in (18 × 24 cm) lengthwise.

Position of patient

- Place the patient in the supine or seated-upright position.
- Place the arms in a comfortable position and adjust the shoulders to lie in the same transverse plane.

Position of part

- Center the cassette to the median sagittal plane of the patient's neck at a point directly below the TMJs.
- Adjust the head so that the median sagittal plane is vertical.
- Flex the neck so that the orbitomeatal line is perpendicular to the plane of the film (Figs. 21-109 to 21-111).
- Place a strip of suitably backed adhesive tape across the chin and anchor the tape to the sides of the grid device or table. This usually furnishes sufficient immobilization. Do not attach adhesive surface directly to patient's skin.
- Ask the patient to suspend respiration for the exposure.

Central ray

- Direct the central ray 35 degrees caudad, centered midway between the temporomandibular joints. It enters at a point approximately 3 inches (7.5 cm) above the nasion.
- Expose one film with the mouth closed, and, when not contraindicated, expose one with the mouth open.

Structures shown

This image shows an AP axial projection of the condyles of the mandible and of the mandibular fossae of the temporal bones (Figs. 21-112 and 21-113).

☐Evaluation criteria

The following should be clearly demonstrated:

- ■ No rotation of the head.
- ■ Minimal superimposition of the petrosa on the condyle in the closed mouth examination.
- ■ Condyle and temporomandibular articulation below the pars petrosa in the open-mouth position.

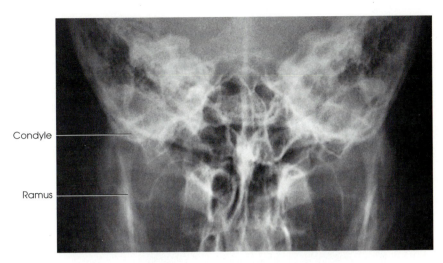

Condyle

Ramus

Fig. 21-112. AP axial TMJs, mouth closed.

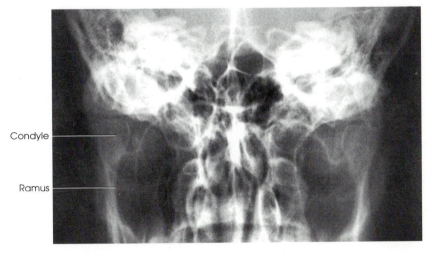

Condyle

Ramus

Fig. 21-113. AP axial TMJs, mouth open.

Temporomandibular articulations

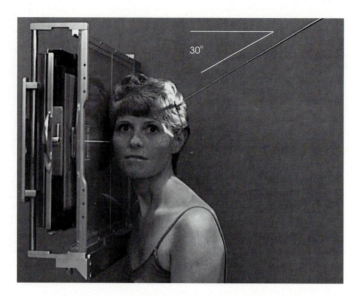

Fig. 21-114. Axiolateral TMJ with mouth closed.

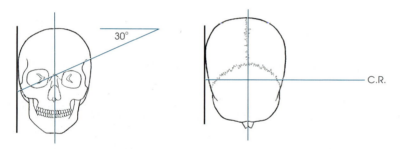

Fig. 21-115. Upright radiography.

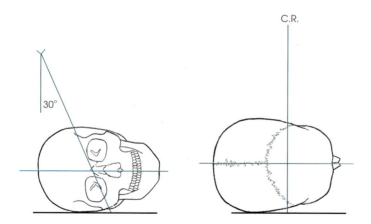

Fig. 21-116. Table radiography.

Temporomandibular Articulations

AXIOLATERAL PROJECTION
R and L positions

Film: 8 × 10 in (18 × 24 cm).

Position of patient

- Put a mark on each cheek at a point ½ inch (1.2 cm) anterior to and 1 inch (2.5 cm) inferior to the external acoustic (auditory) meatus to localize the temporomandibular joint if needed.
- Place the patient in a semiprone position or seated before a vertical grid device.

Position of part

- Center the marked localization point to the cassette and place the head in the lateral position with the affected side closest to the film.
- Adjust the patient's head so that the median sagittal plane is parallel with and the interpupillary line is perpendicular to the film plane (Figs. 21-114 to 21-116).
- Immobilize the head.
- Ask the patient to suspend respiration for the exposure.
- After making the exposure with the patient's mouth closed, change the cassette and, unless contraindicated, have the patient open the mouth wide (Fig. 21-117).
- Recheck the patient's position and make the second exposure.

Central ray

- Direct the central ray to the midpoint of the film at an angle of 25 or 30 degrees caudad. It enters the upper parietal region and passes through the TMJ closest to the film.

Structures shown

These images show the TMJ when the mouth is open and closed (Figs. 21-118 and 21-119). Both sides are examined for comparison.

□ Evaluation criteria

The following should be clearly demonstrated:

- Temporomandibular articulation lying anterior to the external acoustic (auditory) meatus.
- Condyle lying in the mandibular fossa in the closed-mouth examination.
- Condyle lying inferior to the articular tubercle in the open-mouth examination if the patient is normal and able to open the mouth wide.

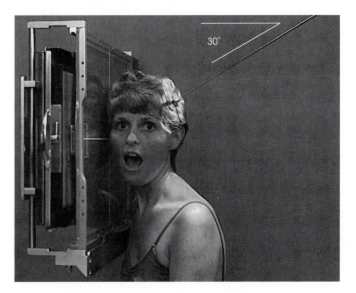

Fig. 21-117. Axiolateral TMJ with mouth open.

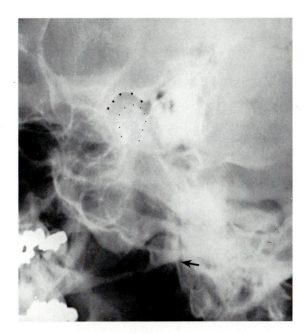

Fig. 21-118. Axiolateral TMJ, mouth closed. Mandibular condyle *(small dots)* and mandibular fossa *(large dots)* are demonstrated. Mandibular condyle of side away from film also seen *(arrow)*.

(Courtesy Lois Baird, R.T.)

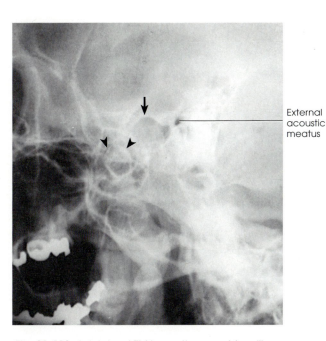

Fig. 21-119. Axiolateral TMJ, mouth open. Mandibular fossa *(arrow)* and mandibular condyle *(arrowheads)* are demonstrated.

(Courtesy Lois Baird, R.T.)

External acoustic meatus

Temporomandibular Articulations

AXIOLATERAL OBLIQUE PROJECTION
R and L positions

Film: 8 × 10 in (18 × 24 cm) crosswise.

Position of patient

- Place the patient in a semiprone position or seated before a vertical grid device.
- In examinations of the temporomandibular joints (TMJs), make one radiograph with the mouth closed and, when not contraindicated, one with the mouth open.
- Use a cassette-changing tunnel or Bucky tray so that it is not necessary to readjust the head between the two exposures.
- Examine both sides for comparison.

Position of part

- Center a point ½ inch (1.2 cm) anterior to the external acoustic (auditory) meatus to the cassette and rest the patient's cheek on the grid device.
- Rotate the median sagittal plane approximately 15 degrees toward the film.
- Do not allow the median sagittal plane to tilt; that is, the plane must be maintained at an equal 15-degree rotation.
- Adjust the flexion of the neck so that the acanthomeatal line is parallel with the transverse axis of the film (Figs. 21-120 to 21-122).
- Immobilize the head.
- Ask the patient to suspend respiration for the exposure.
- After making the exposure with the mouth closed, change the cassette and instruct the patient to open the mouth wide.
- Recheck the position of the acanthomeatal line and make the second exposure.

Central ray

- Direct the central ray 15 degrees caudad, exiting through the TMJ closest to the film.

Structures shown

The images in the open- and closed-mouth positions demonstrate the condyles and necks of the mandible. The images also show the relation between the mandibular fossa and the condyle. The open-mouth position demonstrates the mandibular fossa and the inferior and anterior excursion of the condyle. Both sides are examined for comparison (Fig. 21-123).

The closed-mouth position of this technique is employed for the demonstration of fractures of the neck and condyle of the ramus.

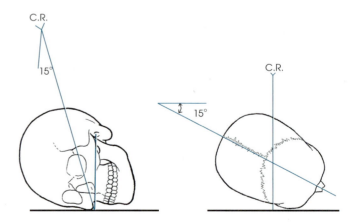

Fig. 21-121. Upright radiography.

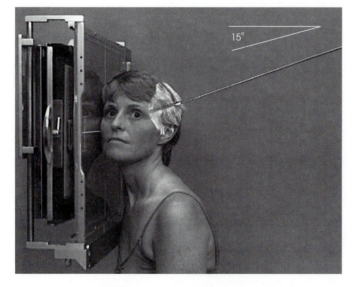

Fig. 21-120. Axiolateral oblique TMJ.

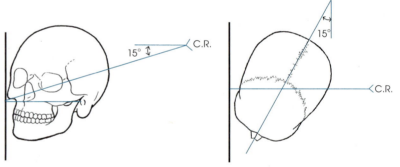

Fig. 21-122. Table radiography.

☐ Evaluation criteria

The following should be clearly demonstrated:

- Temporomandibular articulation.
- Condyle lying in the mandibular fossa in the closed-mouth examination.
- Condyle lying inferior to the articular tubercle in the open-mouth projection if the patient is normal and able to open the mouth wide.

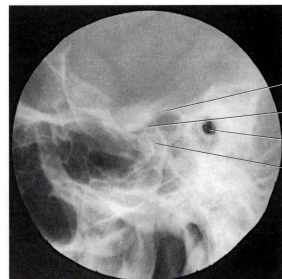

Mandibular fossa

Articular tubercle

External acoustic meatus

Condyle

A

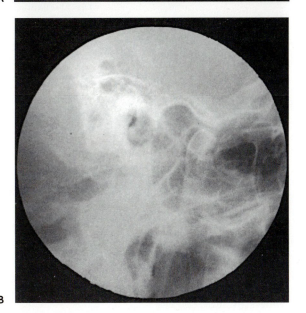

B

Fig. 21-123. Axiolateral TMJ. **A,** Mouth open, right side. **B,** Mouth open, left side on same patient showing more movement on the left side.

Temporomandibular Articulations

AXIOLATERAL OBLIQUE PROJECTION
R and L positions

The semiprone position is especially useful with patients who cannot lie in the prone position. When radiographs are taken with the patient upright, the patient may be more comfortable. Both sides are examined for comparison.

Film: 8 × 10 in (18 × 24 cm).

Position of patient

- With the patient in a recumbent or seated-upright position, turn the body toward the side being examined.
- Adjust the rotation so that the median sagittal plane of the head is approximately parallel to the film.
- Support the elevated hip and shoulder.

Position of part

- Center a point ½ inch (1.2 cm) anterior to and 1 inch (2.5 cm) superior to the external acoustic meatus to the cassette and rest the patient's head on the parietal region.
- Starting with the head in a true lateral position, tilt the head slightly so that the interpupillary line forms a 10- to 15-degree angle from the perpendicular, the chin being farther from the film.
- Turn the face away from the film so that the median sagittal plane forms a 15-degree angle from the plane of the film. This prevents superimposition of the cervical vertebrae over the area of interest (Figs. 21-124 to 21-126).
- Make the first exposure with the mouth closed and, unless contraindicated, change the cassette and make a second exposure with the mouth wide open (Fig. 21-127).
- Immobilize the head.
- Ask the patient to suspend respiration for the exposure.

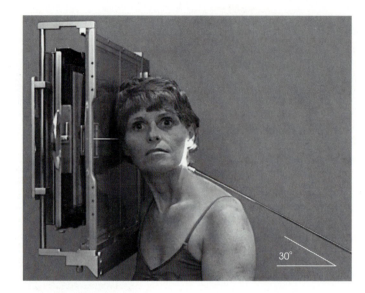

Fig. 21-124. Axiolateral oblique TMJ, mouth closed.

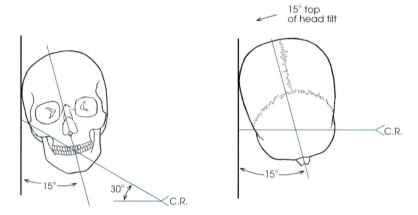

Fig. 21-125. Upright radiography.

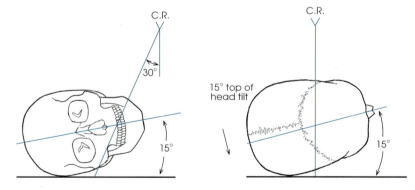

Fig. 21-126. Table radiography.

Central ray

- Direct the central ray at an angle of 30 degrees cephalad entering inferior to the angle of the mandible farthest from the film and passing through the temporomandibular joint (TMJ) closest to the film.

Structures shown

An axiolateral oblique projection of the TMJs in the closed and open positions is shown (Figs. 21-128 and 21-129). Both sides are examined for comparison.

□ Evaluation criteria

The following should be clearly demonstrated:

- No overlap of the temporomandibular region by the opposite side of the mandible.
- No superimposition of the TMJ by the cervical vertebrae.
- Condyle lying in the mandibular fossa in the closed-mouth examination.
- Condyle lying inferior to the articular tubercle in the open-mouth examination if the patient is normal and able to open the mouth wide.

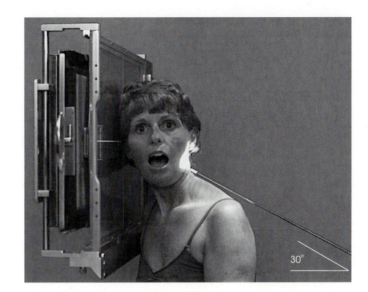

Fig. 21-127. Axiolateral oblique TMJ, mouth open.

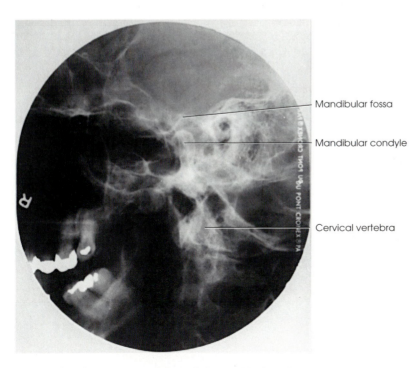

Mandibular fossa

Mandibular condyle

Cervical vertebra

Fig. 21-128. Axiolateral oblique TMJ, mouth closed.

(Courtesy Sharon A. Coffey, R.T.)

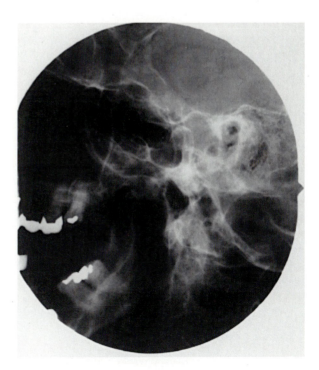

Fig. 21-129. Axiolateral oblique TMJ, mouth open.

(Courtesy Sharon A. Coffey, R.T.)

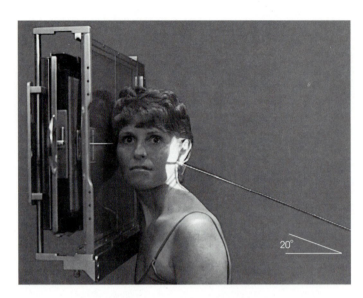

Fig. 21-130. Axiolateral TMJ, mouth closed.

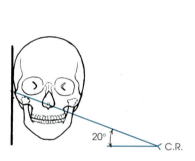

Fig. 21-131. Upright radiography.

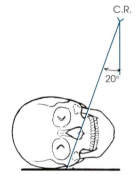

Fig. 21-132. Table radiography.

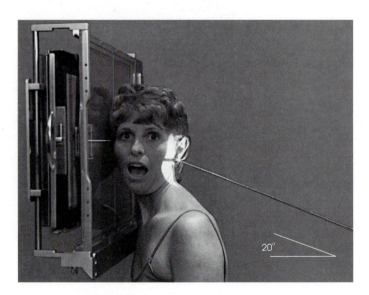

Fig. 21-133. Axiolateral TMJ, mouth open.

Temporomandibular Articulations

AXIOLATERAL PROJECTION
R and L positions
ALBERS-SCHONBERG METHOD

Film: 8 × 10 in (18 × 24 cm).

Position of patient

- Place the patient in a semiprone position or seated before a vertical grid device.

Position of part

- Center the TMJ to the midpoint of the cassette.
- Adjust the patient's head in a true lateral position so that the median sagittal plane is parallel with, and the interpupillary line is perpendicular to, the plane of the film.
- Extend the neck enough so that the infraorbitomeatal line is parallel with the transverse axis of the film (Figs. 21-130 to 21-132).
- Immobilize the head.
- Ask the patient to suspend respiration for the exposure.
- Make the first exposure with the mouth closed and, after changing the cassette, make the second exposure with the mouth wide open unless movement is contraindicated (Fig. 21-133).

Central ray

- Direct the central ray through the TMJ closest to the film at an angle of 20 degrees cephalad.

Structures shown

Axiolateral projections of the TMJs are demonstrated in the closed and open positions. Both sides are examined for comparison (Figs. 21-134 and 21-135).

☐ Evaluation criteria

The following should be clearly demonstrated:

- No overlap of the temporomandibular region by the opposite side of the mandible.
- No superimposition of the TMJ by the cervical vertebrae.
- Condyle lying in the mandibular fossa in the closed-mouth examination.
- Condyle lying below the articular tubercle in the open-mouth examination if the patient is normal and able to open the mouth wide.

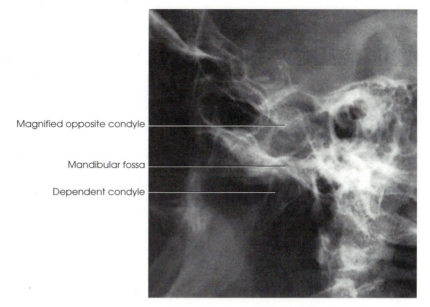

Magnified opposite condyle

Mandibular fossa

Dependent condyle

Fig. 21-134. Axiolateral TMJ, mouth closed.

(Courtesy Karen Cox, R.T.)

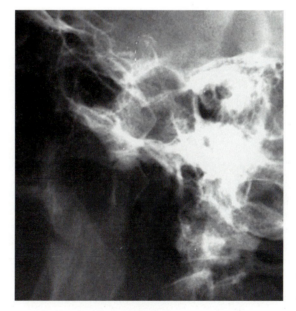

Fig. 21-135. Axiolateral TMJ, mouth open.

(Courtesy Karen Cox, R.T.)

Temporomandibular Articulations

AXIOLATERAL PROJECTION ZANELLI METHOD

Film: 8 × 10 in (18 × 24 cm) crosswise.

Position of patient

- Place the patient in a lateral position, either recumbent or seated, so that the head can be adjusted at a longitudinal angle of 30 degrees to the plane of the film.

Position of part

- Center a point ½ inch (1.2 cm) anterior to the external acoustic (auditory) meatus to the cassette and adjust the patient's head in a lateral position, resting on the parietal region.
- Using a protractor as a guide, adjust the head so that the median sagittal plane forms an angle of 30 degrees to the plane of the film. The interpupillary line will also be 30 degrees from the plane of the film.
- Rotate the chin of the affected side slightly from the lateral position to prevent superimposition of the spine over the TMJ (Figs. 21-136 to 21-138).
- Immobilize the head.
- Ask the patient to suspend respiration for the exposure.
- Make one exposure with the patient's mouth closed and, unless contraindicated, change the cassette, and make a second exposure with the mouth wide open.

Central ray

- Direct the central ray perpendicular to the midpoint of the film entering just distal to the uppermost mandibular angle farthest from the film and emerging at the TMJ closest to the film.

Structures shown

This image demonstrates an axiolateral projection of the temporomandibular joints in the open and closed positions. Both sides are examined for comparison (Figs. 21-139 and 21-140).

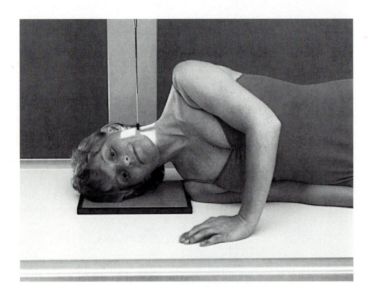

Fig. 21-136. Axiolateral TMJ, Zanelli method.

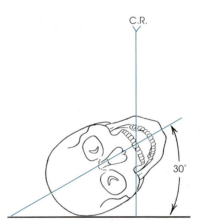

Fig. 21-137. Table radiography.

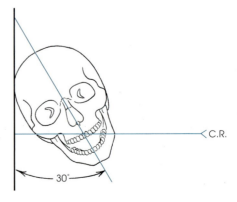

Fig. 21-138. Upright radiography.

□ Evaluation criteria

The following should be clearly demonstrated:

- No overlap of the temporomandibular region by the opposite side of the mandible.
- No superimposition of the TMJ by the cervical vertebrae.
- Condyle lying in the mandibular fossa in the closed-mouth examination.
- Condyle lying inferior to the articular tubercle in the open-mouth examination if the patient is normal and able to open the mouth wide.

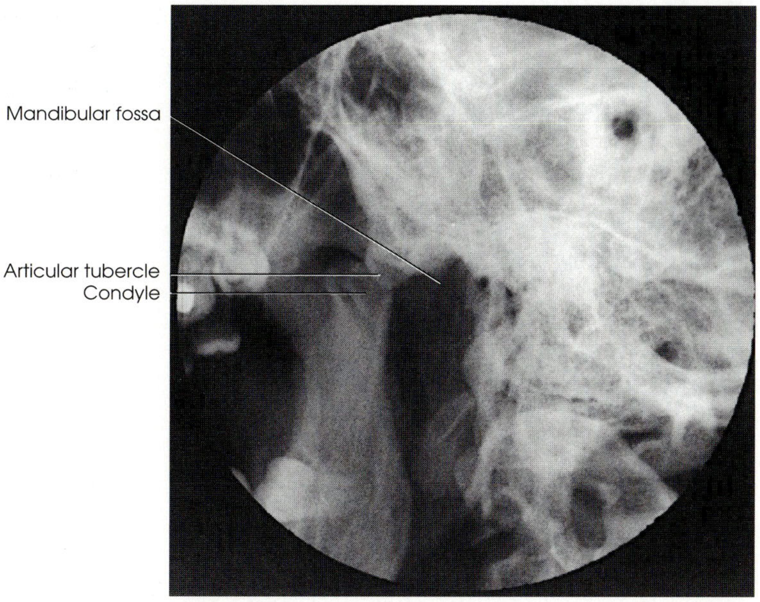

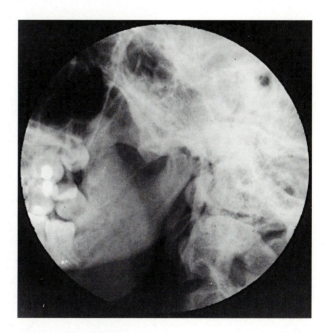

Fig. 21-139. Axiolateral TMJ, mouth open, Zanelli method.

Fig. 21-140. Axiolateral TMJ, mouth closed, Zanelli method.

Panoramic Tomography of Mandible

Panoramic tomography, pantomography, and *rotational tomography* are terms used to designate the technique employed to produce tomograms of curved surfaces. This technique of body-section radiography provides a panoramic image of the entire mandible, including the TMJ, and of both dental arches on one long, narrow film curved to conform to the shape of the patient's jaw. Only the structures near the axis of rotation are sharply defined.

Two types of equipment are available for pantomography. In the first type the patient and the film are rotated before a stationary x-ray tube. This type of machine consists of (1) a specially designed chair mounted on a turntable and (2) a second turntable to support a 4 × 10 in film enclosed in a flexible cassette. The seated and immobilized patient and the film are electronically rotated in *opposite* directions at coordinated speeds. The x-ray tube remains stationary. In one machine the exposure is interrupted in the midline.

In the second type of unit the x-ray tube and the film rotate in the *same direction* about the seated and immobilized patient (Fig. 21-141). The x-ray tube and film drum are attached to an overhead carriage that is supported by the vertical stand-base assembly. The chair of this unit is fixed to the base but can be removed to accommodate wheelchair patients. The attached head holder and radiolucent bite device center and immobilize the patient's head. A scale on the head holder indicates the jaw size. The film, 5 × 12 in or 5 × 14 in as indicated, is placed in a flexible cassette that attaches firmly to the film drum.

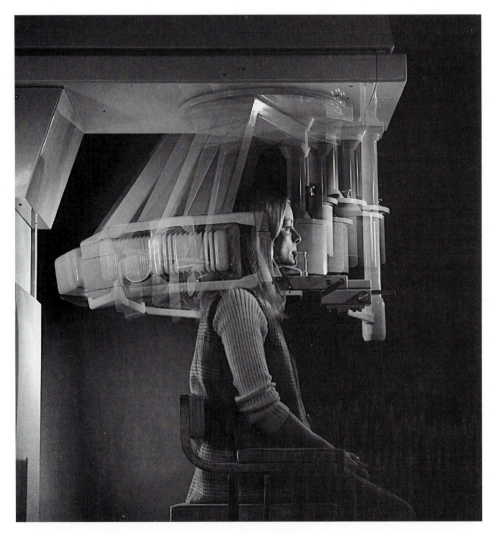

Fig. 21-141. Stroboscopic photograph of Panelipse unit showing movement of x-ray tube and film.

(Courtesy General Electric Co.)

In both types of equipment the beam of radiation is sharply collimated at the tube aperture by a lead diaphragm with a narrow vertical slit. A corresponding slit diaphragm is fixed between the patient and the film, so that the patient and the film (or the tube and the film) rotate; each narrow area of the part is recorded on the film without overlap and without fogging from scattered and secondary radiation.

The rotation time varies from 10 to 20 seconds in different makes of equipment, and this requires a correspondingly long exposure time. Because of the slit diaphragm, however, radiation exposure to the patient at each fraction of a second is restricted to the skin surface passing before the narrow vertical slit aperture.

Panoramic tomography provides a distortion-free lateral image of the entire mandible (Fig. 21-142). It also affords the most comfortable way to position patients who have sustained severe mandibular or TMJ trauma, both before and after splint wiring of the teeth. It must, of course, be supplemented with an AP, PA, or a verticosubmental projection to establish fragment position. This technique of tomography is useful for general survey studies of various dental abnormalities, but it is used to supplement rather than replace conventional periapical radiographs.

NOTE: The reader interested in a more comprehensive and general discussion of basic tomographic principles should refer to Chapter 26, Volume 3.

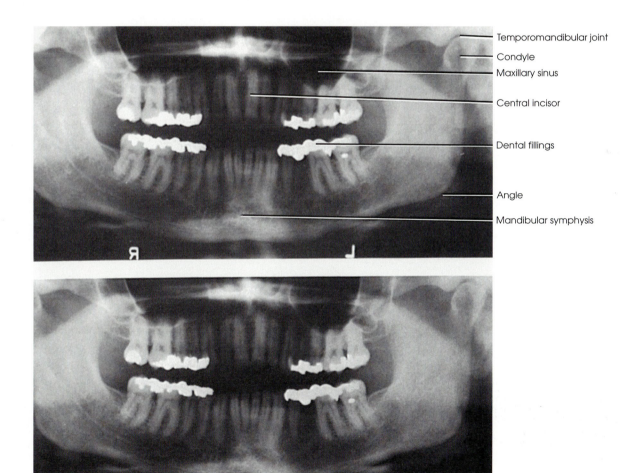

Temporomandibular joint
Condyle
Maxillary sinus
Central incisor
Dental fillings
Angle
Mandibular symphysis

Fig. 21-142. Panoramic tomogram.

Panoramic tomography of mandible

Chapter 22

PARANASAL SINUSES

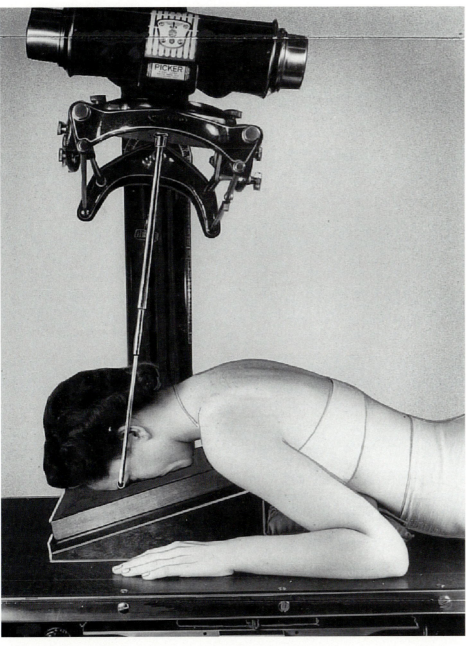

A Granger localizing device for the sella turcica and paranasal sinuses. The Granger device was used until approximately 1950.

The air-containing cavities situated in the frontal, ethmoidal, and sphenoidal bones of the cranium and in the maxillary bones of the face are called the *paranasal* (accessory nasal) *sinuses* because of their formation from the nasal mucosa and their continued communication with the nasal fossae (Figs. 22-1 and 22-2). The function of the sinuses is to provide a resonating chamber for the voice. Additionally, the air-filled cavities serve to decrease the weight of the bones of the head.

The sinuses begin to develop early in fetal life, at first appearing as small sacculations of the mucosa of the nasal meatuses and recesses. As the pouches, or sacs, grow, they gradually invade the respective bones to form the air sinuses and cells. The maxillary sinuses are usually sufficiently well developed and aerated at birth to be demonstrated radiographically. The other groups develop more slowly, so that by age six or seven years the frontal and sphenoidal sinuses (sphenoidal cells) are distinguishable from the ethmoidal air cells, which they resemble in both size and position. The ethmoidal air cells develop during puberty and the sinuses are not completely developed until the seventeenth or eighteenth year of life.

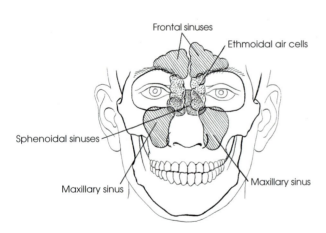

Fig. 22-1. Anterior aspect of paranasal sinuses showing lateral relation to each other and to surrounding parts.

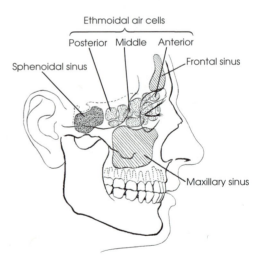

Fig. 22-2. Schematic drawing of paranasal sinuses showing anteroposterior relation to each other and surrounding parts.

The largest sinuses, the *maxillary sinuses* (antra of Highmore), are paired and are located in the body of each maxilla, just lateral to the nasal wall (Figs. 22-1 and 22-2). Although the maxillary sinuses (antra) appear rectangular in the lateral image, they are approximately pyramidal in shape and have only three walls. The apices are directed inferiorly and laterally. The maxillary sinuses vary considerably in size and shape but are usually symmetric. In the adult, the maxillary sinus is approximately 3.5 cm high and between 2.5 and 3 cm wide. The sinus (antrum) is often divided into subcompartments by partial septa, and occasionally it is divided into two sinuses by a complete septum. The sinus (antral) floor usually presents several elevations that correspond to the roots of the subjacent teeth. The maxillary sinuses communicate with the middle nasal meatuses.

The *frontal sinuses,* the second largest sinuses, are paired, pyramidal in shape, and normally located between the tables of the vertical plate of the frontal bone (Figs. 22-1 and 22-2). The frontal sinuses vary greatly in size and form, ranging from complete absence of one or both to as large as approximately 2 to 2.5 cm in either the vertical or lateral dimension. They often extend beyond the frontal region of the bone, most frequently into the orbital plates. The *intersinus septum* is usually deviated from the midline, with the result that the frontal sinuses are rarely symmetric. Because multiple septa are sometimes present, they also vary in number. The sinus walls are usually irregularly marked by incomplete septa, which divide them into pockets, or subcompartments. The frontal sinuses drain into the middle nasal meatuses as do the maxillary sinuses.

The two *ethmoidal labyrinths* (ethmoidal capsules) are located within the lateral masses of the ethmoid bone. The labyrinths are composed of a varying number of air cells. The cells of each capsule are divided into three main groups and are called, in accordance with their position, the anterior, the middle, and the posterior ethmoidal cells (Figs. 22-1 and 22-2). Extralabyrinthine cells are usually present and are described according to their location. The anterior and middle ethmoidal cells vary in number from two to eight, and each group opens into the middle nasal meatus. The posterior cells vary in number from two to six or more and drain into the superior nasal meatus.

The *sphenoidal sinuses* are normally paired and occupy the body of the sphenoid bone (Figs. 22-1 and 22-2). Anatomists state that there is frequently only one but never more than two sphenoidal sinuses. They vary considerably in size and shape, are usually asymmetric, and often present subcompartments formed by ridges, or incomplete septa, projecting from their walls and floor. The sphenoidal sinuses lie immediately below the sella turcica and extend between the dorsum sellae and the posterior ethmoidal air cells. Each sphenoidal sinus opens into the corresponding nasal fossa, the sphenoethmoid recess of the space above the superior ethmoidal concha (turbinate).

The paranasal sinuses vary not only in size and form but also in position. The cells of one group frequently encroach on and resemble those of another group. This characteristic of the sinuses, together with their proximity to the vital intracranial organs, makes accurate radiographic demonstration of their anatomic structure of prime importance. The head must be carefully placed in a sufficient number of positions so that the projections of each group of cavities are as free as possible of superimposed bony structures. The radiographs must be of such quality that the cells of several groups of sinuses can be distinguished, as well as their relationship to the surrounding structures.

Unless sinus radiographs are almost perfect technically, they are of little diagnostic value. For this reason a precise technical procedure is necessary in radiography of the paranasal sinuses. A small focal spot and clean intensifying screens that have perfect contact are the first requisites. The radiographic contrast must similarly distinguish the sinuses from the surrounding structures. The head must be carefully positioned and rigidly immobilized, and respiration must be suspended for the exposures.

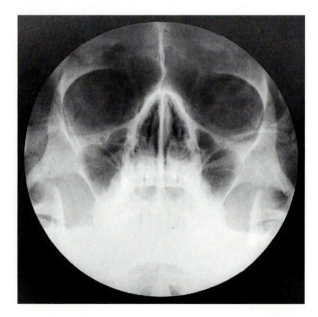

Fig. 22-3. Correctly exposed.

There is probably no region of the body where film density is more critical or more misleading than in sinus radiography (Figs. 22-3 to 22-5). Overpenetration diminishes or completely obliterates existing pathologic conditions, and underpenetration can simulate pathologic conditions that do not exist. A good criterion for properly exposed radiographs is the density of the orbital region; normally aerated, nonpathologic sinuses cast identical density. The correct density of the orbit should be carefully studied in order to accurately judge the density.

Depending on the technique employed, the millampere-second (mAs) and kilovoltage factors should be balanced so that the soft tissue structures, as well as the bony structures, are demonstrated. Although good contrast is desirable, high contrast can result in the inability to visualize soft tissue areas.

Whenever possible, the paranasal sinuses should be radiographed with the patient in the upright position (1) to demonstrate the presence or absence of fluid and (2) to differentiate between fluid and other pathologic conditions. The value of the upright position in sinus examinations was pointed out by Cross[1] and Flecker.[2]

[1]Cross KS: Radiography of the nasal accessory sinuses, Med J Aust 14:569-571, 1927.
[2]Flecker H: Roentgenograms of the antrum (letter), AJR 20:56-57, 1928.

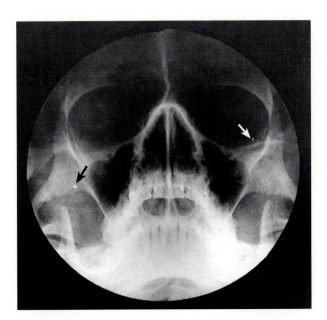

Fig. 22-4. Overexposed sinuses demonstrating two artifacts caused by dirt on screens (arrows).

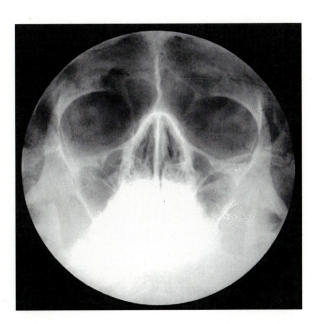

Fig. 22-5. Underexposed sinuses.

The effect of both body position and central ray angulation is clearly demonstrated in the accompanying radiographs of a coconut held in position by head clamps. Fig. 22-6 shows a sharply defined fluid level. This coconut was placed in the vertical position and the central ray directed horizontal. Fig. 22-7 was taken with the coconut still in the vertical position but with the central ray directed upward at an angle of 45 degrees to demonstrate the gradual fading of the fluid line when the central ray is not horizontal. This effect is much more pronounced in actual practice because of structural irregularities. Fig. 22-8 was made with the coconut in the horizontal position and the central ray directed vertically; the resultant film shows a homogeneous density throughout the cavity of the coconut, with no evidence of a fluid level.

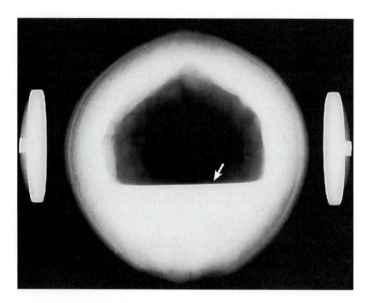

Fig. 22-6. Coconut, vertical position, central ray horizontal, demonstrating air-fluid level *(arrow)*.

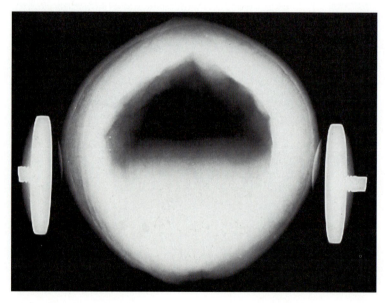

Fig. 22-7. Coconut, vertical position, central ray angled 45 degrees upward. Note fluid level not as sharp.

Exudate contained in the sinuses is not fluid in the usual sense of the word but is commonly a heavy, semigelatinous material. The exudate, rather than flowing freely, clings to the walls of the cavity and takes several minutes, depending on its viscosity, to shift position. For this reason, when the body position is changed, and when the neck is flexed or extended to position the head for special projections, *several minutes should be allowed* for the exudate to gravitate to the desired location before the exposure is made.

Although there are numerous sinus projections, each serving a special purpose, many are employed only when required to demonstrate a specific lesion. The consensus is that five of the standard projections adequately demonstrate all of the paranasal sinuses on a majority of patients, as discussed on the following pages. The following steps are observed in preparing for all of the projections:

- Use a suitable protractor to check and adjust the position of the head to ensure accurate positioning of the patient.
- Have the patient remove dentures, hairpins, and ornaments such as earrings and necklaces before proceeding with the examination.
- Since the patient's face is in contact with the film holder or cassette for many of the radiographs, clean these prior to positioning the patient.

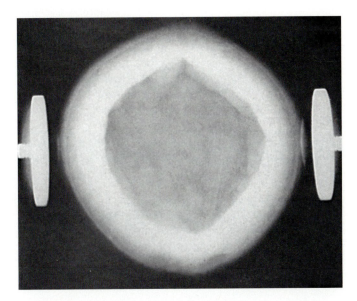

Fig. 22-8. Coconut, horizontal position, central ray vertical. Note evidence of fluid level.

(Courtesy Dr. Ramsay Spillman.)

Radiation Protection

Protection of the patient from unnecessary radiation is a professional responsibility of the radiographer. (See Chapter 1, Volume 1 for specific guidelines.) In this chapter, radiation shielding of the patient is not specified or illustrated because the professional community and the federal government have reported that placing a lead shield over the patient's pelvis does not significantly reduce the gonadal exposure during radiography of the paranasal sinuses.

The *pediatric patient,* however, should be protected by radiation shielding of the thyroid and thymus glands, and gonads. The protective lead shielding used to cover the thyroid and thymus glands can also assist in immobilizing the pediatric patient.

The most effective way to protect the patient from unnecessary radiation is to restrict the radiation beam by using *proper collimation.* Taking care to ensure that the patient is properly instructed and immobilized also reduces the chance of having to repeat the procedure, further limiting the radiation exposure received by the patient.

Paranasal Sinuses

LATERAL PROJECTION
R or L position

Film: 8 × 10 in (18 × 24 cm).

Position of patient

- Seat the patient before a vertical grid device with the body placed in the RAO or LAO position so that the head can be adjusted in a true lateral position.

Position of part

- Center the cassette approximately ½ to 1 inch (1.2 to 2.5 cm) posterior to the outer canthus closest to the film.
- Rest the patient's parietal eminence on the vertical grid device and adjust the head in a true lateral position. The median sagittal plane is parallel with the plane of the film, and the interpupillary line is perpendicular to the plane of the film. Only an exact lateral projection can be used for preoperative measurements (Fig. 22-9).
- Immobilize the head.
- Ask the patient to suspend respiration for the exposure.

Central ray

- Direct the central ray perpendicular entering the patient's head ½ to 1 inch (1.2 to 2.5 cm) posterior to the outer canthus farthest from the film.

Structures shown

A lateral projection shows the anteroposterior and superoinferior dimensions of the paranasal sinuses, their relationship to surrounding structures, and the thickness of the outer table of the frontal bone (Fig. 22-10).

When the lateral projection is to be used for preoperative measurements, it should be made at a 72-inch source–to–image receptor distance to minimize magnification and distortion.

☐ Evaluation criteria

The following should be clearly demonstrated:

- All four sinus groups; sphenoidal sinus is of primary importance.
- No rotation of sella turcica.
- Superimposed orbital roofs.
- Superimposed mandibular rami.
- Sinuses clearly visible.
- Close beam restriction of the sinus area.

NOTE: If the patient is unable to assume the upright body position, a lateral projection can be obtained using a horizontal x-ray beam and a cross-lateral modification.

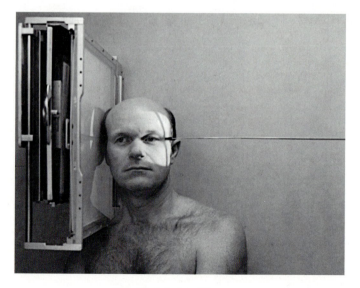

Fig. 22-9. Lateral sinuses.

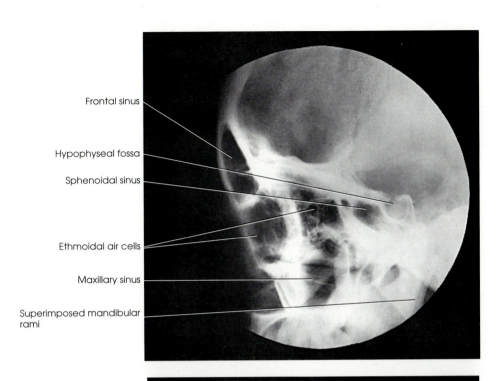

Frontal sinus

Hypophyseal fossa

Sphenoidal sinus

Ethmoidal air cells

Maxillary sinus

Superimposed mandibular
rami

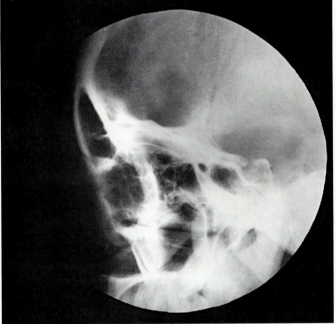

Fig. 22-10. Lateral sinuses.

Frontal and Anterior Ethmoidal Sinuses

PA AXIAL PROJECTION
CALDWELL METHOD

The original method proposed by Caldwell used the glabellomeatal line, an imaginary line extending from the center of the glabella to the external acoustic (auditory) meatus, for the adjustment of the head. The angle between this localization line and the plane of the film depends on the shape of the face and varies from one patient to the next.

Caldwell's modified method uses the orbitomeatal line, which allows the use of a specific central ray angle of 15 degrees caudad to the orbitomeatal line.

Since the glabellomeatal and orbitomeatal lines are separated by an angle, open anteriorly, of 8 degrees, the same projection is obtained when the central ray is angled (1) 23 degrees to the glabellomeatal line or (2) 15 degrees to the orbitomeatal line. The two images are thus identical.

Since sinus images should always be obtained with the patient in the upright body position using a horizontal central ray, the Caldwell method is easily modified when using a head unit or other vertical grid device capable of angular adjustment. For the modification, all of the anatomic landmarks and localization planes remain unchanged.

Film: 8×10 in (18×24 cm).

Position of patient

- With the patient in the preferred upright position, center the median sagittal plane of the body to the midline of the grid.
- Place the patient's arms in a comfortable position and adjust the shoulders to lie in the same transverse plane.

Horizontal central ray technique
Position of part

- Before positioning the patient, tilt the vertical grid device in, so that an angle of 15 degrees is obtained (Fig. 22-11). The central ray is directed horizontal; the 15-degree relationship between the film and radiographic tube remains unchanged.
- With the patient's neck slightly extended, rest the nose and forehead on the vertical grid device and center the nasion to the cassette.
- Adjust the median sagittal plane and orbitomeatal line perpendicular to the plane of the film.
- Immobilize the head.
- Ask the patient to suspend respiration for the exposure.

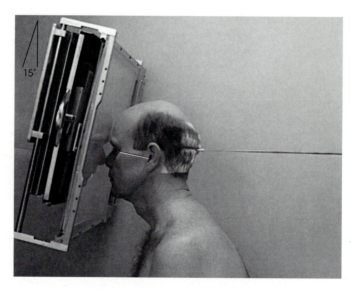

Fig. 22-11. PA axial sinuses with horizontal central ray.

Angled central ray technique
Position of part

When the angulation of the vertical grid device cannot be adjusted, the patient may be positioned as follows. (It must be realized that in this technique, the central ray is not horizontal, so air-fluid interfaces will not exhibit a sharp border.)
- Center the nasion to the cassette.
- Rest the patient's forehead and nose on the vertical grid device and adjust both the median sagittal plane and the orbitomeatal line perpendicular to the plane of the film (Fig. 22-12).

- Immobilize the head.
- Ask the patient to suspend respiration for the exposure.

Central ray

- Direct the central ray to the nasion at an angle of 15 degrees caudad to the orbitomeatal line, which is also 15 degrees to the plane of the film.

Structures shown

Both techniques demonstrate the frontal sinuses, lying superior to the frontonasal suture; the anterior ethmoidal air cells, lying on each side of the nasal fossae and immediately inferior to the frontal sinuses; and the sphenoidal sinuses, projected through the nasal fossae just inferior to or between the ethmoidal air cells (Fig. 22-13). The dense petrosae extend from the inferior third of the orbit inferiorly to obscure the superior third of the maxillary sinus. This projection is used primarily for the demonstration of the frontal sinuses and the anterior ethmoidal air cells.

□ Evaluation criteria

The following should be clearly demonstrated:
- Distance between the lateral border of the skull and the lateral border of the orbits equal.
- Petrous ridge symmetric on both sides.
- Petrous ridge lying in the lower third of the orbit.
- Frontal sinuses lying above the frontonasal suture and the anterior ethmoidal air cells above the petrous ridges.
- Frontal and anterior ethmoidal air cells.
- Close beam restriction of the sinus area.

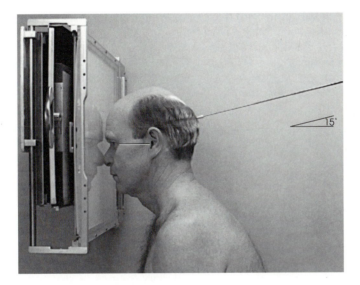

Fig. 22-12. PA axial sinuses with angled central ray.

Frontal sinus

Frontonasal suture

Ethmoidal air cells

Petrous ridge

Sphenoidal air cells

Maxillary sinus

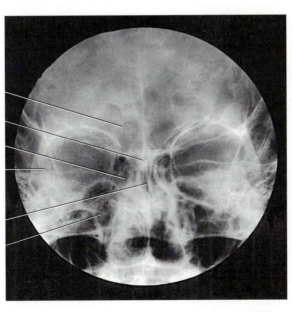
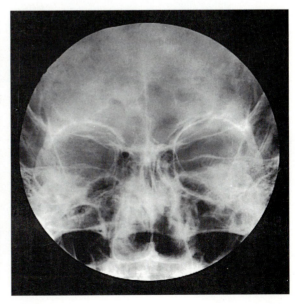

Fig. 22-13. PA axial sinuses.

Maxillary Sinuses

 PARIETOACANTHIAL PROJECTION
WATERS METHOD
OPEN-MOUTH MODIFICATION

Film: 8 × 10 in (18 × 24 cm).

For the Waters[1] method the aim is to extend the patient's neck just enough to place the dense petrosae immediately below the maxillary sinus (antral) floors. When the neck is extended too little, the petrosa are projected over the inferior portions of the maxillary sinuses and thus obscure any underlying pathologic conditions (Fig. 22-16). When the neck is extended too much, the maxillary sinuses are foreshortened, which also results in failure to demonstrate the antral floors.

---

[1]Waters CA: A modification of the occipitofrontal position in the roentgen examination of the accessory nasal sinuses, Arch Radiol Ther 20:15-17, 1915.

Waters specified that the nose should be 1 to 1.5 cm from the film, depending on the shape of the face. The concave-shaped face requires a greater distance than the convex-shaped face. Mahoney[2] found that the petrosa can be correctly placed in a majority of subjects by adjusting the orbitomeatal line at an angle of 37 degrees to the plane of the film. A second advantage of the latter method is that compensations for atypical patients can be calculated from an exact angle.

Position of patient

- Place the patient in an upright position, facing the vertical grid device.
- Center the median sagittal plane of the body to the midline of the grid device.
- Place the arms in a comfortable position and adjust the shoulders to lie in the same transverse plane.

---

[2]Mahoney HO: Head and sinus positions, Xray Techn 1:89-91, 1930.

Position of part

- Extend the patient's neck to approximately the correct position and then center the cassette to the acanthion.
- Rest the chin on the vertical grid device and adjust it so that the median sagittal plane is perpendicular to the plane of the film.
- Using a protractor as a guide, adjust the head so that the orbitomeatal line forms an angle of 37 degrees from the plane of the film. As a positioning check for the average shaped skull, the mentomeatal line is approximately perpendicular to the film plane (Figs. 22-14 to 22-16).
- For the *open-mouth modification,* have the patient first fully open the mouth, then position as described above (Fig. 22-17).
- Immobilize the head.
- Ask the patient to suspend respiration for the exposure.

Central ray

- Direct the central ray perpendicular to the film, entering the vertex and emerging at the acanthion for the original Waters method. For the open-mouth modification, the central ray passes through the sphenoidal sinuses and exits the open mouth of the patient.

Structures shown

A parietoacanthial projection of the maxillary sinuses is demonstrated with the petrous ridges lying inferior to the floor of the maxillary sinus. The frontal and ethmoidal air cells are distorted in this image, and the sphenoidal sinuses are not shown (Fig. 22-18). The sphenoidal sinuses are demonstrated when projected through the open mouth of the patient, as seen in Fig. 22-19. For bilateral demonstration of the posterosuperior wall of the maxillary sinuses, see the PA skull projection described in Chapter 20, page 242.

The Waters method is also used to demonstrate the rotundum foramina, the images of which are seen, one on each side, just inferior to the medial aspect of the orbital floor and superior to the roof of the maxillary sinuses.

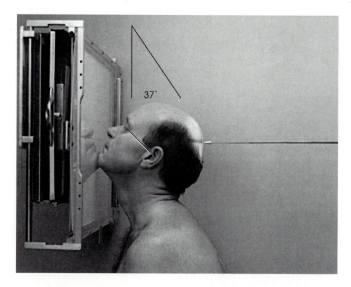

Fig. 22-14. Parietoacanthial sinuses, Waters method.

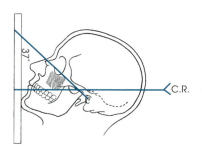

Fig. 22-15. Proper positioning (petrous ridges projected below maxillary sinuses).

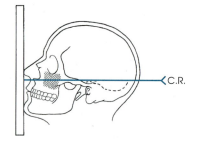

Fig. 22-16. Improper positioning (petrous ridges superimposed on maxillary sinuses).

□Evaluation criteria

The following should be clearly demonstrated:

- Petrous pyramids lying immediately inferior to the floor of the maxillary sinuses.
- Distance between the lateral border of the skull and the lateral border of the orbit equal on both sides.
- Orbits and maxillary sinuses symmetric on each side.
- Maxillary sinuses.
- Close beam restriction of the sinus area.
- Sphenoidal sinuses projected through the open mouth if modification is performed.

NOTE: In order to determine the cause of questionable shadows—those that resemble a fluid level—the head is tilted laterally 30 to 40 degrees. The patient is seated upright for these "tilting projections," and care must be used to maintain the correct object-to-image receptor relationship. Horizontal fluid-level studies are sometimes requested. With the patient laterally recumbent, the head is elevated on a suitable support and adjusted in an exact lateral position. The neck is flexed for a Caldwell method, or it is extended for a Waters method. The cassette is placed vertically, and the central ray is directed horizontally.

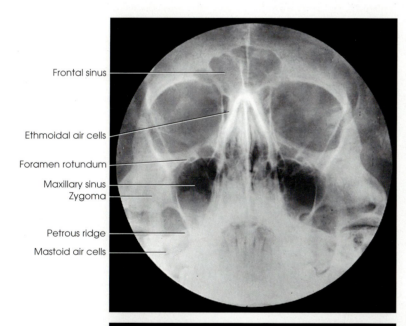

Frontal sinus

Ethmoidal air cells

Foramen rotundum

Maxillary sinus
Zygoma

Petrous ridge

Mastoid air cells

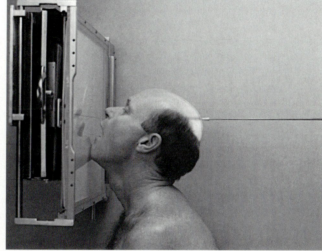

Fig. 22-17. Open mouth parietoacanthial sinuses, Waters method.

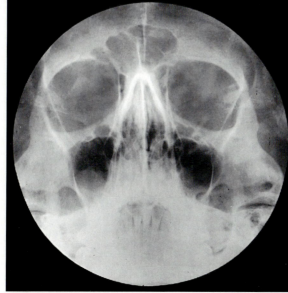

Fig. 22-18. Parietoacanthial sinuses, Waters method.

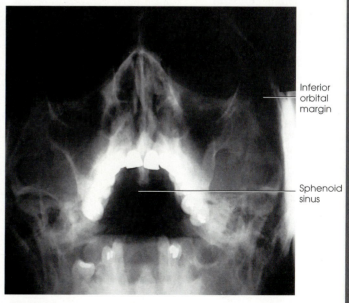

Inferior orbital margin

Sphenoid sinus

Fig. 22-19. Open-mouth parietoacanthial sinuses, Waters method.

(Courtesy Judy McLaughlin, R.T.)

Ethmoidal and Sphenoidal Sinuses

⬥ SUBMENTOVERTICAL PROJECTION

Film: 8 × 10 in (18 × 24 cm).

Position of patient

The success of the submentovertical (SMV) projection depends on (1) placing the infraorbitomeatal line as nearly as possible parallel with the plane of the film and (2) directing the central ray perpendicular to the infraorbitomeatal line.

The upright position is recommended for all paranasal sinus radiographs and is also more comfortable for the patient. The following steps are observed:

- Use a chair that supports the back to obtain greater freedom in positioning the body to place the infraorbitomeatal line parallel with the film.
- Seat the patient far enough away from the vertical grid device so that the head can be adjusted (Fig. 22-20, *A*).
- If possible, examine patients with short necks and hypersthenic patients in the upright position. An advantage of a head unit is that it can be angled from the vertical position (Fig. 22-20, *B*).

When the patient is placed in the supine position, the following steps are observed:

- Elevate the torso on firm pillows or a suitable pad to allow the head to rest on the vertex, with the neck in complete extension.
- Flex the patient's knees to relax the abdominal muscles.
- Center the median sagittal plane of the body to the midline of the grid.
- Place the arms in a comfortable position and adjust the shoulders to lie in the same transverse plane.
- The supine position places considerable strain on the neck; do not keep the patient in the final adjustment longer than absolutely necessary.

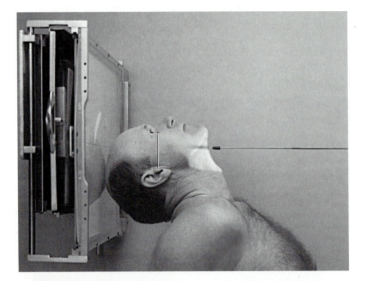

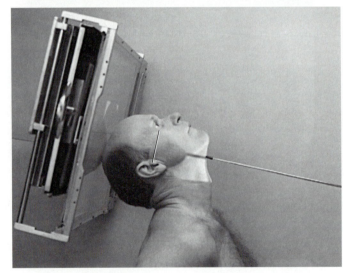

Fig. 22-20. Submentovertical sinuses.

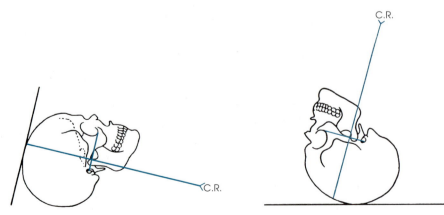

Fig. 22-21. Upright radiography.

Fig. 22-22. Table radiography.

Position of part

- With the median sagittal plane of the body centered to the midline of the vertical grid device, extend the patient's neck as far as possible and rest the head on its vertex.
- Adjust the head so that the median sagittal plane is perpendicular to the midline of the film.
- Adjust the tube so that the central ray is perpendicular to the infraorbitomeatal line and center it to the sella turcica (Figs. 22-20 to 22-22).
- In the absence of a head clamp, if needed, place a suitably backed strip of adhesive tape across the tip of the chin and anchor it to the sides of the radiographic unit. Do not put adhesive surface directly on patient's skin.
- Ask the patient to suspend respiration for the exposure.

Central ray

- Direct the central ray perpendicular to the infraorbitomeatal line through the sella turcica. The central ray enters the midline of the base of the skull approximately ¾ inch (1.9 cm) anterior to the level of the external acoustic (auditory) meatus.

Structures shown

The SMV projection for the sinuses demonstrates a symmetric image of the anterior portion of the base of the skull. The sphenoidal sinus and the ethmoidal air cells are demonstrated (Fig. 22-23).

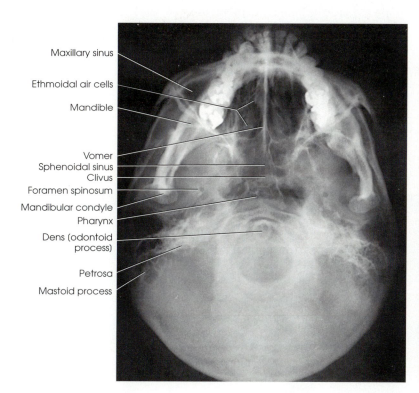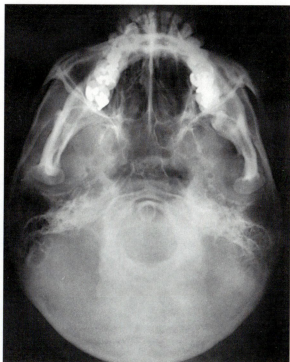

Maxillary sinus
Ethmoidal air cells
Mandible
Vomer
Sphenoidal sinus
Clivus
Foramen spinosum
Mandibular condyle
Pharynx
Dens (odontoid process)
Petrosa
Mastoid process

Fig. 22-23. Submentovertical sinuses.

Ethmoidal and sphenoidal sinuses

385

Ethmoidal, Sphenoidal, and Maxillary Sinuses

 ### PA PROJECTIONS

The patient's head is adjusted for a PA projection for the following three projections. The structures shown depend on the direction of the central ray. Each projection will be considered separately, however, to eliminate the need to refer back to previous descriptions.

Film: 8 × 10 in (18 × 24 cm).

Position of patient

- Place the patient in the seated-upright or the prone position; the former position is preferable, particularly when examining the maxillary sinuses.
- Center the median sagittal plane of the body to the midline of the grid device.
- Place the arms in a comfortable position and adjust the shoulders to lie in the same transverse plane.

Posterior ethmoid sinuses
Position of part

- Center the nasion to the cassette, rest the patient's forehead and nose on the grid device, and adjust the head so that the median sagittal plane is perpendicular to the plane of the film.
- Adjust the flexion of the neck so that the orbitomeatal line is perpendicular to the plane of the film (Fig. 22-24).

- Immobilize the head.
- Ask the patient to suspend respiration for the exposure.

Central ray

- Direct the central ray perpendicular to the film entering the occipital region and emerging at the nasion.

Structures shown

The posterior ethmoidal air cells are projected superior to the anterior air cells (Fig. 22-25).

The following should be clearly demonstrated:
- Posterior ethmoidal air cells just inferior to the cranial bones.
- Distance between the lateral border of the skull and the median sagittal plane equal on both sides.
- Petrous ridges symmetric on each side.
- Close beam restriction of the sinus area.

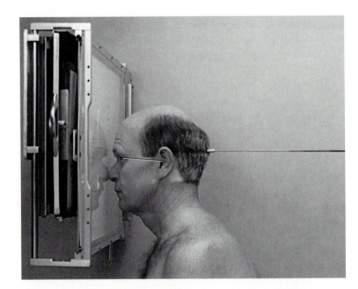

Fig. 22-24. PA for posterior ethmoidal air cells.

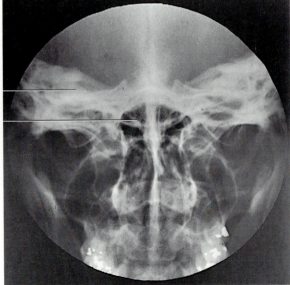
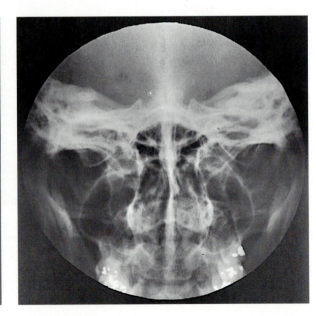

Petrous ridge

Ethmoidal air cells

Fig. 22-25. PA posterior ethmoidal air cells: perpendicular central ray.

Sphenoidal sinuses

Position of part

- Center the glabella to the cassette and rest the patient's forehead and nose on the grid device.
- Adjust the head so that the median sagittal plane is perpendicular to the film.
- Adjust the flexion of the neck so that the orbitomeatal line is perpendicular to the film.
- Immobilize the head.
- Ask the patient to suspend respiration for the exposure.

Central ray

- Direct the central ray to the midpoint of the film at an angle of 10 degrees cephalad passing through the sphenoidal sinuses and emerging at the glabella. (If possible, tilt the head unit so that an angle of 10 degrees, open posterosuperiorly, is obtained, and direct the central ray horizontally.)

Structures shown

The sphenoidal sinuses are projected through the frontal bone (Fig. 22-26). Their images lie superior to those of the frontal sinuses.

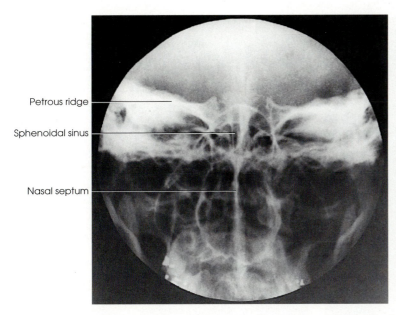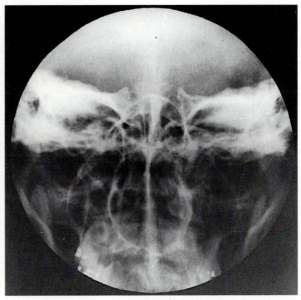

Petrous ridge

Sphenoidal sinus

Nasal septum

Fig. 22-26. PA sphenoidal sinuses: central ray angulation of 10 degrees, cephalad.

Ethmoidal, sphenoidal, and maxillary sinuses

387

Maxillary sinuses
Position of part

- Center the cassette to the median sagittal plane of the head at a point midway between the infraorbital margins and the anterior nasal spine.
- Rest the patient's forehead and nose on the grid device and adjust the head so that the median sagittal plane is perpendicular to the film.
- Adjust the flexion of the neck so that the orbitomeatal line is perpendicular to the film.
- Immobilize the head.
- Ask the patient to suspend respiration for the exposure.

Central ray

- Direct the central ray perpendicular to the film entering the median sagittal plane midway between the infraorbital margins and the anterior nasal spine, through the midregion of the maxillary sinuses.

Structures shown

The maxillary sinuses are projected inferior to the base of the cranium (Fig. 22-27). The posterior ethmoidal air cells are well demonstrated in this projection.

□ Evaluation criteria

The following should be clearly demonstrated:

- Maxillary sinuses below the petrous ridges.
- Distance between the lateral border of the skull and the median sagittal plane equal on both sides.
- Petrous ridges symmetric on each side.
- Close beam restriction of the sinus area.

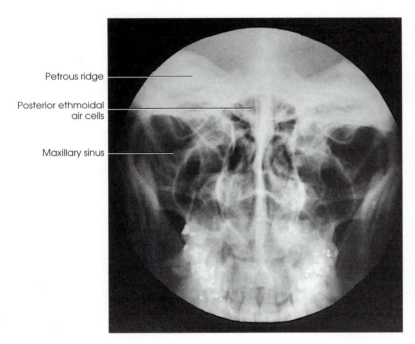
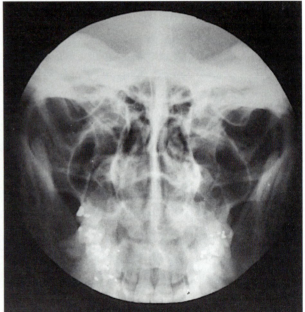

Petrous ridge

Posterior ethmoidal air cells

Maxillary sinus

Fig. 22-27. PA maxillary sinuses: perpendicular central ray.

Sphenoidal Sinuses

VERTICOSUBMENTAL PROJECTION
SCHÜLLER METHOD

The verticosubmental (VSM) projection is also employed to obtain an axial projection of the paranasal sinuses.

Film: 8 × 10 in (18 × 24 cm).

Position of patient

- Place the patient in the seated-upright position or in a prone position that will permit extension of the neck over a horizontally placed cassette.
- Place the arms in a comfortable position and adjust the shoulders to lie in the same transverse plane.

Position of part

- Elevate the side of the cassette adjacent to the patient on a sponge or a small sandbag and adjust the inclination so that the throat can be comfortably extended across the cassette at the minimum object-to-image-receptor distance.
- With the patient's neck fully extended, center the film to the throat at a point midway between the mastoid tips.
- Adjust the head so that the median sagittal plane is perpendicular to the film (Fig. 22-28).
- Immobilize the head.
- Ask the patient to suspend respiration for the exposure.

Central ray

- With the central ray perpendicular to the infraorbitomeatal line, direct it to the intersection of the median sagittal plane and a coronal plane passing through the sella turcica and the angles of the mandible.

Structures shown

The VSM projection shows an axial image primarily of the sphenoidal sinuses and also the posterior ethmoidal air cells, the maxillary sinuses, and the nasal fossae (Fig. 22-29).

The following should be clearly demonstrated:

- Sphenoidal sinuses with the posterior ethmoidal air cells visible just below the mentum of the mandible. (In the submentovertical projection the mandible should be elevated further so that the anterior ethmoidal air cells are not obscured.)
- Distance from the lateral border of the skull to the mandibular condyles equal on both sides.
- Mandible symmetric on both sides.
- Close beam restriction of the sinus area.

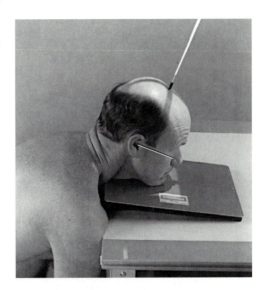

Fig. 22-28. Verticosubmental sinuses.

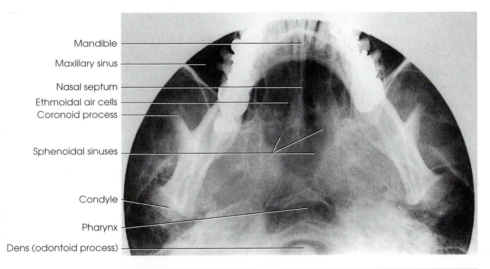

Mandible
Maxillary sinus
Nasal septum
Ethmoidal air cells
Coronoid process
Sphenoidal sinuses
Condyle
Pharynx
Dens (odontoid process)

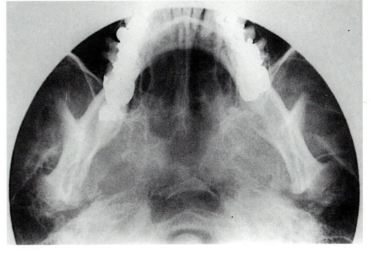

Fig. 22-29. Verticosubmental sinuses.

Sphenoidal sinuses

389

Sphenoidal Sinuses

PA AXIAL PROJECTION (TRANSORAL)
PIRIE METHOD

Film: 8 × 10 in (18 × 24 cm).

Position of patient

- Place the patient in the prone position or preferably seated before a vertical grid device.
- Place the arms in a comfortable position and adjust the shoulders to lie in the same transverse plane.

Position of part

- Clean the grid device or film holder with a disinfectant before use for either body position.
- For the upright position, place the cassette in the vertical holder and adjust the center of the film to the level of the patient's mouth.
- For the prone position, place the cassette on a 15 degree caudally inclined angle sponge and adjust it under the face.
- This position is not comfortable, so do not keep the patient in it longer than is absolutely necessary.
- After centering the film and determining the angulation of the central ray, allow the patient to rest for a few minutes before adjusting the head in the final position.
- Make the final positioning adjustment with the patient's nose and chin firmly resting on the grid device with the mouth wide open and centered on the film.
- Adjust the head so that the median sagittal plane is perpendicular to the film (Fig. 22-30).
- Respiration: Immobilize the head and instruct the patient to phonate "ah-h-h" softly during the exposure, to immobilize the tongue in the floor of the mouth.

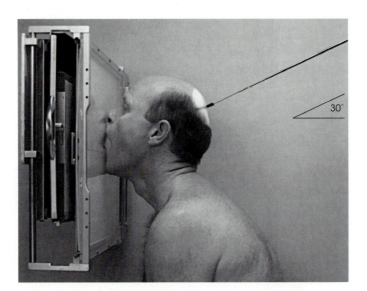

Fig. 22-30. PA axial (transoral) sinuses, Pirie method.

Central ray

- Direct the central ray along a line extending from the sella turcica (¾ inch anterior and ¾ inch superior to external acoustic meatus) to the center of the open mouth. The caudal angulation of the central ray depends on the shape of the face. The angulation of the central ray shown in Fig. 22-30 is 30 degrees caudally.

Structures shown

An axial projection of the sphenoidal sinuses is projected through the open mouth. The maxillary sinuses and the nasal fossae are also demonstrated (Fig. 22-31).

□ Evaluation criteria

The following should be clearly demonstrated:

- Sphenoidal sinuses through the open mouth without overlap from the upper dental arch.
- No superimposition of the sphenoidal sinuses by the tongue.
- Mouth open very wide.
- Distance from the lateral border of the skull to the molars equal on both sides.
- Close beam restriction of the sinus area.

NOTE: A similar image can be obtained when the patient is positioned for the parietoacanthial projection (Waters' method) described on p. 382 with the patient's mouth open wide.

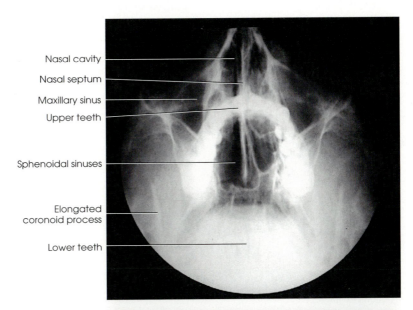

Nasal cavity
Nasal septum
Maxillary sinus
Upper teeth

Sphenoidal sinuses

Elongated coronoid process

Lower teeth

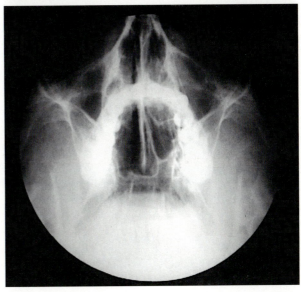

Fig. 22-31. PA axial (transoral) sinuses, Pirie method.

Ethmoidal, Frontal, and Sphenoidal Sinuses
PARIETO-ORBITAL PROJECTION
RHESE METHOD

Film: 8 × 10 in (18 × 24 cm).

Position of patient

- Place the patient in either the preferred seated-upright or the prone position.
- Center the median sagittal plane of the body to the midline of the grid.
- Place the arms in a comfortable position and adjust the shoulders to lie in the same transverse plane.

Position of part

- With the orbit of the affected side centered to the cassette, rest the patient's zygomatic bone (zygoma), nose, and chin on the grid device.
- Adjust the flexion of the neck so that the acanthomeatal line is parallel with the transverse axis of the film.
- Using a protractor as a guide, adjust the rotation of the patient's head so that the median sagittal plane forms an angle of 53 degrees from the plane of the film (Fig. 22-32).
- Immobilize the head.
- Ask the patient to suspend respiration for the exposure.

Central ray

- Direct the central ray perpendicular to the film entering the upper parietal region and emerging at the midorbit resting on the grid device.

Structures shown

This method shows a parieto-orbital projection of the ethmoidal air cells (posterior and anterior) and the frontal and sphenoidal sinuses and the optic canal. Both sides are examined for comparison (Figs. 22-33 and 22-34).

□ Evaluation criteria

The following should be clearly demonstrated:

- Orbit closest to the film projected anterior to the ethmoid sinuses.
- Posterior ethmoidal cells overlapping the inferior portion of the orbit.
- Optic canals in the inferior and lateral portion of the orbit.
- Close beam restriction of the sinus area.

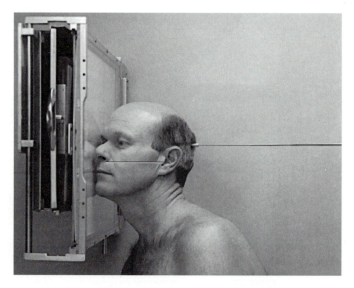

Fig. 22-32. Parieto-orbital sinuses, Rhese method.

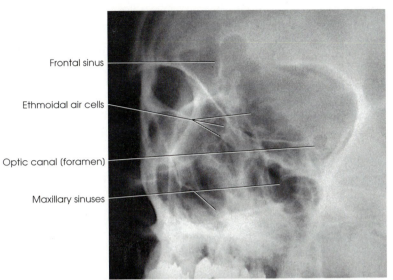

Frontal sinus

Ethmoidal air cells

Optic canal (foramen)

Maxillary sinuses

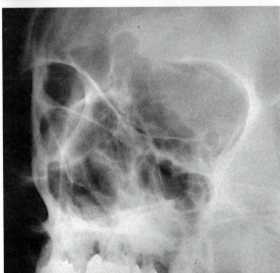

Fig. 22-33. Parieto-orbital sinuses, Rhese method.

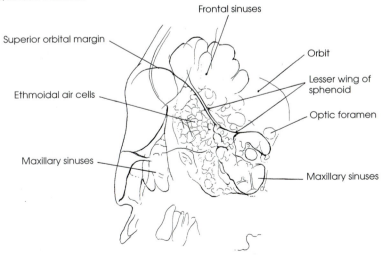

Frontal sinuses

Superior orbital margin

Orbit

Ethmoidal air cells

Lesser wing of sphenoid

Optic foramen

Maxillary sinuses

Maxillary sinuses

Fig. 22-34. PA oblique sinuses, Rhese method.

Relationship of Teeth to Maxillary Sinuses' Floor

PA AXIAL OBLIQUE PROJECTION
LAW METHOD

Film: 8 × 10 in (18 × 24 cm).

Position of patient

- Place the patient in the seated-upright or prone position.

Position of part

- Place the region of the maxillary sinus of interest centered to the cassette.
- Fully extend the patient's neck and rest the chin, the nose, and the zygomatic bone on the grid device (Fig. 22-35). When properly positioned, the acanthomeatal line forms an approximate angle of 20 degrees from the perpendicular; the median sagittal plane is rotated approximately 35 degrees from being perpendicular; and the head is tilted so that the median sagittal plane is angled 20 degrees.
- Immobilize the head.
- Ask the patient to suspend respiration for the exposure.

Central ray

- Direct the central ray to the midpoint of the film at an angle of 25 to 30 degrees cephalad. It enters posterior to the uppermost angle of the mandible and emerges from the opposite maxillary sinus.

Structures shown

A PA axial oblique projection of the floor of the maxillary sinus (antrum) is seen, showing its relationship to the teeth, from the molars to the canine. Both sides are examined for comparison (Fig. 22-36).

□ Evaluation criteria

The following should be clearly demonstrated:
- Maxillary sinus without superimposition from the opposite maxillary sinus.
- Teeth projected below the maxillary sinus.
- Close beam restriction of the sinus area.

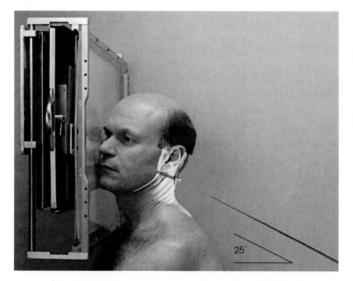

Fig. 22-35. PA axial oblique sinuses, Law method.

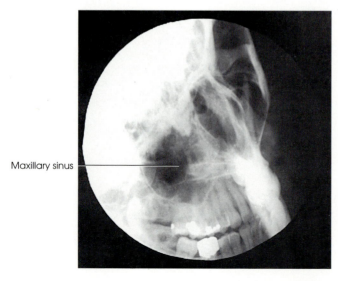
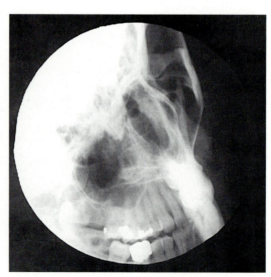

Maxillary sinus

Fig. 22-36. PA axial oblique sinuses, Law method.

Chapter 23

TEMPORAL BONE

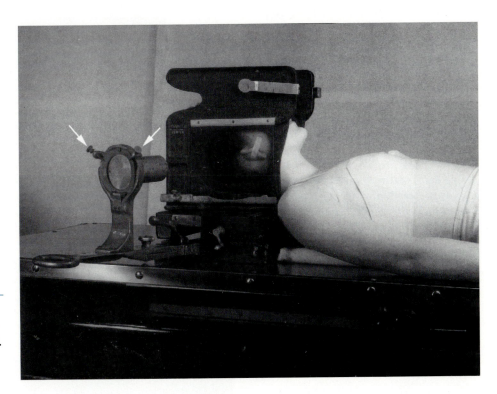

A Bullitt mastoid localizer device. The x-ray tube was attached to the end of the round tube port *(arrows)*. The patient's head was positioned as shown.

Temporal Bone Anatomy

For a complete description of the anatomy of the temporal bone, see the beginning of Chapter 20 in this volume.

Radiation Protection

Protection of the patient from unnecessary radiation is a professional responsibility of the radiographer. (See Chapter 1, Volume 1 for specific guidelines.) In this chapter, radiation shielding of the patient is neither specified nor photographically shown because the professional community and the federal government have reported that placing a lead shield over the patient's pelvis does not significantly reduce the gonadal exposure when obtaining radiographs of the temporal bone. The exception to this is the pediatric patient. The pediatric patient should be protected by shielding the thyroid and thymus glands and gonads. The protective lead shielding used to cover the thyroid and thymus glands can assist in immobilizing the pediatric patient while also providing improved radiation protection.

The most effective way to protect the patient from unnecessary radiation is to restrict the radiation beam by using proper collimation. Taking care to ensure that the patient is properly instructed about the procedure and immobilized also reduces the chance of having to repeat the procedure. This further limits the radiation exposure received by the patient.

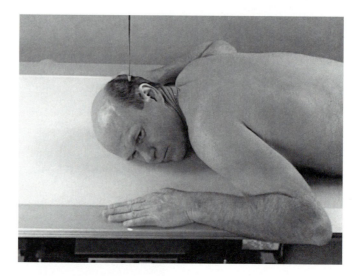

Fig. 23-1. Median sagittal rotation of 15 degrees for mastoid process.

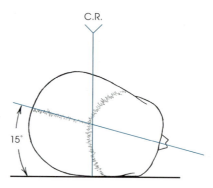

Fig. 23-2. Median sagittal rotation of 15 degrees.

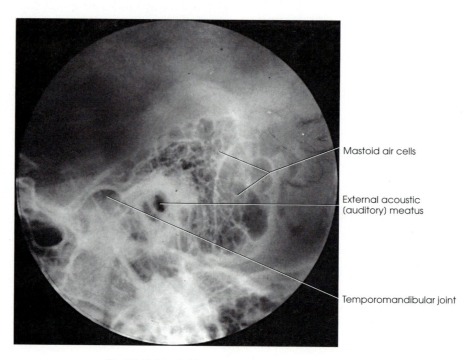

Mastoid air cells

External acoustic (auditory) meatus

Temporomandibular joint

Fig. 23-3. Mastoid process.

Temporal bone

TEMPORAL BONE

RADIOGRAPHY

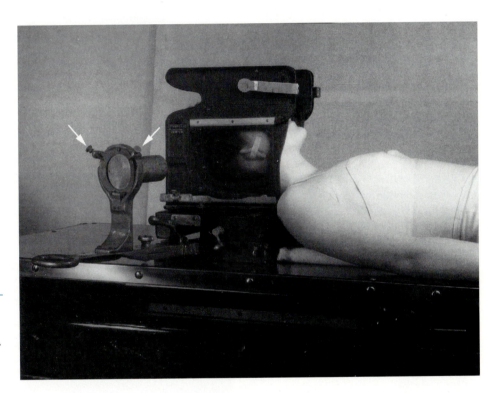

A Bullitt mastoid localizer device. The x-ray tube was attached to the end of the round tube port *(arrows)*. The patient's head was positioned as shown.

Temporal Bone Anatomy

For a complete description of the anatomy of the temporal bone, see the beginning of Chapter 20 in this volume.

Radiation Protection

Protection of the patient from unnecessary radiation is a professional responsibility of the radiographer. (See Chapter 1, Volume 1 for specific guidelines.) In this chapter, radiation shielding of the patient is neither specified nor photographically shown because the professional community and the federal government have reported that placing a lead shield over the patient's pelvis does not significantly reduce the gonadal exposure when obtaining radiographs of the temporal bone. The exception to this is the pediatric patient. The pediatric patient should be protected by shielding the thyroid and thymus glands and gonads. The protective lead shielding used to cover the thyroid and thymus glands can assist in immobilizing the pediatric patient while also providing improved radiation protection.

The most effective way to protect the patient from unnecessary radiation is to restrict the radiation beam by using proper collimation. Taking care to ensure that the patient is properly instructed about the procedure and immobilized also reduces the chance of having to repeat the procedure. This further limits the radiation exposure received by the patient.

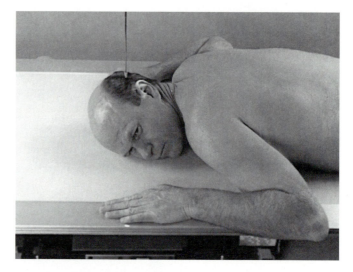

Fig. 23-1. Median sagittal rotation of 15 degrees for mastoid process.

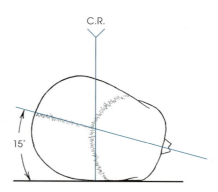

Fig. 23-2. Median sagittal rotation of 15 degrees.

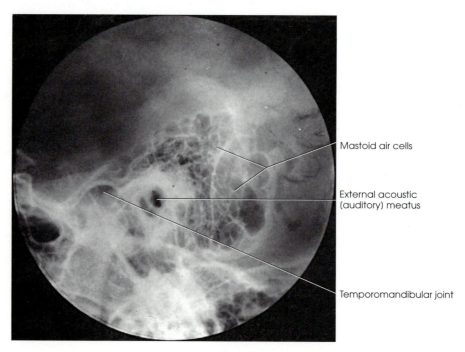

Mastoid air cells

External acoustic (auditory) meatus

Temporomandibular joint

Fig. 23-3. Mastoid process.

Petromastoid Portion
Mastoid Process

In an AP or lateral projection of the cranium, the mastoid process is obscured by superimposition of the dense petrosa or the contralateral mastoid process. To obtain an unobstructed lateral projection of the mastoid process, it is necessary to obtain the projection in a slightly oblique orientation by angling either the head or the central ray to prevent objectionable superimposition (Figs. 23-1 to 23-3). The degrees of angulation that are recommended for this purpose by various authors cover a considerable range in both the single-angle and the double-angle techniques of examination. The 15-15-degree double-angle technique, and the 15-degree and the 25-degree single-angle techniques are most commonly employed.

Both mastoid processes are always examined for comparison purposes, and it is essential that the radiographs be exact duplicates in both part position and technical quality. Likewise, radiographs made in follow-up examinations must be exact duplicates of those made in preceding examinations. Every effort must be made to establish an exact procedure in centering and adjusting the part according to the specific localization points and planes used in the particular image. Errors in centering the part can be minimized by first adjusting the patient's head and then checking the position with a protractor.

The auricles of the ears may be folded forward to prevent the relatively dense margins cast by the ear cartilages from obscuring the superimposed mastoid cells. Taping each auricle forward with a narrow strip of adhesive tape ensures keeping it in place, and, at the same time, causes a minimum of discomfort to the patient by eliminating the necessity of repeated handling of a part that is often inflamed and tender. To prevent the adhesive strip from overlapping the mastoid cells, it should be placed so that it will not extend beyond the posterior junction of the auricle and the head. Compare the auricle images in Figs. 23-4 and 23-5.

The visualization of sharp outlines of the thin, fragile walls of the mastoid cells depends on the following factors:

1. An x-ray tube having a small effective focal-spot size of not more than 0.6 mm must be used.
2. High-resolution intensifying screens are required to demonstrate the small mastoid structures.
3. Perfect film-screen contact and clean screens are essential.
4. The collimator must be adjusted to the smallest possible field size. Limiting the radiation area reduces the amount of secondary radiation reaching the film.
5. During the exposure, complete immobilization of the head and cessation of respiration are needed. The slightest movement, although not enough to cause visible blurring of the outlines of the comparatively gross surrounding structures, can diffuse the outlines of the thin cell walls. Unfortunately, when confined to the cellular structure, the diffusion cannot always be recognized as motion. For this reason the head must be rigidly immobilized.

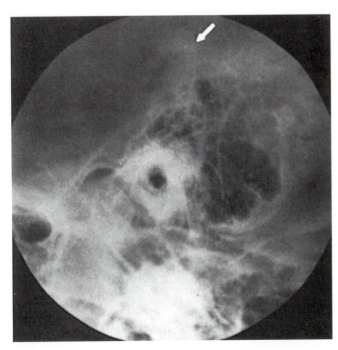

Fig. 23-4. Mastoid process: auricle folded forward (arrow).

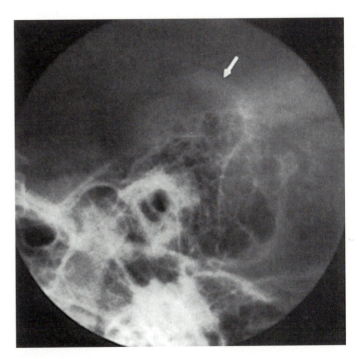

Fig. 23-5. Mastoid process: auricle not folded forward (arrow).

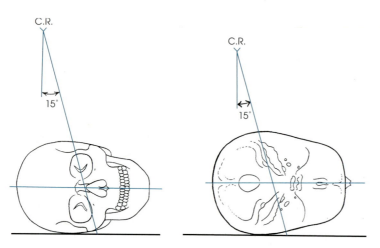

Fig. 23-6. Axiolateral oblique petromastoid portion, original Laws method: nongrid, double-tube angulation. Table radiography.

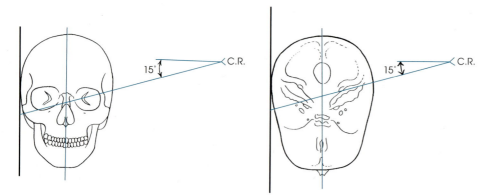

Fig. 23-7. Axiolateral oblique petromastoid portion, original Laws method: nongrid, double-tube angulation. Upright radiography.

LAW METHODS

Positioning to demonstrate the mastoid process, or the axiolateral oblique projection, was originally performed using a nongrid technique. The original position, as described by Law, used a double tube angulation as shown in Figs. 23-6 and 23-7. Grid techniques are commonly used today and, therefore, two modifications of the axiolateral projection are also described. These two projections do not require a sideways central ray angulation into the grid. One modification uses rotation of the median sagittal plane and a caudal central ray. The second modification uses rotation of the median sagittal plane and an angled interpupillary line with a perpendicular central ray. The radiographic images from all three projections are almost identical in appearance.

Petromastoid Portion

AXIOLATERAL OBLIQUE PROJECTION
Double-tube angulation
ORIGINAL LAW METHOD

Film: 8 × 10 in (18 × 24 cm).

Position of patient

• Place the patient on the radiographic table in the prone body position or seated before a *nongrid cassette*.

Position of part

• Position the patient with the head in a true lateral position.
• Adjust the flexion of the head so that the interpupillary line is perpendicular to, and the infraorbitomeatal line and the median sagittal plane are parallel with, the plane of the film (Figs. 23-6 and 23-7).
• Immobilize the head.
• Ask the patient to suspend respiration for the exposure.

Central ray

• Direct the central ray to the film at an angle of 15 degrees caudad and 15 degrees anteriorly. It enters approximately 2 inches (5 cm) posterior to, and 2 inches (5 cm) above, the uppermost external acoustic (auditory) meatus.

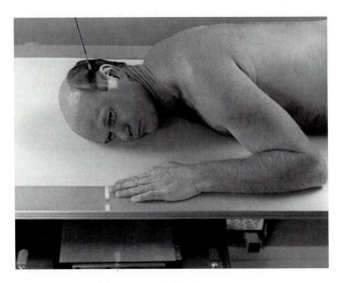

Fig. 23-8. Axiolateral petromastoid portion, modified Law method. Single-tube angulation.

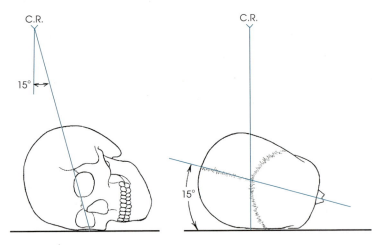

Fig. 23-9. Table radiography; single-tube angulation.

AXIOLATERAL PROJECTION
Single-tube angulation
MODIFIED LAW METHOD

Film: 8 × 10 in (18 × 24 cm).

Position of patient

- Place the patient on the table in the prone position or seated before a vertical grid device.

Position of part

- To ensure accurate centering of the part, make a mark on each mastoid process at a point 1 inch (2.5 cm) directly posterior from the center of the external acoustic (auditory) meatus.
- Tape each auricle forward with a narrow strip of adhesive tape.
- Center the marked localization point to the cassette, and rest the patient's head in a true lateral position.
- Adjust the flexion of the head so that the infraorbitomeatal line is parallel with, and the interpupillary line perpendicular to, the film.
- Rotate the affected side of the patient's chin toward the film until the median sagittal plane is adjusted to an angle of 15 degrees (Figs. 23-8 to 23-10).
- When the patient is recumbent, place a support under the side of the mandible to prevent rotation.
- Check the position of the head with a protractor.
- Immobilize the head.
- Ask the patient to suspend respiration for the exposure.

Central ray

- Direct the central ray to the midpoint of the grid at an angle of 15 degrees caudad. The central ray enters approximately 2 inches (5 cm) posterior to, and 2 inches (5 cm) superior to, the uppermost external acoustic (auditory) meatus.

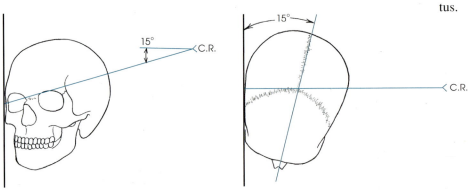

Fig. 23-10. Upright radiography; single-tube angulation.

Structures shown

The axiolateral projection demonstrates the mastoid cells, the sigmoid sinus, the lateral portion of the pars petrosa, the tegmen tympani, the superimposed internal and external acoustic (auditory) meatuses, and, when present, the mastoid emissary vessel (Fig. 23-11).

□ Evaluation criteria

The following should be clearly demonstrated:

- Mastoid closest to the film with the air cells centered to the film.
- Opposite mastoid not superimposing but lying inferior and slightly anterior to the mastoid of interest.
- Auricle of the ear not superimposing the mastoid.
- Superimposition of the internal and external acoustic (auditory) meatuses.
- Temporomandibular joint visible anterior to the mastoid.
- Close beam restriction of the mastoid region.

A

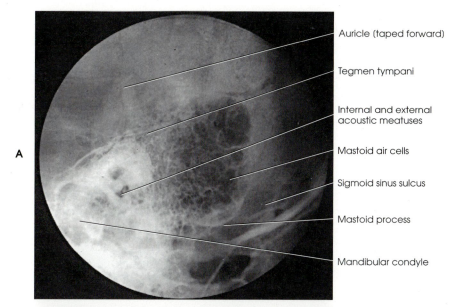

Auricle (taped forward)

Tegmen tympani

Internal and external acoustic meatuses

Mastoid air cells

Sigmoid sinus sulcus

Mastoid process

Mandibular condyle

B

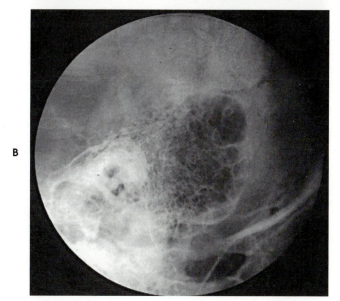

Fig. 23-11. Axiolateral petromastoid portion, modified Law method.

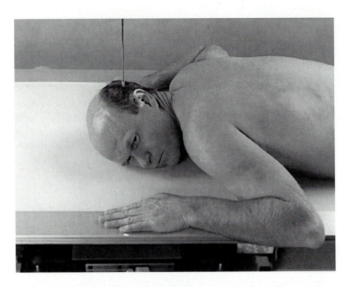

Fig. 23-12. Axiolateral oblique, petromastoid portion: part-angulation technique.

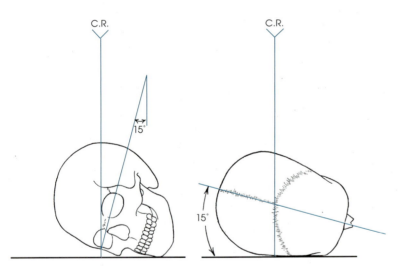

Fig. 23-13. Table radiography.

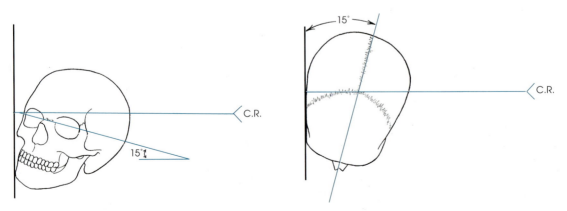

Fig. 23-14. Upright radiography.

Petromastoid Portion

AXIOLATER.AL OBLIQUE PROJECTION
Part-angulation
MODIFIED LAW METHOD

The part-angulation technique of examining the mastoid processes is especially useful where immobilization is limited. Because the head rests on the broad surface of the cheek in a natural and comfortable position, motion as a result of discomfort or lack of support is reduced to a minimum.

Film: 8 × 10 in (18 × 24 cm).

Position of patient

- Place the patient in the prone position or seated before a vertical grid device.

Position of part

- Place a mark on each mastoid process at a point 1 inch (2.5 cm) directly posterior to the center of the external acoustic (auditory) meatus.
- Tape the auricles forward.
- Center the localization mark to the cassette and rest the head on the flat surface of the cheek.
- Using a protractor as a guide, rotate the face towards the cassette so that the median sagittal plane is angled 15 degrees toward the cassette. Tilt the head so that the interpupillary line forms a 15-degree angle from the vertical (Figs. 23-12 to 23-14).
- Immobilize the head.
- Ask the patient to suspend respiration for the exposure.

Central ray

• Direct the central ray perpendicular to the film, entering the head at a point approximately 2 inches (5 cm) posterior to, and 2 inches (5 cm) superior to, the uppermost external acoustic (auditory) meatus.

Structures shown

This image demonstrates the mastoid cells, the sigmoid sinus, the superimposed internal and external acoustic (auditory) meatuses, the lateral part of the pars petrosa, the tegmen tympani, and, when present, the mastoid emissary vessel (Fig. 23-15).

The following should be clearly demonstrated:

■ Mastoid closest to the film, including the air cells.

■ Opposite mastoid not superimposing but lying inferior and slightly anterior to the mastoid of interest.

■ Auricle of the ear not superimposing the mastoid.

■ Superimposition of the internal and external acoustic (auditory) meatuses.

■ Temporomandibular joint visible anterior to the mastoid.

■ Close beam restriction of the mastoid region.

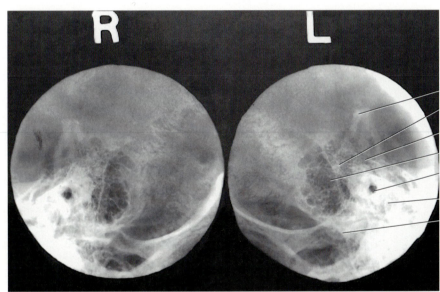

Auricle (taped forward)

Mastoid antrum

Tegmen tympani

Mastoid air cells

Superimposed internal and external acoustic meatuses

Mandibular condyle

Mastoid process

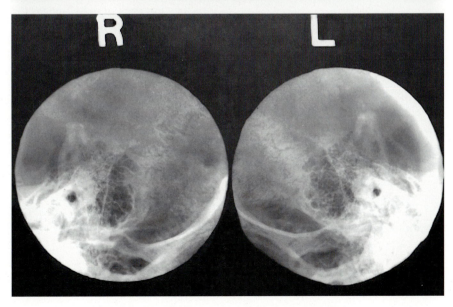

Fig. 23-15. Axiolateral oblique petromastoid portion.

Petromastoid portion

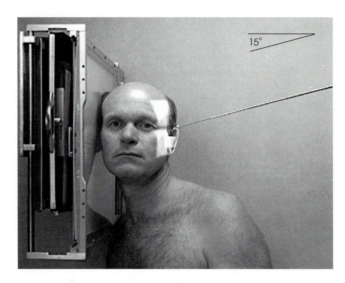

Fig. 23-16. Axiolateral petromastoid portion: Henschen method, 15 degrees.

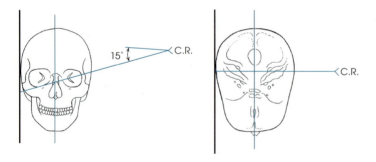

Fig. 23-17. Upright radiography, Henschen method.

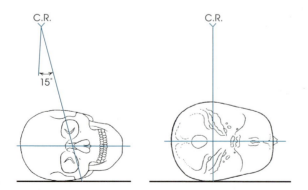

Fig. 23-18. Table radiography, Henschen method.

Petromastoid Portion

AXIOLATERAL PROJECTION
HENSCHEN, SCHÜLLER, AND LYSHOLM METHODS

Film: 8 × 10 in (18 × 24 cm).

Position of patient

- Place the patient in the prone position, or, preferably, seated before a vertical grid device.

Position of part

- Place a mark on each mastoid process at the junction of the auricle and the head immediately behind the external acoustic (auditory) meatus.
- When the mastoid cells are the point of interest, tape the auricles forward.
- Position the patient's head in the lateral position.
- Center the marked localization point either to the midline, or ¾ inch (1.9 cm) superior to the midline, of the film, depending on the central ray angulation used.
- Place the patient's head in the true lateral position with the median sagittal plane parallel with, and the interpupillary line perpendicular to, the film plane.
- Adjust the flexion of the neck so that the infraorbitomeatal line is parallel with the transverse axis of the film.
- Immobilize the head.
- Ask the patient to suspend respiration for the exposure.

Central ray

For each of these images the central ray is directed through the external acoustic (auditory) meatus closest to the film at the following caudal angles:

1. Henschen method: 15 degrees (Figs. 23-16 to 23-18)
2. Schüller method: 25 degrees (Fig. 23-19)
3. Lysholm method: 35 degrees (Fig. 23-20)

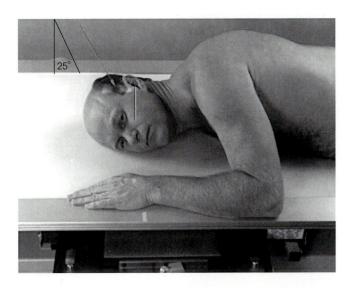

Fig. 23-19. Axiolateral petromastoid portion: Schüller method, 25 degrees.

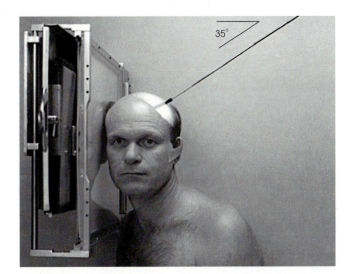

Fig. 23-20. Axiolateral petromastoid portion: Lysholm method, 35 degrees.

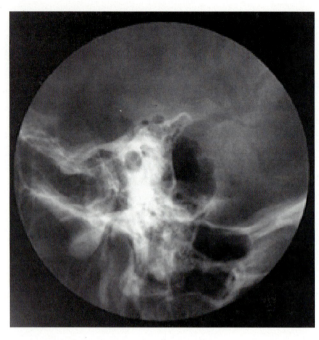

Fig. 23-21. Axiolateral petromastoid portion: Henschen method, 15 degrees.

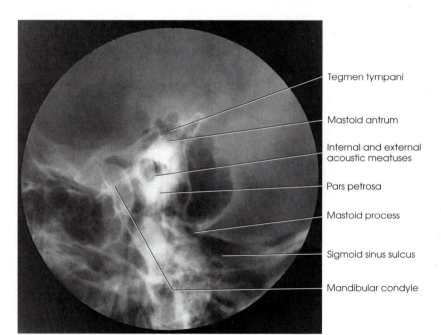

Tegmen tympani

Mastoid antrum

Internal and external acoustic meatuses

Pars petrosa

Mastoid process

Sigmoid sinus sulcus

Mandibular condyle

Fig. 23-22. Axiolateral petromastoid portion: Schüller method, 25 degrees.

Structures shown

The Henschen 15-degree method (Fig. 23-21) demonstrates the mastoid cells, the mastoid antrum, the internal and external acoustic (auditory) meatuses, and the tegmen tympani. This approach was recommended by Henschen,[1] and later by Cushing,[2] for the demonstration of tumors of the acoustic nerve.

The Schüller 25-degree method (Fig. 23-22) demonstrates the pneumatic structure of the mastoid process, the mastoid antrum, the tegmen tympani, the internal and external acoustic (auditory) meatuses, the sinus and dural plates, and, when present, the mastoid emissary vessel.

The Lysholm 35-degree method[3] (sometimes referred to as the Runström II method) seen in Fig. 23-23 demonstrates the mastoid cells, the mastoid antrum, the external acoustic (auditory) meatus, the tegmen tympani, the labyrinthine area, and the carotid canal.

Runström[4] recommends that the exposures be made with the mouth open for visualization of the petrous apex between the anterior wall of the external acoustic (auditory) meatus and the mandibular condyle.

[1]Henschen F: Die Akusticustumoren, eine neue Gruppe radiographisch darstellbar Hirntumoren, Fortschr Roentgenstr 18:207, 1912.
[2]Cushing H: Tumors of the nervus acusticus, Philadelphia, 1917, WB Saunders.
[3]Lyshom E: Apparatus and technique for roentgen examination of the skull, Acta Radiol 12(suppl):83-85, 1931.
[4]Runström G: A roentgenological study of acute and chronic ototis media, Acta Radiol 17(suppl):1-88, 1933.

□ Evaluation criteria

The following should be clearly demonstrated:

- Mastoid and petrous regions in the center of the radiograph.
- Mastoid air cells lying posterior to the petrous region.
- Temporomandibular joint lying anterior to the petrous region.
- Opposite mastoid and petrous region not superimposing the side of interest and projecting to a more inferior location as the angulation of the central ray increases.
- Close beam restriction of the mastoid and petrous region.

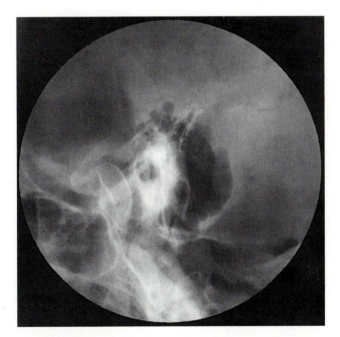

Fig. 23-23. Axiolateral petromastoid portion: Lysholm method, 35 degrees.

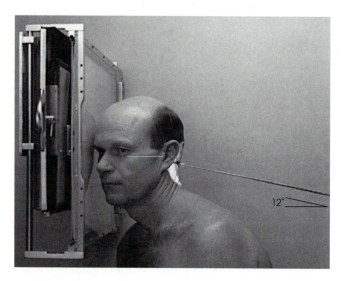

Fig. 23-24. Axiolateral oblique petromastoid portion. Posterior profile, Stenvers method.

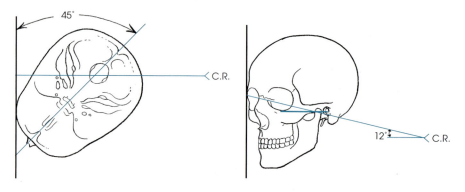

Fig. 23-25. Upright radiography.

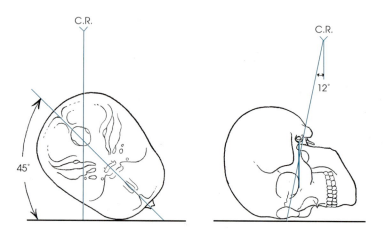

Fig. 23-26. Table radiography.

Petromastoid Portion

AXIOLATERAL OBLIQUE PROJECTION (POSTERIOR PROFILE)
STENVERS METHOD

Film: 8 × 10 in (18 × 24 cm).

Position of patient

- Place the patient in the prone position or seated before a vertical grid device.

Position of part

- Place a mark on each cheek at a point 1 inch (2.5 cm) directly anterior to the external acoustic (auditory) meatus. When the head is correctly adjusted, this point will be inferior to the arcuate eminence.
- Center the localization point to the midpoint of the cassette and rest the head on the forehead, the nose, and the zygomatic bone (zygoma).
- Adjust the flexion of the neck so that the infraorbitomeatal line is parallel with the transverse axis of the film.
- Using a protractor as a guide, rotate the face away from the side being examined until the median sagittal plane forms an angle of 45 degrees with the plane of the film (Figs. 23-24 to 23-26).
- In patients with brachycephalic (short front-to-back) skulls, the petrous ridges form an angle of approximately 54 degrees with the median sagittal plane. Patients with this skull type will require less-than-normal rotation of the median sagittal plane to place the petrous ridge parallel with the film. In patients with dolichocephalic (long front-to-back) skulls, the petrous ridges form an angle of approximately 40 degrees with the median sagittal plane. Patients with this skull type will require more rotation of the median sagittal plane to place the petrous ridges parallel with the film.
- Immobilize the head.
- Ask the patient to suspend respiration for the exposure.

Central ray

- Direct the central ray 12 degrees cephalad to exit 1 inch (2.5 cm) anterior to the external acoustic (auditory) meatus closest to the film.

Structures shown

The Stenvers method shows a profile image of the pars petrosa closest to the film. When the patient is correctly positioned, the petrosa of interest is parallel with the plane of the film (Fig. 23-27). It demonstrates the petrous ridge, the cellular structure of the mastoid process, the mastoid antrum, the area of the tympanic cavity, the bony labyrinth, the internal acoustic (auditory) canal, and the cellular structure of the petrous apex.

□Evaluation criteria

The following should be clearly demonstrated:
- Petrosa and petrous ridge in profile without distortion.
- Lateral border of the skull to the lateral border of the orbit.
- Petrous ridge extended to a point approximately two thirds of the way up the lateral border of the orbit.
- Mastoid process in profile below the margin of the cranium. (Air cells are not well visualized when the internal aspects of the petrosa are properly exposed.)
- Posterior margin of mandibular ramus superimposing lateral border of cervical column.
- Mandibular condyle projecting over the first cervical vertebra near the petrosa.
- Close beam restriction to the petrosa and mastoid region.

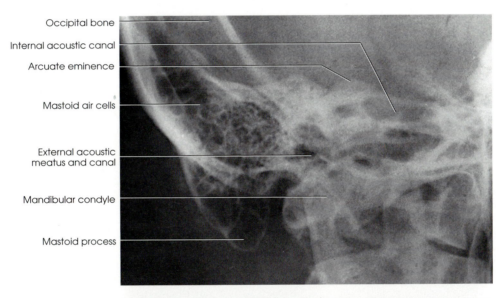

Occipital bone
Internal acoustic canal
Arcuate eminence
Mastoid air cells
External acoustic meatus and canal
Mandibular condyle
Mastoid process

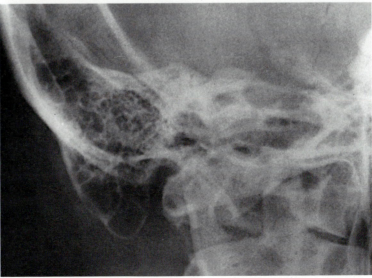

Fig. 23-27. Axiolateral oblique petromastoid portion. Posterior profile, Stenvers method.

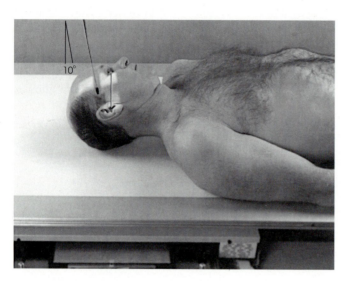

Fig. 23-28. Axiolateral oblique petromastoid portion. Anterior profile, Arcelin method.

Petromastoid Portion

 ## AXIOLATERAL OBLIQUE PROJECTION (ANTERIOR PROFILE)
ARCELIN METHOD

The Arcelin method is particularly useful with children and with adults who cannot be placed in the prone or seated-upright position for the Stenvers method described on the previous page.

Film: 8 × 10 in (18 × 24 cm).

Position of patient

- Center the median sagittal plane of the patient's body to the midline of the table, place the arms along the sides of the body, and adjust the shoulders to lie in the same transverse plane.

Position of part

- Make a mark on each cheek at a point 1 inch (2.5 cm) directly anterior to the external acoustic (auditory) meatus.
- Rotate the patient's face approximately 45 degrees away from the side being examined.
- Center the cassette directly below the marked localization point.
- Adjust the head so that the median sagittal plane forms an angle of 45 degrees with the plane of the film.
- Adjust the flexion of the neck so that the infraorbitomeatal line is perpendicular to the plane of the film (Figs. 23-28 to 23-30).

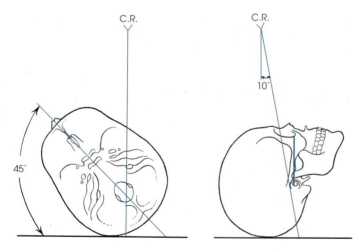

Fig. 23-29. Table radiography.

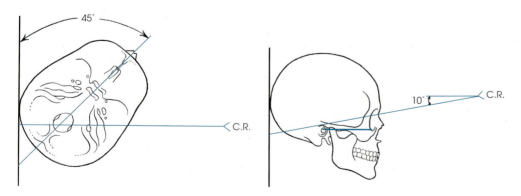

Fig. 23-30. Upright radiography.

- In patients with brachycephalic (short front-to-back) skulls, the petrous ridges form an angle of approximately 54 degrees with the median sagittal plane. Patients with this skull type will require less-than-normal rotation of the median sagittal plane to place the petrous ridge parallel with the film. In patients with dolichocephalic (long front-to-back) skulls, the petrous ridges form an angle of approximately 40 degrees with the median sagittal plane. Patients with this skull type will require more rotation of the median sagittal plane to place the petrous ridges parallel with the film.
- Immobilize the head.
- Ask the patient to suspend respiration for the exposures.

Central ray

- Direct the central ray to the film at an angle of 10 degrees caudad. It enters the temporal area at a point approximately 1 inch (2.5 cm) anterior to, and ¾ inch (1.9 cm) above, the external acoustic (auditory) meatus.

Structures shown

The anterior profile Arcelin method (Fig. 23-31), the exact reverse of the Stenvers method, demonstrates the petrous portion of the temporal bone farthest from the film. With the Arcelin method, the object-to-image receptor distance increases approximately 2 cm, which is not sufficient to cause appreciable magnification.

□ **Evaluation criteria**

The following should be clearly demonstrated:
- Petrosa and petrous ridge in profile.
- Lateral border of the skull to the lateral border of the orbit.
- Petrous ridge lying horizontally and at a point approximately two thirds of the way up the lateral border of the orbit.
- Mastoid process in profile below the margin of the cranium. (Air cells are not well visualized when petrosa is properly exposed.)

- Posterior surface of mandibular ramus parallel to the lateral surface of cervical vertebrae.
- Mandibular condyle projected over the first cervical vertebra near the petrosa.
- Close beam restriction to the petrosa and mastoid region.

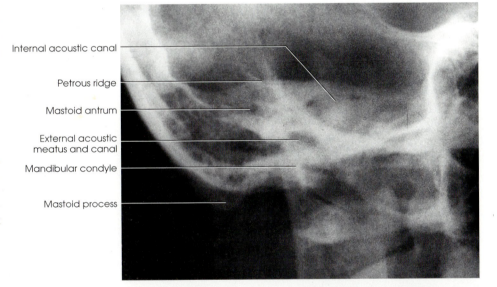

Internal acoustic canal
Petrous ridge
Mastoid antrum
External acoustic meatus and canal
Mandibular condyle
Mastoid process

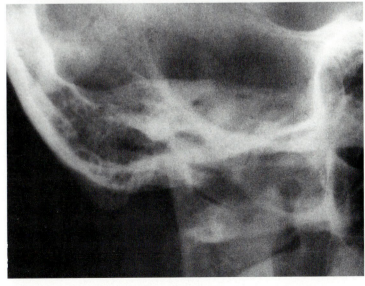

Fig. 23-31. Axiolateral oblique petromastoid portion. Anterior profile, Arcelin method.

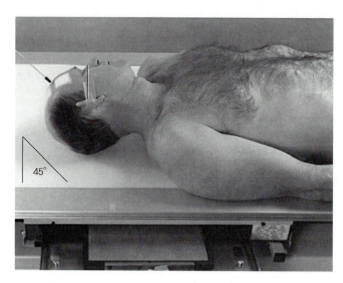

Fig. 23-32. Axiolateral oblique petromastoid portion, Mayer method.

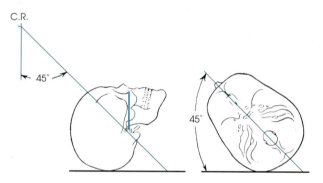

Fig. 23-33. Table radiography.

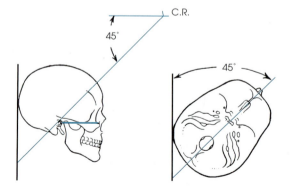

Fig. 23-34. Upright radiography.

Petromastoid Portion

For Acoustic Ossicles and Attic-Aditus-Antrum
AXIOLATERAL OBLIQUE PROJECTION
MAYER METHOD

NOTE: The axiolateral oblique projection or Mayer method, was originally described using a non-grid technique. The original technique has been modified to use a grid for improved radiographic quality.

Film: 8 × 10 in (18 × 24 cm).

Position of patient

- Place the patient in the supine position or seated laterally before a vertical grid device.

Position of part

- Make a mark directly behind each external acoustic (auditory) meatus at the junction of the auricle and the head.
- Tape the auricles forward.
- With the ear of interest adjacent to the film, adjust the median sagittal plane at an angle of 45 degrees from the film plane.
- Center the localization point behind the auricle to the cassette.
- Depress the patient's chin enough to place the mastoid process close to the grid device. This usually places the infraorbitomeatal line parallel with the transverse axis of the film (Figs. 23-32 to 23-34).

Central ray

- Direct the central ray through the dependent external acoustic (auditory) meatus at an angle of 45 degrees caudad.

Structures shown

An axiolateral oblique projection of the petrosa in the direction of its long axis demonstrates the external acoustic (auditory) meatus, the tympanic cavity and ossicles, the epitympanic recess (attic), the aditus, and the mastoid antrum closest to the film (Fig. 23-35).

The following should be clearly demonstrated:

- Petrosa inferior to the mastoid air cells.
- External acoustic (auditory) meatus visible adjacent and anterior to the petrosa.
- Temporomandibular joint visible anterior to the external acoustic (auditory) meatus.
- Auricle of the ear not superimposing the petrosa or mastoid air cells.
- Close beam restriction of the petrosal region.

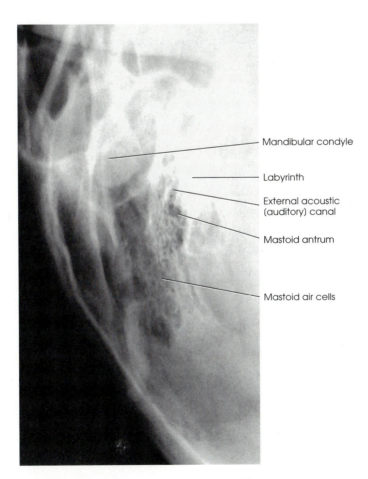

— Mandibular condyle

— Labyrinth

— External acoustic (auditory) canal

— Mastoid antrum

— Mastoid air cells

Fig. 23-35. Axiolateral oblique petromastoid portion, Mayer method.

(Courtesy Norma Harman, R.T.)

Petromastoid portion

413

Modifications

Mayer,[1] and later Owen,[2] stated that it is sometimes an advantage to vary the rotation of the head and/or the central ray angulation. Many modifications of the Mayer method, each attributed to Owen, have been used. A few modifications are illustrated.

In the Owen modification cited by Pendergrass, Schaeffer, and Hodes,[3] the patient's head is adjusted so that the median sagittal plane is 40 degrees from the film. The tabletop film and the head are angled 10 degrees caudally, and the central ray is angled 28 degrees caudally (a total caudal angulation of 38 degrees) (Fig. 23-36).

In the Owen modification described by Etter and Cross,[4] the median sagittal plane of the head is adjusted at an angle of 30 degrees to the film. The central ray is then directed 25 to 30 degrees caudally (Fig. 23-37). In the Owen modification described by Compere,[5] the head rotation is varied from 30 to 45 degrees to the plane of the film, and the central ray is directed caudally at an angle of 30 degrees.

[1]Mayer EG: The technic of the roentgenologic examination of the temporal bone, Radiology 7:306-317, 1926.

[2]Owen GR: A simplified method of producing the axial view of Mayer in chronic mastoiditis and attic cholesteatoma, AJR 57:260-263, 1947.

[3]Pendergrass EP, Schaeffer JP, and Hodes PJ: The head and neck in roentgen diagnosis, ed 2, Springfield, Ill, 1956, Charles C Thomas, Publisher.

[4]Etter LE and Cross LC: Projection angle variations required to demonstrate the middle ear, Radiology 80:255-257, 1963.

[5]Compere WE: The roentgenologic aspects of tympanoplasty, AJR 81:956-963, 1959.

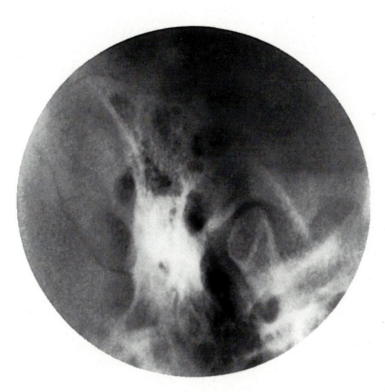

Fig. 23-36. Axiolateral oblique petromastoid region, Owen-Pendergrass modification. Head rotated 40 degrees with total caudal central ray angulation of 38 degrees.

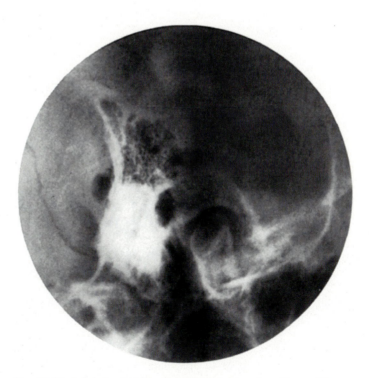

Fig. 23-37. Axiolateral oblique petromastoid region, Owen-Etter-Cross modification. Head rotated 30 degrees with caudal central ray angulation of 30 degrees.

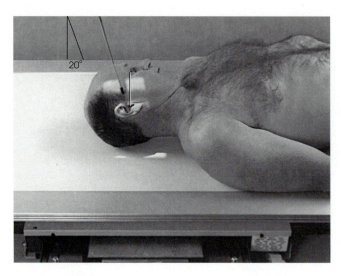

Fig. 23-38. AP axial oblique for petromastoid region.

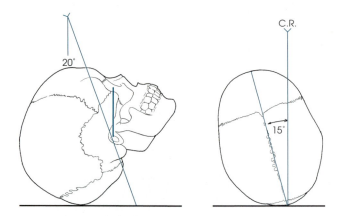

Fig. 23-39. Table radiography.

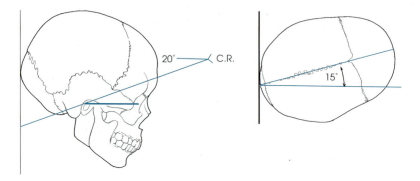

Fig. 23-40. Upright radiography.

Petromastoid Portion
Middle Ear Region
AP AXIAL OBLIQUE PROJECTION
CHAUSSÉ III METHOD

Chaussé[1] specifies that (1) the head be adjusted for the AP projection with the orbitomeatal line perpendicular to the plane of the film, and (2) the central ray be directed through the middle ear at an eccentric angle of 20 degrees caudally and from 10 to 20 degrees medially. With grid technique, head rotation has been substituted for the medial angulation of the central ray as originally described.

Film: 8 × 10 in (18 × 24 cm).

Position of patient

- Place the patient in either the supine or the seated-upright position.

Position of part

- Rotate the face away from the side being examined until the median sagittal plane is 15 (10 to 20) degrees.
- Adjust the position of the patient or the film so that a point 1 inch (2.5 cm) medial to the tragus is centered to the midline.
- Adjust the flexion of the neck so that the orbitomeatal line is parallel with the transverse axis of the film (Figs. 23-38 to 23-40).
- Recheck for rotation and immobilize the head.
- Ask the patient to suspend respiration for the exposure.

[1]Chaussé C: Trois incidences pour l'examen du rocher, Acta Radiol 34:274-287, 1950.

Central ray

• Direct the central ray to a point midway between the lateral margin of the orbit and the tragus at an angle of 20 degrees caudad. The central ray parallels a line passing through the external acoustic (auditory) meatus.

Structures shown

A slightly oblique image of the petrosa, demonstrating the epitympanic recess, the aditus ad antrum, and the mastoid antral areas, is shown (Fig. 23-41).

□ Evaluation criteria

The following should be clearly demonstrated:
■ Epitympanic recess, aditus ad antrum, and mastoid antrum (middle ear region) near the lateral margin of the orbit.
■ Skull only slightly obliqued.
■ Petrous ridge extending to the superior margin of the orbit.
■ Entire petrosal region.
■ Close beam restriction of the petrosal region.

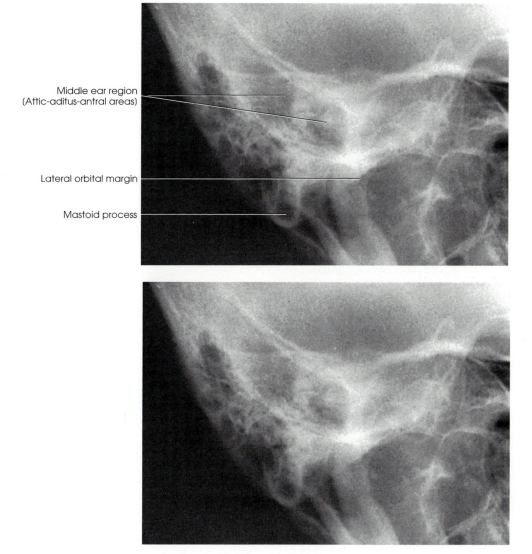

Middle ear region
(Attic-aditus-antral areas)

Lateral orbital margin

Mastoid process

Fig. 23-41. AP axial oblique petromastoid portion, Chaussé III method.

Petromastoid portion

417

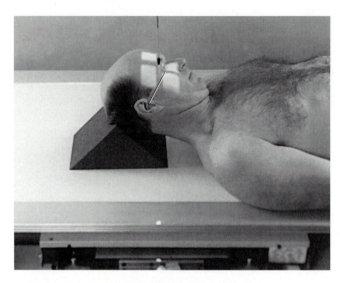

Fig. 23-42. AP axial oblique petromastoid portion: Sansregret modification of Chaussé III method.

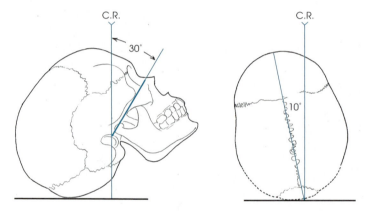

Fig. 23-43. Table radiography.

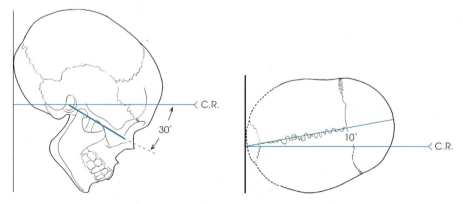

Fig. 23-44. Upright radiography.

Petromastoid Portion

Middle Ear Region
AP AXIAL OBLIQUE PROJECTION
SANSREGRET MODIFICATION OF CHAUSSÉ III METHOD

Film: 8 × 10 in (18 × 24 cm).

Position of patient

- Place the patient in the supine position with the head elevated on an angle sponge or seated at a vertical grid device.

Position of part

- Rotate the patient's face to adjust the median sagittal plane 10 (8 to 12) degrees away from the side being examined.
- Adjust the position so that a point 1 inch (2.5 cm) medial to the external acoustic (auditory) meatus is centered to the midline of the grid.
- Center the cassette longitudinally at the level of the tragus.
- Adjust the flexion of the neck so that the infraorbitomeatal line is at an angle of 30 degrees from the vertical (Figs. 23-42 to 23-44).
- Recheck for rotation and immobilize the head.
- Ask the patient to suspend respiration for the exposure.

Central ray

- Direct the perpendicular central ray to enter slightly superior and lateral to the superolateral margin of the orbit and to parallel a line passing through the tragus.
- Because of the increased object-image-receptor distance, the source-to-image receptor distance (SID) may be increased about 8 inches (20 cm).

Structures shown

A slightly oblique image of the petrosa is demonstrated, showing the epitympanic recess, aditus ad antrum, and mastoid antrum (middle ear region) (Fig. 23-45). Sansregret[1] states that this method gives an excellent tangential projection of the edge of the attic epitympanic recess wall. Because of individual variations, he recommends that three films be taken with slight (2-degree) variations in head rotation.

---

[1]Sansregret A: Technique for the study of the middle ear, AJR 90:1156-1166, 1963.

The following should be clearly demonstrated:

- Epitympanic recess, aditus ad antrum, and mastoid antrum near the lateral margin of the orbit.
- Skull only slightly obliqued.
- Petrous ridge extending to the superior margin of the orbit.
- Entire petrosal region.
- Close beam restriction of the petrosal region.

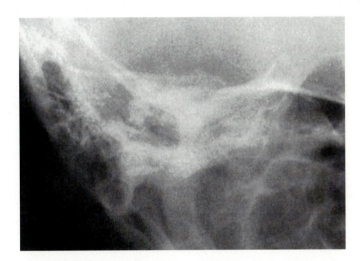

Fig. 23-45. AP axial oblique petromastoid portion. Sansregret modification of Chaussé III method.

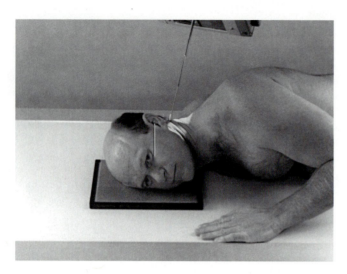

Fig. 23-46. Axiolateral oblique petromastoid portion, Löw-Beer method.

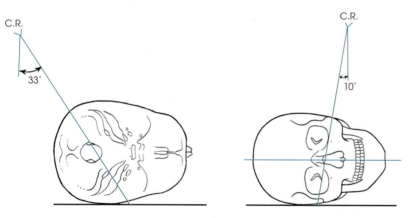

Fig. 23-47. Table radiography.

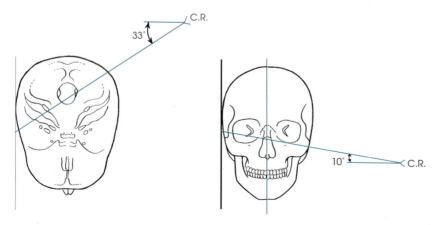

Fig. 23-48. Upright radiography.

Petromastoid Portion

AXIOLATERAL OBLIQUE PROJECTION
LÖW-BEER METHOD

Film: 8 × 10 in (18 × 24 cm) nongrid.

Position of patient

- Make a mark on each cheek at a point 1½ inches (3.7 cm) directly anterior to the external acoustic (auditory) meatus.
- Place the patient in a semiprone position.
- Adjust the rotation of the body so that the median sagittal plane of the head is horizontal.
- Have the patient rest on the forearm and flexed knee.

Position of part

- Center the marked localization point to the midpoint of the film, and rest the head in a lateral position.
- Adjust the flexion of the neck so that the infraorbitomeatal line is parallel with the transverse axis of the film.
- Adjust the head so that the median sagittal plane is parallel with, and the interpupillary line is perpendicular to, the film (Figs. 23-46 to 23-48).
- Support the mandible to prevent rotation.
- Immobilize the head.
- Ask the patient to suspend respiration for the exposure.

Central ray

- Direct the central ray to exit a point 1½ inches (3.7 cm) anterior to the lower external acoustic (auditory) meatus at an angle of 33 degrees anteriorly and 10 degrees cephalad.

Structures shown

An image that is somewhat similar to the posterior profile Stenvers method is demonstrated. The petrous apex, the labyrinthine and sinus (antral) areas, the internal acoustic (auditory) canal, and the mastoid cells are demonstrated (Fig. 23-49).

□ Evaluation criteria

The following should be clearly demonstrated:

- Lateral border of the skull to the lateral border of the orbit.
- Petrous ridge extending to a point approximately two thirds of the way up the lateral border of the orbit.
- Most of the mastoid process projected onto the skull because of the cephalic angulation.
- Mandibular condyle projected over the first cervical vertebra near the petrosa.
- Close beam restriction to the petrosa and mastoid region.

Petromastoid portion

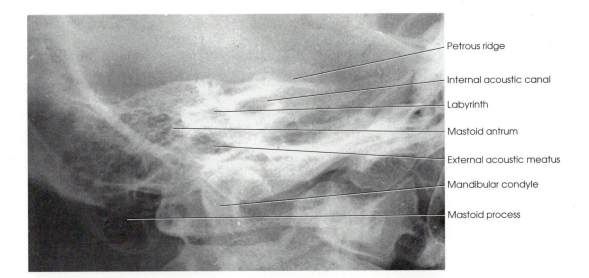

Petrous ridge

Internal acoustic canal

Labyrinth

Mastoid antrum

External acoustic meatus

Mandibular condyle

Mastoid process

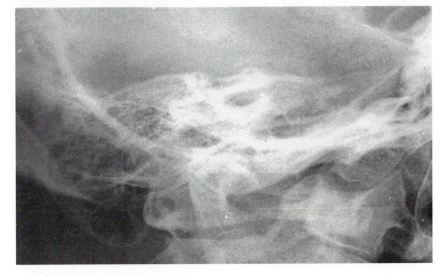

Fig. 23-49. Axiolateral oblique petromastoid portion, Löw-Beer method.

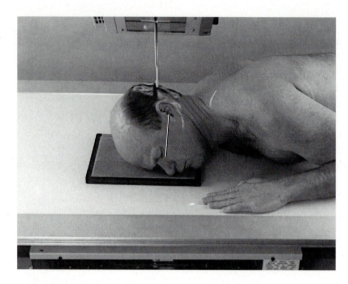

Fig. 23-50. Parietotemporal petromastoid portion, Lysholm method.

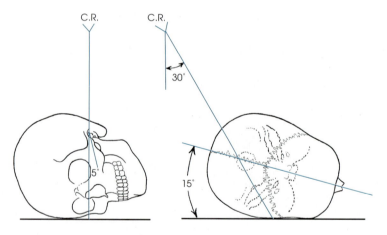

Fig. 23-51. Table radiography.

Petromastoid Portion

PARIETOTEMPORAL PROJECTION
LYSHOLM METHOD

Film: 8×10 in (18×24 cm) nongrid.

Position of patient

- Make a mark on each cheek at a point 1½ inches (3.7 cm) directly anterior to the external acoustic (auditory) meatus.
- Place the patient in a semiprone position, resting on the forearm and flexed knee of the elevated side.
- Place the arms in a comfortable position.
- Adjust the shoulders to lie in the same transverse plane.

Position of part

- Center the marked localization point to the cassette, and rest the temple on the nongrid placed cassette.
- Adjust the flexion of the neck so that the infraorbitomeatal line is at an angle of 5 degrees, open cranially, to the transverse axis of the film.
- Adjust the forward rotation of the head so that the median sagittal plane forms an angle of 15 degrees from the plane of the film (Figs. 23-50 and 23-51).
- Immobilize the head.
- Ask the patient to suspend respiration for the exposure.

Central ray

• Direct the central ray to exit at a point 1½ inches (3.7 cm) anterior to the dependent external acoustic (auditory) meatus at an angle of 30 degrees anteriorly.

Structures shown

A profile image of the petrosa, showing the apex, the sinus (antral) and labyrinthine areas, the internal acoustic (auditory) canal, the carotid canal, and the mastoid cells is demonstrated (Fig. 23-52).

□ Evaluation criteria

The following should be clearly demonstrated:

■ Lateral border of the skull to the lateral border of the orbit.
■ Petrous ridge extending to a point approximately two thirds of the way up the lateral border of the orbit.
■ Mastoid process in profile inferior to the margin of the cranium. (Air cells are not well visualized when the inner aspects of the petrosa are properly exposed.)
■ Mandibular condyle near the mastoid process.
■ Close beam restriction to the petrosa and mastoid region.

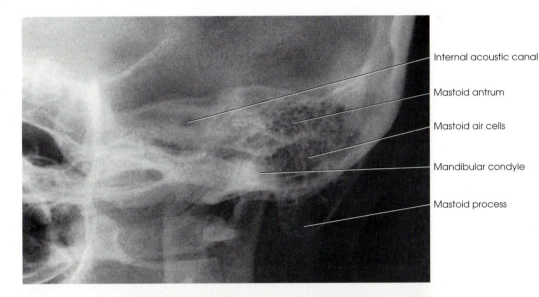

Internal acoustic canal

Mastoid antrum

Mastoid air cells

Mandibular condyle

Mastoid process

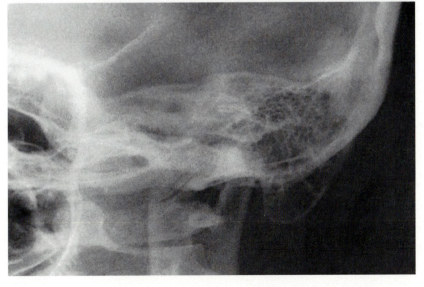

Fig. 23-52. Parietotemporal petromastoid portion, Lysholm method.

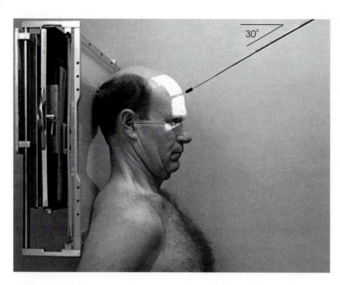

Fig. 23-53. AP axial petromastoid portion, Towne method.

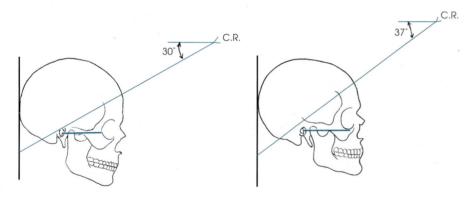

Fig. 23-54. Upright radiography.

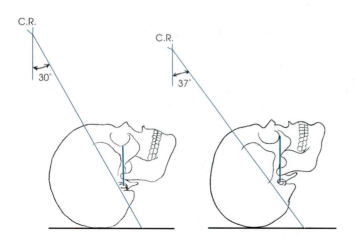

Fig. 23-55. Table radiography.

Petromastoid Portion

AP AXIAL PROJECTION
TOWNE METHOD

Film: 8×10 in (18×24 cm) lengthwise.

Position of patient

- Place the patient in either the supine or the seated-upright position.
- Center the median sagittal plane of the body to the midline of the grid device.
- Place the patient's arms in a comfortable position.
- Adjust the shoulders to lie in the same transverse plane to prevent rotation of the head.

Position of part

- Adjust the head to place the median sagittal plane perpendicular to the midline of the grid.
- Flex the neck enough to place the orbitomeatal line perpendicular to the plane of the film.
- When the patient's head cannot be flexed to this extent, adjust it to place the infraorbitomeatal line perpendicular to the film and then compensate with a 7-degree increase in the caudal angulation of the central ray (Figs. 23-53 to 23-55).
- Adjust the position of the cassette so that the midpoint of the film coincides with the central ray.
- Immobilize the head.
- Ask the patient to suspend respiration for the exposure.

Central ray

- Direct the central ray to the intersection of the median sagittal plane of the head and a line extending through the external acoustic (auditory) meatuses at a caudal angle of (1) 30 degrees to the orbitomeatal line or (2) 37 degrees to the infraorbitomeatal line. It enters approximately 2½ inches above the nasion.

Structures shown

This projection shows the petrosae projected above the base of the skull (Fig. 23-56). It demonstrates the internal acoustic (auditory) canals, the arcuate eminences, the labyrinths, the mastoid antrums, and the middle ears. The dorsum sellae is seen within the shadow of the foramen magnum.

□ Evaluation criteria

The following should be clearly demonstrated:

- Entire petrous and mastoid regions visible.
- Distance from the lateral border of the skull to the lateral margin of the foramen magnum equal on both sides.
- Petrous pyramids symmetric.
- Dorsum sellae visible within the foramen magnum.
- Close beam restriction to the petrous and mastoid region.

NOTE: Tomography, radiographic or computed, is often employed in examinations of the ear. These studies may be made with the patient's head adjusted for the AP projection. When indicated, further studies may be made in the lateral position or in another selected petrosal position. For additional information regarding radiographic tomography, including radiographs of the inner ear, see Chapter 26, in this volume. For additional information on computed tomography, see Chapter 34, in Volume 3.

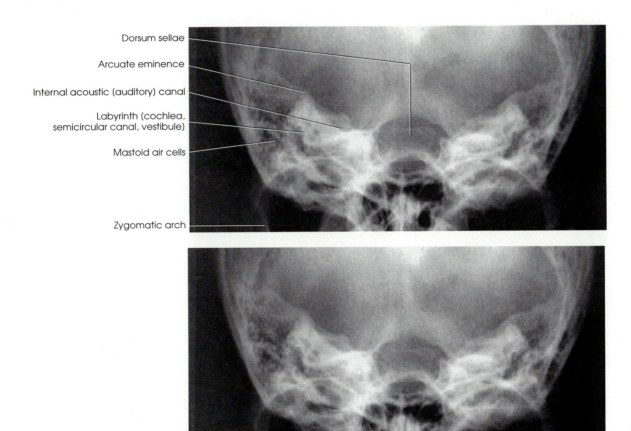

Dorsum sellae
Arcuate eminence
Internal acoustic (auditory) canal
Labyrinth (cochlea, semicircular canal, vestibule)
Mastoid air cells
Zygomatic arch

Fig. 23-56. AP axial petromastoid portion, Towne method.

Petromastoid portion

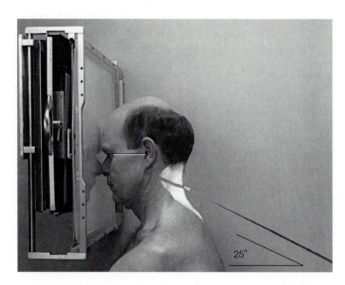

Fig. 23-57. PA axial petromastoid portion, Haas method.

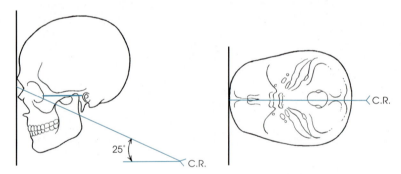

Fig. 23-58. Upright radiography.

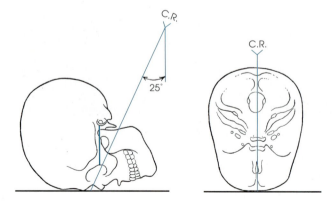

Fig. 23-59. Table radiography.

Petromastoid Portion

PA AXIAL PROJECTION
HAAS METHOD

Film: 8×10 in (18×24 cm) lengthwise.

Position of patient

- Place the patient in the seated-upright or the prone position.
- Center the median sagittal plane of the body to the midline of the grid.
- Place the arms in a comfortable position.
- Adjust the shoulders to lie in the same transverse plane to prevent rotation of the head.

Position of part

- Rest the patient's forehead and nose on the table, and adjust the head so that the median sagittal plane and orbitomeatal line are perpendicular to the plane of the film.
- Center the cassette 1 inch (2.5 cm) superior to the nasion (Figs. 23-57 to 23-59).
- Immobilize the head.
- Ask the patient to suspend respiration for the exposure.

Central ray

- Direct the central ray through the nasion at an angle of 25 degrees cephalad.

Structures shown

This projection shows a symmetric, PA axial image of the petrous portions projected above the base of the skull (Fig. 23-60). This demonstrates the internal acoustic (auditory) canals, the labyrinths, the mastoid antrums, the middle ears, and, within the shadow of the foramen magnum, the dorsum sellae. The image obtained of the petrosal structures is comparable to that obtained with the AP axial projection (Fig. 23-61). For this reason, this radiographic approach is employed with patients who cannot be satisfactorily adjusted for the AP axial projection.

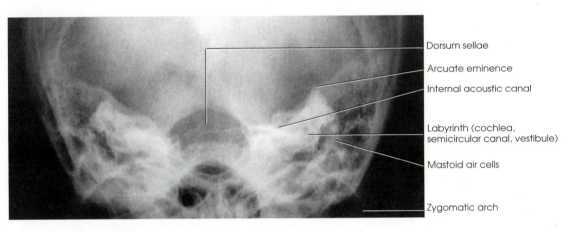

Dorsum sellae

Arcuate eminence

Internal acoustic canal

Labyrinth (cochlea, semicircular canal, vestibule)

Mastoid air cells

Zygomatic arch

Fig. 23-60. PA axial petromastoid portion, Haas method.

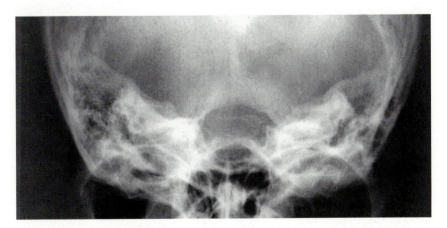

Fig. 23-61. AP axial petromastoid portion, Towne method, for comparison.

Petromastoid portion

427

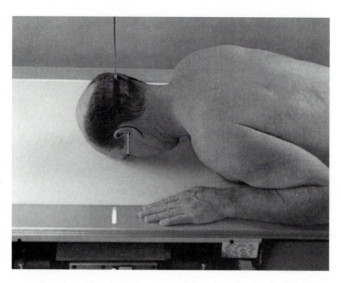

Fig. 23-62. PA (transorbital) petromastoid region with perpendicular central ray.

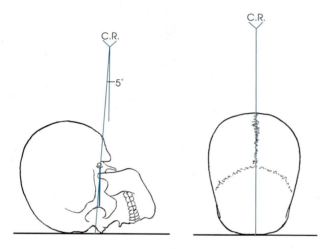

Fig. 23-63. Table radiography showing 5-degree cephalad angulation, if needed.

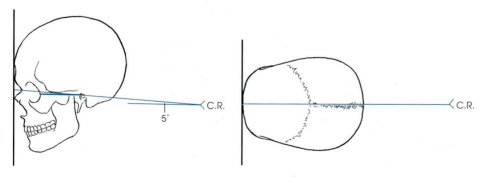

Fig. 23-64. Upright radiography showing 5-degree cephalad angulation, if needed.

Petromastoid Portion
PA PROJECTION (TRANSORBITAL)

Because the petrous portion of the temporal bone, containing the internal acoustic (auditory) canal, is located in the center of the skull in the anteroposterior dimension, a tightly collimated AP or PA projection is often of value. The image obtained is the only projection available in which the two internal acoustic (auditory) canals are symmetrically imaged and compared on one radiograph with one radiation exposure.

If the patient condition permits, the PA projection is recommended instead of the AP because of the reduced radiation dose received by the lens of the eye; dose reductions of greater than 90% have been reported.[1]

Film: 8 × 10 in (18 × 24 cm).

Position of patient

- Place the patient in either the prone or the seated-upright position.
- Center the median sagittal plane of the body to the midline of the grid device.
- Flex the patient's elbows.
- Place the arms in a comfortable position.
- Adjust the shoulders to lie in the same transverse plane.

Position of part

- Rest the patient's forehead and nose on the table, with the median sagittal plane perpendicular to the midline of the grid.
- Adjust the flexion of the neck so that the orbitomeatal line is perpendicular to the plane of the film (Fig. 23-62).
- With the cassette in the Bucky tray, center it at the nasion. The x-ray beam must be very tightly collimated to reduce scatter radiation.
- Immobilize the head.
- Ask the patient to suspend respiration for the exposure.

---

[1]Frank ED et al: Use of the posteroanterior projection: a method of reducing x-ray exposure to specific radiosensitive organs, Radiol Technol 54:343-347, 1983.

Temporal bone

Central ray

- Direct the central ray perpendicular to exit the nasion. In patients with brachycephalic (short front-to-back) skulls, the petrosae lie somewhat higher. Therefore, a caudad angulation of approximately 5 degrees is often needed to project the acoustic canals within the orbits. In patients with dolichocephalic (long front-to-back) skulls, the internal structures are generally lower and therefore need an approximate 5-degree cephalic angulation of the central ray as shown in Figs. 23-63 and 23-64.

Structures shown

The PA projection demonstrates the internal acoustic (auditory) canals projected through the orbits as seen in Fig. 23-65. The distance between the floor and roof of each internal acoustic (auditory) canal should be equal. A height difference of 2 mm or more may suggest a pathologic condition such as an acoustic neuroma.

☐ Evaluation criteria

The following should be clearly demonstrated:

- Petrous ridges inferior to the superior margin of the orbits.
- No sagittal rotation as evidenced by an equal distance between the lateral margins of the skull and the orbitals.
- Close collimation enabling visualization of the internal acoustic (auditory) canals.

Internal acoustic canal (superior margin)

Semicircular canals

Vestibule and cochlea

Internal acoustic canal (inferior margin)

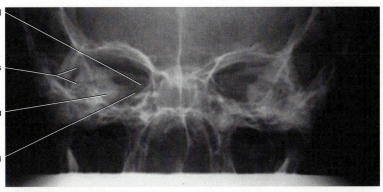

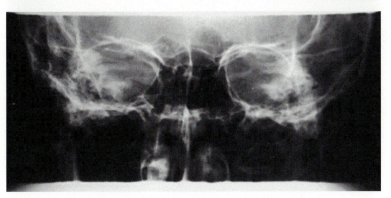

Fig. 23-65. PA (transorbital) petromastoid region.

(Courtesy Cheryl Stillberger, R.T.)

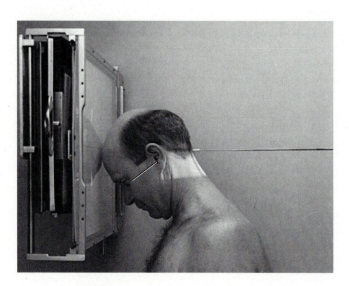

Fig. 23-66. PA axial petromastoid region.

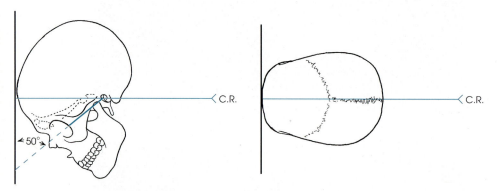

< C.R.

< C.R.

Fig. 23-67. Upright radiography.

50°

C.R.

C.R.

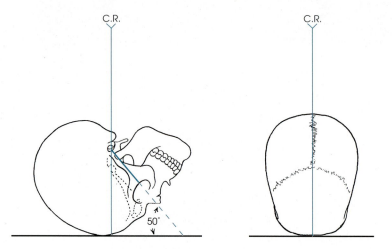

50°

Fig. 23-68. Table radiography.

Petromastoid Portion

PA AXIAL PROJECTION
VALDINI METHOD

Film: 8×10 in (18×24 cm) lengthwise.

Position of patient

- Seat the patient before a vertical grid device or place in the prone position with the thorax elevated on several firm pillows to permit complete flexion of the neck.
- Center the median sagittal plane of the body to the midline of the grid.
- Place the patient's arms in a comfortable position.
- Adjust the shoulders to lie in the same transverse plane.

Position of part

- Rest the patient's head on the upper frontal region and adjust it so that the median sagittal plane is perpendicular to the midline of the grid.
- Place a protractor beside the face and adjust the flexion of the neck (1) to place the *infraorbitomeatal* line at a 50-degree angle from the plane of the film for the demonstration of the labyrinths and the internal acoustic (auditory) canals (Fig. 23-66) and (2) to place the *orbitomeatal* line at a 50-degree angle from the plane of the film for the demonstration of the external acoustic (auditory) canals, the tympanic cavities, and the bony part of the eustachian tube (Figs. 23-67 and 23-68).
- Center the film at, or a little above, the level of the external acoustic (auditory) meatuses.
- Immobilize the head.
- Ask the patient to suspend respiration for the exposure.

Central ray

- Direct the central ray perpendicular through the foramen magnum at, or slightly superior to, the level of the external acoustic (auditory) meatuses.

Structures shown

Because of the absence of angular distortion, the Valdini method gives an excellent image of the vestibulocochlear organ (of hearing). The labyrinth and the internal acoustic (auditory) canal are best shown when the head is adjusted by the infraorbitomeatal line (Fig. 23-69). The external auditory canal, the tympanic cavity, and the bony part of the eustachian tube are shown to best advantage when the head is adjusted by the orbitomeatal line (Figs. 23-70).

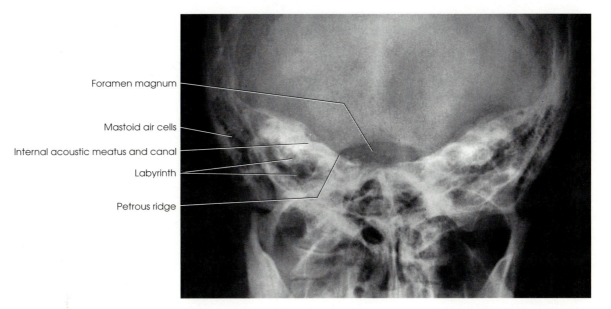

Foramen magnum

Mastoid air cells

Internal acoustic meatus and canal

Labyrinth

Petrous ridge

Fig. 23-69. PA axial petromastoid portion: infraorbitomeatal line 50 degrees.

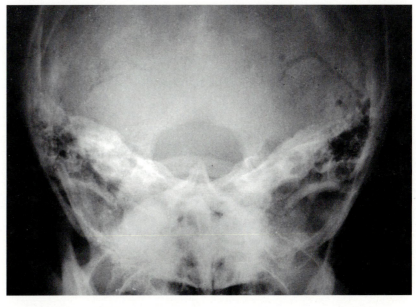

Fig. 23-70. PA axial petromastoid portion: orbitomeatal line 50 degrees.

Petromastoid portion

431

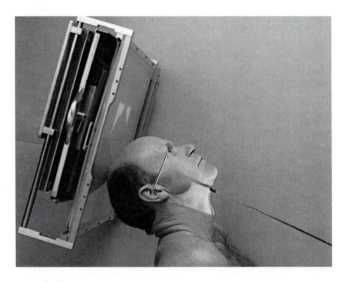

Fig. 23-71. Upright: submentovertical (subbasal) petromastoid portion. Central ray perpendicular to orbitomeatal line.

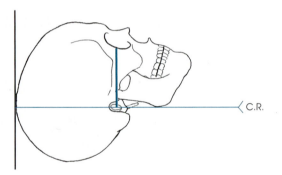

Fig. 23-72. Upright: central ray perpendicular to orbitomeatal line.

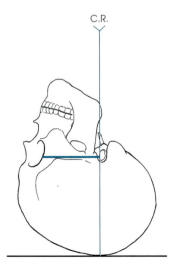

Fig. 23-73. Table: central ray perpendicular to orbitomeatal line.

Petromastoid Portion
SUBMENTOVERTICAL PROJECTIONS

In the submentovertical (SMV) basilar projection used for examination of the ear structures, the head is adjusted or the central ray is angled to obtain less superimposition of the structures than is obtained with the basilar projection used for general survey examinations of the base of the cranium. (Recall that for the basilar cranium projection, the central ray is perpendicular to the infraorbitomeatal line.) The goal of the basilar projection for the petromastoid portion is to project the long axis of the external acoustic (auditory) meatuses, the tympanic cavities, and the osseous part of the auditory (eustachian) tubes immediately behind the mandibular condyles.

Film: 8 × 10 in (18 × 24 cm).

Position of patient

- Seat the patient before a vertical grid device or place in the supine position with the trunk elevated enough to permit full extension of the neck. When the patient is in the supine position, the knees should be flexed to relax the abdominal muscles.

Position of part

- Center the median sagittal plane of the body to the midline of the grid.
- With the patient's arms placed in a comfortable position, adjust the shoulders to lie in the same transverse plane to prevent rotation of the head.
- Rest the head on the vertex and adjust it so that the median sagittal plane is perpendicular to the midline of the grid.
- Position the patient using either of two basic approaches:
  - Adjust the extension of the neck so that the orbitomeatal line is parallel with the plane of the film (Figs. 23-71 to 23-73). When the neck cannot be fully extended, the central ray should be angled anteriorly until it is perpendicular to the orbitomeatal line (Fig. 23-74).
  - An alternate method is to adjust the extension of the neck so that the supraorbitomeatal line is parallel with the plane of the film (Figs. 23-75 and 23-76).
- Adjust the position of the cassette so that the midpoint will coincide with the central ray.
- Immobilize the head.
- Ask the patient to suspend respiration for the exposure.

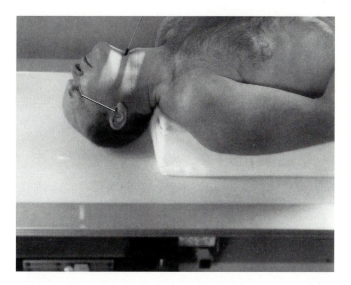

Fig. 23-74. Supine: Submentovertical petromastoid portion. Central ray perpendicular to orbitomeatal line.

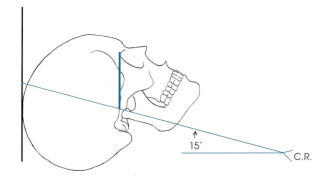

Fig. 23-75. Upright: supraorbitomeatal line parallel with film plane.

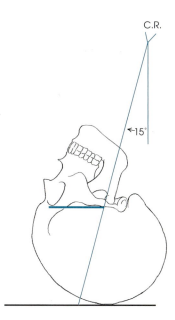

Fig. 23-76. Table: supraorbitomeatal line parallel with film plane.

Petromastoid portion

433

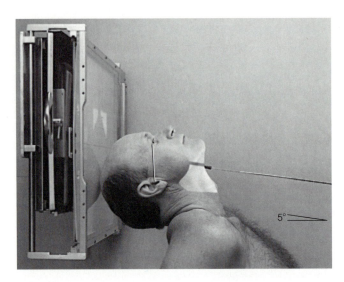

Fig. 23-77. Upright submentovertical petromastoid portion. Hirtz method. Central ray 5 degrees to orbitomeatal line.

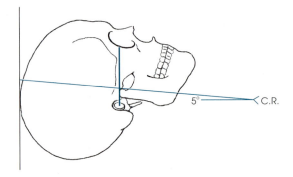

Fig. 23-78. Upright: Hirtz method.

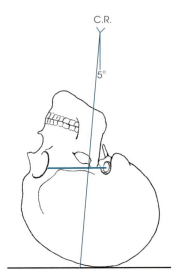

Fig. 23-79. Table: Hirtz method.

Central ray

- For the general submentovertical projection, direct the central ray (1) perpendicular to the orbitomeatal line (Figs. 23-71 to 23-74) and center it midway between the external acoustic (auditory) meatuses, or (2) through the median sagittal plane of the throat at a point 1 inch (2.5 cm) anterior to the level of the external acoustic (auditory) meatuses at an anterior angle of 15 to 20 degrees to the supraorbitomeatal line (Fig. 23-75 and 23-76).

- For the Hirtz method,[1] direct the central ray to a point midway between, and 1 inch (2.5 cm) anterior to, the external acoustic (auditory) meatuses at an anterior angle of 5 degrees (Figs. 23-77 to 23-79).

- As in all examinations, the basic central ray angulations are varied according to the requirements of the individual patient.

---

[1]Hirtz EJ: Quelques nouveaux détails sur la radiographie de la base du crane, Bull Soc Radiol Med Paris 10:110-113, 1922.

Structures shown

A symmetric axial projection of the petrosae demonstrates the mastoid processes, the labyrinths, the external acoustic (auditory) meatuses, the tympanic cavities, and the acoustic (auditory) ossicles (Fig. 23-80).

□ Evaluation criteria

The following should be clearly demonstrated:
- Mandibular condyles anterior to the external acoustic (auditory) canals and the petrous pyramids.
- Organs of hearing within the petrosae.
- Distance from the lateral border of the skull to the mandibular condyles equal on both sides.
- Petrosae symmetric.
- Close beam restriction of the petrosal region.

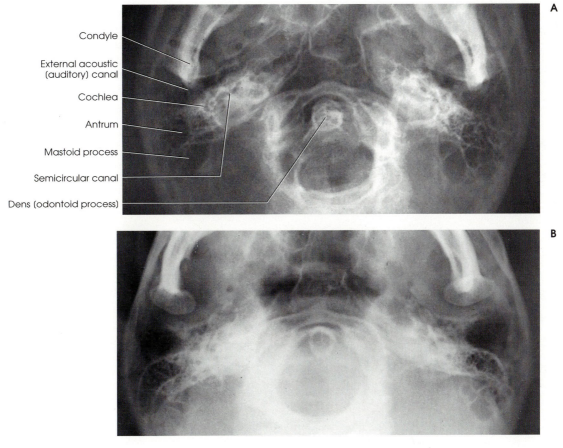

Condyle
External acoustic (auditory) canal
Cochlea
Antrum
Mastoid process
Semicircular canal
Dens (odontoid process)

A

B

Fig. 23-80. Submentovertical petromastoid region.

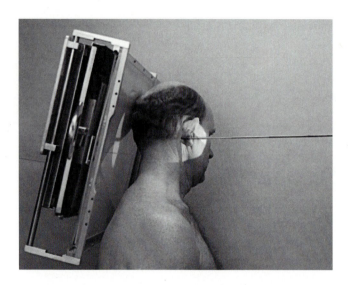

Fig. 23-81. AP tangential mastoid process (modified).

Mastoid Process
AP TANGENTIAL PROJECTION
MODIFIED HICKEY METHOD

Film: 8 × 10 in (18 × 24 cm).

Position of patient

- Place the patient in the supine or the seated-upright position.
- Center the median sagittal plane to the center of the grid.

Position of part

- Tape the auricles forward.
- Center the cassette 1 inch (2.5 cm) above the palpable tip of the mastoid process.
- Using a protractor, rotate the face away from the side being examined so that the median sagittal plane forms a 55-degree angle from the plane of the film.
- Adjust the head so that the infraorbitomeatal line is horizontal (upright) or vertical (supine). (Figs. 23-81 to 23-83).
- Immobilize the head.
- Ask the patient to suspend respiration for the exposure.

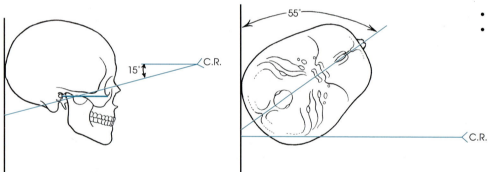

Fig. 23-82. Upright radiography.

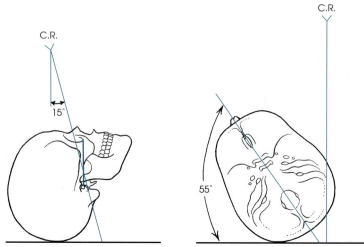

Fig. 23-83. Table radiography.

Central ray

- Direct the central ray 15-degrees caudad to the midpoint of the cassette. It enters the anterior border of the mastoid process at the junction of the auricle of the ear and the head 1 inch superior to the palpable tip of mastoid process.

Structures shown

A tangential projection of the mastoid process is demonstrated, projected free of superimposition of the adjacent bony structures (Fig. 23-84).

□ Evaluation criteria

The following should be clearly demonstrated:

- Mastoid process visible below the shadow of the occipital bone.
- Low contrast showing the two bone densities of the antrum and tip equally well.
- Auricle of the ear not superimposing the mastoid.
- Close beam restriction of the mastoid region.

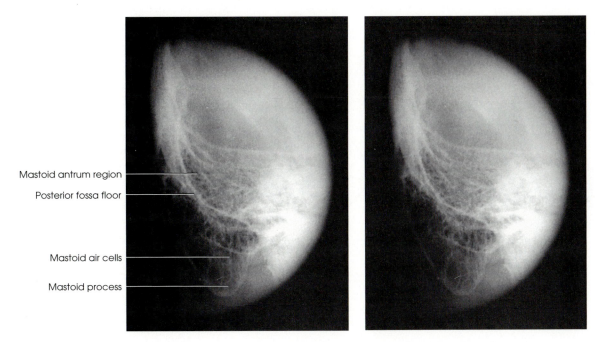

Mastoid antrum region

Posterior fossa floor

Mastoid air cells

Mastoid process

Fig. 23-84. AP tangential mastoid process.

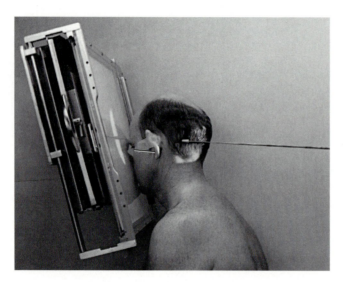

Fig. 23-85. PA tangential mastoid process.

Mastoid Process

PA TANGENTIAL PROJECTION

Film: 8 × 10 in (18 × 24 cm).

Position of patient

- Place the patient in the seated-upright or prone position.
- With the patient in the prone position, elevate the chest on a firm pillow to enable the head to be placed on a 15-degree inclined angle sponge.

Position of part

- Make a mark at a point 1 inch (2.5 cm) superior to the palpable tip of each mastoid process.
- Tape the auricles forward.
- For the upright position, tilt the top of the grid device 15 degrees away from the patient. Place the front of the head against the grid device.
- For the prone patient, place the cassette on the inclined 15-degree–angle sponge and adjust it under the patient's head (Fig. 23-87).
- Immobilize the cassette with sandbags to prevent it from slipping during the adjustment of the head.

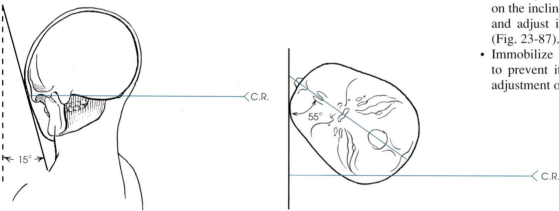

Fig. 23-86. Upright radiography.

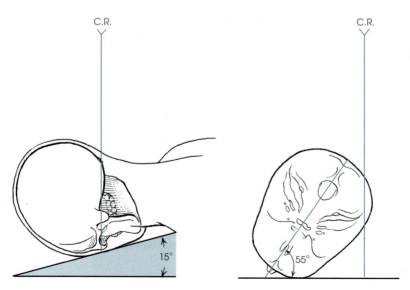

Fig. 23-87. Table radiography.

- Rest the patient's cheek on the grid device with the localization point centered to the cassette.
- Adjust the head so that the infraorbitomeatal line is perpendicular to the plane of the film.
- Using a protractor as a guide, rotate the face away from the side of interest until the median sagittal plane forms an angle of 55 degrees to the plane of the film (Figs. 23-85 to 23-87).
- Immobilize the head.
- Ask the patient to suspend respiration for the exposures.

Central ray

- Direct the central ray to the midpoint of the film. It enters the posterior border of the dependent mastoid process at the junction of the auricle of the ear and the head 1 inch superior to the palpable tip of the mastoid process.
- If necessary, adapt this projection to the seated-upright position by angling the central ray 15 degrees cephalad instead of the film.

Structures shown

This image demonstrates a PA tangential projection of the mastoid process, projected free of superimposition shadows of adjacent structures (Fig. 23-88).

The following should be clearly demonstrated:

- Mastoid process visible below the occipital bone and above the mandibular condyle.
- Low contrast showing the two bone densities of the antrum and tip equally well.
- Auricle of the ear not superimposing the mastoid.
- Close beam restriction of the mastoid region.

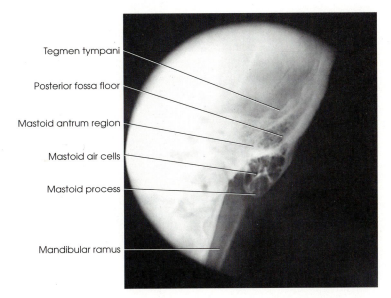
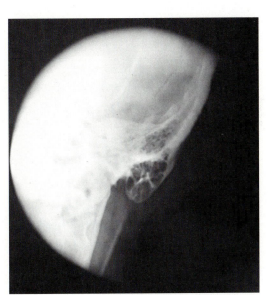

Tegmen tympani
Posterior fossa floor
Mastoid antrum region
Mastoid air cells
Mastoid process
Mandibular ramus

Fig. 23-88. PA tangential mastoid process.

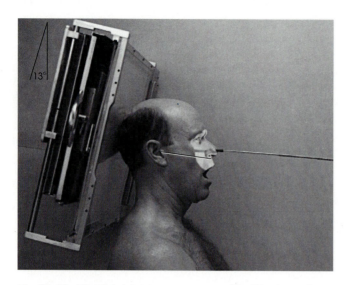

Fig. 23-89. AP axial styloid processes, modified Fuchs method.

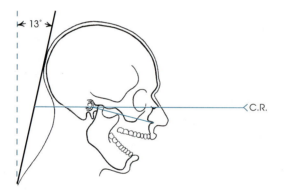

Fig. 23-90. Upright radiography.

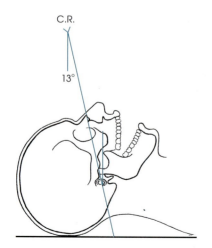

Fig. 23-91. Table radiography.

Styloid Processes
AP PROJECTION
MODIFIED FUCHS METHOD[1]

Film: 8 × 10 in (18 × 24 cm).

Position of patient

- Place the patient in the seated-upright or supine position.
- The grid device is angled 13 degrees with the top inward toward the patient.
- Center the median sagittal plane to the midline of the grid.
- Place the arms in a comfortable position and adjust the shoulders to lie in the same transverse plane.

Position of part

- Center the cassette to the median sagittal plane of the head at the level of the external acoustic (auditory) meatuses.
- With the median sagittal plane aligned, extend the neck to place the acanthomeatal line perpendicular to the plane of the film.
- Immobilize the head and instruct the patient to open the mouth (Figs. 23-89 to 23-91).
- Recheck the position of the acanthomeatal line.
- Have the patient hold the mouth open during the exposure to prevent the coronoid processes of the mandible from being superimposed on those of the styloid processes.
- Ask the patient to suspend respiration for the exposure.

[1]In the original method the central ray is directed vertically and the cassette is placed on a 13-degree caudally inclined angle block.

Central ray

• The central ray is directed 13 degrees caudally from being perpendicular to the plane of the film. It is directed through the median sagittal plane and parallel with a line extending through the external acoustic (auditory) meatuses. For the supine position, direct the central ray 13 degrees caudad.

Structures shown

A symmetric image of the styloid processes of the temporal bone is projected within the shadows of the maxillary sinus (Fig. 23-92).

□Evaluation criteria

The following should be clearly demonstrated:

■ Occipital bone and coronoid processes of the mandible superimposing the temporal styloid processes.
■ No rotation of the head.

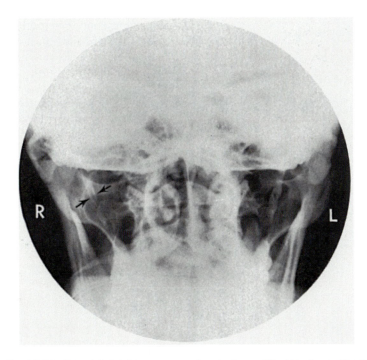

Fig. 23-92. AP axial styloid processes *(arrows)*, modified Fuchs method.

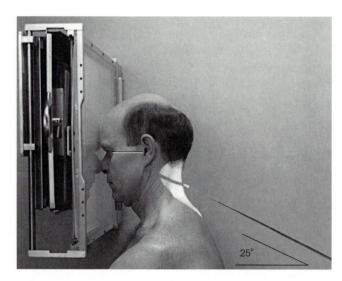

Fig. 23-93. PA axial styloid processes, Cahoon method.

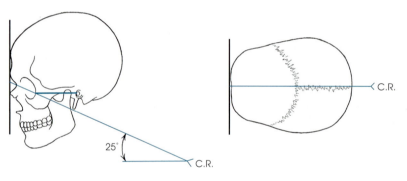

Fig. 23-94. Upright radiography.

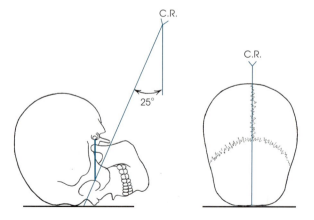

Fig. 23-95. Table radiography.

Styloid Processes
PA AXIAL PROJECTION
CAHOON METHOD

Film: 8 × 10 in (18 × 24 cm).

Position of patient

- Place the patient in the seated-upright or prone position.
- Center the median sagittal plane of the body to the midline of the grid.
- Have the patient flex the elbows.
- Place the arms in a comfortable position and adjust the shoulders to lie in the same transverse plane.

Position of part

- Rest the patient's forehead and nose on the grid device and adjust it so that the median sagittal plane is perpendicular to the midline of the grid.
- Center the cassette to the nasion.
- Adjust the flexion of the neck so that the orbitomeatal line is perpendicular to the plane of the film (Figs. 23-93 to 23-95).
- Immobilize the head.
- Ask the patient to suspend respiration for the exposure.

Central ray

- Direct the central ray to the nasion at an angle of 25 degrees cephalad.

Structures shown

The Cahoon method demonstrates a symmetric image of the styloid processes of the temporal bones projected within or just above the maxillary sinuses (Fig. 23-96).

The following should be clearly demonstrated:

- Temporal styloid processes free of superimposition from the frontal bone, occipital bone, and the coronoid processes of the mandible.
- No rotation of the head.

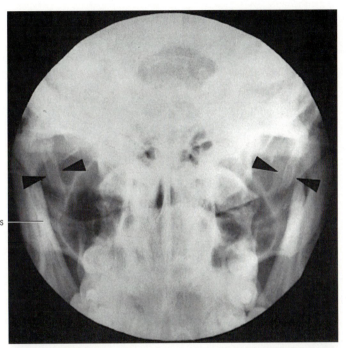

Coronoid process

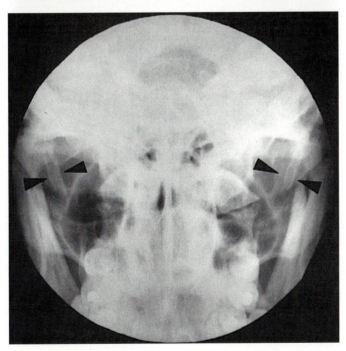

Fig. 23-96. PA axial styloid processes *(arrows)*, modified Cahoon method.

443

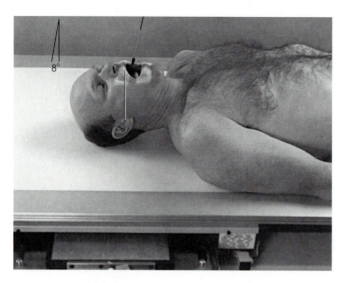

Fig. 23-97. AP oblique styloid process, Wigby-Taylor method.

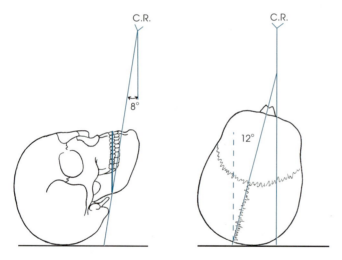

Fig. 23-98. Table radiography.

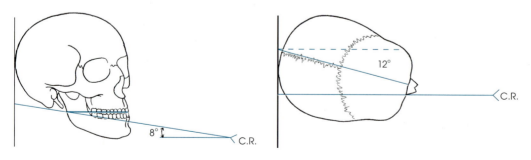

Fig. 23-99. Upright radiography.

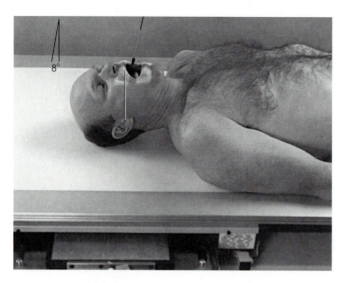

Styloid Process

AP OBLIQUE PROJECTION
WIGBY-TAYLOR METHOD

Film: 8×10 in (18×24 cm).

Position of patient

- Make a mark on each side of the posterior surface of the neck at a point 1 inch (2.5 cm) lateral to the median sagittal plane at the level of the mastoid tip.
- Place the patient in the supine position.
- Align the body so that the marked localization point of the side being examined is centered to the midline of the grid.
- Place the arms along the sides of the body and adjust the shoulders to lie in the same transverse plane.

Position of part

- With the localization point centered to the midline of the grid, rest the patient's head on the occiput.
- Using a protractor as a guide, rotate the median sagittal plane 12 degrees from the perpendicular toward the side being examined.
- Extend the neck enough so that the occlusal plane of the upper teeth is perpendicular to the plane of the film (Figs. 23-97 to 23-99).
- After immobilizing the head, instruct the patient to open the mouth wide and then recheck the position of the occlusal plane.
- Have the patient hold the mouth open during the exposure in order to move the coronoid process of the mandible inferiorly.

Temporal bone

- Center the cassette to a point 1 inch (2.5 cm) above the tip of the mastoid process.
- *Respiration:* Most patients mouths can be immobilized in the open position by softly phonating "ah-h-h." If not, ask the patient to suspend respiration for the exposure.

Central ray

- With the central ray at an angle of 8 degrees cephalad, direct it along a line passing approximately ¼ inch (0.6 cm) distal to the tip of the mastoid process of the side adjacent to the film.

Structures shown

This image shows an oblique projection of the styloid process overlying the soft tissues of the neck (Fig. 23-100). Both sides are examined for comparison.

□ Evaluation criteria

The following should be clearly demonstrated:

- Temporal styloid process not superimposing the teeth, occipital bone, or the coronoid process of the mandible.
- Styloid process with a soft tissue density.

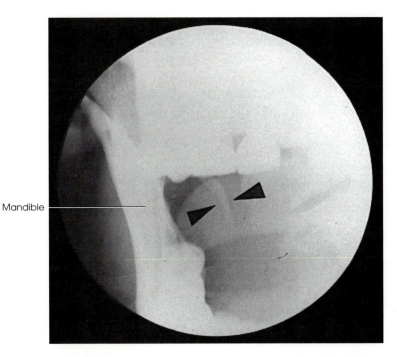

Mandible

Fig. 23-100. AP oblique styloid process *(arrows)*, Wigby-Taylor method.

Styloid Process

AXIOLATERAL OBLIQUE PROJECTION
FUCHS METHOD

Film: 8 × 10 in (18 × 24 cm) nongrid.

Position of patient

- Place the patient in a semiprone position.
- Adjust the rotation of the body to place the median sagittal plane of the head horizontal.
- Instruct the patient to rest on the forearm and flexed knee.
- Place the arms in a comfortable position and adjust the shoulders to lie in the same transverse plane.

Position of part

- Center the external acoustic (auditory) meatus to the cassette and rest the head in a lateral position.
- Adjust the head so that the median sagittal plane is parallel with, and the interpupillary line is perpendicular to, the plane of the film.
- Adjust the flexion of the neck so that the acanthomeatal line is parallel with the transverse axis of the film.
- After immobilizing the head, instruct the patient to open the mouth wide to move the coronoid processes of the mandible inferiorly (Figs. 23-101 and 23-102).
- Recheck the position of the head after the mouth is opened.
- Ask the patient to suspend respiration for the exposure.

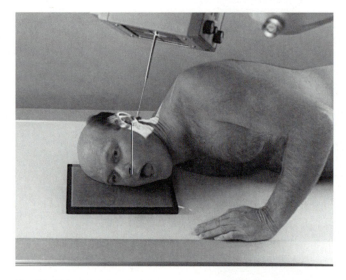

Fig. 23-101. Axiolateral oblique styloid process, Fuchs method.

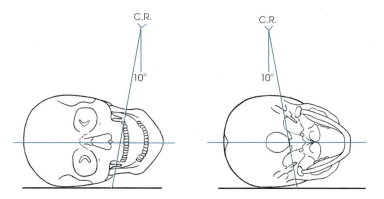

C.R. 10°   C.R. 10°

Fig. 23-102. Table radiography.

Central ray

- Direct the central ray to exit the external acoustic (auditory) meatus closest to the film at an angle of 10 degrees cephalad and 10 degrees anteriorly.

Structures shown

A lateral image of the styloid process projected into the space superior to the mandibular notch is demonstrated (Fig. 23-103). Both sides are usually examined for comparison.

The following should be clearly demonstrated:

- Styloid process free of superimposition from the cervical vertebrae, mandible, or the styloid process from the opposite side.

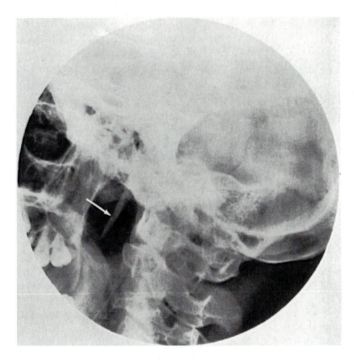

Fig. 23-103. Axiolateral oblique styloid process *(arrow)*, Fuchs method.

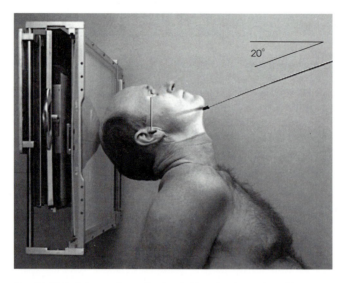

Fig. 23-104. Submentovertical axial jugular foramina, Kemp Harper method.

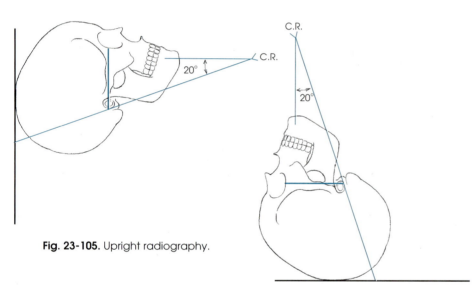

Fig. 23-105. Upright radiography.

Fig. 23-106. Table radiography.

Jugular Foramina

SUBMENTOVERTICAL AXIAL PROJECTION
KEMP HARPER METHOD[1]

Film: 8×10 in (18×24 cm).

Position of patient

- For the submentovertical (SMV) axial projection, place the patient in the supine or seated-upright position. In the supine position, it may be necessary to elevate the patient's trunk to permit full extension of the head. The head can be extended more fully and more comfortably from the seated-upright position.

Position of part

- Center the median sagittal plane of the body and head to the midline of the grid device.
- Rest the patient's head on the vertex and adjust it so that the orbitomeatal line is parallel with the plane of the film.
- Recheck the perpendicular median sagittal plane (Figs. 23-104 to 23-106).
- Adjust the position of the film so that its midpoint will coincide with the central ray.
- Immobilize the head.
- Ask the patient to suspend respiration for the exposure.

Central ray

- Direct the central ray to a point 1 inch (2.5 cm) distal to the mandibular symphysis at a 20-degree posterior angle. It should parallel a line passing through, or just distal to, the external acoustic (auditory) meatuses (Fig. 23-107).

[1]Kemp Harper RA: Glomus jugulare tumors of the temporal bone, J Fac Radiologists 8:325-334, 1957.

Coronoid process

Mandibular angle

Dens (odontoid process)

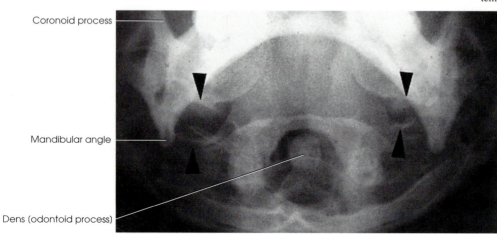

Fig. 23-107. Submentovertical axial jugular foramina *(arrowheads)*, Kemp Harper method.

Temporal bone

ERASO MODIFICATION[1]

The Eraso modification is not as demanding a position for the patient to assume as the SMV Kemp Harper method.

Position of part

- Place the patient similarly to the Kemp Harper position with the orbitomeatal line placed at an angle of 25 degrees from the plane of the film (Figs. 23-108 to 23-110).
- With the median sagittal plane perpendicular to the film, center the film 1 inch (2.5 cm) below the level of the external acoustic (auditory) meatuses.

Central ray

- Direct the central ray perpendicular to the midpoint of the film entering approximately 2 inches (5 cm) distal to the mandibular symphysis.

Structures shown

Both submentovertical axial projections (Figs. 23-107 and 23-111) demonstrate the jugular foramina projected at or near the level of the angles of the mandible. When examining a patient who has a prominent mandible, the central ray angle may be increased from 5 to 10 degrees caudally.

□ Evaluation criteria

The following should be clearly demonstrated:

- Jugular foramina free of superimposition from the mandible.
- Distance from the angle of the mandibles to the lateral border of the skull equal on both sides.
- The Eraso modification will project the jugular foramen at an angle 5 degrees greater than the Kemp Harper method.

NOTE: Strickler[2] suggests a modification of the Eraso method wherein the neck is extended until a line passing through the infratragal notch and a point 2 cm distal to the mandibular symphysis is perpendicular to the plane of the film. The central ray coincides with this line.

[1]Eraso ST: Roentgen and clinical diagnosis of glomus jugulare tumors, Radiology 77:252-256, 1961.
[2]Strickler JM: New and simple techniques for demonstration of the jugular foramen, AJR 97:601-606, 1966.

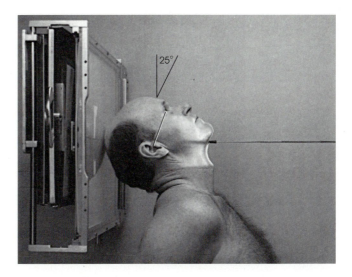

Fig. 23-108. Eraso modification of Kemp Harper method.

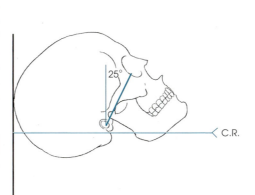

Fig. 23-109. Eraso modification: upright radiography.

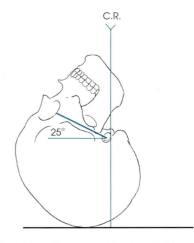

Fig. 23-110. Eraso modification: table radiography.

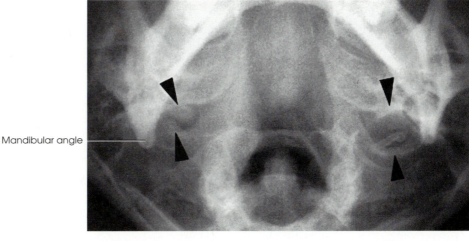

Mandibular angle

Fig. 23-111. Eraso modification of Kemp Harper method, demonstrating jugular foramina (arrows).

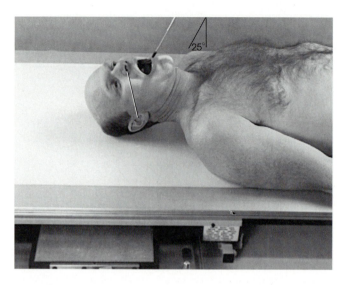

Fig. 23-112. AP axial (transoral) jugular foramina, Chaussé II method.

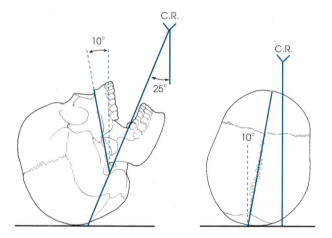

Fig. 23-113. Table radiography.

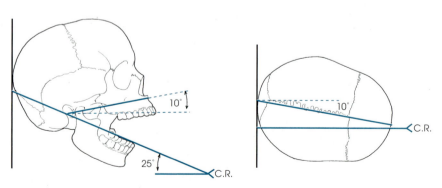

Fig. 23-114. Upright radiography.

Jugular Foramina

AP AXIAL PROJECTION (TRANSORAL)
CHAUSSÉ II METHOD[1]

Film: 8 × 10 in (18 × 24 cm) crosswise.

Position of patient

- Place the patient in the supine position. In the examination of a short-necked subject, it may be necessary to elevate the shoulders on a pillow to obtain adequate extension of the neck.

Position of part

- Rotate the median sagittal plane 10 degrees toward the side being examined.
- Adjust the position so the inner canthus of the lowermost side is centered to the midline of the grid.
- Adjust the extension of the neck to place the acanthomeatal line at an angle of 10 degrees, open cranially, from the vertical.
- After adjusting the central ray angulation and the position of the film, recheck the position of the patient's head and, while holding it in position, ask the patient to open the mouth as wide as possible (Figs. 23-112 to 23-114).
- *Respiration:* Most patients' mouths can be immobilized in the open position by softly phonating "ah-h-h." If not, ask the patient to suspend respiration for the exposure.

---

[1]Chaussé C: Trois incidences pour l'examen du rocher, Acta Radiol 34:274-287, 1950.

Central ray

- The central ray is directed through the open mouth at an angle of 25 degrees cephalad. It parallels a line passing just distal to the tragus and is in line with the inner canthus of the eye to the side closest to the film.

Structures shown

The jugular foramen on the side closest to the table is seen through the open mouth between the shadows of the upper and lower molars (Fig. 23-115). The contralateral jugular foramen is clearly delineated through the superjacent mandibular ramus.

□ Evaluation criteria

The following should be clearly demonstrated:

- Jugular foramen on the side closest to the table free of superimposition from the upper and lower molars or the mandibular ramus.
- Jugular foramen on the contralateral side visible through the superimposing mandibular ramus.

NOTE: Strickler[1] suggests two transoral positions, one bilateral and one unilateral. The patient is placed in the supine position, the shoulders elevated on a pillow and the median sagittal plane of the body centered to the midline of the table. The patient is asked to open the mouth wide, and the head is then adjusted until the gap between the upper and lower molars and the infratragal notch is aligned on a vertical axis. The central ray traverses this axis. For a bilateral radiograph the head is adjusted so that the median sagittal plane is vertical. The central ray passes through the midline. For a unilateral radiograph the patient's head is rotated 10 degrees or less away from the side being examined; this centers the uppermost jugular foramen to the central ray.

[1]Strickler JM: New and simple techniques for demonstration of the jugular foramen, AJR 97:601-606, 1966.

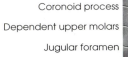

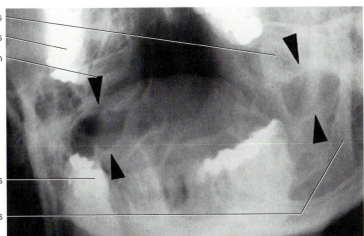
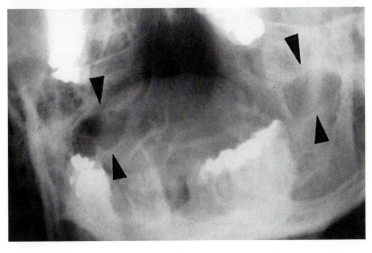

Coronoid process
Dependent upper molars
Jugular foramen
Lower molars
Mandible ramus

Fig. 23-115. AP axial (transoral) jugular foramina, Chaussé II method.

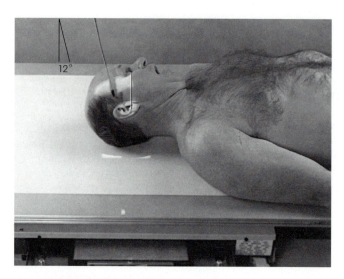

Fig. 23-116. Axiolateral oblique hypoglossal canal. Anterior profile, Miller method.

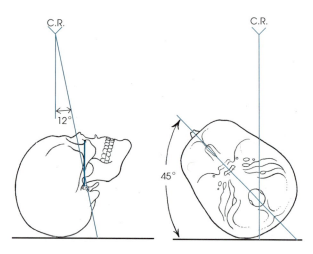

Fig. 23-117. Table radiography.

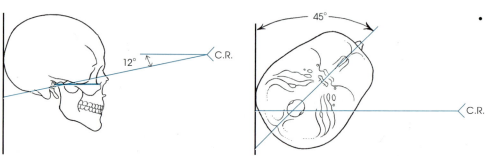

Fig. 23-118. Upright radiography.

Hypoglossal Canal

AXIOLATERAL OBLIQUE PROJECTION (ANTERIOR PROFILE) MILLER METHOD

The Miller method is used to delineate the hypoglossal canal in cases of hypoglossal (twelfth cranial) nerve tumor. The hypoglossal canals, one on each side, pass through the lateral part of the occipital bone at the base of the anterior limb of the occipital condyle. These canals transmit the twelfth cranial nerves, which are the motor nerves of the tongue.

Film: 8 × 10 in (18 × 24 cm).

Position of patient

- Place the patient in the supine position or seated before a vertical grid device.

Position of part

- Make a mark on each cheek at a point 1 inch (2.5 cm) directly anterior to, and ½ inch (1.2 cm) inferior to, the level of the external acoustic (auditory) meatus.
- Rotate the median sagittal plane 45 degrees away from the side being examined.
- Adjust the position of the patient so that the localization mark is centered over the midline of the grid.
- Adjust the cassette tray to center the film ¾ inch (1.9 cm) below the localization mark.
- Using a protractor, check the 45-degree obliquity of the head.
- Ask the patient to open the mouth as wide as possible.
- Adjust the flexion of the neck so that the infraorbitomeatal line is parallel with the transverse axis of the film (Figs. 23-116 to 23-118).
- Immobilize the head and have the patient softly phonate "ah-h-h" to immobilize the mouth in the open position.
- If respiration cannot be controlled by having the patient phonate "ah-h-h," ask the patient to suspend respiration for the exposure.

452

Central ray

- Direct the central ray at an angle of 12 degrees caudad to enter 1 inch (2.5 cm) directly anterior to, and ½ inch (1.2 cm) inferior to, the level of the external acoustic (auditory) meatus on the side farthest from the film.

Structures shown

A profile, or image of the hypoglossal canal is shown (Figs. 23-119). The mandibular condyle is projected inferior and anterior to that of the canal when the patient can open the mouth wide enough. Because of normal anatomic variations, the ideal image is not always obtained. Compare the accompanying radiographs.

The following should be clearly demonstrated:
- Hypoglossal canal in profile inferior to the petrous bone.
- Mandibular condyle not superimposing the hypoglossal canal.

NOTE: Kirdani[1] and Valvassori and Kirdani[2] recommend that the hypoglossal canal be examined by tomographic sectioning in the submentovertical, semiaxial anteroposterior, and Stenvers positions. These studies also provide excellent demonstration of the jugular foramina.

---

[1]Kirdani MA: The normal hypoglossal canal, AJR 99:700-704, 1967.
[2]Valvassori E and Kirdani MA: The abnormal hypoglossal canal, AJR 99:705-711, 1967.

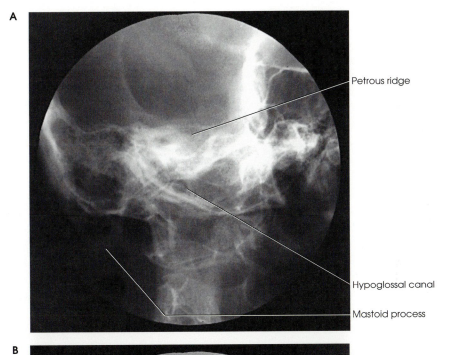

A

Petrous ridge

Hypoglossal canal

Mastoid process

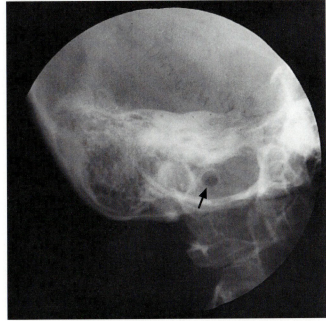

B

Fig. 23-119. Axiolateral oblique hypoglossal canal *(arrow)*. Anterior profile, Miller method.

Chapter 24

MAMMOGRAPHY

ROME V. WADLINGTON

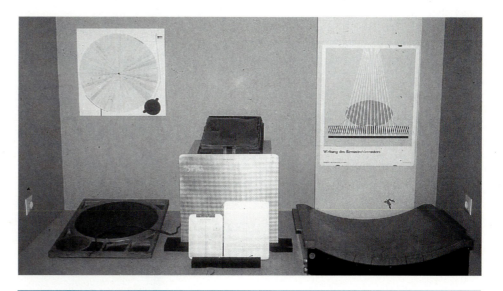

Radiographic grids and a wooden tabletop. Note the circular (rotating) grid device on the left.

Introduction and Historical Development*

Mammography is the single most important innovation in breast cancer control since the introduction of the *radical mastectomy.*** in 1898. Mammography has done more to influence the detection and management of breast cancer than any other development since that time, and the importance of mammography is directly related to its value in the detection and management of breast cancer. If breast cancer did not exist, there would be few indications for mammography. Until 1984, breast cancer was the leading cause of death from cancer among American women, and 1 of every 9 American women will develop breast cancer in her lifetime. (In 1984 lung cancer became the leading cancer killer of women.) Although breast cancer is more common in older than in middle-aged women, the most common cause of death of women between the ages of 39 and 45 is breast cancer.

---

*Appreciation is extended to John O. Olsen, M.D., for his work in revising earlier editions of this chapter.
**All italicized terms are defined at the end of this chapter.

Before the development of the radical mastectomy operation by William Stewart Halstead, breast cancer was considered a hopeless and invariably fatal disease. Less than 5% of patients survived 4 years after the diagnosis, and the local recurrence rate of surgically treated breast cancer was over 80%. The 1898 Halstead procedure raised the 4-year survival rate to 40% and reduced the rate of local recurrence to approximately 10%. This was certainly a great step forward; however, over the next 60 years there was no additional improvement in breast cancer survival. Some principles of breast cancer management became clear, and those principles remain valid today. The patients who responded well to extensive surgery were those who had an early stage of the disease. Patients with advanced disease did poorly. The earlier the diagnosis of breast cancer is made, the better the chances of survival. The concept of removing all palpable breast masses in hopes of finding earlier cancers was developed, and it was recognized that careful physical examination of the breast could lead to the detection of some early breast cancers. However, most patients with breast cancer were not being diagnosed until their disease was advanced. This fact and the still dismal breast cancer survival statistics illustrated the need for a tool that would aid in the early detection of breast cancer. That need is filled by mammography (Fig. 24-1).

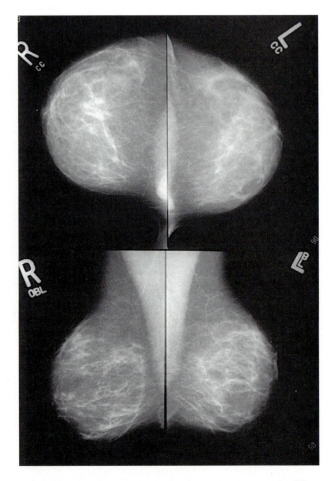

Fig. 24-1. A four-image, bilateral mammogram of a 37-year-old woman. Craniocaudal and mediolateral oblique projections demonstrate normal, symmetric breast parenchyma.

In 1913 a German physician named Soloman reported the radiographic appearance of breast cancers and described the mechanism of how breast cancer spread, based on x-ray studies of cancerous breasts removed at surgery. The first published radiograph of a living person's breast was made by Kleinschmidt, and it appeared in a 1927 German medical textbook on malignant tumors. During the 1930s there were publications on mammography from South America, the United States, and Europe, but there was little clinical interest in mammography for breast cancer diagnosis. A few pioneers, including LeBorgne in Uruguay, Gershon-Cohen in the United States, and Gros in Germany, published excellent comparisons of mammographic and pathologic anatomy and developed some of the clinical techniques of mammography. The significance of breast *microcalcifications* was well understood by that time. By the mid-1950s mammography was refined to the point of being a reliable clinical tool. Refinements included low kilovoltage x-ray tubes with molybdenum targets and high-detail, industrial-grade x-ray film. In the mid-1950s Egan in the United States and Gros in Germany popularized the application of mammography for the diagnosis and evaluation of breast cancer. Breast xerography was introduced in the 1960s and popularized by Wolfe and Ruzicka. Xerography substantially lowered the radiation dose received by the patient, compared with industrial grade x-ray film. Many practitioners found the xerographic images easier to understand and evaluate, and xeromammography was widely applied to the evaluation of breast disease. The first attempts at widespread population screening began at this time.

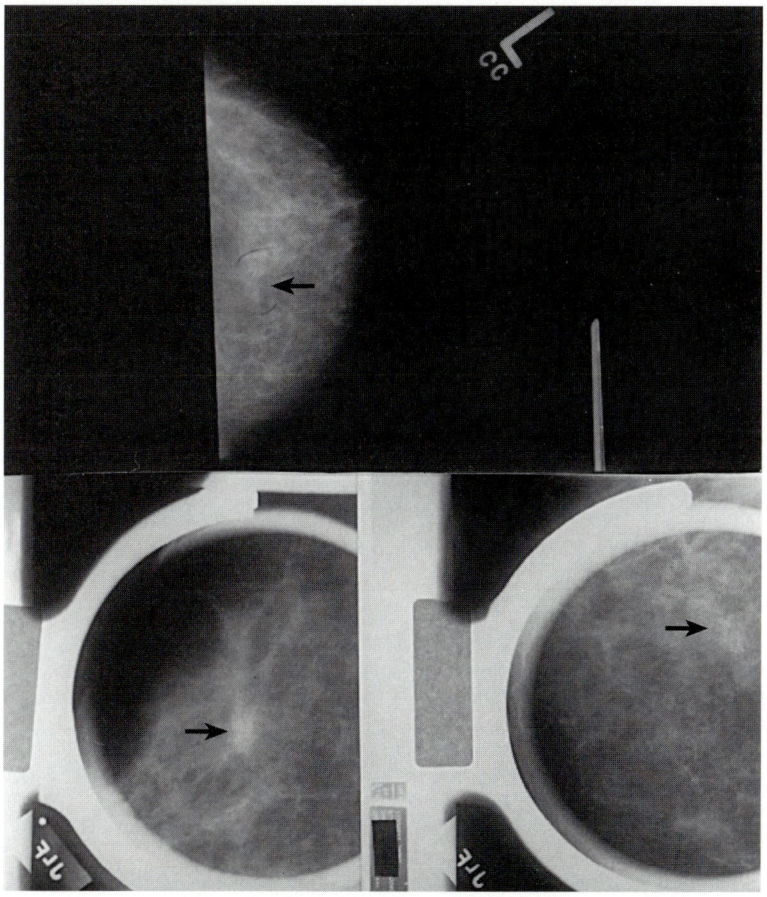

Higher-resolution, faster-speed x-ray film used in combination with an intensifying screen was first introduced by the Du Pont Company in 1970, again substantially reducing radiation exposure to the patient. Improved film-screen combinations were developed by both Kodak and Du Pont in 1975, and by this time extremely high-quality mammography images could be produced with very low patient radiation exposures. Even faster lower-dose films, magnification techniques, and grids for scatter rejection have since been introduced. It is now widely recognized that high-quality mammography, careful physical examination, and monthly breast self-examination (BSE) can lead to detection of breast cancer at an early stage when it is most curable (Fig. 24-2).

In 1973 the Breast Cancer Detection Demonstration Project (BCDDP) was implemented. In this project 280,000 women underwent annual screening for breast cancer at 29 locations throughout the United States for 5 years. This project, organized by the American Cancer Society and the National Cancer Institute, demonstrated unequivocally that a program of screening, physical examination, mammography, and breast self-examination leads to the earlier diagnosis of breast cancer. In the project over 41% of all the cancers were found only with mammography, and an even greater proportion of *early* breast cancers were found only with mammography. This study was not designed to demonstrate that early detection of breast cancer would lead to increased survival rates, but there is now definite evidence from carefully controlled studies in other countries, including the Netherlands, Sweden, and Germany, that the early diagnosis of breast cancer leads to an increase in its curability. In the United States, the HIP (Health Insurance Plan) study in New York City showed the same reduction in mortality from breast cancer through mammography screening in women over age 50.

Fig. 24-2. Microcalcifications are an early sign of breast cancer. A mass with calcifications (*arrow*, top illustration) is best visualized with two right angle projections (*arrows*, bottom illustration).

Risk Versus Benefit

In the mid-1970s a major controversy over mammography arose in which many members of the public developed the perception that the radiation exposure from diagnostic x-rays would cause breast cancer and would actually induce more breast cancers than would be detected. This is not the case, but fear of radiation exposure still causes some women to refuse mammography, and many women who undergo the examination are rightfully concerned about exposure levels and the resultant risk of carcinogenesis. For this reason it is necessary to understand the relationship between breast irradiation and breast cancer and to understand the relative risks of mammography in light of the natural incidence of breast cancer and the potential benefit of the examination. There is no direct evidence to suggest that the small doses of diagnostic x-rays used in mammography can induce the development of breast cancer. It has been demonstrated, however, that large doses of radiation can lead to an increased incidence of breast cancer and that the risk is dose dependent. The evidence that breast irradiation can increase the risk of breast cancer comes from three studies of groups of women who developed increased incidences of breast cancer after being exposed to large doses of radiation: (1) the population exposed to the atom bomb at Hiroshima and Nagasaki; (2) a group of women with tuberculosis who received multiple fluoroscopic examinations of the chest; and (3) a group of women who were treated with radiation for *postpartum mastitis*. In each case, the radiation received by the women was many times higher than that from mammography. Based on experience with large doses of radiation and using a linear dose response relationship, estimates of possible risks at lower levels of radiation can be made (Fig. 24-3). It can be estimated that 1 rad of radiation to the breast tissue will cause a 1% increase in the incidence of breast cancer over the natural incidence. The natural incidence of breast cancer is 8%, or 8 breast cancers for every 100 women, over their lifetime. An increase of 1% over the natural incidence would lead to a total incidence of 8.08% or almost 8.1 cancers in 100 women over their lifetime. This is the worst-case estimate because it assumes a direct linear relationship. The actual risk from 1 rad of radiation to the breast might be much lower, and it is definitely not higher. When scientists argue over whether the risk is low or very low, the uncertainty can confuse the public into thinking that the risk is unknown and therefore might be very high.

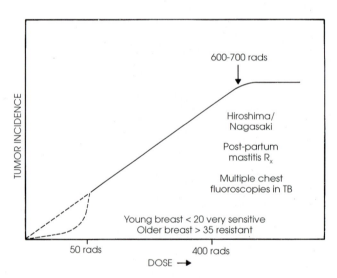

Fig. 24-3. Dose response curve for radiation-induced breast cancers. The *solid line* represents a summary of known data from three different populations exposed to large doses of radiation. Since there is no population data available that shows an increased incidence of breast cancer of doses under 50 rads, the *dotted lines* indicate estimated incidence of lower doses. The *upper straight-line* estimate is a direct extrapolation from the known data. This model is the one used in all calculations of radiation risk. The *lower curved line* is the pattern actually observed in all experimental animal studies of radiation-induced tumors. Although the curved model would predict a lower level of risk at lower levels of radiation, this model is not used in any patient risk calculations.

Today, the average radiation dose to the breast parenchyma in a high-quality xerographic or mammographic examination is actually much lower than 1 rad. The average mid-breast dose for a typical xerogram exposure in the BCDDP was 0.37 rad, and the average mid-breast dose for a typical film-screen mammogram exposure in the BCDDP was 0.04 rad. In comparison with other risks of living, the risk of having an x-ray film-screen mammogram is equivalent to the risk of smoking several cigarettes, driving 60 miles in an automobile, or being a 60-year-old man for 10 minutes.

Based on the success of the national BCDDP project in finding early breast cancer, it is possible to conservatively calculate that the *risk versus benefit* ratio of mammography is well over 25 to 1 for women who begin breast *screening* at age 50. That means that at least 25 cancers can be found and successfully treated for every cancer induced. In women 35 years of age who enroll in lifetime annual screening mammography, at least 10 cancers can be found and successfully treated for every cancer induced.

The current recommendations from the American Cancer Society and the American College of Radiology concerning screening mammography are that all women over the age of 50 should have an annual mammogram. Women between the ages of 40 and 50 should have an annual or biannual mammogram. A baseline examination made sometime before the onset of menopause is useful for subsequent evaluation of the breast.

An important observation in the previously mentioned population studies illustrating the potential sensitivity of breast tissue to radiation is that the breast tissue of women in their teens to early twenties seems to be much more sensitive to radiation than the breast tissue of women over the age of 30. We must be concerned with breast irradiation, and we need to conduct our examinations with as little radiation exposure as possible consistent with accurate detection.

Let us distinguish between *diagnosis* and detection. The mammogram is an excellent tool for the detection of breast cancer, but it does not diagnose breast cancer. Some lesions seen on the mammogram may appear consistent with malignant disease but turn out to be completely benign conditions. Breast cancer can therefore be diagnosed only by a pathologist evaluating a tissue sample from the lesion. However, mammography can detect lesions that may be cancerous. Once a lesion is detected, a more specific diagnostic evaluation of the patient, which might include aspiration, breast biopsy, or ultrasound examination, is indicated.

The preceding discussion addresses the screening of patients who do not have significant breast symptoms. All patients with clinical evidence of significant or potentially significant breast disease should undergo mammography, and all patients who are going to have a breast biopsy should have a mammogram (Fig. 24-4).

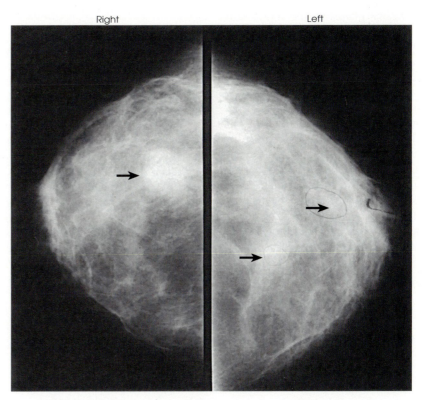

Fig. 24-4. Craniocaudal projections of the right and left breasts in a 28-year-old woman 4 months postpartum and not breast feeding. The right breast contains a large mass *(arrow)* palpable on physical examination. The left breast contains two smaller nonpalpable masses *(arrows)* with microcalcifications. All three lesions were breast cancers.

Anatomy and Physiology of the Breast

The terms *breast* and *mammary gland* are often used as synonyms. Anatomy textbooks tend to use the term mammary gland, whereas radiography texts tend to favor the term breast. The breasts (mammary glands) are lobulated glandular structures located within the superficial fascia of the anterolateral surface of the thorax of both males and females. The mammary glands divide the superficial fascia into anterior and posterior components, so the mammary tissue is completely surrounded by fascia and is enveloped between the anterior and posterior layers of superficial fascia. In the female, the breasts represent one of the secondary sex characteristics and function as accessory glands to the reproductive system by producing and secreting milk during lactation. In the male, the breasts are rudimentary and without function. Rarely, they are subject to abnormalities, such as neoplasm, which require radiologic evaluation.

The female breast varies considerably in size and shape, depending on the amount of fat and glandular tissue and the condition of the suspensory ligaments. Each breast is usually cone-shaped, with the base or posterior surface of the breast overlying the pectoralis major and serratus anterior muscles. These muscles extend from the second or third rib inferiorly to the sixth or seventh rib and from near the lateral margin of the sternum laterally toward the anterior axillary plane. An additional portion of breast tissue called the axillary prolongation or axillary "tail" of the breast extends from the upper lateral base of the breasts into the axillary fossa (Fig. 24-5).

The breast tapers anteriorly from the base, ending in the nipple, which is surrounded by a circular area of pigmented skin called the *areola*. The breasts are supported by suspensory ligaments extending from the posterior layers of the superficial fascia through the anterior fascia into the subcutaneous tissue and skin. These ligaments are called Cooper's ligaments. It is the condition of these ligaments and not relative fat content that gives the breasts firmness or lack of firmness.

The adult female breast consists of 15 to 20 lobes. The lobes are distributed so that there are more lobes superiorly and laterally than inferiorly and medially. Each lobe is divided into many lobules, which are the basic structural units of the breast. The lobules contain the glandular elements, or *acini*. Each lobule consists of several acini, draining ducts, and interlobular stroma or connective tissue. All these elements are part of the breast parenchyma and participate in hormonal changes. During the late teens to early twenties, each breast contains several hundred lobules. The lobules tend to decrease in size with increasing age and particularly after pregnancy. This normal process is called *involution*.

The openings of each *acinus* join to form lactiferous ductules that drain the lobules, which in turn join to form 15 to 20 lactiferous ducts, one for each lobe. Several lactiferous ducts may combine before emptying directly into the nipple, so there are usually fewer duct openings on the nipple than there are breast ducts and lobes. The individual lobes are incompletely separated from each other by the Cooper's ligaments. The space between the lobes also contains fatty tissue and additional connective tissue. A layer of fatty tissue surrounds the gland, except in the area immediately under the areola and nipple (Fig. 24-6).

The lymphatic vessels of the breast drain laterally into the axillary lymph nodes and medially into the internal mammary chain of lymph nodes. Approximately 75% of the lymph drainage is toward the axilla, and 25% of the drainage is toward the internal mammary chain. The axillary nodes vary in number from 12 to 30 or more. The axilla is occasionally radiographed during breast examinations to evaluate these nodes. The internal mammary nodes are situated behind the sternum and manubrium and, if enlarged, are occasionally visible on a lateral chest radiograph.

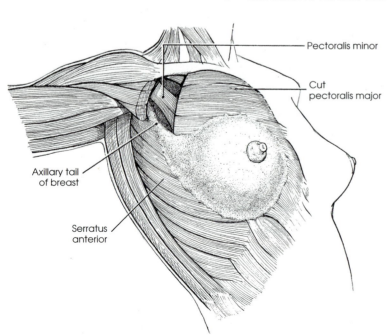

Fig. 24-5. Relationship of the breast to the chest wall is demonstrated. Note the extension of breast tissue posteriorly into the axilla.

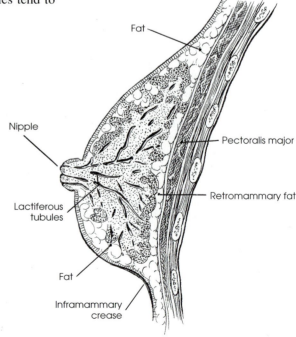

Fig. 24-6. Sagittal section through the female breast illustrating structural anatomy.

TISSUE VARIATIONS

The glandular and connective tissues of the breasts are soft tissue–density structures. The ability to demonstrate radiographic detail within the breast depends on the fat within and between the breast lobules and the fat surrounding the breasts. The postpubertal adolescent breast contains primarily dense connective tissue and casts a relatively homogeneous radiographic image with little tissue differentiation (Fig. 24-7). Increasing development of glandular tissue does not increase radiographic contrast except to the extent that the increased fat is also accu-

mulated by the breasts. Fat accumulation varies markedly among individuals. During pregnancy, significant hypertrophy of glands and ducts within the breasts occurs. This change causes the breasts to become extremely dense and opaque. Following the end of lactation, there usually is considerable involution of glandular and parenchymal tissues, which are replaced with increased amounts of fat. This normal fat accumulation significantly increases the natural radiographic contrast within the breasts (Fig. 24-8). Patients with some forms of fibrocystic parenchymal condition may not show this involution (Fig. 24-9).

The glandular and connective tissue elements of the breast can regenerate as needed for subsequent pregnancies. After menopause, the glandular and stromal elements undergo gradual atrophy (Fig. 24-10). Major external factors such as surgical menopause and ingestion of hormones may retard this normal process. From puberty through menopause, the breast is influenced by mammotrophic hormones that induce cyclic changes. Thus the glandular and connective tissues are in a state of constant change (Figs. 24-11 to 24-15).

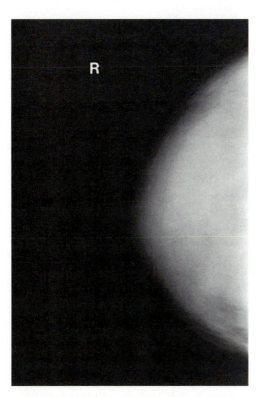

Fig. 24-7. Craniocaudal projection of normal breast in a 19-year-old woman who has never been pregnant. Note dense glandular tissues with small amounts of fat. For women who do not become pregnant, breasts may remain dense for many years.

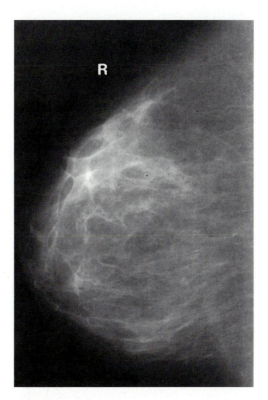

Fig. 24-8. Mediolateral projection of normal breast in a 24-year-old woman who has had two pregnancies. Note decreased volume of glandular tissue and increased amount of fat.

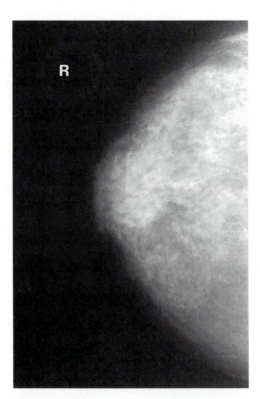

Fig. 24-9. Craniocaudal projection of the breast of a 42-year-old woman with fibrocystic condition illustrating prominent dilated ducts.

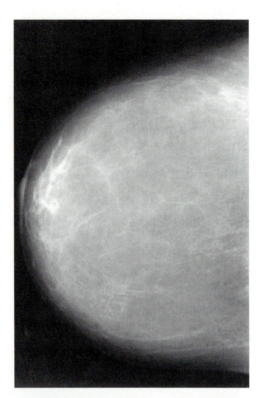

Fig. 24-10. Craniocaudal projection of the normal breast of a 68-year-old woman. Most of the glandular tissue is atrophic. Some glandular tissue remains in the lateral breast posteriorly and in the retroareolar area.

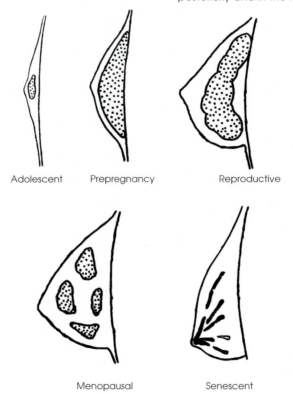

Adolescent   Prepregnancy   Reproductive

Menopausal   Senescent

Fig. 24-11. Diagrammatic profile drawings of breast illustrating the most likely variation and distribution of radiographic density *(shaded areas)* related to the normal life cycle from adolescence to senescence. This normal sequence may be altered by external factors such as pregnancy, hormone medications, surgical menopause, and fibrocystic breast condition.

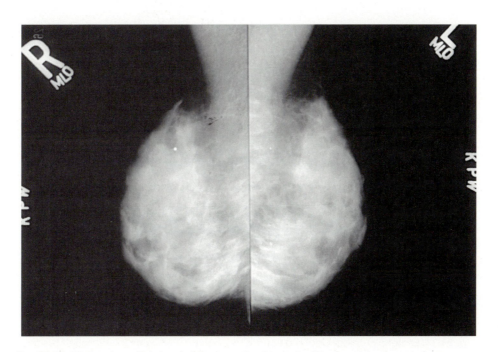

Fig. 24-12. Bilateral mediolateral oblique projections of a 27-year-old woman who stopped breast feedings 2 months before having this mammogram. Dense parenchyma with multinodularity throughout all quadrants is demonstrated bilaterally. A lead marker in the upper quadrant of the right breast marks a palpable mass that was proved by ultrasound to be solid.

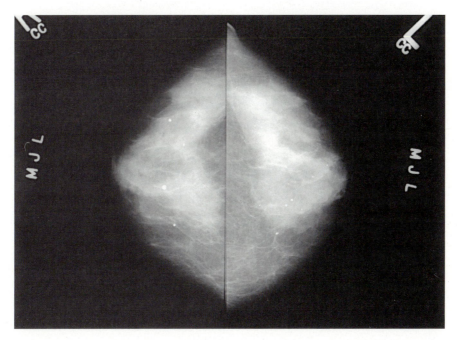

Fig. 24-13. Bilateral craniocaudal projections that demonstrate multiple, bilateral, benign calcifications.

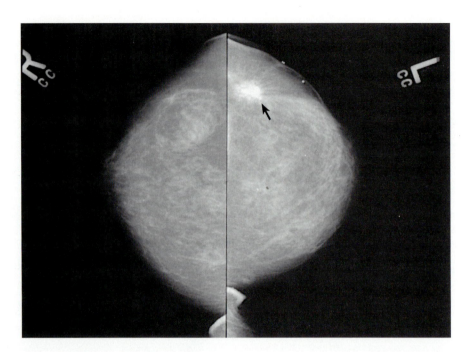

Fig. 24-14. Bilateral craniocaudal projections of a 55-year-old woman whose left breast has been surgically altered as a result of previous breast cancer. A lumpectomy scar is visible on the left breast *(arrow)*. Surgical scars can mimic characteristics of breast cancer.

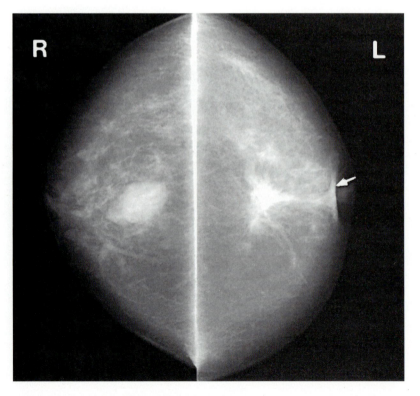

Fig. 24-15. Craniocaudal projections of bilateral breast masses. *L*, Left breast contains irregular carcinoma producing considerable spiculation and nipple retraction *(arrow)* skin thickening. *R*, Right breast contains fibroadenoma.

Breast Imaging

There are two basic recording systems available for displaying x-ray images of the breast. One system uses a dry electrophotographic process called xerography and is referred to as *xeromammography.* This system was preferred before the improvement in film-screen combinations; however, it is rapidly being replaced. The other system employs x-ray film and is referred to as *film-screen mammography.* Today, film-screen mammography is the preferred system because of its ability to capture more detailed information, use less radiation, and employ a faster processing time. Because of these major differences in technical requirements, equipment designed to work well with one image recording system is entirely inappropriate for the other.

FILM-SCREEN MAMMOGRAPHY

The most commonly used film-screen recording systems available from different manufacturers employ one high-resolution intensifying screen and a single-emulsion fine-grain film. Double-emulsion film-screen systems designed for mammography have been developed but are not widely used because of the added noise or grainy appearance of the processed radiographs. The cassettes are designed to achieve a nearly perfect film-screen contact. The current film-screen combinations result in a 30- to 150-fold reduction in breast radiation dose compared with industrial film mammography. Film-screen systems can provide excellent images with a total absorbed radiation dose for the examination of well under 1 rad to the breast. For example, the average mid-breast radiation dose from a typical exposure used in film-screen mammography in the BCDDP was 0.04 rad, which is significantly less than the similar dose of 0.37 rad for the xerographic examination. Before the successful introduction of fine-detail intensifying screens, industrial-grade nonscreen film or single-emulsion fine-grain nonscreen medical film was required to demonstrate the fine structures of the breast. These obsolete systems resulted in an excessive radiation dose to the breast of approximately 4 to 16 rads per examination, and sometimes doses were even higher. Since satisfactory film-screen combinations are available, nonscreen films should not be employed except in very limited circumstances. Any imaging system, whether film-screen or xerographic, that results in a breast dose greater than 1 rad per entire examination is not acceptable.

Although film-screen mammography might seem to have more in common with general radiography in terms of using x-ray film, high-quality film-screen mammograms cannot be made with standard x-ray equipment. Nearly all of the image contrast on a film-screen mammogram is the result of the difference in the attenuation coefficients of fat and soft tissue. The maximum difference between fat and soft tissue attenuation of the x-ray beam occurs in the low kilovoltage range. With increasing kilovoltage, attenuation coefficients of fat and soft tissue become similar and the natural radiographic contrast between these two substances decreases. Film-screen mammograms are usually made in the 22 to 28 kilovoltage range. The standard generators found in a radiology department cannot produce reliable exposures at this low kilovoltage. Transformers designed for low kilovoltage are required for film-screen mammography.

The standard target material used in x-ray tubes is tungsten. Qualities such as heat tolerance and a smaller percentage of low kilovoltage photons make tungsten a desirable target material for most diagnostic radiographic applications. However, tungsten is *not* desirable for film-screen mammography. *Molybdenum targets* are more efficient at producing a low-energy x-ray beam in the kilovoltage appropriate for mammography. Molybdenum target x-ray tubes produce a high percentage of 17.5 keV characteristic molybdenum K-edge x-rays that are ideally suited for soft tissue radiography. With the exception of mammography, molybdenum target x-ray tubes have limited applications in radiology and are entirely unacceptable for xeromammography, which is best performed using a tungsten target x-ray tube.

The particular requirements of film-screen breast imaging led to the development of dedicated mammography systems. The first such unit was the CGR Senographe introduced in 1969 (Fig. 24-16). Specialized units have many common design features, such as transformers that operate in the low kilovolt range and molybdenum target x-ray tubes. Usually filtration material of 0.03 mm of additional molybdenum (0.5 mm aluminum equivalent) is added to the x-ray beam to produce some minimal hardening and to further increase the proportion of 17.5 keV characteristic x-rays. X-ray tubes with small focal spot targets improve geometric sharpness and produce better definition of small structures. The original dedicated units had focal spots of 0.5 to 0.6 mm. Focal spots of 0.3 to 0.4 mm are currently available. Some units are designed for magnification studies, and these units feature target focal spots of 0.1 mm.

It is essential that the cathode of the x-ray tube be placed closest to and aligned with the plane of the patient's anterior chest wall and that the anode end be away from the patient. Technically, the entire cathode side of the triangular x-ray beam is eliminated by design of the unit. By orientating and designing the x-ray tube as described, the *perpendicular* x-rays that are parallel to the plane of the chest wall can be projected through the more dense posterior breast (closest to the chest wall) and the entire breast tissue can be included on the image.

Compression devices are built into mammographic units. One of the basic problems with breast imaging, particularly with film-screen systems, relates to the variation in thickness of the breast from front to back (Fig. 24-17). Uniform compression of the entire breast equalizes the great difference of front-to-back thickness. As the maximum thickness of the breast is decreased by compression, exposure time is shortened. In addition to reducing radiation exposure, the compression technique produces a radiograph of more uniform density. Compression pushes all of the contents of the breast closer to the x-ray film, further decreasing geometric distortion. Spreading the breast out over a greater area of the film decreases the summation effects of overlying structures (Fig. 24-17). Compression can also reduce the motion of the breast during relatively long mammographic exposures, and it can enhance the demonstration of any architectural distortion produced by small tumors. The wide latitude of xeromammography allows adequate exposure of the entire breast without the extreme compression necessary for film-screen mammography. Compression is still useful to reduce motion, decrease overlap, and enhance recognition of architectural distortion produced by tumors. Compression should be considered an important aid to xeromammography and absolutely essential for film-screen mammography.

Some patients may feel considerable discomfort with adequate compression. The patient will be better able to cooperate for the examination and tolerate the compression if she understands why compression is necessary for a satisfactory examination. Some mammographers recommend that patients go on a low-caffeine diet for several days before the mammogram. This is thought to increase some patients' tolerance of compression.

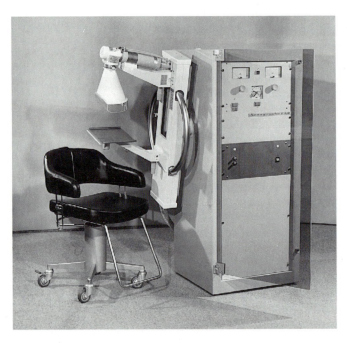

Fig. 24-16. The Senographe by CGR was the first dedicated mammography system.

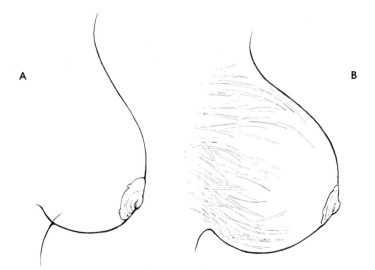

Fig. 24-17. A, Lateral profile of the breast demonstrating inadequate compression and a drooping breast. **B,** Lateral profile of a properly compressed breast. Note how compression has overcome the effect of gravity and the breast is spread out over a greater area.

The use of any type of compression requires a firm, nonyielding, film-holding surface on which the breast can be supported. Most units achieve compression by use of a motorized compression plate attached to the C-arm located above the film-holding device. Fig. 24-18 illustrates the effect of compression, focal spot size, and targeted film distance on image sharpness. The target-to-film distance of a dedicated mammography system should be at least 24 inches (60 cm).

There is considerable variability in the tissue density of breasts of different patients related to the varying amounts of fat-density material and soft tissue–density material contained within the breast. The tone and firmness of the breast result from the tone of the supporting suspensory (Cooper's) ligaments and not from the relative proportions of fat and soft tissue–density tissue. It is not possible to evaluate the relative proportion of fat and soft tissue–density in the breast based on physical examination of the breast. Therefore accurate exposures in mammography can best be achieved with automatic exposure control. Most dedicated mammography units have an automatic exposure control built into the film holder. As with all automatic exposure systems, it is important to position the most dense part of the breast over the detector so that the exposure does not prematurely terminate.

Dedicated mammography systems all have *apertures* that ensure proper collimation and projection of the useful x-ray beam. These systems are compact and allow for all images of the breast or axilla with the patient in the standing or seated position. The convenience, speed, and small space required by these units are all advantages, particularly when a large number of patients are to undergo radiography. One perceived disadvantage of the dedicated mammography film-screen unit is that the chest wall is not visualized. Some physicians report this as a drawback because a deeply seated tumor may not be identified. However, with due care, it is usually possible to pull the breast forward into the field of view so that all of the posterior mammary tissue is examined.

Most mammography systems have moving grids available for reducing the amount of scattered x-radiation reaching the film. Only moving grids are acceptable, because visible grid lines produced by stationary grids will compromise the image quality. The specially designed grids usually have a 5:1 or 6:1 grid ratio.

The use of grids in mammography requires an increase in the amount of radiation exposure required to obtain a properly exposed image. Authorities still debate the merits of routine grid use for imaging a breast that measures less than 2 cm when compressed, contrasting the improved image quality against the increased radiation received by the patient. It is generally accepted, however, that grids do significantly improve image quality in dense breasts and in breasts that cannot be compressed to 6 cm or less. Grids yield little improvement in image quality when radiographing fatty breasts that can be compressed to 6 cm or less.

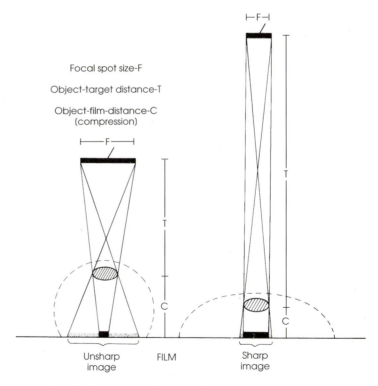

Focal spot size-F

Object-target distance-T

Object-film-distance-C
(compression)

Unsharp image   FILM   Sharp image

Fig. 24-18. Technical factors affecting image sharpness.

467

Some institutions confine the use of grids to breasts that cannot be compressed to less than 6 cm and to breasts that are known to be dense or are shown to be dense after the initial image is reviewed. A grid system that is easily mounted and dismounted makes such flexibility possible.

For any imaging system there must be strict attention to quality assurance. At least once a year a qualified physicist should calibrate the exposure timer's accuracy and reproducibility, the linearity of milliamperage settings, and the uniformity of exposure over the x-ray field. All interlocks need to be checked for proper function, and the unit should be checked for radiation leakage from the x-ray tube housing. At least every 6 months measurements should be taken of the absolute exposures at the breast surface. Measure-

ments of the focal spot size should be taken, the beam quality should be evaluated, and the integrity of the filters should be tested. Exposures of a standard phantom should be made and evaluated at least monthly. Fig. 24-19 illustrates a standard mammography phantom with which an evaluation of line pair resolution, densitometry, and contrast resolution can be made.

With film-screen mammography, close attention must be paid to the temperature of the x-ray film processor. The processor must be cleaned at frequent intervals. Single-emulsion film is nonforgiving, and processor insults to the film that would go completely unnoticed with a standard double-emulsion film can severely compromise a mammogram. Xerographic processors also deserve frequent preventive maintenance.

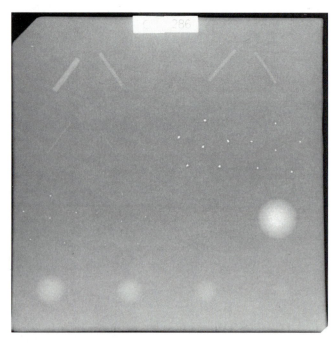

Fig. 24-19. Radiograph of the RMI (Radiation Measurements, Inc.) breast phantom containing a series of fibers, specks, and masses. A minimum of four fibers, three specks, and three masses should be readily visible if the mammography and film processing systems are working properly.

XEROMAMMOGRAPHY

Xeromammography is a specialized radiography processing system employing a dry, electrophotographic technique. The system uses a charged aluminum plate coated with selenium powder instead of traditional x-ray film. A thin layer of the selenium powder is carefully deposited on an electrically conductive plate. The powder is then charged by applying an electrical voltage; the charge remains uniformly distributed over the plate. When exposed to x rays, the plate discharges in proportion to the quantity of radiation deposited. The remaining charge on the plate contains the latent x-ray image. This electrostatic image is made visible by dusting the selenium layer with a fine layer of charged powder, which brings out a fine-grain image. For a permanent image, the powder image is electrostatically transferred to paper. The entire developing and recharging process is performed automatically in a special Xerox processor.

There are several major differences between xeromammography and film mammography. The relative contrast demonstrated between fat and soft tissue–density is much lower in xerography than in film recording systems. However, whenever a sharp change in density occurs, the change is intensified on the xerogram by an edge enhancement effect. This effect exaggerates the actual contrast of borders and helps delineate areas of nearly equal x-ray density by accentuating edges. The xerogram has a much wider range of exposure latitude. (Latitude and contrast are reciprocal.) Because the technique depends on edge enhancement rather than natural contrast, the study should be conducted using 55 kVp and a tungsten target x-ray tube. This means using a different target tube material and a much higher peak kilovoltage than that used for film-screen mammography. Xerograms taken with kVp much lower than 50 to 55 result in substantially more radiation to the breast without any advantage in image quality. Xeromammography dosimetry to the breast is approximately 1 rad or less for an entire examination consisting of mediolateral and craniocaudal projections. The average mid-breast dose for a typical xerogram exposure in the BCDDP was 0.37 rad. Xerography should be performed using x rays generated from a tungsten target x-ray tube with 0.2 to 0.3 mm of aluminum filtration. Molybdenum target x-ray tubes used in dedicated state-of-the-art film-screen mammographic equipment today produce a longer wavelength (softer) x-ray beam and are not appropriate for xerography.

The xerographic image contains less overall information than does a film image, but it demonstrates the important features, and the resolution is sufficient to show fine microcalcifications. The final image can be displayed in a positive or a negative mode. The negative mode has some advantage, because it requires less radiation exposure than the positive mode (Figs. 24-20 to 24-22).

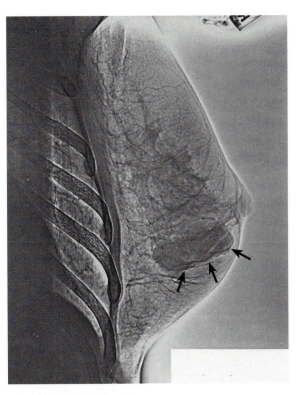

Fig. 24-20. Xeromammogram. Mediolateral projection of the breast in a 48-year-old woman. Several large cysts are visible in the inferior portion of the breast (arrows).

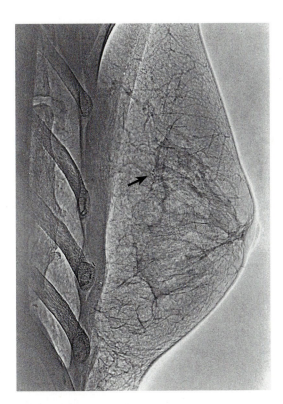

Fig. 24-21. Xeromammogram. Mediolateral projection of the breast in a 39-year-old woman. A small cluster of microcalcifications (arrow) indicates the presence of a carcinoma.

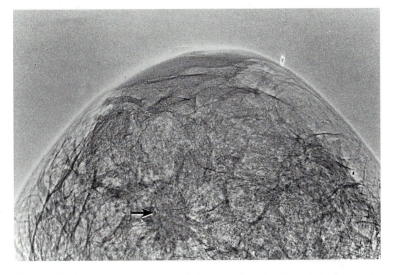

Fig. 24-22. Xeromammogram. Craniocaudal projection of the breast in a 51-year-old woman with carcinoma (arrow).

Method of Examination

The patient should be dressed in an open-front gown. The breast must be bared for the examination because the mammogram will record the slightest wrinkle in any cloth covering. Before the breast is radiographed, a careful physical examination is performed, and all biopsy scars, palpable masses, suspicious thickenings, skin abnormalities, and nipple alterations are noted. Both breasts are routinely radiographed obtaining craniocaudal and mediolateral oblique images. Occasionally additional projections, including a 90-degree true lateral, axillary, lateromedial, and exaggerated craniocaudal, are useful. In addition, two magnified right-angle images are obtained to better characterize lesions and calcifications.

In a symptomatic patient the examination should not be limited to the symptomatic breast. Both breasts should be examined, both for comparison and because significant lesions may be demonstrated in a clinically normal breast.

ROUTINE PROJECTIONS

In this section, techniques for conducting mammographic examinations on dedicated systems are described.

- For each of the two basic breast projections, ensure that the breast is firmly supported and adjusted so that the nipple is directed straightforward.
- If possible, profile the nipple. Imaging the posterior breast tissue should be the primary consideration, however, and an additional projection to profile the nipple can be obtained if necessary. The use of nipple markers, clearly locating the nipple that is not in profile, can prevent the need for this additional radiograph.
- Use a rigid, radiolucent compression paddle to compress the surface of the breast. This compression tends to spread the breast so that the tissue thickness is more equally distributed over the film and better separation of the glandular elements is achieved. Compression is one of the most important components of achieving a high quality mammogram. The primary objective of compression is to produce uniform breast thickness from the nipple to the most posterior aspect of the breast.
- Perform positioning of the breast consistently so that any lesion can be accurately localized in the gland and so that a valid comparison can be made between periodic examinations.
- Place the identification markers according to the following standard convention:

     For the oblique and mediolateral projections, place markers along the upper border of the breast; and for craniocaudal projections, place markers along the lateral side of the breast. The marker denotes the portion of the breast closest to the axilla.

CRANIOCAUDAL PROJECTION

- Have the patient stand or be seated on an adjustable stool facing the film holder.
- Elevate the affected breast using all of its natural mobility.
- Raise the edge of the film holder to meet the elevated inframammary fold.
- Place the breast on the film holder, and center it with the nipple in profile.
- Ensure that the edge of the film cassette is flush against the chest wall under the breast.
- Instruct the patient to press her thorax against the film holder so that the inferior margin of the breast will be on the film.
- Ask the patient to relax her shoulder to permit projection of the lateral quadrants of the breast on the film.
- Turn the patient's head away from the side being examined.
- After informing the patient that compression of the breast will be used, bring the compression paddle into contact with the breast, and slowly apply compression (Fig. 24-23).
- Instruct the patient to indicate when compression becomes uncomfortable. Compression is adequate when palpation of the patient's breast reveals tenseness of the breast tissue and firmness of the skin. The compression should feel tight and uncomfortable but not painful.
- When full compression is achieved, instruct the patient to suspend breathing.
- Make the exposure.

In a properly positioned craniocaudal radiograph, the image should demonstrate all of the medial breast tissue and the nipple should be centered on the film. Demonstration of the pectoral muscle is seen on approximately 20% of all craniocaudal radiographs (Fig. 24-24).

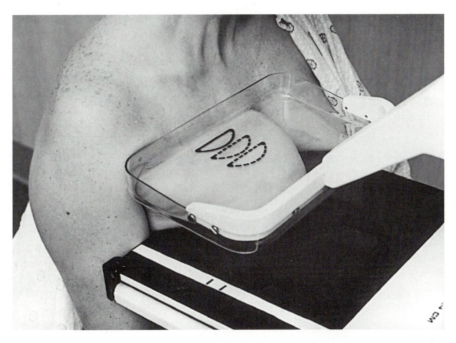

Fig. 24-23. Breast in proper position and compression paddle in place for a craniocaudal projection.

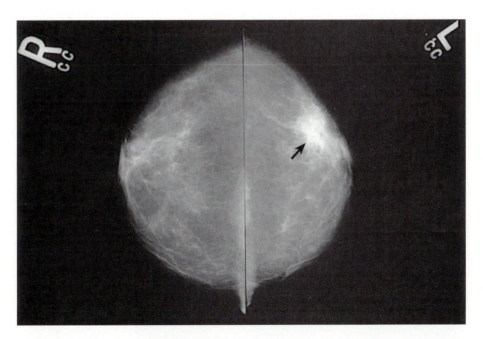

Fig. 24-24. Bilateral craniocaudal projections of a 63-year-old woman that demonstrate proper positioning. The craniocaudal projection should include maximum medial breast tissue with the nipples centered. Breast cancer (left, *arrow*) is marked by a lead marker placed over the palpable mass.

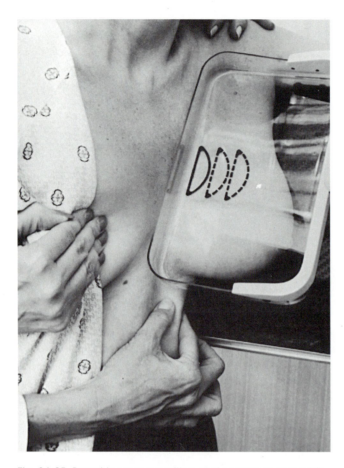

Fig. 24-25. Breast in proper position and compression paddle in place for a mediolateral oblique projection. Note radiographer smoothing inframammary folds.

MEDIOLATERAL OBLIQUE PROJECTION

The second standard projection is an oblique, with the central ray directed from the superomedial to the inferolateral portion of the breast. For this position the following steps are observed:

- Instruct the patient to raise the arm of the side being examined and rest the hand on the handgrip adjacent to the film holder.
- Place the film holder as high as possible into the axilla between the pectoral and latissimus dorsi muscles so that the film is behind the pectoral fold.
- With the patient relaxed and the shoulder leaning slightly anterior, turn the patient to face the film holder while gently pulling the breast superiorly and anteriorly away from the chest and then apply the compression paddle.
- Direct the central ray to pass through the breast at an angle between 30 and 60 degrees. The actual angle will depend on the angle of the pectoral muscle, which varies from patient to patient depending upon the body habitus.
- Place the film holder parallel with the pectoral muscle to visualize the maximum amount of breast tissue.

In a properly aligned oblique position (Fig. 24-25), the pectoral fold will extend from the axilla to at least as far as the nipple level of the breast. Additionally, a small portion of abdomen will be projected onto the film just inferior to the breast (Fig. 24-26). Including the abdomen ensures that the patient was as far against the film holder as possible and the maximum amount of posterolateral breast and axilla has been included on the radiograph. The breast is supported by the film holder and the compression plate for the separation of deep and superficial tissue. The breast will not droop on the image, and the upper contour of the breast will be bulging rather than sagging.

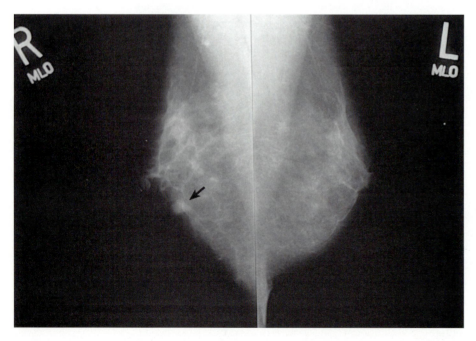

Fig. 24-26. Bilateral mediolateral oblique projections that demonstrate proper positioning. Images should include pectoral muscle to the level of the nipple, visualization of posterior breast tissue, and the inframammary fold/abdominal skin junction. Images of a 42-year-old woman demonstrates a benign nodule located inferior to the right nipple *(arrow)*.

SUPPLEMENTAL PROJECTIONS

Occasionally additional images are used to supplement the standard radiographs.

Mediolateral projection

The mediolateral projection is useful in confirming and localizing abnormalities that are seen in only one of the standard projections.

Upright position

- Rotate the C-arm assembly 90 degrees, with the x-ray tube placed on the medial side of the breast.
- Turn the patient slightly to bring the nipple into profile.
- Instruct the patient to bend slightly forward and to grasp the handgrip on the unit with the hand of the side being examined; gently push the film carrier as high as possible into the axilla.
- Ask the patient to relax the shoulder.
- Ensure that the lateral rib margin is pressed firmly against the edge of the film holder.
- Elevate the breast into its normal form, gently pull the breast superiorly and inferiorly, and compress it as much as possible between the film holder and the compression paddle.
- Position the nipple as far laterally toward the cassette as possible. Demonstration of the retromammary space and the breast lying in close contact with the thoracic walls and ribs is difficult to achieve in this upright lateral position. Pulling the breast anteriorly is essential to bring the posterior breast tissue off the chest wall and into the radiation field (Fig. 24-27).

Recumbent position

- Instruct the patient to lie on her side on the examining table with the arm of the side that is being examined placed as high as possible under the head.
- Place the film holder as far as possible into the axilla beneath the breast.
- Elevate the film holder until the breast is elevated with the nipple in exact profile.
- Bring the arm forward until it forms a right angle to the long axis of the body.
- Flex the forearm, and supinate the hand under the head.
- Pull the opposite breast and shoulder posteriorly.
- Use the compression paddle to compress the breast being examined.

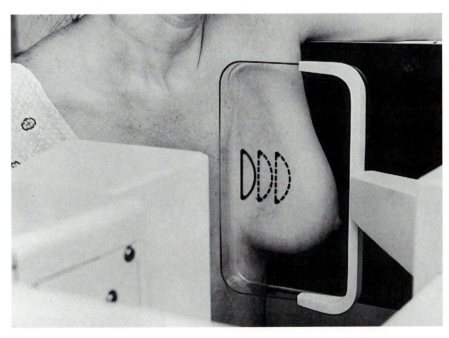

Fig. 24-27. Breast in proper position and compression paddle in place for a mediolateral projection.

Lateromedial projection

The lateromedial projection is used to bring abnormalities in the medial part of the breast closer to the film for improved resolution. The following steps are observed:

- Rotate the film holder and tube 180 degrees from the mediolateral projection for the same breast. Note that any markers affixed to the film holder will now appear at the bottom of the film.
- Position the patient so that the film holder is against the patient's sternum.
- Elevate the arm of the side being examined.
- Center the x-ray tube and film holder midway between the superior and inferior portions of the breast.
- Have the patient grasp the handgrip, pulling herself forward so that the sternum is placed firmly against the edge of the film holder.
- Position the breast by gently pulling it anteriorly and superiorly.
- Apply compression (Fig. 24-28).

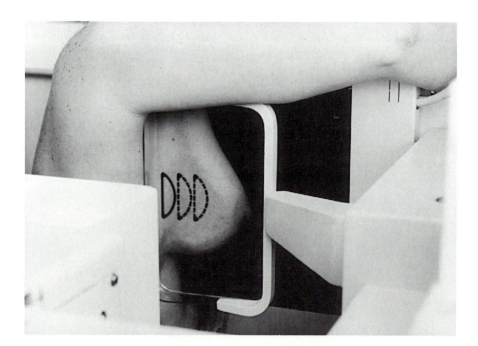

Fig. 24-28. Breast in proper position and compression paddle in place for a lateromedial projection.

Axillary projection for axillary tail

If it is desirable to evaluate the axillary lymph nodes and the axillary tail, this special projection can be taken. The following steps are observed:

- Depending on the design of the mammography unit, conduct this position in the supine or the upright body position.
- In the supine position, have the patient hold the upper arm at a right angle to the body, flex the forearm, and place the hand under the head in supination.
- Place the film under the axilla in such a way that the upper arm and axillary tail will be included on the image.
- Pull the breast medially, direct the central ray of the x-ray tube to the axillary tail, and apply breast compression (Fig. 24-29).
- Increase the exposure by approximately 2 kVp.
- To demonstrate the axilla in the upright body position, instruct the patient to drape the arm over the top of the film holder, flex the elbow, and hold on to the handgrip.
- Position the patient so that the axilla overlies the film, and pull the axilla and superior breast forward to be included in the image.
- Direct the central ray through the axillary tail and apply compression (Fig. 24-30).
- The exact patient position and placement of the central ray will vary among patients. Experienced mammographers will be able to palpate the axillary tail area, position the patient, and direct the central ray precisely.

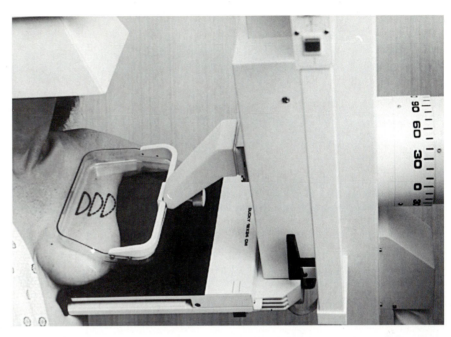

Fig. 24-29. Breast in proper position and compression paddle in place for an axillary projection.

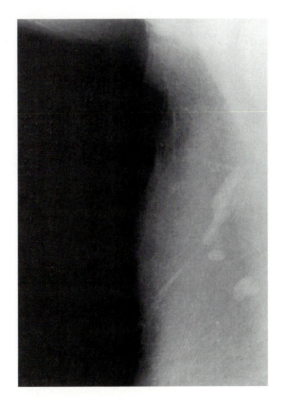

Fig. 24-30. Axillary tail projection containing several enlarged lymph nodes.

(Courtesy Sylvia L. Cousins, R.T.)

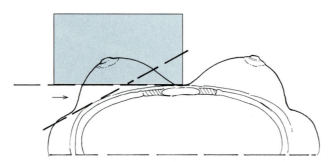

Fig. 24-31. Superior profile illustrating how placement of the flat edge of the cassette against the curved chest wall will exclude a portion of the breast tissue *(arrow)*. Dashed line indicates placement of cassette for exaggerated position.

Exaggerated craniocaudal projection (for lateral aspect of breast)

Because the anterior thoracic wall curves posteriorly as it extends laterally, and since the edge of the cassette is flat, it is often not possible to project all of the *lateral* breast tissue onto the film during the craniocaudal projection (Fig. 24-31). A modified craniocaudal projection can be obtained to accentuate the lateral portion of the breast. When a questionable abnormality is suspected on the standard images, an additional craniocaudal image taken with lateral angulation of the patient can be helpful (Fig. 24-32). The use of a 5-degree tube angulation may be necessary to eliminate the overlapping of the humeral head.

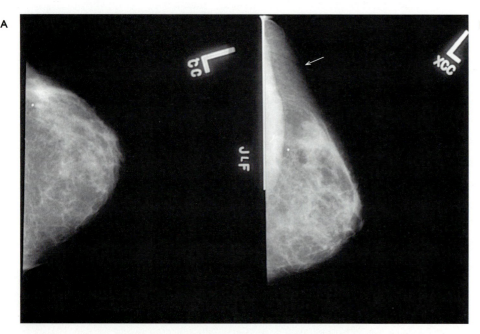

A   B

Fig. 24-32. Two projections of the left breast. **A,** Craniocaudal. **B,** Exaggerated craniocaudal. This projection is exaggerated laterally in order to demonstrate the axillary tail *(arrow)*. Note also the visualization of the pectoral muscle.

Caudocranial projection

The caudocranial projection, or reverse craniocaudal, is used to demonstrate lesions located in the *superior* aspect of the breast. This reverse technique allows the breast lesion to be placed closer to the film, thus decreasing magnification and improving visibility of a possible breast lesion on the image. Additionally, the caudocranial projection allows a larger amount of tissue to be imaged in the kyphotic or male patient. The following steps are observed:

- To position the patient, rotate the C-arm assembly 180 degrees.
- Elevate the film holder to be in contact with the superior aspect of the breast (Fig. 24-33).
- Place the compression paddle to be in contact with the inferior and posterior aspect of the breast from below.

Craniocaudal projection (cleavage view) for medial breast tissue

- Have the patient lean forward as far as possible, pressing the rib cage just beneath the breasts against the film holder and supporting herself by grasping the handgrip.
- Distribute the medial portion of both breasts over the film to obtain a craniocaudal projection of the cleavage area (Fig. 24-34).
- If desired, instead of combining the medial portions of both breasts on one film, examine the breasts individually on separate films.
- With the combined projection, manually control the exposure, since the breasts do not lie over the automatic exposure control detector.

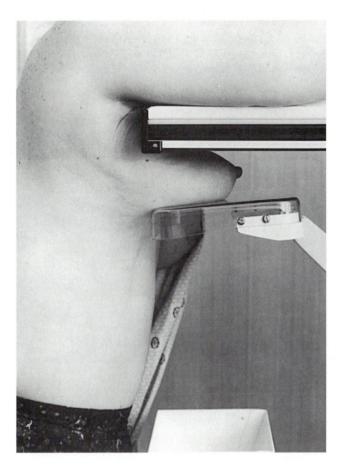

Fig. 24-33. Breast in position and compression paddle in place for a caudocranial projection. Note 180-degree rotation of the tube/film assembly.

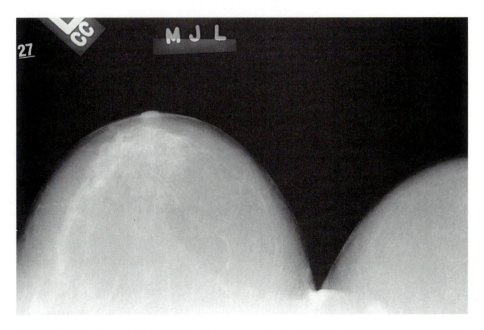

Fig. 24-34. Craniocaudal projection (cleavage view) of both breasts. For demonstration of the deep medial breast tissue.

MAGNIFICATION TECHNIQUES

If the x-ray tube has a 0.1 mm focal spot target, magnification techniques can be used. Magnification is useful in evaluating the characteristics of breast calcification and the margins of breast masses to deter- mine whether breast lesions are likely to be benign or malignant. If other projec- tions have been used to indicate the possi- ble presence of a lesion, magnification may clarify whether a lesion is or is not present.

All magnification techniques require the use of a firm radiolucent device, which elevates the breast above the film holder to increase the OFD (object-film dis- tance). Increasing the OFD requires using an additional piece of equipment that is at- tached above the film holder (Figs. 24-35 and 24-36). The amount of magnification is determined by the distance between the breast and the film. The magnification usually ranges from 1.5× to 2× but is a fixed quantity as determined by the di- mension of the magnification surface.

A nongrid film holder can be used for magnification imaging of breast tissue. An increase in radiation exposure occurs in magnification radiography, and radiation exposure would be further increased by the use of a grid. The increased OFD re- quired for magnification studies decreases scatter radiation, which also reduces the need to use a grid.

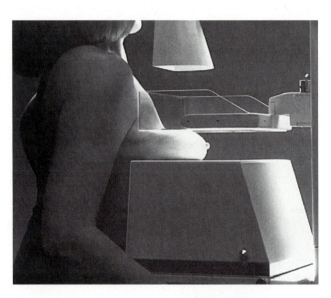

Fig. 24-35. A radiolucent platform has been placed between the breast and the film holder. This will cause the breast tissue to be enlarged.

(Courtesy Picker International.)

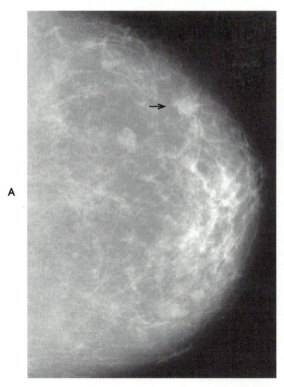
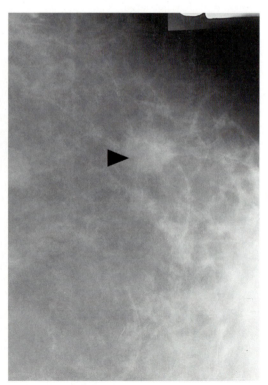

Fig. 24-36. A, Craniocaudal projection showing possible lesion in right breast *(arrow).* **B,** Same patient with 2× magnification and convincingly demonstrating the lesion with irregular margin *(arrowhead).* Note smooth noninvasive benign lesion *(arrowhead).*

The Augmented Breast

Mammography is clearly the preferred technique and most reliable method of screening for breast cancer. While mammography has an 80% to 90% true-positive rate for diagnosing cancer in breasts that do not contain implants, over 2 million women in the United States have received augmentation mammoplasty (implants) for cosmetic or reconstructive purposes. The true-positive (pathologic-mammographic) diagnostic rate for cancer decreases to approximately 60% for the augmented breast patient because the implant can obscure up to 85% of breast structures, potentially hiding a small cancer that could normally be detected with mammography at an early and curable stage.

Successful radiography of the augmented breast requires a highly skilled radiographer. Precautions must be taken during the examination to avoid rupture of the augmentation device.

Mammography of the augmented breast presents a challenge that cannot be met with the standard two-image examination of each breast. An eight-radiograph examination is preferred whenever possible. The posterior and superior aspects of the augmented breast can be satisfactorily evaluated using the craniocaudal and mediolateral oblique projections (Fig. 24-37). However, these four images will not adequately demonstrate the surrounding breast parenchyma. The initial two projections may be combined with the Eklund, or implant displaced, technique (Fig. 24-38). For the Eklund method, the implant is pushed posteriorly against the chest wall so it is excluded from the image, while the breast tissue surrounding the implant is pulled anteriorly and compressed. This positioning improves both compression of breast tissue and visualization of breast structures (Fig. 24-39). Craniocaudal and mediolateral oblique projections are often performed using the implant displaced technique.

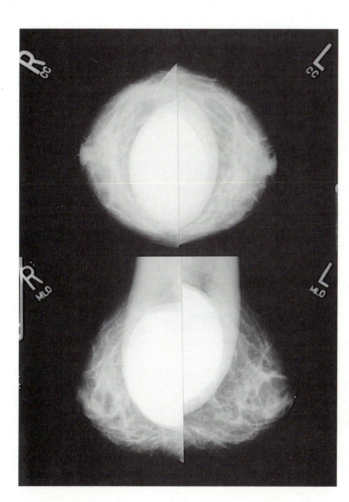

Fig. 24-37. Bilateral, four-image examination of the augmented breasts of a 37-year-old woman. Implants have been surgically placed behind the pectoral muscle. Radiographs should be obtained using the Eklund technique (see Fig. 24-38).

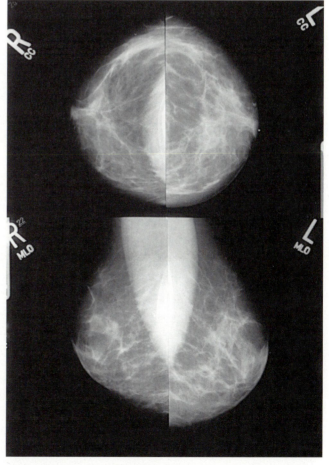

Fig. 24-38. Bilateral, four-image examination of the same patient in Fig. 24-37 using the Eklund, or implant displaced, technique. The implants are pushed back for better visualization of the surrounding breast tissue.

Complications often associated with breast augmentation include fibrosis, increase of fibrous tissue surrounding the implant, shrinking, hardening, leakage, and pain. Mammography alone cannot fully demonstrate all complications; therefore, both ultrasound and magnetic resonance imaging (MRI) are also considered for patients with symptomatic implants.

Ultrasound of the breast has proven useful in identifying implant leakage in cases where implant rupture is suggested by mammographic findings and/or clinical examination and in a few cases where leakage is not suspected. Ultrasound has also successfully identified leakage that has migrated to the axillary lymph nodes. Although ultrasound is not yet recommended as a screening modality for implant leakage, it has somewhat enhanced the mammographic examination.

MRI of the augmented breast is currently the most common modality for evaluating the augmented breast. Although MRI offers several diagnostic advantages, the cost and timely nature of the procedure inhibits its use as a screening modality. MRI has proven useful as a preoperative tool in locating the position of the implant, identifying the contour of the deformity, and confirming rupture and leakage migration patterns, and its sensitivity will be further defined in the future.

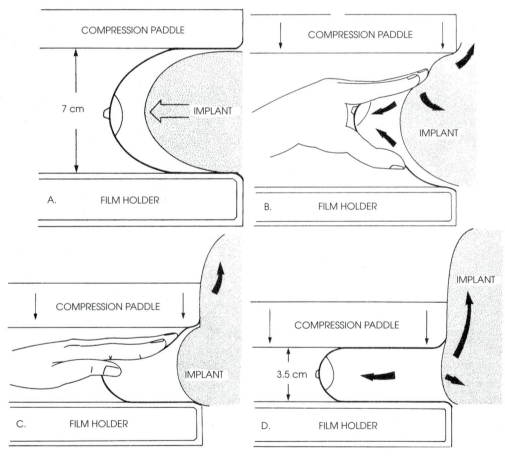

Fig. 24-39. A, Breast with implant and normal positioning technique. **B, C, D,** Ecklund technique of pushing the implant posteriorly against the chest wall and pulling the breast anteriorly and compressing.

(Reprinted courtesy of Eklund GW et al: Improved imaging of the augmented breast, AJR, 151:469-473, 1988.)

Localization of Nonpalpable Lesions for Biopsy

When mammography identifies a nonpalpable lesion, the radiology team must accurately locate the abnormality for the surgeon so that only a small amount of tissue needs to be removed for microscopic examination, and trauma to the breast can be minimized. In this way the maximal amount of normal breast tissue can be preserved unless the biopsy indicates that more extensive surgery is required.

The most popular technique of preoperative localization uses a needle that contains a hooked guidewire. The four most common needle-wire localization systems are the Frank, Kopans, Hawkins, and Homer biopsy guides. With each system, a long needle containing a hooked wire is pushed into the breast so that the tip approximates the lesion. The needle is then withdrawn over the wire, leaving the hooked wire in position. The hook on the end of the wire keeps the wire fastened in the breast tissue (Fig. 24-40).

The surgeon cuts along the guidewire and removes the breast tissue around the hooked end of the guidewire. The hooked end of the wire is completely contained within the Kopans and Homer needles (18-gauge) and the 20-gauge Hawkins needle. The narrow Frank needle (21-gauge) cannot accommodate the folded wire, so the hook of the wire folds back over the outside of the needle tip. The Frank needle has two minor disadvantages because of the small-diameter design. The needle cannot be pushed directly through the skin and subcutaneous tissue. It is necessary to use a scalpel blade to make a 1 to 2 mm incision in the skin at the site of needle insertion. Because the hook is outside the needle tip, the localization wire cannot be withdrawn and repositioned. The other available needle-wire localization systems can be inserted without a skin incision and can be repositioned until the needle is pulled back from the end of the wire. In practice, all four systems work well. The localization procedure can be performed several hours before surgery or it can be performed as part of an outpatient breast biopsy procedure.

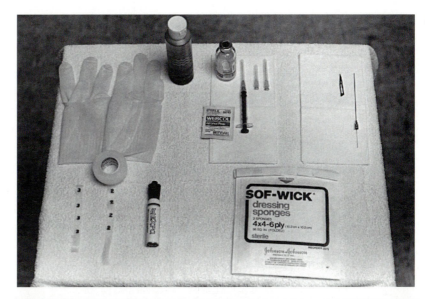

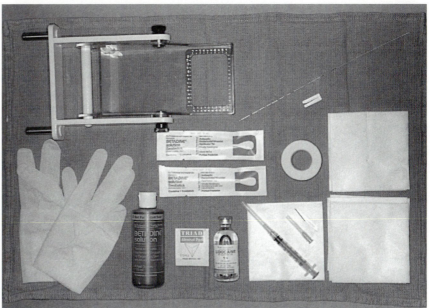

Fig. 24-40. A, Material for breast localization without a specialized compression plate: sterile gloves, topical antiseptic, local anesthetic, 5-ml syringe for anesthetic, 25-gauge needle for administering skin anesthesia, 18-gauge needle, alcohol swab, scalpel blade, needle-wire localization system, lead skin markers on tape, magic marker, and sterile gauze. **B,** Material for breast localization using a specialized compression plate: alphanumeric localization compression plate, sterile gloves, topical antiseptic, alcohol wipe, local anesthetic, 5-ml syringe, 25-gauge needle, scalpel blade, sterile gauze, tape, and needle-wire localization system.

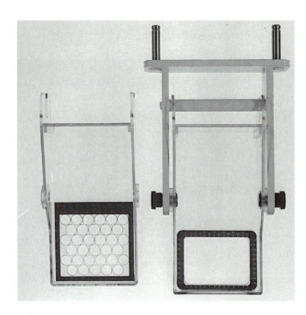

Fig. 24-41. Compression plates specifically designed for breast localization procedure. Fenestrated plate *(left)* and open-hole plate attached to frame *(right)*.

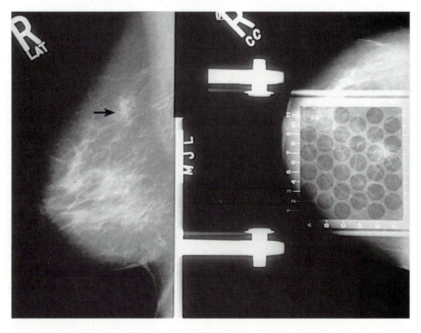

Fig. 24-42. Preliminary projections for breast localization procedure. The lateral projection *(left)* is obtained to determine the depth of the lesion *(arrow)*. The compressed plate *(right)* immobilizes the breast for needle-wire insertion. Note: the alphanumeric grid demonstrates that the lesion is located nearest to the E-7 junction. The needle-wire will be inserted through the posterior aspect of the hole E-7.

BREAST LESION LOCALIZATION WITH A SPECIALIZED COMPRESSION PLATE

Many mammography units have an optional compression plate with an opening that can be positioned over a breast lesion and through which a localizing wire and needle can be introduced into the breast. The initial mammogram and the mediolateral projection are reviewed to determine the shortest distance from the skin to the breast lesion; for example, a lesion in the inferior region of the breast would be approached either from the inferior surface of the breast or from the medial or lateral surface, but not from the superior surface. An estimate is also made regarding the approximate depth of the lesion to the closest surface.

The opening in the compression plate may consist of a rectangular cutout with radiopaque alphanumeric grid markings along at least two adjacent sides, or it may contain several rows of holes, each of which is large enough to clear the hub of the localization needle (Fig. 24-41).

The following steps are observed:

- Clean the skin of the breast over the lesion with a topical antiseptic.
- Position the patient so that the compression plate is as close to the lesion as possible, usually with the x-ray tube oriented along the verified (superior or inferior approach) or horizontal (lateral or medial approach) plane.
- Make a preliminary exposure using compression (Fig. 24-42).
- Process the film without removing the breast from between the compression plate and film holder. The film will show where the lesion lies in relation to the compression plate opening.

- The localizing needle and guidewire are inserted into the breast perpendicular to the compression plate and parallel to the chest wall directly toward the underlying lesion. The needle is advanced to the estimated depth of the lesion; it is better to pass beyond the lesion than it is to be short of the lesion. It also must be remembered that the breast is flattened and compressed in the direction of needle travel when the needle is introduced.
- With the needle in position, an exposure is made (Fig. 24-43). The compression plate is then released, leaving the needle-wire system in place, and an additional projection is obtained following a 90-degree shift (Fig. 24-44). From these two radiographs, the position of the end of the needle-wire system relative to the lesion is determined. If necessary the needle and wire can be repositioned and the exposures repeated. When the needle is satisfactorily placed in the lesion, the needle is withdrawn, leaving the hooked guidewire in place. A gauze bandage is placed over the breast, and the patient is transported to surgery along with the final localization radiographs.

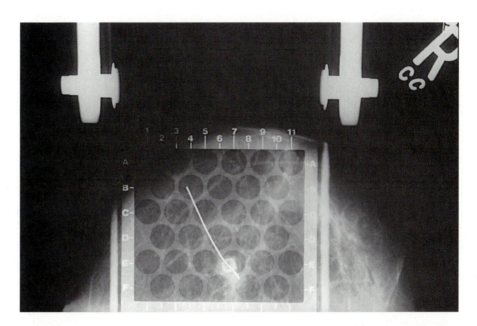

Fig. 24-43. The needle-wire localization device has been advanced through the hole in the compression plate to the approximate location of the lesion in the craniocaudal projection.

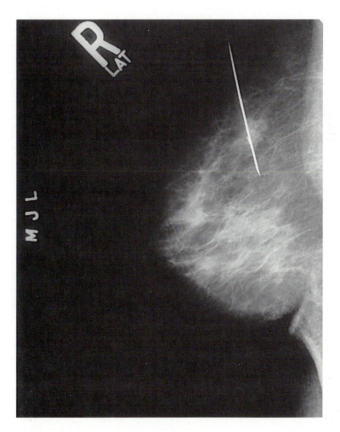

Fig. 24-44. A second projection is obtained after the x-ray tube is rotated 90 degrees. This projection allows the depth of the needle-wire localization systems to be determined. The fenestrated compression plate is replaced with a standard compression plate.

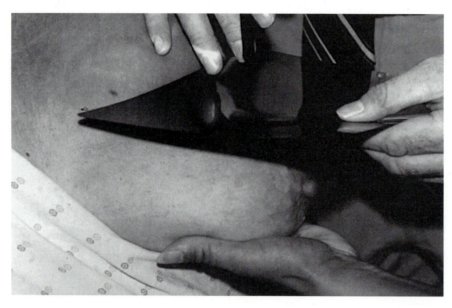

Fig. 24-45. The radiographer supports the breast while the physician superimposes the craniocaudal projection mammogram over the breast, used to locate the breast lesion in reference to the skin surface.

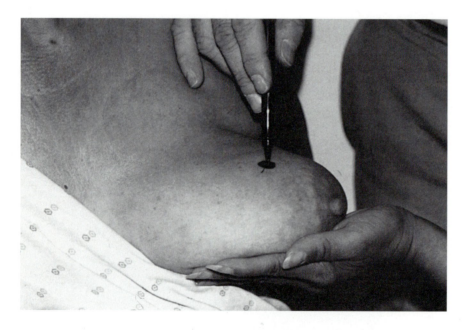

Fig. 24-46. An ink mark is placed on the breast surface directly over the breast lesion, locating the lesion in the superoinferior aspect. The same technique is used to place a mark over the lesion using the mediolateral projection to locate the lesion in the mediolateral aspect.

BREAST LESION LOCALIZATION WITHOUT A SPECIALIZED COMPRESSION PLATE

Preliminary craniocaudal and 90-degree lateral projections are taken of the abnormal breast. Using these preliminary radiographs, an ink mark is placed on the breast surface relating the position of the lesion in each image. Taping alphanumeric lead markers to the breast for the preliminary radiographs can aid in relating the position of the lesion on the radiograph to the breast surface in each projection. Because the breast is compressed for the exposures, the breast must approach the compressed position to accurately place the ink marks. The radiographer assists by reproducing the compressed position of the breast with his or her hands while the physician orients the radiograph to the breast and marks the surface of the breast at the appropriate site (Figs. 24-45 and 24-46).

Triangulation of the two surface marks fixes the three-dimensional location of the lesion within the breast. The needle can be inserted either perpendicular to the chest wall or parallel to the chest wall. The breast is washed with a topical antiseptic, and the selected site for needle insertion is anesthetized with lidocaine. The needle is inserted toward the lesion for the predetermined distance (Figs. 24-47 and 24-48). With the Frank guidewire system, a preliminary small incision is made in the skin and the needle is withdrawn after insertion, leaving only the guidewire in place. With the other needle-wire localization systems, the needle and wire are left in place. The breast is again radiographed in the craniocaudal and 90-degree lateral projections so that the exact site of the wire relative to the lesion can be determined.

Repositioning may be necessary if the original location is unsatisfactory. If repositioning of the guidewire is not necessary, a sterile gauze bandage is placed over the breast and the patient is referred to the surgical area for excision of the lesion (Fig. 24-49).

With the Kopans system, some practitioners insert the needle without the wire and, after checking the position, inject 0.3 ml of a colored dye, such as methylene blue. This further helps the surgeon immediately locate the lesion.

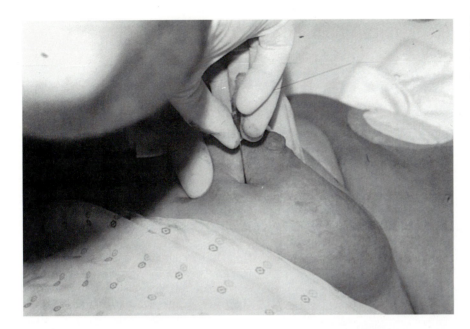

Fig. 24-47. A Frank biopsy needle and guide wire is inserted into the breast perpendicular to the chest wall at a site directly anterior to the lesion. The site and depth of insertion is selected by triangulation using the external skin marks.

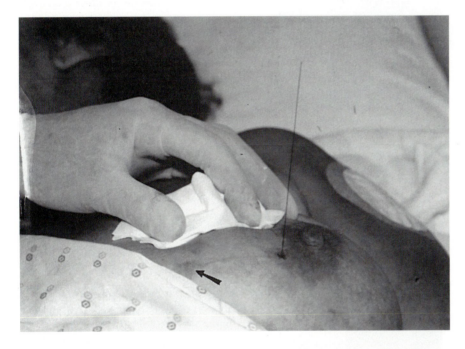

Fig. 24-48. After inserting the needle and guide wire to the depth of the lesion, the needle is removed leaving the guide wire in place. The lateral skin mark used for selecting needle insertion site is seen (arrow).

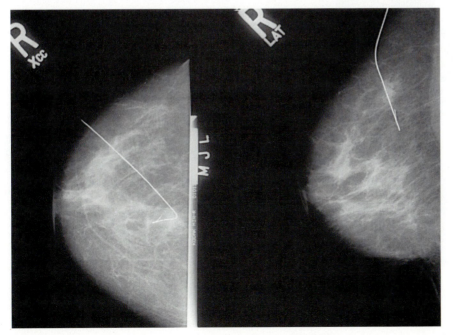

Fig. 24-49. Craniocaudal and true lateral right-angle projections demonstrate the relationship of the wire to the lesion. The needle has been removed.

Localization of nonpalpable lesions for biopsy

485

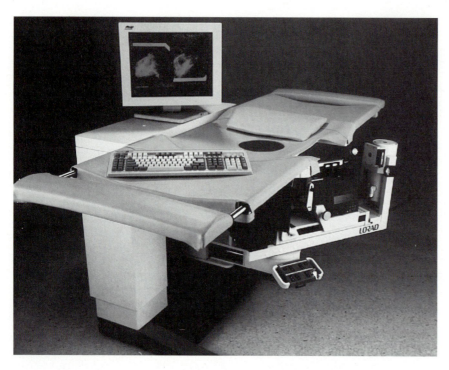

Fig. 24-50. Prone stereotactic biopsy system with digital imaging.

(Courtesy Delta Medical Systems, Inc.)

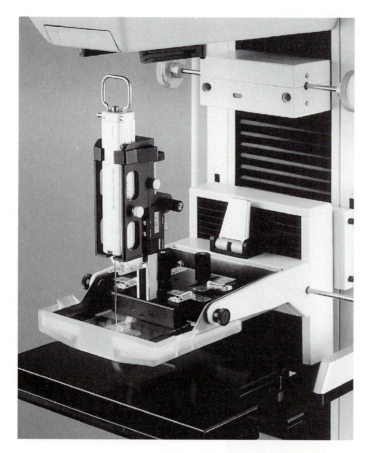

Fig. 24-51. Upright stereotactic system attached to a dedicated mammography unit.

(Courtesy LORAD Medical Systems, Inc.)

STEREOTACTIC PROCEDURES

Approximately 85% of all nonpalpable breast lesions identified by mammography are not malignant. However, the results are not definite until the breast lesion has been microscopically evaluated. Stereotactic intervention, or *stereotaxis,* is a minor surgical procedure used in determining the benign or malignant nature of suspicious breast lesions. Stereotaxis, guided by mammographic imaging, is the preferred technique of obtaining biopsy specimens of nonpalpable breast lesions. Increasing interest in this technique of breast biopsy, due primarily to the accurate diagnostic results produced by wide screening mammography, has caused it to be more widely used throughout the modern world. More women are becoming candidates for stereotactic breast biopsies because the eligibility criterion is mammographic evidence of a nonpalpable breast lesion.

Stereotaxis is used to differentiate between benign and malignant breast lesions. The benefit of stereotaxis compared with surgical biopsy is that there is less pain, scarring, recovery time, and cost for the patient, as well as less anxiety.

Stereotaxis can expedite pathology results, enabling potential surgical decisions, such as those regarding lumpectomy or mastectomy, to be made with minimal delay.

Stereotactic breast biopsy requires a team approach involving a radiologist, radiographer, cytologist or histologist, and surgeon. The radiologist, radiographer, and occasionally the surgeon perform the procedure. In the best-case scenario, the cytologist is present to offer immediate breast specimen analysis.

Stereotactic prone biopsy tables and upright, add-on devices used for breast biopsy intervention are both commercially available (Figs. 24-50 and 24-51). The upright, add-on system has disadvantages which include limited working space, potential for patient motion, lack of patient cooperation due to patient's ability to observe the procedure, and fainting. Both biopsy systems are capable of performing three procedures, but because of the disadvantages, the upright system will not be discussed at the same level of detail as the prone biopsy system.

Stereotactic prone biopsy tables are the most popular and most widely used. The patient is in the prone position, unable to see the procedure, which maximizes patient cooperation and minimizes motion, two crucial components in measuring the success of the procedure. The breast being examined hangs freely through the open aperture of the prone biopsy table, which enables increased flexibility in positioning (Fig. 24-52).

Stereotactic breast biopsy uses the concept of three-dimensional triangulation to identify the exact location of a breast lesion. A digitizer, an electronic instrument capable of calculating the triangulation coordinates, is commercially available and when used, reduces the procedure time significantly (Fig. 24-53). The digitizer transmits the lesion coordinates to the stage, or "brain," of the prone biopsy table where dialing-in of the triangulation coordinates occurs. The stage of the system also supports the biopsy gun, a mechanism that houses the biopsy needle and provides the force needed to project the biopsy needle into the breast tissue (Fig. 24-54). The digitizer calculates X, Y, and Z triangulation coordinates used by the radiographer and/or surgeon to determine the direction of the biopsy needle. The X coordinate identifies the transverse location (from right to left), the Y coordinate identifies the height of the lesion (from top to bottom), and the Z coordinate designates the depth (front to back) the needle will be inserted to reach the breast lesion. Two exposures on a single film are taken at a difference of 30 degrees, one exposure at +15 degrees and the other at −15 degrees from the perpendicular. The resulting image localizes the breast lesion in three dimensions. The "double exposed" image is referred to as a stereo image (Fig. 25-55). Using the stereo image, the physician determines the appropriate approach needed to reach the breast lesion. The time needed to perform any one of the three stereotactic procedures is 30 minutes to 1 hour.

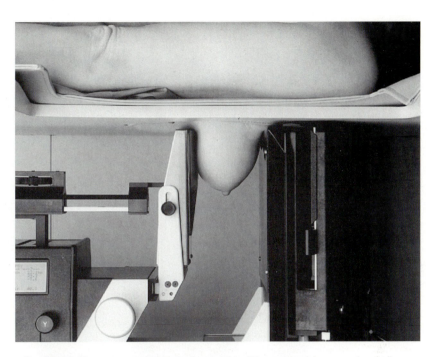

Fig. 24-52. The open aperture in the table of the prone biopsy system allows the breast to be positioned beneath the table.

(Courtesy LORAD Medical Systems, Inc.)

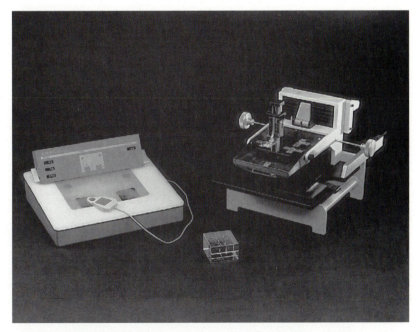

Fig. 24-53. The digitizer (*left*) calculates and transmits the X, Y, and Z coordinates to the stage of the biopsy system, where the biopsy gun is attached. This information is used to determine placement of the biopsy needle.

(Courtesy LORAD Medical Systems, Inc.)

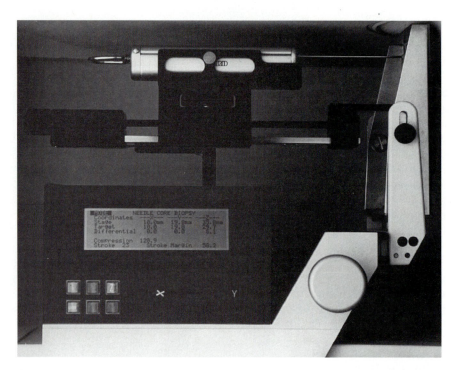

Fig. 24-54. The stage, or "brain," of the biopsy system supports the biopsy gun. The X, Y, and Z coordinates are displayed here.

(Courtesy Delta Medical Systems, Inc.)

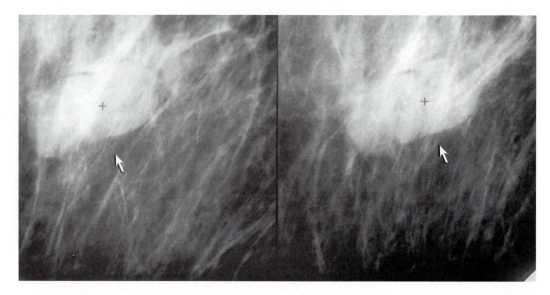

Fig. 24-55. Stereo images demonstrating 3-dimensional visualization of a breast lesion prior to intervention *(arrows)*.

(Courtesy Ross J. Wright, Baldwin.)

Before beginning the procedure, the physician reviews the initial mammographic images to determine the shortest distance from the surface of the skin to the breast lesion. Identification of the exact lesion location permits the biopsy needle to travel through the least amount of breast tissue, therefore minimally traumatizing the breast. For example, a lesion located in the lateral aspect of the upper outer quadrant would be approached from the lateral aspect, whereas a lesion located in the medial and superior portion of the breast would be approached from above. After a successful approach has been determined, the patient is placed in the prone position with the affected breast positioned through the open aperture, permitting the breast to fall freely away from the chest wall. The breast is compressed and a single scout image is taken to localize the breast lesion. Once the breast lesion has been localized, stereo images are taken to triangulate the lesion so that proper coordinates can be calculated and dialed into the biopsy table stage. The breast is aseptically cleansed to minimize infectious complications. Pain, another complication, can be effectively managed using a local anesthetic to numb the skin at the area where the biopsy needle enters.

The physician's preference generally determines which of the three procedures will be performed. Fine needle aspiration biopsy (FNAB) employs a hollow needle to extract tissue cells from a suspicious lesion. Large core needle biopsy (LCNB) uses a needle with a groove adjacent to the tip of the needle to obtain small amounts of tissue. Needle-wire localization places a hooked guidewire at a lesion to aid in biopsy by excision. All three procedures can be accomplished using the prone or upright stereotactic breast biopsy systems.

The physician decides where the first and subsequent peripheral passes (travel of the biopsy needle to reach the breast lesion) will occur. Five passes are commonly obtained to ensure multiple tissue samples for FNAB or LCNB procedures. The travel, or throw, of the biopsy needle occurs through use of the biopsy gun. The biopsy gun projects the hollow biopsy needle into the breast tissue, using force determined by the preset X, Y, and Z coordinates. A 2-mm incision is made in the skin and the tip of the needle is placed just beneath the skin line and directed toward the breast lesion.

The needle-wire localization procedure is performed in an attempt to locate the breast lesion using only one hooked guidewire and needle. In place of the biopsy gun, an apparatus called a needle guide, which is attached to the stage in a clip-on fashion, is used to guide the needle into place. Craniocaudal and true lateral images are obtained for placement of the needle. When the needle is correctly placed, the wire is inserted through the needle to the breast lesion location and the needle then withdrawn, leaving the wire in place. Following needle-wire localization, the patient is properly bandaged and referred to the surgical area for excisional biopsy.

After the 2-mm incision is made in the breast for FNAB and LCNB, the tip of the needle is placed just beneath the skin and directed toward the breast lesion. A set of stereo images is obtained to confirm correct direction of the needle. The first biopsy pass is made by placing the biopsy needle within the lesion and obtaining a "post-fire" image to confirm correct placement of the needle (Fig. 24-56). This image determines the course of subsequent passes. Redigitization, or using the digitizer to repeat the steps needed to calculate the new triangulation coordinates, can be done at this time to obtain additional samples, or a similar goal can be achieved by estimating where to move the biopsy needle based on the initial location within the breast lesion. The biopsy needle must make a clean pass through the lesion to the opposite side and be pulled back through the lesion to ensure adequate sampling. This procedure is repeated, based on the discretion of the physician, four or five times.

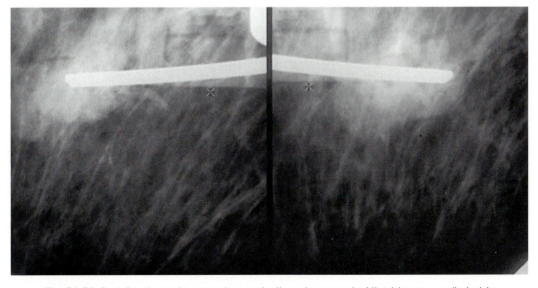

Fig. 24-56. Post-fire stereo images demonstrating placement of the biopsy needle inside the lesion.

(Courtesy Ross J. Wright, Baldwin.)

The FNAB tissue sample is obtained using the negative pressure, or suction, of a syringe to aspirate lesion cells into the hollow of the needle. The aspirated cells are managed in one of two ways. The cells can remain inside the needle, still attached to the syringe, and the needle can be sent to the pathology lab for the pathologist to put the cells on a slide there; or the cells may be placed on a slide in the area where the procedure is performed, and the slide can then be transported to the lab. LCNB tissue samples are obtained using a needle with a groove adjacent to the needle tip. With the needle located inside the lesion, a sheath or needle covering slides over the groove, capturing a small amount of tissue inside the groove of the needle. The sheath holds the tissue sample in place while the needle is withdrawn. When the needle is outside the breast, the sheath is pulled back, exposing the tissue sample. The sample is then transferred to a specimen container for transportation to the lab.

At the completion of five needle passes for the FNAB and LCNB procedures and correct placement of the wire for needle-wire localization, the breast is cleansed and appropriately bandaged using sterile technique. To aid the process of healing, it may be beneficial to apply Steri-strips to the incision site. Compression may be applied to prevent excessive bleeding, and ice may be applied to minimize discomfort and swelling of the related tissues.

Breast Specimen Radiography

Of equal importance with regard to accurate preoperative localization of the site for excisional biopsy is the need to confirm that the suspected lesion is contained in its entirety in the tissue removed during the biopsy. Often very small lesions are characterized only by tissue irregularity or microcalcifications that are nonpalpable in the excised specimen and may not be detectable on visual inspection. Compression of the specimen is necessary to identify lesions, especially lesions that do not contain calcifications. Magnification images can help to better visualize microcalcifications. Specimen radiography is often done in an immediate postexcision procedure while the patient is still under anesthesia. Speed is therefore imperative. The selection of film type, technical factors, and the procedure for handling the specimen must be established ahead of time. The cooperation of the radiologist, radiographer, surgeon, and pathologist is a necessity. Extremely fine-grain non-screen film may be used because exposure to the patient is no longer a factor. Exposure factors used depend on the thickness of the specimen and the film employed (Fig. 24-57).

It may be helpful to obtain two images of the breast specimen, one for the radiologist for interpretation and the second for the pathologist. The pathologist often uses the specimen radiograph to precisely locate the area of concern. The second step is to match the actual specimen to the specimen radiograph just prior to dissection. Marking the area of concern by placing a radiopaque object, such as a 1- or 2-inch needle, directly at the area of concern will assist the pathologist to more accurately locate the abnormality.

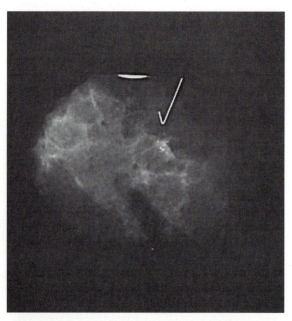

Fig. 24-57. Radiograph of a surgical specimen containing suspicious microcalcifications.

Examination of Milk Ducts

Occasionally, when a nipple discharge is localized in one of the multiple duct openings on the nipple, the milk duct can be studied with opaque contrast medium. The purpose of the examination is to seek evidence of an intraductal mass as the cause of the discharge.

Equipment and supplies needed for the examination are a sterile hypodermic syringe; a 30-gauge needle with a specially prepared, smooth round tip; a skin cleansing agent; sterile gauze sponges or cotton balls; a waste basin; and an organic, water-soluble, iodinated contrast medium.

After the nipple is cleansed, the round-tipped needle is inserted into the orifice of the duct and the contrast medium is injected. To prevent unnecessary discomfort and possible extravasation, the injection is terminated as soon as the patient experiences a sense of fullness. Usually, less than 1 ml of contrast medium is needed. Occasionally, when ducts are very distended, as much as 3 ml can be used. The following guidelines are observed:

- Immediately take radiographs with the patient positioned for the craniocaudal and lateral projections (Fig. 24-58).
- Employ the exposure techniques used in general mammography.
- Do not apply compression, because it would expel the contrast medium.

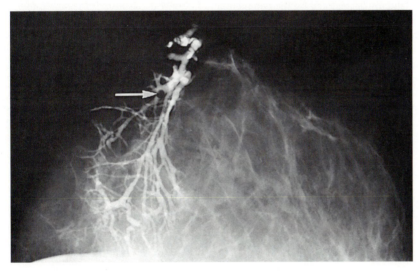

Fig. 24-58. Craniocaudal projection of opacified milk ducts.

Summary

Radiographic examination of the breast is a technically demanding procedure. Success is extremely dependent on the skills of the radiographer, more so than in most other areas of radiology. In addition to skill, the radiographer must have a strong desire to perform high quality mammography and be willing to work with the patient to allay qualms and obtain cooperation. In the course of taking the patient's history and physically examining and radiographing the breasts, the radiographer may be asked questions about breast disease, breast self-examination (BSE), and breast radiography that the the patient has been reluctant to ask other health professionals. The knowledge, skill, and attitude imparted to the patient may be lifesaving. Although most patients will not have significant breast disease when first examined, the statistics show that over 8% of the patients will develop breast cancer at some time during their life. An early positive mammography encounter may make the patient more willing to undergo mammography in the future. Breast radiography properly done is safe, and at present the application of mammography offers the best hope for significantly reducing the mortality of breast cancer.

Definition of Terms

acinus One of multiple small, saclike structures found within the breast parenchyma capable of dilatation.

aperture An interchangeable device used to constrict the imaging field, enabling a smaller, more defined image.

areola The circular area of increased pigmentation surrounding the nipple.

early Breast cancer found at its most curable stage. Early breast cancers can be seen by mammography approximately 2 years before they can be clinically detected.

film-screen mammography A breast imaging process in which the radiographic densities are recorded on special single-emulsion radiographic film using high-detail intensifying screens.

involution A normal process or stage in the development of the mature breast in which the volume of glandular tissue and supporting connective tissue stroma decreases. The process starts at variable times after the initial maturing of the breast. The process is substantially accelerated by the completion of a pregnancy.

microcalcifications Tiny calcifications found in the breast. Some patterns of microcalcifications are commonly associated with breast cancer; others are rarely associated with cancer.

molybdenum target A hard, silvery white metallic element (Mo) most suitable for producing a low energy x-ray beam in the kilovoltage range appropriate for film-screen mammography.

orthogonal coned magnification Two radiographic images obtained at right angles using a coning aperture and magnification of 1.5 to 2 times the size of the original image. These images better characterize the borders and architecture of nodules and size, shape, and configuration of breast calcification.

postpartum mastitis A bacterial infection in the breast appearing after pregnancy, usually as a complication of breast feeding.

radical mastectomy A surgical procedure in which the breast and underlying pectoralis major and pectoralis minor muscles are removed, usually with full removal of lymph nodes from the axilla.

risk versus benefit A comparison of the potential harm from a specific action with the potential benefit to be derived from the action.

screening Testing for evidence of disease in an asymptomatic population.

xeromammogram A radiographic study of the breast in which the radiographic densities of the breast are reflected in discharges of a charged plate. The discharge pattern is made visible by depositing toner powder on the plate. The powder is transferred to a paper, producing a permanent image. The plate is used again after recharging.

SELECTED BIBLIOGRAPHY

American College of Radiology: Mammography quality control: radiologic technologists manual, Chicago, 1992.

Anderson I et al: Breast cancer screening with mammography by population-based, randomized trial with mammography as the only screening mode, Radiology 132:273-276, 1979.

Anderson I et al: Radiographic patterns of the mammary parenchyma; variation with age at examination and age at first birth, Radiology 138:59-62, 1981.

Baker LH: Breast cancer detection demonstration project: five-year summary report, CA 32:194-225, 1982.

Bassett LW et al: Reduced-dose magnification mammography, Radiology 141:665-670, 1981.

Bassett LW et al: Breast radiography using the oblique projection, Radiology 149:585-587, 1983.

Bassett LW and Gold RH: The evolution of mammography, AJR 150:493-498, 1988.

Eklund GW et al: Improved imaging of the augmented breast, AJR 151:469-473, 1988.

Egan RL: Early breast cancer. In Gallager HS, editor: Mammography: a historical perspective, early breast cancer detection and treatment, New York, 1975, John Wiley & Sons.

Egan RL et al: Intramammary calcifications without an associated mass in benign and malignant diseases, Radiology 137:1-7, 1980.

Egan RL et al: Grids in mammography, Radiology 146:359-362, 1983.

Fajardo LL and Westerman BR: Mammography equipment: practiced considerations for the radiologist, Applied Radiol 19(5):12-15, 1990.

Feig SA: Assessment of the hypothetical risk from mammography and evaluation of the potential benefit, Radiol Clin North Am 21:173-183, 1983.

Feig SA: Radiation risk for mammography: is it clinically significant? AJR 143:469-475, 1984.

Feig SA: Mammography equipment: principles, features, selection, Radiol Clin North Am 25:897-911, 1987.

Fox S: Benefit/risk analysis of aggressive mammography screening, Radiology 128:359-365, 1978.

Gisrold JJ et al: Prebiopsy localization of nonpalpable breast lesions, AJR 143:477-481, 1984.

Goodrich WA: The Cleopatra view in xeromammography, Radiology 128:811-812, 1978.

Hammerstein GR et al: Absorbed radiation dose in mammography, Radiology 130:485-491, 1979.

Hayes-Macaluso MK et al: Imaging the augmented breast, Applied Radiol 22(12):21-26, 1993.

Hoeffken W and Langi M: Mammography: technique, diagnosis, differential diagnosis, results, Philadelphia, 1977, WB Saunders.

Homer MJ: Percutaneous localization of breast lesions: experience with the Frank Breast Biopsy Guide, J Can Assoc Radiol 30:238-241, 1979.

Jackson VP: The status of mammographically guided fine needle aspiration biopsy of nonpalpable breast lesions, Radiol Clin North Am 30(1):155-166, 1992.

Jackson VP, Lex AM, and Smith DJ: Patient discomfort during screen-film mammography, Radiology 168:421-423, 1988.

Jensen SR et al: Wire localization of nonpalpable breast lesions (technical note), Radiology 132:484-485, 1979.

Kimme Smith C, Bassett LW, and Gold RH: Evaluation of radiation dose, focal spot, and automatic exposure of newer film-screen mammography units, AJR 149:913-917, 1987.

Kopans DB et al: Modified needle-hookwire technique to simplify preoperative localization of occult breast lesions (technical note), Radiology 134:781, 1980.

Law J and Kirkpatrick AE: Films, screens and cassettes for mammography, Br J Radiol 62:163-167, 1989.

Linden SS and Sullivan DC: Breast skin calcifications: localization with a stereotactic device, Radiology 171:570-571, 1989.

Loh CK et al: Improved method of localization of nonpalpable breast lesions (technical note). Radiology 130:244-245, 1979.

Mammography 1982: a statement of The American Cancer Society, CA 32:226-228, 1982.

Martin JE: A demonstration comparing film mammography with the new high sensitivity xeromammography, Radiographics 9:153-168, 1989.

Miller SH et al: Improved imaging of the augmented breast, AJR 151:469-473, 1988.

Moskowitz M: Mammographic screening significance of minimal breast cancers, AJR 136:735, 1981.

Moskowitz M: Mammography to screen asymtomatic women for breast cancer, AJR 143:457-459, 1984.

Moskowitz M et al: Mammographic patterns as markers for high-risk benign breast disease and incident cancers, Radiology 134:293-295, 1980.

Moskowitz M et al: Evidence of breast cancer mortality reduction aggressive screening in women under age 50, AJR 138:911, 1982.

Muntz EP et al: Mammography at reduced doses: present performance and future possibilities, AJR 141:665, 1981.

Pennes DR and Homer MJ: Disappearing breast masses caused by compression during mammography, Radiology 165:327-328, 1987.

Sickles EA: Microfocal spot magnification mammography using xeroradiographic and screen-film recording systems, Radiology 131:599-607, 1979.

Sickles EA et al: Controlled single-blind clinical evaluation of low-dose mammographic screen-film systems, Radiology 130:347-351, 1979.

Skolnick AA: Ultrasound may help detect breast implant leaks, JAMA 267(6):786, 1992.

Stanton L et al: Study of mammographic exposure and detail visibility using three systems: Xerox 125, Min-R and Zonics XERG, Radiology 132:455-462, 1979.

Tabar L et al: Screening for breast cancer, the Swedish trial, Radiology 138:219-222, 1981.

Tabar L et al: Galactography: the diagnostic procedure of choice for nipple discharge, Radiology 149:31, 1983.

Selected bibliography

493

Chapter 25

CENTRAL NERVOUS SYSTEM

NINA KOWALCZYK

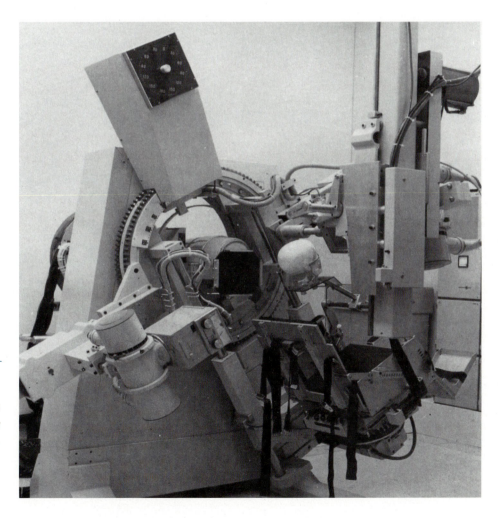

A somersault chair for pneumoen-cephalograms. When air was injected into a patient's ventricles, the patient was somersaulted so that air could rise to the highest point. Radiographs were taken in order to show any space-occupying lesions in the brain.

For descriptive purposes, the central nervous system is divided into two parts: (1) the *brain* (encephalon), which occupies the cranial cavity, and (2) the *spinal cord* (medulla spinalis), which is suspended within the vertebral canal.

The brain is composed of an outer portion of gray matter called the cortex and an inner portion of white matter. The brain consists of the *cerebrum* (telencephalon), the *cerebellum,* and the *brain stem,* which is continuous with the spinal cord (Fig. 25-1). The brain stem consists of the *diencephalon, midbrain* (mesencephalon), *pons,* and *medulla oblongata.*

The cerebrum comprises the largest part of the brain and is referred to as the *forebrain.* The surface of the cerebral hemispheres is convoluted by many fissures and grooves that make them into lobes and lobules. The stemlike portion that connects the cerebrum to the pons and the cerebellum is termed the *midbrain.* The cerebellum, the pons, and the medulla oblongata make up the *hindbrain.*

A deep cleft, called the longitudinal fissure, separates the cerebrum into *right* and *left hemispheres,* which are closely connected by bands of nerve fibers or commissures. The main commissure between the cerebral hemispheres is the *corpus callosum.* Each cerebral hemisphere contains a fluid-filled cavity called a *lateral ventricle.* At the diencephalon, the cerebral hemispheres surround the *third ventricle.* Extending inferiorly from the diencephalon is the *hypophysis cerebri* (pituitary gland). This endocrine gland resides in the hypophyseal fossa of the sella turcica.

The cerebellum, the largest part of the hindbrain, is separated from the cerebrum by a deep transverse cleft. The hemispheres of the cerebellum are connected by a median constricted area called the *vermis.* The surface of the cerebellum contains numerous transverse fissures that account for its laminated appearance. The tissues between the curved fissures are called *folia.* The pons, which forms the upper part of the hindbrain, is the commissure (coming together across the midline) between the cerebrum, the cerebellum, and the medulla. The medulla, which extends between the pons and the spinal cord, forms the lower portion of the hindbrain.

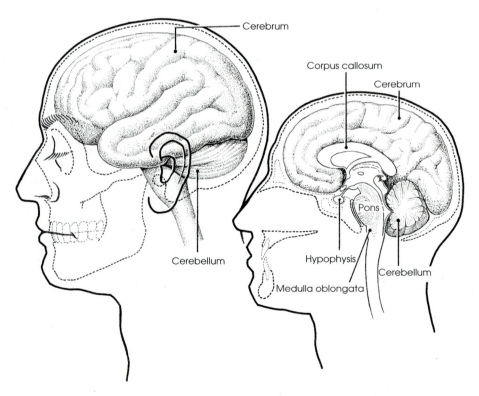

Fig. 25-1. Lateral surface and midsection of brain.

The spinal cord is a slender, elongated structure consisting of an inner, gray, cellular substance, which has an H shape on transverse section, and an outer, white, fibrous substance (Figs. 25-2 and 25-3). The cord extends from the brain, being connected to the medulla oblongata at the level of the foramen magnum, to the approximate level of the space between the first and second lumbar vertebrae. The spinal cord ends in a pointed extremity called the *conus medullaris*. A delicate, fibrous strand extending from the conus medullaris attaches the cord to the upper coccygeal segment. There are 31 pairs of spinal nerves, each arising from two roots at the sides of the spinal cord. The nerves are transmitted through the intervertebral and sacral foramina. Spinal nerves below the termination of the spinal cord extend inferiorly through the vertebral canal. These nerves resemble a horse's tail and are referred to as the cauda equina.

The brain and spinal cord are enclosed by three continuous, protective membranes called *meninges*. The inner sheath, called the *pia mater* (L., tender mother), is highly vascular and closely adherent to the underlying brain and cord structure.

The delicate central sheath is called the *arachnoid*. This membrane is separated from the pia mater by a comparatively wide space called the *subarachnoid space,* which is widened in certain areas. These areas of increased width are called cisternae, the widest of which is the *cisterna cerebellomedullaris* (cisterna magna). This cavity is triangular and is situated at the posterosuperior part of the subarachnoid space between the base of the cerebellum and the dorsal surface of the medulla oblongata. The subarachnoid space is continuous with the ventricular system of the brain and communicates with it by way of the *median aperture* (foramen of Magendie) and by *lateral apertures* (foramina of Luschka) located between the cisterna cerebellomedullaris and the fourth ventricle. The ventricles of the brain and the subarachnoid space contain cerebrospinal fluid (CSF). The cisterna cerebellomedullaris is sometimes used as a point of entry into the subarachnoid space.

The outermost sheath, called the *dura mater* (L., hard mother), forms the strong, fibrous covering of the brain and spinal cord. The dura is separated from the arachnoid by the *subdural space* and from the vertebral periosteum by the *epidural space*. These spaces do not communicate with the ventricular system. The dura mater is composed of two layers throughout its cranial portion. The outer (endosteal) layer lines the cranial bones, thus serving as periosteum to their inner surface. The inner (meningeal) layer serves to protect the brain and to support the blood vessels. The meningeal layer also sends out four partitions for the support and protection of the various parts of the brain. The dura mater extends below the spinal cord, to the level of the second sacral segment, to enclose the spinal nerves, which are prolonged inferiorly from the cord to their respective exits. The lower portion of the dura mater is called the *dural sac*.

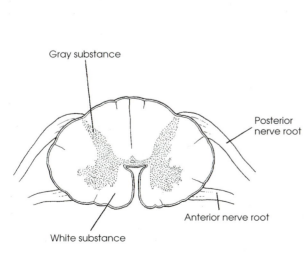

Fig. 25-2. Transverse section of spinal cord.

Gray substance

Posterior nerve root

Anterior nerve root

White substance

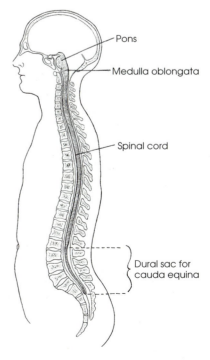

Fig. 25-3. Sagittal section showing spinal cord.

Pons

Medulla oblongata

Spinal cord

Dural sac for cauda equina

The ventricular system of the brain consists of four irregular, fluid-containing cavities that communicate with each other through connecting channels (Figs. 25-4 to 25-6). The two upper cavities are an identical pair and are simply called *right* and *left lateral ventricles.* They are situated, one on each side of the median sagittal plane, in the inferior, medial part of the corresponding hemisphere of the cerebrum.

Each lateral ventricle consists of a central portion called the *body* of the cavity. The body is prolonged anteriorly, posteriorly, and inferiorly into hornlike portions that give the ventricle an approximate U shape. The prolonged portions are known as the *anterior* (frontal), the *posterior* (occipital), and the *inferior* (temporal) *horns* (cornua). Each lateral ventricle is connected to the third ventricle by a channel called the *interventricular foramen* (foramen of Monro), through which it communicates directly with the third ventricle and indirectly with the opposite lateral ventricle.

The *third ventricle* is a slitlike cavity with a somewhat quadrilateral shape. It is situated in the median sagittal plane just inferior to the level of the bodies of the lateral ventricles. This cavity extends anteroinferiorly from the pineal gland, which produces a recess in its posterior wall, to the optic chiasm, which produces a recess in its anteroinferior wall.

The interventricular foramina, one from each lateral ventricle, open into the anterosuperior portion of the third ventricle. The cavity is continuous posteroinferiorly with the fourth ventricle by a passage known as the *cerebral aqueduct* (aqueduct of Sylvius).

The *fourth ventricle* is diamond shaped and is the cavity of the hindbrain. It is also a midline structure located anterior to the cerebellum and posterior to the pons and upper portion of the medulla oblongata. The distal, pointed end of the fourth ventricle is continuous with the central canal of the medulla oblongata. The fourth ventricle communicates with the subarachnoid space via the *median aperture* and the *lateral apertures,* as discussed earlier in this chapter.

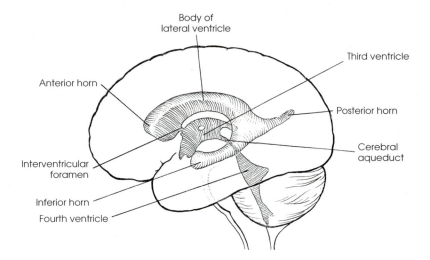

Fig. 25-4. Lateral aspect of cerebral ventricles in relation to surface of brain.

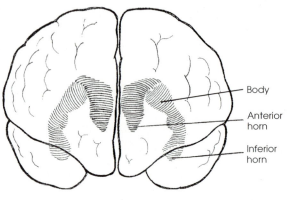

Fig. 25-5. Anterior aspect of lateral cerebral ventricles in relation to surface of brain.

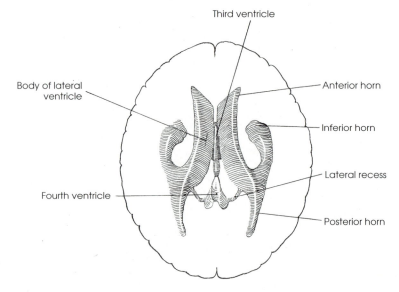

Fig. 25-6. Superior aspect of cerebral ventricles in relation to surface of brain.

Plain Radiographic Examination

Radiographs of the cerebral and visceral cranium and of the vertebral column may be employed to demonstrate bony anatomy. In the case of trauma, radiographs are obtained to detect bony injury, subluxation, or dislocation of the vertebral column and to determine the extent and stability of the bony injury.

When radiographing a traumatized patient with possible central nervous system involvement, a cross-table lateral cervical spine radiograph must be obtained first to rule out fracture or misalignment of the cervical spine. Approximately two thirds of significant spine pathologic conditions can be detected on this initial radiograph. Care must be taken to adequately demonstrate the entire cervical spine, to include the C7-T1 articulation. It may be necessary to employ the Twining (Swimmers) method (see Chapter 8, Volume 1) to demonstrate radiographically this anatomic region.

Once the cross-table lateral radiograph has been checked and cleared by a physician, it is necessary to obtain the following cervical spine projections: AP projection, bilateral AP oblique projections (trauma technique may be necessary), and an AP projection of the dens (odontoid process). A vertebral arch, or pillar radiograph (see Chapter 8, Volume 1) of the cervical spine may be used to provide additional information regarding the posterior portions of the cervical vertebrae. An upright lateral cervical spine radiograph may also be requested to better demonstrate the alignment and assess the normal lordotic curvature of the vertebrae.

Tomography (see Chapter 29, Volume 3) may be used to supplement spine radiographs for initial screening purposes. However, tomography has been largely replaced with computed tomography (CT; see Chapter 33, Volume 3) in many institutions. Tomography may be employed to demonstrate long, continuous areas of the spine, whereas CT is limited because of the design and reconstruction limitations of the equipment. Disadvantages of tomography include a lack of soft tissue detail and the difficulty in positioning a traumatized patient for lateral tomographic radiographs.

Myelography

Myelography (Gr., *myelos,* marrow; the spinal cord) is the general term applied to radiologic examination of the central nervous system structures situated within the vertebral canal. These examinations are performed by introducing a contrast medium into the subarachnoid space by spinal puncture, most commonly at the L2-3 or L3-4 interspace or at the cisterna cerebellomedullaris. Myelography is employed to demonstrate extrinsic spinal cord compression caused by a herniated disk, bone fragments, or tumors, as well as spinal cord swelling resulting from traumatic injury. These encroachments appear radiographically as a deformity in, or an obstruction of the passage of the column of contrast medium within the subarachnoid space. Myelography is also useful in identifying the narrowing of subarachnoid space by evaluating the dynamic flow patterns of the CSF.

CONTRAST MEDIA

A non–water-soluble iodinated ester (Pantopaque) was introduced in 1942. It was used for many years for myelography, but is no longer commercially available. Disadvantages of this contrast material included poor visualization of the nerve root sheaths and the fact that it had to be removed from the subarachnoid space after the myelogram was completed.

The first water-soluble nonionic iodinated contrast agent, metrizamide, was introduced in the late 1970s. Following its introduction, water-soluble contrast media quickly became the medium of choice. Nonionic water-soluble contrast agents provide good visualization of nerve roots (Fig. 25-7), provide good enhancement for follow-up CT of the spine, and are readily absorbed by the body. One disadvantage of metrizamide was its tendency to be absorbed very quickly, requiring radiographs to be performed promptly and accurately. Further research has lead to the development of improved nonionic contrast agents such as iohexol, iopamidol, and ioversol. Improvements in nonionic contrast agents have resulted in fewer side effects, rendering them the contrast media of choice in performing myelography and CT of the spine. CT examinations of the spine are performed without contrast. Postmyelogram CT studies are done with the contrast already in the thecal sac.

Gas myelography uses air or oxygen but these negative contrast agents are rarely used today. Because of the different weights of gaseous and opaque contrast agents, they move in opposite directions when the patient is moved. The gas rises as the patient's head is elevated, whereas the opaque medium gravitates downward. Gas myelography is not performed with any regularity at most health care facilities. (For additional information, see Volume 3, p. 96 of the sixth edition of this atlas.) When used, the gaseous contrast medium is introduced by way of lumbar puncture.

Preparation of examining room

One of the responsibilities of the radiographer is the preparation of the examining room before the patient's arrival. The radiographic equipment should be checked, and, because the procedure involves aseptic technique, the table and overhead equipment must be cleaned. The footboard should be attached, and the padded shoulder supports should be placed and ready for adjustment to the patient's height. The spot-filming device should be locked so that it cannot accidentally come in contact with the spinal needle.

The spinal puncture and injection of the contrast medium are performed in the radiology department. Under fluoroscopic observation, placement of the spinal needle is verified to be in the subarachnoid space, and then the contrast medium is injected. The sterile tray and the nonsterile items required for the spinal puncture and injection of the contrast medium should be ready for convenient placement.

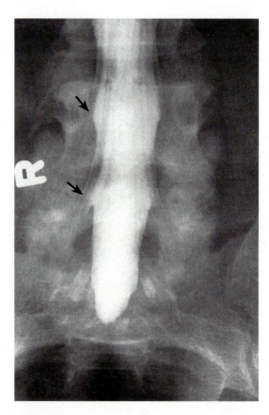

Fig. 25-7. Myelogram using water-soluble (metrizamide) contrast medium. Nerve roots seen at arrows.

EXAMINATION PROCEDURE

To reduce apprehension and to prevent alarm at unexpected maneuvers during the procedure, the details of performing the myelogram should be explained to the patient before the examination begins. The patient should be informed that there will be repeated and acute changes in the angulation of the examining table (Figs. 25-8 and 25-9) and also told why the head must be maintained in a fully extended position when the table is tilted to the Trendelenburg position. The patient must be assured of his or her safety when the table is acutely angled, and he or she must be assured that everything possible will be done to avoid causing unnecessary discomfort.

Some physicians prefer to have the patient placed on the table in the prone position for the spinal puncture. Most, however, have the patient adjusted in the lateral position with the spine flexed to widen the interspinous spaces for easier introduction of the needle.

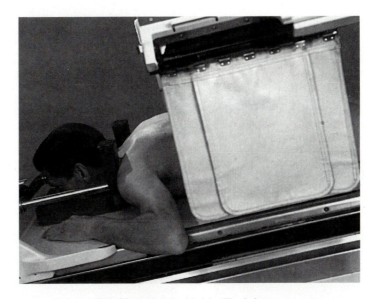

Fig. 25-8. Head of table tilted down.

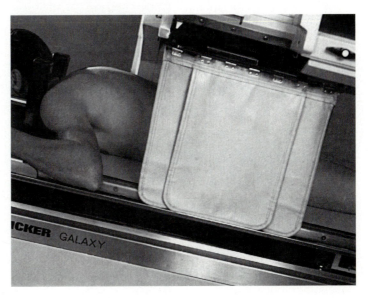

Fig. 25-9. Foot end of table tilted down.

The physician usually withdraws spinal fluid for laboratory analysis and injects an equal amout of contrast medium. After the injection has been completed, the spinal needle is removed. The traveling of the contrast medium column is observed fluoroscopically, and the direction of its flow is controlled by varying the angulation of the table. Spot radiographs are taken at the level of any blockage of or distortion in the outline of the contrast column. Conventional radiographic studies, with the central ray directed vertically or horizontally, may be taken as requested by the radiologist. Cross-table lateral radiographs are obtained with grid-front cassettes or a stationary grid, and they must be closely collimated (Figs. 25-10 to 25-15).

The position of the patient's head must be guarded as the contrast column nears the cervical area to prevent the medium from passing into the cerebral ventricles. Acute extension of the head compresses the cisterna cerebellomedullaris (cisterna magna) and thus prevents further ascent of the medium. Because the cisterna cerebellomedullaris is situated posteriorly, neither forward nor lateral flexion of the head will compress the cisternal cavity.

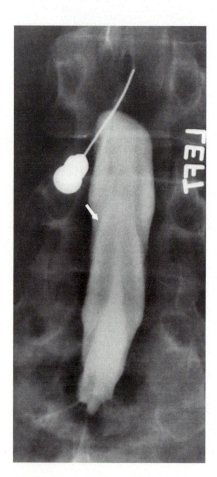

Fig. 25-10. Lumbar myelogram. AP projection with non water-soluble iodinated contrast medium, showing axillary pouches and corresponding nerve roots (arrow).

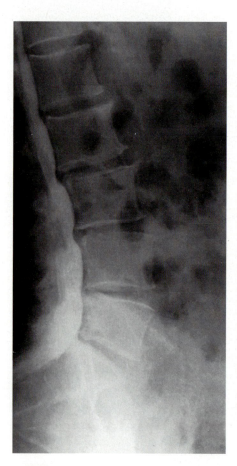

Fig. 25-11. Lumbar myelogram. Lateral projection with water-soluble (metrizamide) contrast medium.

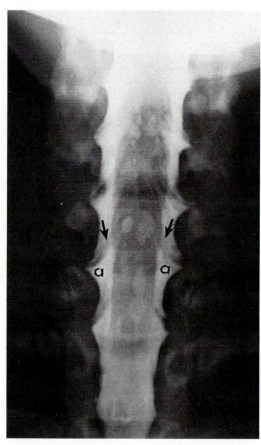

Fig. 25-12. Cervical myelogram. AP projection showing symmetrical nerve roots (arrows) and axillary pouches (a) on both sides, as well as spinal cord.

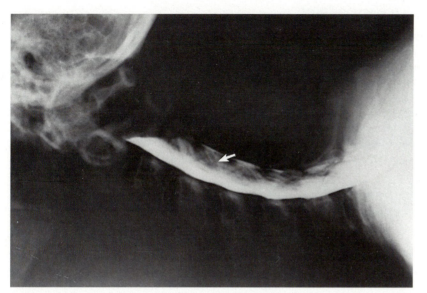

Fig. 25-13. Myelogram. Prone, cross-table lateral projection showing dentate ligament and posterior nerve roots *(arrow).*

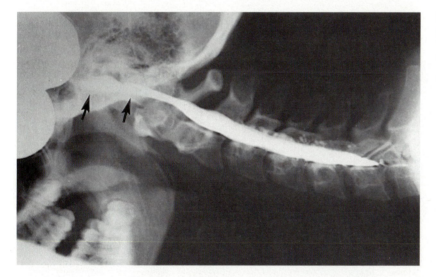

Fig. 25-14. Myelogram. Prone, cross-table lateral projection showing contrast medium passing through the foramen magnum and lying against the lower clivus *(arrows).*

(Courtesy Dr. K. Y. Chynn.)

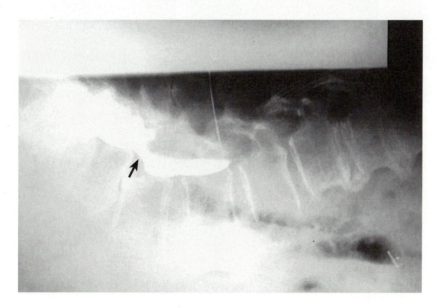

Fig. 25-15. Myelogram. Cross-table lateral projection showing subarachnoid space narrowing *(arrow).*

COMPUTED TOMOGRAPHY

Computed tomography is a rapid, noninvasive technique of imaging the central nervous system. It is particularly useful in the evaluation of head trauma to rule out hematomas (Fig. 25-16). CT of the brain is also quite helpful in the diagnosis and treatment of primary and metastatic neoplastic diseases of the brain and the management of hydrocephalus.

The myelographic procedure is usually followed by a CT examination of the spine (Fig. 25-17). The CT examination is generally limited to specific regions of the spine and performed while the contrast agent is still within the subarachnoid space. Because CT has the ability to distinguish between relatively small contrast differences, the contrast agent may be visualized up to 4 hours after the myelogram.

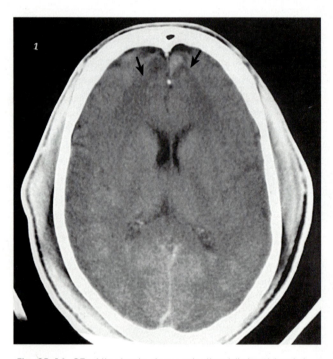

Fig. 25-16. CT of the brain demonstrating bilateral frontal and right temporal lobe brain contusions *(arrows)* following trauma.

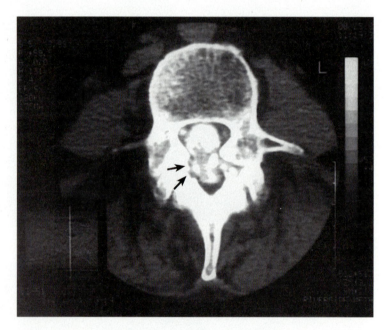

Fig. 25-17. CT myelogram of the lumbar spine demonstrating subarachnoid space narrowing *(arrows).*

CT myelography demonstrates the size, shape, and position of the spinal cord and the nerve roots. It is an excellent modality in cases of compressive injuries or in determining the extent of dural tears resulting in extravasation of the CSF.

CT of the spine without myelography may be performed in cases of spinal trauma (Fig. 25-18). Preoperatively, it can clearly demonstrate the size, number, and location of the fracture fragments. This information can greatly assist physicians during surgery. Postoperatively, CT may be utilized to assess the outcome of the surgery. See Chapter 33, Volume 3 for an in-depth discussion of CT imaging.

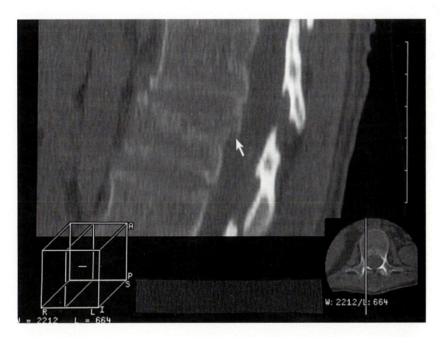

Fig. 25-18. Sagittal CT lumbar spine. Reconstruction of axial images showing a compression fracture of L1 following trauma *(arrow)*.

Diskography

Diskography and *nucleography* are terms used to denote the radiologic examination of individual intervertebral disks. The exam is performed by injection of a small quantity of one of the water-soluble, iodinated media into the center of the disk by way of a double-needle entry. This procedure was introduced by Lindblom[1] in 1950, and it has been further detailed by Cloward[2,3] and by Butt.[4]

---

[1]Lindblom K: Technique and results in myelography and disc puncture, Acta Radiol 34:321-330, 1950.
[2]Cloward RB and Buzaid LL: Discography, AJR 68:552-564, 1952.
[3]Cloward RB: Cervical discography: a contribution to the etiology and mechanism of neck, shoulder, and arm pain, Ann Surg 150:1052-1064, 1959.
[4]Butt WP: Discography—some interesting cases, J Can Assoc Radiol 17:167-175, 1966.

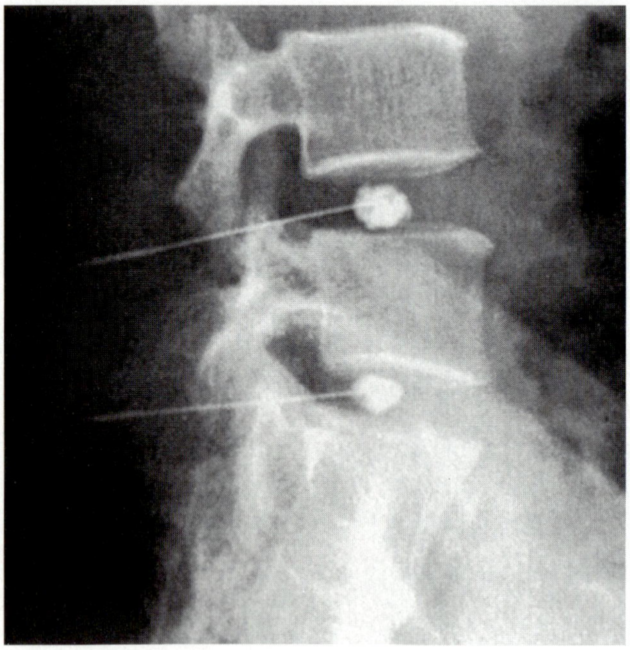

Diskography is used in the investigation of internal disk lesions, such as rupture of the nucleus pulposus, that cannot be demonstrated by myelographic examination (Fig. 25-19). Diskography may be performed separately, or it may be combined with myelography. The patient is given only a local anesthetic so that he or she will be fully conscious and therefore able to inform the physician as to the location of pain when the needles are inserted and the injection is made.

Magnetic resonance imaging (MRI) and CT myelography have largely replaced the use of diskography. (For more information regarding diskography, see Chapter 29, Volume 3, p. 109 of the seventh edition of this atlas.)

Fig. 25-19. Lumbar diskogram demonstrating normal nucleus pulposus of round contour type.

Chemonucleolysis

Begun in the early 1980s, *chemonucleolysis* is an alternative technique to conventional laminectomy for the treatment of lumbar herniated nucleus pulposus. This procedure employs a *chymopapain* enzyme, derived from the papaya, to dissolve the herniated disk.

Chemonucleolysis is generally performed after a CT myelogram confirms the presence and location of the herniated nucleus pulposus. The procedure is generally performed in the surgical area under fluoroscopic control. The patient is placed in a lateral position, and an 18-gauge needle is inserted into the nucleus pulposus. Diskography is routinely performed to ensure proper needle placement before the chymopapain injection. Once the enzyme is injected, the needle is kept in place for approximately 5 minutes before being removed.

Chemonucleolysis does not generally result in scarring, which is often associated with a conventional laminectomy procedure. However, post-treatment stiffness and spasm are often associated with chemonucleolysis, especially during the first few weeks after this treatment procedure.

Magnetic Resonance Imaging

Magnetic resonance imaging provides excellent anatomic detail of the brain, spinal cord, intervertebral disks, and subarachnoid space. Additionally, MRI can be performed without the need for intrathecal injection (into the subarachnoid space) of contrast media. Image reconstruction may be performed in a variety of planes (such as axial, sagittal, and coronal) to aid in the diagnosis and treatment of neurologic disorders (Figs. 25-20 to 25-22). Brain stem lesions as small as 3 mm in diameter can be identified on thin-slice axial images. MRI is the imaging modality of choice in the diagnosis of multiple sclerosis (MS). See Chapter 36, Volume 3 for a discussion of MRI.

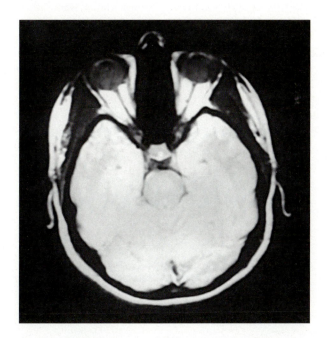

Fig. 25-20. Axial MRI section through the brain.

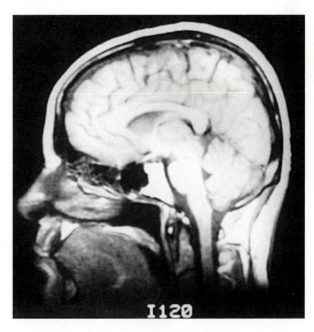

Fig. 25-21. Sagittal MRI section through the brain.

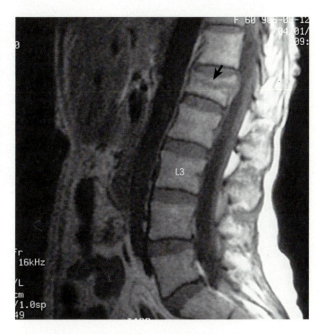

Fig. 25-22. Sagittal MRI section of the lumbar spine demonstrating a compression fracture of L1 following trauma *(arrow)*.

Cerebral Pneumonography/ Ventriculography

Since the introduction of CT scanners, cerebral pneumonography/ventriculography is seldom, if ever, performed in radiology departments; thus the discussion included in this chapter has been reduced. For additional information regarding cerebral pneumonography, see the Bibliography in this volume and Volume 3, pp. 872 to 888 in the fourth edition of this atlas.

Cerebral pneumonography is a general term applied to the radiologic examination of the brain by means of the introduction of a gaseous medium into the ventricular system. Because of the radiographic homogeneity of the brain substance and fluid-filled channels, noncalcified lesions of intracranial structures cannot be satisfactorily demonstrated without the use of a contrast agent. A gaseous medium—air, oxygen, or carbon dioxide—is generally used for this purpose in preference to opaque media, because the gases produce less irritation in the ventricular system. In addition, they are readily absorbed in the subarachnoid spaces.

Cerebral pneumonography is employed to demonstrate space-occupying, intracranial lesions as shown by filling defects or deformations in the shadow outline of the gas-filled ventricular system or the subarachnoid cisternae and channels. *Pneumoventriculography* (Fig. 25-23) and *pneumoencephalography* are the two specific terms used, respectively, to denote the direct and indirect routes of injection. These terms also indicate the extent of structural delineation obtained by each injection route.

Direct injection of the gas into the central ventricular system (pneumoventriculography) delineates only the inner, or ventricular, surfaces of the brain. Indirect introduction of the contrast agent by way of the subarachnoid route (pneumoencephalography) delineates the subarachnoid spaces of the brain as well as the ventricular system. Each procedure has specific indications and contraindications, so that the injection route is determined according to the type and location of the intracranial disorder.

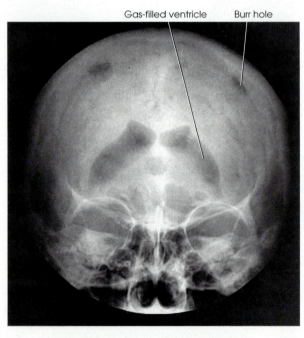

Gas-filled ventricle   Burr hole

Fig. 25-23. Pneumoventriculogram.

(Courtesy Dr. Ernest H. Wood.)

Stereotactic Surgery

Stereotactic surgery and *stereotrophic surgery* are terms used to denote a highly specialized neurosurgical therapeutic technique for the precise three-dimensional guidance of a slender surgical instrument through a burr hole in the cranium to a predetermined point deep within the brain. The first practical stereotactic instrument was introduced in the late 1940s for use with pneumoencephalography (Fig. 25-24). Stereotactic surgery is used in the treatment of various diseases of the nervous system, some of which cause a loss of control of body movement and some of which cause intractable pain. The most frequent use of this surgical technique may be for the treatment of Parkinson's disease. Other uses are to obtain a biopsy of a deep tumor within the brain and to drain abscesses. Stereotactic surgery is often the preferred technique for treatment of such conditions because the diseased structure can be reached and surgically destroyed with a slender, specialized instrument guided through a small burr hole in the cranium, thus eliminating the need for open surgery.

The tip of the surgical instrument must be placed in the target area with an accuracy of 1 mm deviation from the target point. This precise placement requires a specialized instrument-guidance system known as a stereotactic frame or stereotactic device (Fig. 25-25). Numerous types of stereotactic devices are currently in use. Basically, they consist of a frame into which the surgeon immobilizes the patient's head with attached fixation screws. The frame incorporates an external reference system and an adjustable instrument device.

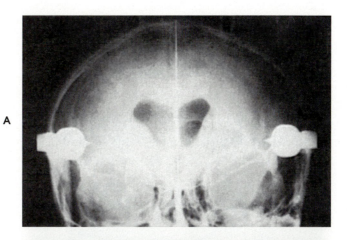

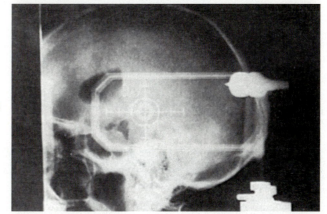

Fig. 25-24. Patient's head fixed in frame. Air has been injected into ventricles. **A**, frontal, and **B**, lateral centering devices aligned.

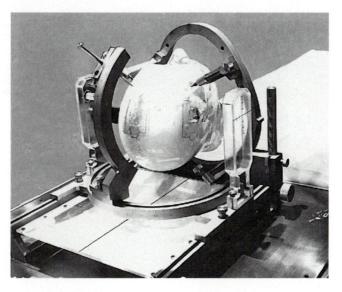

Fig. 25-25. Stereotactic frame with dry skull in place.

(Courtesy Dr. Harold L. Stitt.)

Currently, stereotactic localization is performed with the assistance of CT. Early CT stereotactic devices used metal to fix the device to the skull, resulting in computer-generated artifacts on the CT image. Newer stereotactic devices contain carbon graphite posts and fine metal skull pins surrounded by plastic bushings (Figs. 25-26 and 25-27). Computer programs are available that aid in the guidance of the needle for biopsy procedures. The data processing necessary to determine frame coordinates and probe depth can be performed with a programmable calculator. A software system transforms the two-dimensional coordinates obtained on the CT image to three-dimensional coordinates used by the surgeon. These coordinates are checked using a phantom simulator before the actual surgical procedure is performed.

A metal head ring is fixed to the skull with an attached localizing system consisting of three sets of vertical and diagonal rods. These rods visualize on the CT images and are used to determine spatial relationships. On completion of the CT examination, the patient is transported to the operating room where the localizing rods are removed and replaced by an arc-guidance system to allow passage of the surgical instruments. The stereotactic frame is removed following the surgical procedure, and a postoperative CT examination may be performed to check the biopsy site.

The use of MRI in conjunction with stereotactic surgery is still in its infancy. Stereotactic frames must be constructed of nonferromagnetic components and must be constructed so that eddy currents are not induced. The coordinate markers must be constructed of paramagnetic materials that visualize on the MRI. MRI-assisted stereotactic procedures should prove useful for pathologic conditions that do not visualize well on CT images. Additional research into MRI applications is currently under investigation.

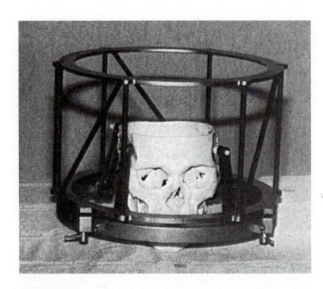

Fig. 25-26. Localizing system attached to head ring.

(From Haaga JR: Computed tomography, St Louis, 1983, Mosby.)

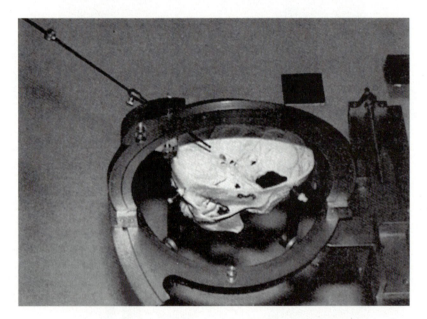

Fig. 25-27. Stereotactic instrument arc guidance system.

(From Haaga JR: Computed tomography, St Louis, 1983, Mosby.)

SELECTED BIBLIOGRAPHY

Brown RA, Roberts TS, and Osborn AB: Stereotaxic frame and computer software for CT-directed neurosurgical localization, Invest Radiol 15:308-312, 1980.

Cooper PR and Cohen W: Evaluation of cervical spinal injuries with metrizamide myelography–CT scanning, J Neurosurg 61:281-289, 1984.

Donovon-Post MJ et al: Spinal infection: evaluation with MR imaging and interoperative ultrasound, Radiology 169:765-771, 1988.

Gehweiler JA, Osborn RL, and Becker RF: The radiology of vertebral trauma, Philadelphia, 1980, WB Saunders.

Haaga JR and Alfidi RJ: Computed tomography of the whole body, ed 2, St Louis, 1988, Mosby, vols. I and II.

Javid MJ: Signs and symptoms after chemonucleolysis: a detailed evaluation of 214 worker's compensation and noncompensation patients, Spine 13:1428-1437, 1988.

Katirji MB, Agrawal R, and Kantra TA: The human cervical myotomes: an anatomical correlation between electromyography and CT/myelography, Muscle Nerve 11:1070-1073, 1988.

Lemansky E: Contrast agents used for myelography: an historical perspective, Radiol Technol 60:489-496, 1989.

Maravilla KR, Cooper PR, and Sklar FH: The influence of thin section tomography on the treatment of cervical spine injuries, Radiology 127:131-139, 1978.

Marymount JV and Shapiro WM: Vertebral hemangioma associated with spinal cord compression, South Med J 81:1586-1587, 1988.

Russin LD and Guinto FC: Multidirectional tomography in cervical spine injury, J Neurosurg 45:9-11, 1976.

Stark D and Bradley W: Magnetic Resonance Imaging, ed 2, St Louis, 1992, Mosby, vols. I & II.

Zee CS et al: MR imaging of neurocysticercosis, J Comput Assist Tomogr 12:927-934, 1988.

Selected bibliography

Chapter 26

CIRCULATORY SYSTEM

MICHAEL G. BRUCKNER

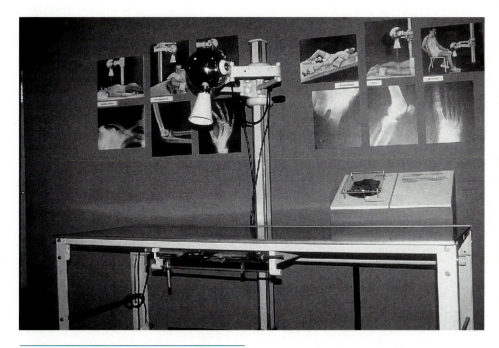

A radiographic table from 1930.

The circulatory system comprises two complex systems of intimately associated vessels through which fluid is transported throughout the body in a continuous, unidirectional flow. The major portion of the circulatory system transports blood and is called the blood-vascular system (Fig. 26-1). The minor portion, called the lymphatic system, collects from the tissue spaces the fluid that is filtered out of the blood vessels and conveys it back to the blood-vascular system. The fluid conveyed by the lymphatic system is called lymph. Together, the blood-vascular and lymphatic systems carry oxygen and nutritive material to the tissues and collect and transport carbon dioxide and other waste products of metabolism from the tissues to the organs of excretion: the skin, the lungs, the liver, and the kidneys.

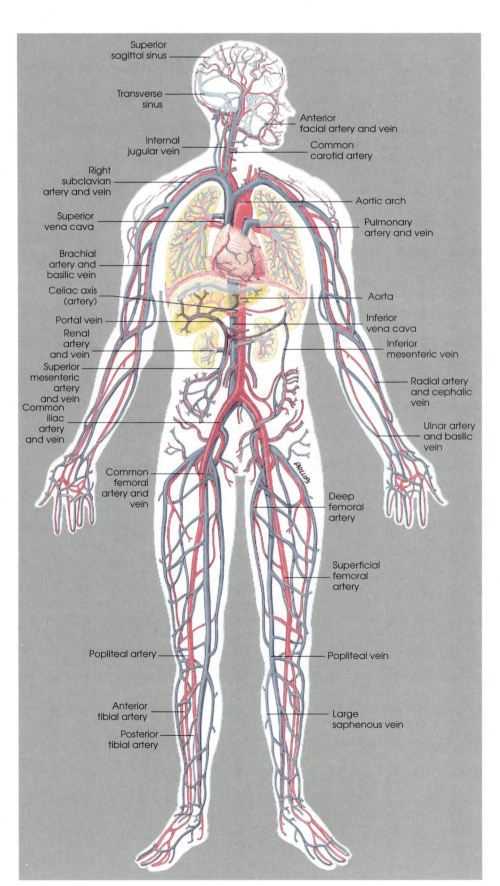

Superior sagittal sinus

Transverse sinus

Internal jugular vein

Right subclavian artery and vein

Superior vena cava

Brachial artery and basilic vein

Celiac axis (artery)

Portal vein

Renal artery and vein

Superior mesenteric artery and vein

Common iliac artery and vein

Common femoral artery and vein

Popliteal artery

Anterior tibial artery

Posterior tibial artery

Anterior facial artery and vein

Common carotid artery

Aortic arch

Pulmonary artery and vein

Aorta

Inferior vena cava

Inferior mesenteric vein

Radial artery and cephalic vein

Ulnar artery and basilic vein

Deep femoral artery

Superficial femoral artery

Popliteal vein

Large saphenous vein

Fig. 26-1. Major arteries and veins. *Red,* arterial; *blue,* venous; *purple,* portal.

Blood-Vascular System

The blood-vascular system consists of the heart and two circulatory systems that branch out from and return blood back to the heart. One of these systems traverses the lungs to discharge carbon dioxide and take up oxygen for delivery to the remainder of the body tissues; this system of vessels is known as the pulmonary circulation. The second system branches throughout the body to the various organs and tissues and is called the systemic circulation. The heart serves as a pumping mechanism to keep the blood in constant circulation throughout the vast system of blood vessels. Arteries convey the blood away from the heart. Veins convey the blood back toward the heart for redistribution.

From the main trunk vessels arising at the heart—the pulmonary artery for the pulmonary circulation and the aorta for the systemic circulation—the arteries progressively diminish in size as they divide and subdivide along their course, finally ending in minute branches called arterioles. The arterioles divide to form the capillary vessels, and the branching process is then reversed: the capillaries unite to form venules, the beginning branches of the veins, which in turn unite and reunite to form larger and larger vessels as they approach the heart. The pulmonary veins end in four trunks opening into the left atrium of the heart, two trunk veins leading from each lung. The systemic veins are arranged in a superficial set and in a deep set with which the superficial veins communicate; both sets converge toward a common trunk vein. The systemic veins end in two large vessels opening into the heart: the superior vena cava leads from the upper portion of the body, and the inferior vena cava leads from the lower portion.

The capillaries connect the arterioles and venules to form networks that pervade most organs and all other tissues supplied with blood. The capillary vessels have exceedingly thin walls through which the essential functions of the blood-vascular system take place—the blood constituents are filtered out, and the waste products of cell activity are absorbed. The exchange takes place through the medium of tissue fluid, which is derived from the blood plasma and is drained off by the lymphatic system for return to the blood-vascular system. The tissue fluid undergoes modification in the lymphatic system and is then called lymph.

The heart is the central organ of the blood-vascular system and functions solely as a pump to keep the blood in circulation. It is shaped somewhat like a cone and measures approximately 12 cm in length, 9 cm in width, and 6 cm in depth. It is situated obliquely in the middle mediastinum, largely to the left of the median sagittal plane. The base of the heart is directed superiorly, posteriorly, and to the right. Its apex rests on the diaphragm and against the anterior chest wall and is directed anteriorly, inferiorly, and to the left.

The muscular wall of the heart is called the myocardium, and, because of the force required to drive blood through the extensive systemic vessels, it is about three times as thick on the left side as on the right. The membrane that lines the heart interior is called the endocardium. The heart is enclosed in the double-walled pericardial sac, the exterior wall being fibrous. The thin, closely adherent membrane that covers the heart is referred to as the epicardium or, because it also serves as the serous inner wall of the pericardial sac, the visceral pericardium. The narrow, fluid-containing space between the two walls of the sac is called the pericardial cavity.

The cavity of the heart is divided by septa into right and left halves, and each half is subdivided by a constriction into two cavities, or chambers. The two upper chambers are called atria, and each atrium consists of a principal cavity and of a lesser one called the auricula. The two lower chambers of the heart are called ventricles. The opening between the right atrium and the right ventricle is controlled by the right atrioventricular (tricuspid) valve, and the opening between the left atrium and the left ventricle is controlled by the left atrioventricular (mitral or bicuspid) valve. The atria function as re-ceiving chambers and the ventricles as distributing chambers. The right side of the heart handles the venous, or deoxy-genated, blood, and the left side handles the arterial, or oxygenated, blood. The left ventricle pumps oxygenated blood through the aortic valve into the aorta. The right ventricle pumps deoxygenated blood through the pulmonary valve into the pulmonary artery. The pulmonary veins, two right and two left, open into the left atrium. The superior and inferior ve-nae cavae open into the right atrium (Fig. 26-2).

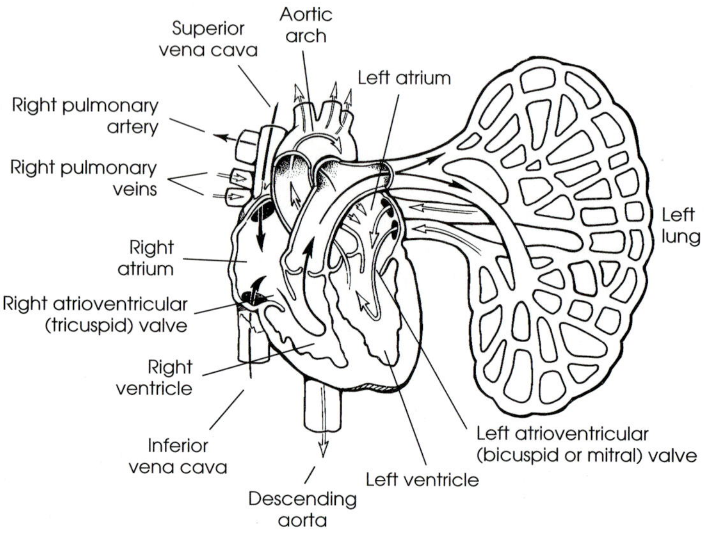

Blood is supplied to the myocardium by the right and left coronary arteries. They arise in the aortic sinus immediately superior to the aortic valve. Most of the cardiac veins drain into the coronary sinus on the posterior aspect of the heart, which drains into the right atrium (Figs. 26-3 and 26-4).

The aorta arises from the superior por-tion of the left ventricle and passes superi-orly and to the right for a short distance. It then arches posteriorly and to the left and descends along the left side of the verte-bral column to the level of the fourth lum-bar vertebra, where it divides into the right and left common iliac arteries. The common iliac arteries diverge from each other as they pass to the level of the lum-bosacral junction, where each ends by di-viding into the internal iliac, or hypogas-tric, artery and the external iliac artery. The internal iliac artery passes into the pelvis. The external iliac artery passes to a point about midway between the anterior superior iliac spine and the symphysis pu-bis and then enters the thigh to become the femoral artery.

The arteries are usually named accord-ing to their location. The several portions of the aorta—the ascending aorta, the arch of the aorta, and the descending aorta—are described according to direction. The last division, the descending aorta, has thoracic and abdominal portions. The sys-temic arteries branch out, treelike, from the aorta to all parts of the body. The sys-temic veins usually lie parallel to their re-spective arteries and are given the same names.

Fig. 26-2. The heart and great vessels. *Black arrows* indicate deoxygenated blood flow. *White arrows* indicate oxy-genated blood flow.

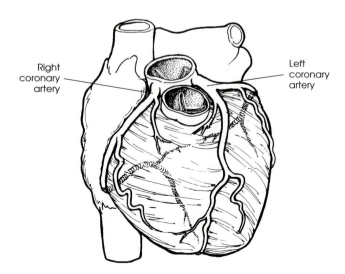

Fig. 26-3. Anterior view of coronary arteries.

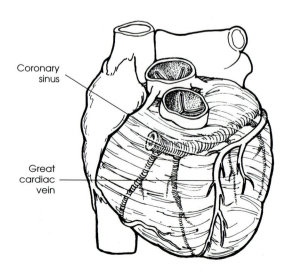

Fig. 26-4. Anterior view of coronary veins.

Each organ has its own vascular circuit that, arising from the trunk artery, leads back to the trunk vein for return to the heart. The veins returning blood from the abdominal viscera do not join the systemic venous system directly but rather join to form the portal vein, which drains into the liver. After the blood is processed in the liver it flows via the hepatic veins into the inferior vena cava.

The pulmonary artery, the main trunk of the pulmonary circulation, arises from the right ventricle of the heart, passes superiorly and posteriorly for a distance of about 5 cm, and then divides into two branches, the right and left pulmonary arteries. These vessels enter the root of the respective lung and, following the course of the bronchi, divide and subdivide to form a dense network of capillaries surrounding the alveoli of the lungs. Through the thin walls of the capillaries, the blood discharges carbon dioxide and absorbs oxygen from the air contained in the alveoli. The oxygenated blood passes onward through the pulmonary veins for return to the heart. In the pulmonary circulation, the deoxygenated blood is transported by the arteries, and the oxygenated blood is transported by the veins.

As shown in Fig. 26-5, the oxygenated (arterial) blood leaves the left ventricle by way of the aorta and is carried through the arteries to all parts of the body except the lungs. The deoxygenated (venous) blood is collected by the veins and returned to the right atrium, through the superior vena cava from the upper part of the body and through the inferior vena cava from the lower part of the body. This circuit, from the left ventricle to the right atrium, is called the systemic circulation. The venous blood passes from the right atrium into the right ventricle and out through the pulmonary artery and its branches to the lungs. After being oxygenated in the capillaries of the lungs, the blood is conveyed to the left atrium of the heart through the pulmonary veins. The circuit from the right ventricle to the left atrium is called the pulmonary circulation. The pathway of venous drainage from the abdominal viscera to the liver is called the portal system.

The heart contracts (systole) in pumping blood into the arteries and relaxes or dilates (diastole) in receiving blood from the veins. One phase of contraction (referred to as the heartbeat) and one phase of dilation are called a cardiac cycle. In the average adult one cycle lasts ⁸⁄₁₀ second. However, the heart rate, or number of pulsations per minute, varies with size, age, and sex, being faster in small persons, young individuals, and females. The heart rate is also increased with exercise, food, and emotional disturbances.

The velocity of blood circulation varies with the rate and intensity of the heartbeat, as well as in the different portions of the system in accordance with their distance from the initial pressure of the intermittent waves of blood issuing from the heart. The speed of flow is thus highest in the large arteries arising at or near the heart because these vessels receive the full force of each wave of blood pumped out of the heart. The arterial walls expand during the pressure of receiving each wave. They then rhythmically contract, gradually diminishing the pressure of the advancing wave from point to point until the flow of blood is normally reduced to a steady, nonpulsating stream through the capillaries and veins. The beat, or contraction and expansion of an artery, which may be felt with the fingers at a number of points, is called the pulse.

It has been calculated that a complete circulation of the blood through both the systemic and pulmonary circuits, from a given point and back again, requires about 23 seconds and an average of 27 heartbeats. In certain contrast examinations of the cardiovascular system, tests are made on each subject to determine the circulation time from the point of injection of the contrast medium to the site of interest. The circulation time is influenced by body position, that is, whether the patient is upright or recumbent.

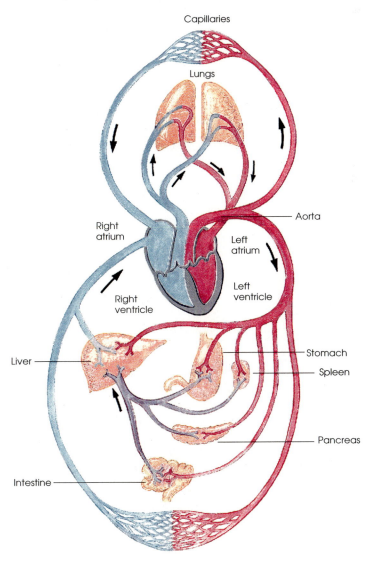

Fig. 26-5. The pulmonary, systemic, and portal circulation, depicting oxygenated (red), deoxygenated (blue), and nutrient-rich (brown) blood.

517

Lymphatic System

The lymphatic system consists of an elaborate arrangement of closed vessels that collect fluid from the tissue spaces and transport it to the blood-vascular system. Almost all lymphatic vessels are arranged in two sets—a superficial set that lies immediately under the skin and accompanies the superficial veins and a deep set that accompanies the deep blood vessels and with which the superficial lymphatics communicate (Fig. 26-6). Unlike the blood-vascular system, the lymphatic system has no pumping mechanism. The conducting vessels are richly supplied with valves to prevent backflow, whereas the movement of the lymph through the system is believed to be maintained largely by extrinsic pressure from the surrounding organs and muscles.

The lymphatic system begins in complex networks of thin-walled, absorbent capillaries situated in the various organs and tissues. The capillaries unite to form larger vessels, which in turn form networks and unite to become still larger vessels as they approach the terminal collecting trunks. The terminal trunks communicate with the blood-vascular system.

The lymphatic vessels are small in caliber and have delicate, transparent walls. Along their course the collecting vessels pass through one or more nodular structures called lymph nodes. The nodes occur singly but are usually arranged in chains or groups of 2 to 20. The nodes are situated so that they form strategically placed centers toward which the conducting vessels converge. The nodes vary from the size of a pinhead to the size of an almond or larger. They may be spherical, oval, or kidney-shaped. Each node has a hilum through which the arteries enter and veins and efferent lymph vessels emerge; the afferent lymph vessels do not enter at the hilum. In addition to the lymphatic capillaries, blood vessels, and supporting structures, each lymph node contains masses, or follicles, of lymphocytes that are arranged around its circumference and from which cords of cells extend through the medullary portion of the node.

A number of conducting channels, here called afferent lymph vessels, enter the node opposite the hilum and break into wide capillaries that surround the lymph follicles and form a canal known as the peripheral or marginal lymph sinus. The network of capillaries continues into the medullary portion of the node, widens to form medullary sinuses, and then collects into several efferent vessels that leave the node at the hilum. The conducting vessels may pass through several nodes along their course, each time undergoing the process of widening into sinuses. Lymphocytes, a variety of white blood cells formed in the lymph nodes, are added to the lymph while it is in the nodes. It is thought that a majority of the lymph is here absorbed by the venous system and that only a small part is passed on through the conducting vessels.

The absorption and interchange of tissue fluids and of cells take place through the thin walls of the capillaries. The lymph passes from the beginning capillaries through the conducting vessels, which eventually empty their contents into terminal lymph trunks for conveyance to the blood-vascular system. The main terminal trunk of the lymphatic system, the lower, dilated portion of which is known as the cisterna chyli, is called the thoracic duct. This duct receives the lymphatic drainage from all parts of the body below the diaphragm and from the left half of the body above the diaphragm. The thoracic duct extends from the level of the second lumbar vertebra to the base of the neck, where it ends by opening into the venous system at the junction of the left subclavian and internal jugular veins. Three terminal collecting trunks—the right jugular, the subclavian, and the bronchomediastinal trunks—receive the lymphatic drainage from the right half of the body above the diaphragm. These vessels open into the right subclavian vein separately or occasionally after uniting to form a common trunk called the right lymphatic duct.

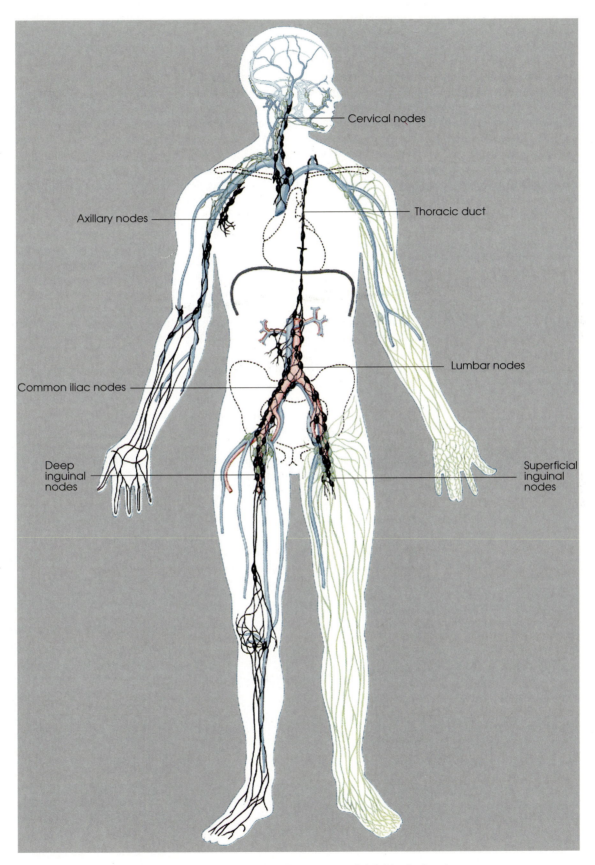

Cervical nodes

Axillary nodes

Thoracic duct

Lumbar nodes

Common iliac nodes

Deep
inguinal
nodes

Superficial
inguinal
nodes

Fig. 26-6. Lymphatic system (*green,* superficial; *black,* deep).

Blood vessels are not normally visualized in conventional radiography because no natural contrast exists between them and the other adjacent soft tissues of the body. Therefore it is necessary to fill vessels with a radiopaque contrast medium to delineate them for radiography. *Angiography** is a general term that describes the radiologic examination of vascular structures within the body after the introduction of an iodinated contrast medium.

The visceral and peripheral angiography procedures identified in this chapter can be categorized generally as either *arteriography* or *venography.* Examinations are more precisely named for the specific blood vessel opacified and for the method of injection. For example, for intravenous digital vascular imaging of the right renal artery, a contrast medium is injected into a vein but images are obtained of the renal artery (see Chapter 35). Producing images of the right renal artery by injecting a contrast medium directly into the artery is accomplished by performing a selective right renal arteriogram.

---

*All italicized words on succeeding pages are defined at the end of this chapter.

Angiography is used mainly to identify the anatomy or pathologic process of the vessels being studied. For example, the lower limb venogram, probably the most common of all angiograms, is usually performed to determine if deep venous *thrombosis* is the cause of a patient's leg swelling or pain. Chronic cramping leg pain following physical exertion, a condition known as claudication, may prompt a physician to order an arteriogram of the lower extremities to determine if *atherosclerosis* is diminishing the blood supply to the leg muscles. Detection of a *stenosis,* most often caused by atherosclerosis, is the purpose of many arteriograms. Detecting and verifying the existence and exact position of an *aneurysm* are the purposes of cerebral angiography (which is presented in the next section of this chapter). Although most angiographic examinations are performed to investigate anatomic variances, some evaluate the motion of the part. Certain cardiac catheterization procedures (see Chapter 31), for example, visualize the interior anatomy of the heart and the motion of the cardiac valves. Other vascular examinations evaluate suspected tumors by opacifying the organ of concern. Angiography for therapeutic rather than diagnostic purposes is discussed in a later section of this chapter.

The broad term *angiography* also encompasses examinations involving other vessels of the body. For example, lymphangiography is discussed in a later section of this chapter and cholangiography is described in Chapter 16, Volume 2.

HISTORICAL DEVELOPMENT

Angiography was conceived just 10 weeks after the announcement of Roentgen's discovery when, in January 1896, Haschek and Lindenthal announced that they had produced a radiograph demonstrating the blood vessels of an amputated hand using Teichman's mixture, a thick emulsion of chalk, as the contrast agent. The potential for this new type of examination to delineate vascular anatomy was immediately recognized. The advancement of angiography was hindered by a lack of suitable contrast media and by a lack of low-risk techniques to deliver the contrast medium to the desired location. By the 1920s researchers had used sodium iodide as a contrast medium to produce lower limb studies that were comparable in quality to studies seen in modern angiography. However, limitations still existed. Until the 1950s, contrast medium was most commonly injected through a needle that punctured the vessel or through a ureteral catheter that passed into the body through a surgically exposed peripheral vessel. Then in 1952, shortly after the development of a flexible thin-walled catheter, Seldinger announced a *percutaneous* method of catheter introduction. The Seldinger technique eliminated the surgical risk associated with the exposure of tissues and made a much smaller wound (see catheterization section of this chapter for a description).

Early angiograms consisted of single radiographs or the visualization of vessels by fluoroscopy. Because the advantage of serial filming was recognized, cassette changers, roll film changers, cut film changers, and cine and serial spot-filming devices were developed. Pumps to inject contrast media were also developed to allow more rapid and precise control of injection rates and volumes than was possible by hand. Early mechanical injectors were powered by pressurized gas, and the injection rate was a function of the pressure setting. Electrically powered automatic injectors were subsequently developed that allowed the injection rate to be set directly.

CONTRAST MEDIA

A wide variety of opaque contrast media are used in angiographic studies. All materials currently in use are organic iodine solutions. Although usually tolerated, the injection of iodinated contrast medium causes undesirable consequences. Iodinated contrast medium is filtered out of the bloodstream by the kidneys but is nephrotoxic. It causes physiologic cardiovascular side effects including peripheral vasodilation, blood pressure decrease, and cardiotoxicity. It also produces an uncomfortable burning sensation in muscular artery branches and nausea in roughly 1 out of 10 patients. Most significantly, the injection of iodinated contrast medium may invoke allergic reactions. They may be minor, such as hives or a slight difficulty in breathing, and not require any treatment, or they may be severe and require immediate medical intervention. Severe reactions are characterized by a state of shock in which the patient exhibits shallow breathing and a high pulse rate and may lose consciousness. Historically, 1 out of every 14,000 patients suffers a severe allergic reaction. The administration of contrast medium is clearly one of the significant risks in angiography.

At the kilovoltages used in angiography, iodine is slightly more radiopaque, atom for atom, than lead. The iodine is incorporated into water-soluble molecules formed as tri-iodinated benzene rings. These molecules vary in exact composition. Some forms are organic salts that dissociate in solution and are therefore ionic. The iodinated anion is diatrizoate iothalamate or ioxaglate. The radiolucent cation is meglumine, sodium, or a combination of both. These ionic forms yield two particles in solution for every three iodine atoms (a 3:2 ratio) and are six to eight times as osmolar as plasma. Other tri-iodinated benzene rings are created as nonionic molecules. These forms have three iodine atoms on each particle in solution (a 3:1 ratio) because they do not dissociate and are only two to three times as osmolar as plasma. Studies indicate that these properties of nonionic contrast media result in decreased chemotoxicity to the kidneys. Nonionic contrast media also cause decreased physiologic cardiovascular side effects, fewer sensations, and fewer allergic reactions. They are, however, much more expensive than ionic media.

One form of ionic contrast medium is a dimer; two benzene rings are bonded together as the anion. This results in six iodine atoms for every two particles in solution, which yields the same 3:1 ratio as a nonionic contrast medium. The ionic dimer has advantages over the ionic monomeric molecule but lacks some of the properties of the nonionic molecule.

All forms of iodinated contrast media are available in a variety of iodine concentrations. The agents of higher concentration are more opaque. Typically, 30% iodine concentrations are used for cerebral and limb arteriography, whereas 35% concentrations are used for visceral angiography. Peripheral venography may be performed with 30% or lower concentrations. The ionic agents of higher concentration and the nonionic agents are more viscous and produce greater resistance in the catheter during injection. The choice of contrast medium may vary with the patient and is usually made by the examining physician.

INJECTION TECHNIQUES

Contrast medium may be introduced into a vessel through a "direct stick," which is simply the process of placing a needle tip into the desired vessel and injecting through the needle. This technique is acceptable in limited situations. A flush injection through a catheter involves placing the catheter tip into a large proximal vessel so that the vessel and its major branches are opacified. In a selective injection the catheter tip is positioned into a specific artery orifice so that only that artery is injected. This has the advantage of more densely opacifying the vessel and of limiting the superimposition of vessels.

Contrast medium may be injected by hand with a syringe, but ideally an automatic injector is used. The major advantage of an automatic injector is to control the injection of a known quantity of the contrast medium during a predetermined period. Automatic injectors have controls to set the injection rate, injection volume, and maximum pressure to be allowed to occur inside a catheter or other injection pathway. Another useful feature is a control to set a time interval during which the injector gradually achieves the set injection rate. This may prevent a catheter or needle from being dislodged by whiplash.

Because the opacifying contrast medium is often carried away from the area of interest by blood flow, the injection and filming of the opacified vessels usually occur simultaneously. The injector, therefore, is often electronically connected to the rapid filming equipment to coordinate the timing between the injector and filming. Such accurate timing is required when the filming is to begin slightly before or after the injection begins.

EQUIPMENT

Most angiograms record flowing contrast medium in a series of radiographs, which requires rapid *film changers* and/or cinefluorography devices. Less complex angiographic procedures such as peripheral arteriography and venography may be performed with a conventional Bucky tray.

A number of rapid film changers are available from different manufacturers. All these devices move the film and permit exposures at intervals of a fraction of a second; one device is capable of changing as many as 12 films per second, although most film changers have a maximum speed of six films or fewer per second. These rapid film changers transport films from a supply magazine to a position between screens that come into close contact with the film during exposure and then retract so that the film can be transported into a receiving magazine. Cut film changers that can move twenty or thirty 14 × 14 inch (35 × 35 cm) films are common. Rapid film changers may be used either singularly or in combination at right angles to obtain simultaneous frontal and lateral images of the vascular system under investigation with one injection of contrast medium. This arrangement of units is called a *biplane* rapid film-changing system.

Lower limb angiograms are the most likely to use cassette changers. Cassette changers specialized for these procedures move large cassettes containing 11 × 48 inch (30 × 120 cm) or 14 × 51 inch (35 × 130 cm) film, depending on the manufacturer, into and out of the exposure field. Because these devices move heavy objects, they operate at slower maximum speeds, usually one film per second.

Cinefluorography apparatus essentially consists of a movie or cine camera that photographs the output phosphor of an image-intensification system. Almost all image-intensification devices used for vascular procedures include television monitoring. Such equipment allows angiographic examinations to be viewed on a television screen and simultaneously videotaped in conjunction with obtaining the cine recording.

A cine camera uses 16 or 35 mm roll film and usually can achieve sequential exposure rates of up to 60 frames or more per second, with the resultant true motion picture radiography. The photographic resolution achieved with cine units is not as great as that seen with rapid film changers. However, many more events can be photographed with the cine attachment, and dynamic function can be more satisfactorily evaluated with cinefluorography.

Serial radiographic filming requires large focal spot x-ray tubes capable of withstanding a high heat load. Magnification studies, however, require fractional focus tubes with focal spot sizes of between 0.1 and 0.3 mm. X-ray tubes may have to be specialized to satisfy these extreme demands.

Rapid serial filming also necessitates radiographic generators with high-power output. Since short exposure times are needed to compensate for all patient motion, the generators must be capable of producing high-milliampere output. The combination of high kilowatt-rated generators and rare earth film-screen technology significantly aids in decreasing the radiation dose to the patient while producing radiographs of improved quality with the added advantage of prolonging the life of such high-powered generators and x-ray tubes.

A comprehensive angiographic room contains a great amount of equipment other than specifically radiologic devices. Monitoring systems record patient electrocardiographic data and blood pressure readings from within vessels. Emergency equipment may include resuscitators, a defibrillator for the heart, and anesthesia apparatus. The radiographer must be familiar with the use of each piece of equipment (Fig. 26-7).

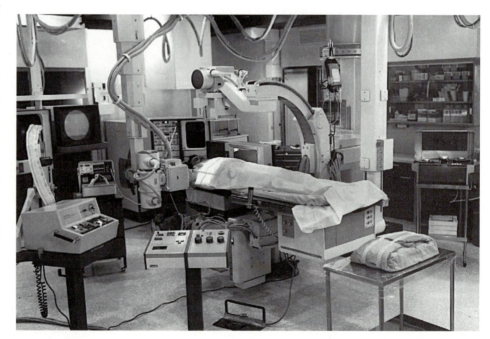

Fig. 26-7. Angiographic suite demonstrating equipment used to perform vascular procedures.

MAGNIFICATION

Magnification occurs both intentionally and unintentionally in angiographic imaging sequences. Intentional use of magnification can result in a significant increase in resolution of fine vessel recorded detail. Fractional focal spot tubes of 0.3 mm or less are necessary for direct radiographic magnification techniques. The selection of a fractional focal spot necessitates the use of low milliamperage. Short exposure time is maintained by the use of the air gap rather than the grid to control scatter radiation.

The formula for magnification is:

$$M = \frac{SID}{SOD} \text{ or } \frac{SID}{SID - SOD}$$

The SID is source-to-image receptor distance, SOD is source-to-object distance, and OID is object-to-image receptor distance. For a 2:1 magnification study using 100 cm SID, both the focal spot and the film changer are positioned 50 cm from the area of interest. A 3:1 magnification study using a 100 cm SID is accomplished by placing the focal spot 33 cm from the area of interest and the film changer 67 cm from the area of interest (Figs. 26-8 to 26-10).

Unintentional magnification occurs when the area of interest cannot be placed in direct contact with the image receptor.

This is a problem particularly in a biplane imaging sequence, where the need to center the area of interest in the first plane may create some unavoidable distance of the body part to the image receptor in the second plane. Even in single plane imaging, vascular structures are separated from the image receptor by some distance. The magnification that occurs as a result of these circumstances is frequently 20% to 25%. For example, a 25% magnification occurs when a vessel within the body is 20 cm from the film, an OID of 20 cm, while the SID is 100 cm. Angiographic film series therefore do not represent vessels at their actual size. This must be taken into account when direct measurements are made from angiographic cut films. Unintentional magnification can be reduced by increasing the SID while maintaining the OID. Increasing SID may not be an option, however, if the increase in technical factors would exceed tube output capacity or exposure time maximum.

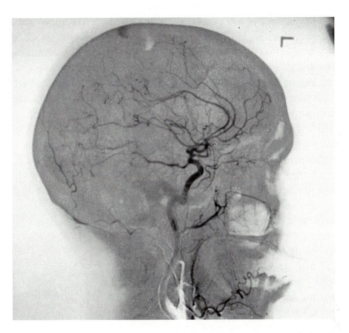

Fig. 26-8. Nonmagnified, photographically subtracted, lateral selective common carotid arteriogram.

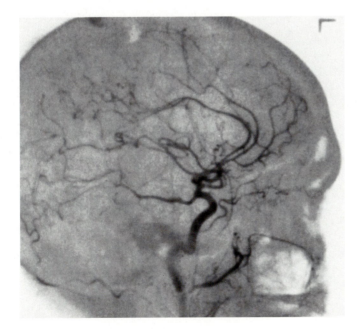

Fig. 26-9. 2:1 magnified, photographically subtracted, lateral selective common carotid arteriogram.

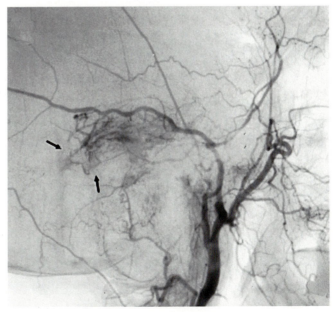

Fig. 26-10. 3:1 magnified, photographically subtracted, lateral selective external carotid arteriogram. *Arrows* indicate visualization of fine tumor neovascularity.

FILM PROGRAMMING

Film programming is the task of controlling the rate and number of serial exposures made with a film changer. This is accomplished either through manipulation of the device intimately associated to the film changer known as the film programmer or through a combination of precisely patterning films in the film changer's supply magazine and setting the film programmer to operate the film changer at specific rates for specific amounts of time. Film programmers instruct the film changers at which rate to cycle, but every cycle does not necessarily transport and expose a film. When two film changers operate together for simultaneous *biplane* imaging, exposures in both planes cannot be made at the same moment because scatter radiation would fog the films; yet biplane changers must cycle exactly together so that synchronization can be electronically controlled. Therefore it is necessary to alternate the cycles that transport film in the two planes. In the first cycle, even though both changers are cycling, only one changer is allowed to transport and expose a film. In the second cycle, the changer that transported film in the first cycle will be allowed to cycle empty while the other changer transports and exposes a film. This process of changers alternating between transporting and not transporting film during opposite cycles must continue throughout the series. The maximum exposure rate of a film changer operated in the biplane mode is one half of its maximum cycle rate because only every other cycle transports and exposes a film.

The most sophisticated film programmers automatically control the alternating of film in the biplane mode. The radiographer selects single-plane or biplane mode and enters the number of exposures to be made in each second interval of the series. With less sophisticated programming systems the radiographer has control of the cycle rate and rate duration but must manually select which cycles will transport film. For a biplane program with manually loaded equipment, the film supply magazine for the AP changer is loaded with film in the odd-numbered spaces. The even-numbered spaces are left empty. The lateral film supply magazine is loaded in the even-numbered spaces. The film programmer must then be set to cycle the changers at a rate double to the film rate for each plane. The rate duration, however, remains the same. The time interval in which the film remains motionless for exposure must be known for every cycle rate so that a cycle rate with a motionlessness interval less than the radiographic exposure time can be selected.

CATHETERIZATION

Catheterization for filling vessels with contrast media is a technique that is preferred over the injection of the media through a needle. The advantages of catheterization are that the risk of *extravasation* is reduced, most body parts can be reached for selective injection, the patient can be positioned as needed, and the catheter can be safely left in the body while radiographs are being examined. The femoral, axillary, and brachial arteries are the ones most frequently catheterized. The femoral site is preferred because it is associated with the fewest risks.

The most widely used method of catheterization is the modern Seldinger technique, the steps of which are described in Fig. 26-11. It is performed under sterile conditions. The catheterization site is suitably cleaned and then surgically draped. The conscious patient is given local anesthesia at the catheterization site.

With this percutaneous technique an arteriotomy or venotomy is no larger than the catheter itself. Hemorrhage, therefore, is minimized. Usually the patient can resume normal activity within 24 hours. The risk of infection is lower than in surgical procedures because tissues are not exposed.

After a catheter is introduced into the blood-vascular system, it can be maneuvered by pushing, pulling, and turning the part of the catheter still outside the patient so that the part of the catheter inside the patient travels to a specific location. The wire is sometimes positioned inside the catheter to help manipulate and guide the catheter to the desired location. Whenever the wire is removed from the catheter, the catheter is infused with sterile solution to help prevent clot formation. Infusing the catheter and assisting the physician in the catheterization process may be the radiographer's responsibility.

When the examination is complete, the catheter or needle is removed. Pressure is applied to the site until hemorrhage ceases. Blood flow through the vessel, however, is maintained. The physician often prescribes complete patient bed rest and orders to be alert for the development of a *hematoma*.

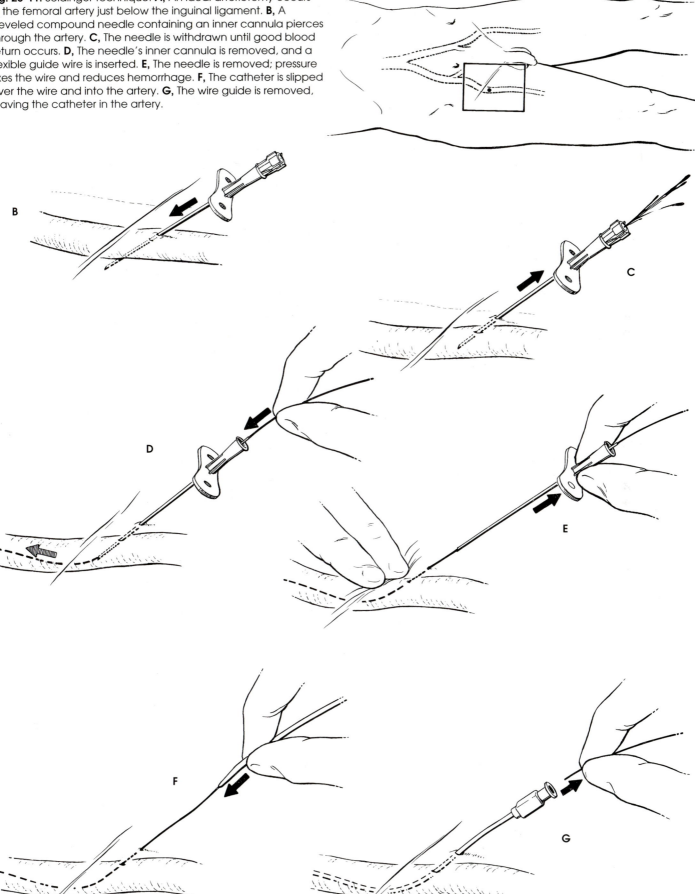

Fig. 26-11. Seldinger technique. **A,** An ideal arteriotomy occurs in the femoral artery just below the inguinal ligament. **B,** A beveled compound needle containing an inner cannula pierces through the artery. **C,** The needle is withdrawn until good blood return occurs. **D,** The needle's inner cannula is removed, and a flexible guide wire is inserted. **E,** The needle is removed; pressure fixes the wire and reduces hemorrhage. **F,** The catheter is slipped over the wire and into the artery. **G,** The wire guide is removed, leaving the catheter in the artery.

When the peripheral artery sites are unavailable, a catheter may sometimes be introduced into the aorta using the translumbar approach. For this technique the patient is positioned prone and a special catheter introducer system is inserted percutaneously through the posterolateral aspect of the back and directed superiorly so that the catheter enters the aorta around the T11 to T12 level. This method is used primarily for aortography and rarely for selective studies.

Catheters are produced in various forms, each with a particular advantage in shape, maneuverability, or maximum injection rate (Fig. 26-12). Angiographic catheters are made of pliable plastic that allows them to straighten for insertion over the wire guide. They normally reassume their original shape after the wire guide is withdrawn. The reverse-curve catheter, which has a bend of 180 degrees a few centimeters from the tip, usually requires manipulation from the angiographer to resume its original shape. Catheters with a bent tip are designed for maneuverability into artery origins for selective injections. They may have only an end hole, or they may have two additional side holes near the tip. The side holes stabilize the catheter tip by reducing the whiplash that occurs from the rapid ejection of contrast medium from the end hole. Some catheters have multiple side holes to facilitate high injection rates but are used only in large vascular structures for flush injections. A "pigtail" catheter is a special multiple side hole catheter that has a circular tip to further reduce the amount of contrast that exits the end hole.

Common angiographic catheters range in size from 4 Fr. (0.05 inch) to 7 Fr. (0.09 inch), although even smaller or larger sizes may be used. Most have inner lumens allowing them to be inserted over wire guides ranging from 0.032 to 0.038 inches in size.

PATIENT CARE

Before the initiation of an angiographic procedure it is appropriate to explain the process and the potential complications to the patient. Written consent is often obtained after such an explanation. Potential complications include a vasovagal reaction; stroke; bleeding at the catheterization site; nerve, blood vessel, or tissue damage; and an allergic reaction to the contrast medium. Bleeding at the arteriotomy or venotomy site is usually easily controlled with pressure to the site. Blood vessel and tissue damage may require a surgical procedure to correct. A vasovagal reaction is characterized by sweating and nausea caused by a drop in blood pressure. The patient's legs should be elevated, and intravenous fluids may be administered to help restore blood pressure. Minor allergic reactions to iodinated contrast media, such as hives and congestion, are usually controlled with medications and may not require any treatment. Severe allergic reactions may result in shock, which is characterized by shallow breathing, high pulse rate, and possibly loss of consciousness. The examining physician must be immediately notified of any change in patient status. Of course, angiography is performed only if the benefits of the examination outweigh the risks.

Patients are usually restricted to clear liquid intake and routine medications before undergoing angiography. Adequate hydration from liquid intake may minimize damage to the kidneys from iodinated contrast media. Solid food intake is restricted so that the chance of aspiration from the nausea that occurs in 10% of patients from iodinated contrast media is reduced. Contraindications to the examination will be determined by physicians and include previous severe allergic reaction to iodinated contrast media, severely impaired renal function, impaired blood clotting factors, and the inability to undergo a surgical procedure or general anesthesia.

Because general anesthesia is more of a risk than most angiographic procedures, adult patients are usually conscious for the examination. Just before the procedure, most are given a sedative to reduce anxiety and discomfort. Thoughtful communication from the radiographer and physician will also calm and reassure the patient. It is important that either the radiographer or physician warn the patient about the sensations that the contrast medium will cause and the noise produced by the filming equipment. This information also reduces the patient's anxiety and helps ensure a good radiographic series free from patient motion.

ANGIOGRAPHIC TEAM

The angiographic team consists of the physician, usually a radiologist, the radiographer, and other specialists such as an anesthetist and a nurse.

The radiographer often assists in performing procedures that require sterile technique and may be responsible for operating monitoring devices and emergency equipment, in addition to operating the radiographic equipment. When the radiographer is required to operate the supporting apparatus, he or she must be provided adequate directions for proper use of the equipment. Instruction in patient care techniques and sterile procedure, however, is included in the basic preparation of the radiographer.

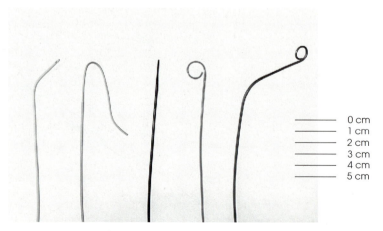

0 cm
1 cm
2 cm
3 cm
4 cm
5 cm

Fig. 26-12. Selected catheter shapes used for angiography.

Visceral Angiography
AORTOGRAPHY

The most satisfactory method for visualizing the aorta is achieved by placing a catheter into the aorta at the desired level. This is commonly accomplished with the Seldinger technique from the right or left femoral artery sites using a multiple side hole catheter. Aortography is usually accomplished with the patient in the supine position for simultaneous frontal and lateral imaging with the central ray perpendicular to the film. Translumbar catheter introduction is an alternative for aortography and requires that the patient is in the prone position.

Thoracic aortography

Thoracic aortography may be performed to rule out an aortic aneurysm, for *aortic dissection,* or to evaluate congenital or postsurgical conditions. Biplane film changers are recommended so that AP or PA and lateral projections can be obtained with one contrast medium injection. The radiographer observes the following guidelines:

- For lateral projections, move the patient's arms superiorly to move them out of the image.
- For best results, increase the lateral SID, usually to 60 inches, so that magnification is reduced.
- If biplane equipment is not available, use a single-plane 45-degree RPO or LAO position, which will often produce an adequate study of the aorta.
- For all projections, direct the perpendicular central ray to the center of the chest at the level of T6. This should allow visualization of the entire thoracic aorta including the proximal brachiocephalic, carotid, and subclavian vessels.

Injection of contrast medium is made at rates ranging from 25 to 35 ml/sec for a total volume of 50 to 70 ml. The radiographer then performs the following steps:

- Begin filming simultaneously with the injection.
- Make exposures in each plane at rates ranging from one and one-half to three exposures per second for 3 to 4 seconds; exposures may then slow to one film or less per second for an additional 3 to 5 seconds.
- Make the exposures at the end of suspended inhalation (Figs. 26-13 and 26-14).

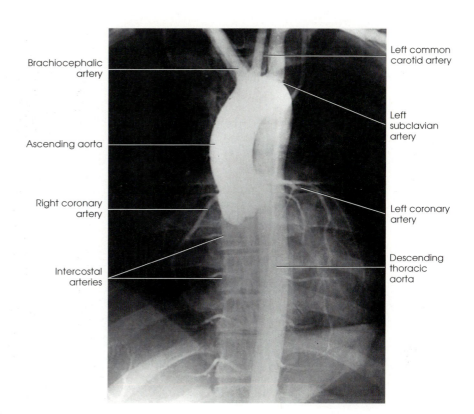

Brachiocephalic artery

Left common carotid artery

Ascending aorta

Left subclavian artery

Right coronary artery

Left coronary artery

Intercostal arteries

Descending thoracic aorta

Fig. 26-13. AP thoracic aorta that also demonstrates right and left coronary arteries.

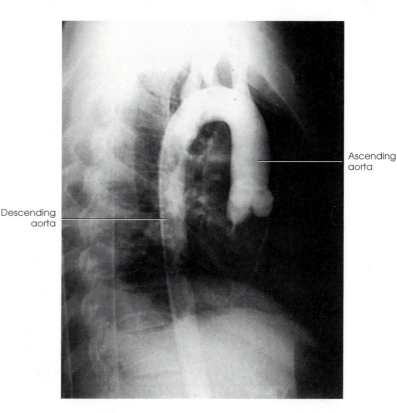

Descending aorta

Ascending aorta

Fig. 26-14. Lateral thoracic aorta.

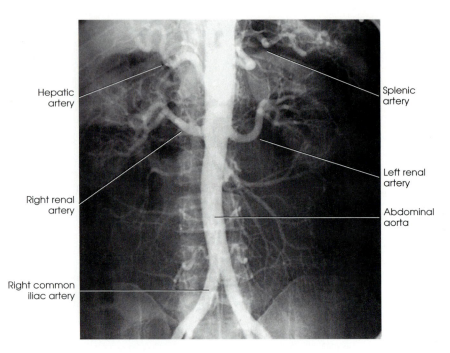

Hepatic artery

Splenic artery

Left renal artery

Right renal artery

Abdominal aorta

Right common iliac artery

Fig. 26-15. AP abdominal aorta.

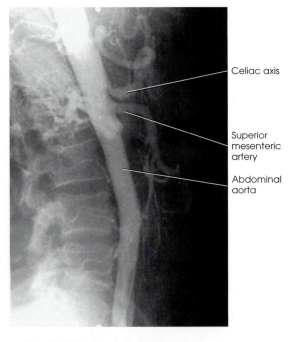

Celiac axis

Superior mesenteric artery

Abdominal aorta

Fig. 26-16. Lateral abdominal aorta.

Abdominal aortography

Abdominal aortography may be performed to evaluate abdominal aortic aneurysm, occlusion, or atherosclerotic disease. Simultaneous AP and lateral projections are recommended. The radiographer observes the following guidelines:

- For the lateral projection, move the patient's arms superiorly to move them out of the image field.
- Usually, collimate the field in the anteroposterior aspect.
- Direct the perpendicular central ray at the level of L2 so that the aorta is visualized from the diaphragm to the aortic bifurcation. The AP projection will best demonstrate the renal artery origins, the aortic bifurcation, and the course and general condition of all of the abdominal visceral branches, whereas the lateral projection best demonstrates the celiac and superior mesenteric artery origins because the celiac and superior mesenteric arteries arise from the anterior abdominal aorta.
- Make the exposures. Representative injection and film programs are 25 ml/sec for 60 ml total volume and two films per second for 4 seconds followed by one film per second for 4 seconds in each plane.
- Begin exposures simultaneously with the beginning of the injection and at the end of suspended expiration (Figs. 26-15 and 26-16).

Pulmonary Arteriography

Under fluoroscopic control, a catheter is passed from a peripheral vein through the vena cava and right side of the heart and into the pulmonary arteries. This technique is usually employed for a selective injection, and the examination is primarily performed for the evaluation of embolic disease.

Simultaneous AP and lateral projections of the supine patient are recommended for this procedure. The suggested SID for the lateral projection is 60 inches. The radiographer observes the following guidelines:

- Move the patient's arms superiorly to move them out of the field of view.
- When biplane projections are not possible, use a single-plane 35-degree RAO or LPO position to usually achieve satisfactory results for both the right and left pulmonary arteriograms.
- Direct the central ray perpendicular to the film for all of these radiographs.
- Use a compensating (trough) filter on the AP projection to obtain a radiograph with more uniform density between the vertebrae and the lungs if needed.
- In studies of the pulmonary arteries, lengthen the time of the filming program to reveal the opacified left atrium, left ventricle, and thoracic aorta.
- Make the exposures. Representative injection and film programs are 25 ml/sec for 50 ml total volume and two to four films per second for 4 seconds followed by one film per second for an additional 4 seconds in each plane (Figs. 26-17 to 26-20).

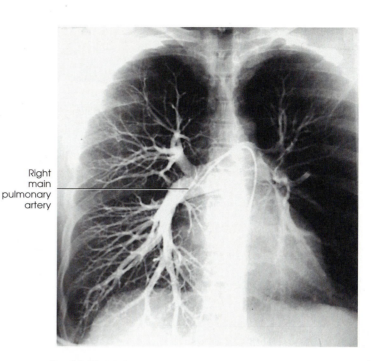

Fig. 26-17. AP right main pulmonary artery during early phase of injection.

Right main pulmonary artery

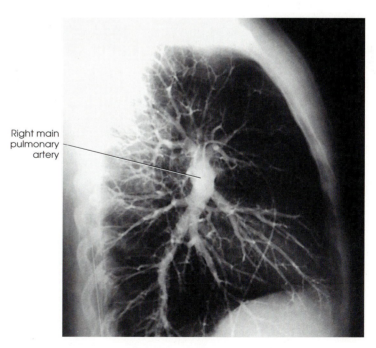

Fig. 26-18. Lateral right pulmonary artery during early phase of injection.

Right main pulmonary artery

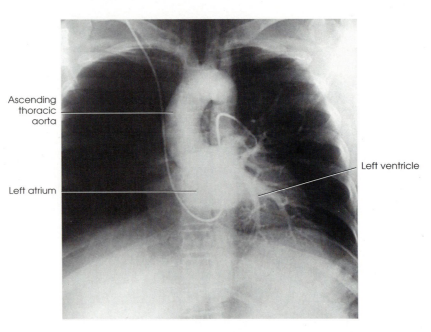

Fig. 26-19. Late-phase AP pulmonary arteriogram demonstrates left atrium, left ventricle, and thoracic aorta.

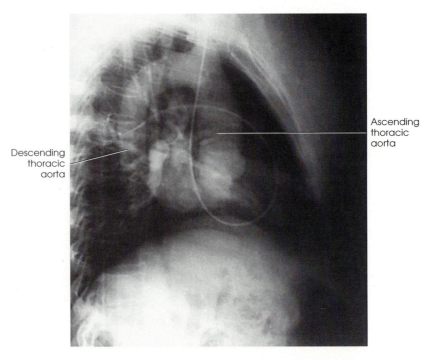

Fig. 26-20. Late phase lateral pulmonary artery injection showing aorta.

SELECTIVE ABDOMINAL VISCERAL ARTERIOGRAPHIC STUDIES

Abdominal visceral arteriographic studies are usually performed to rule out atherosclerotic disease, thrombosis, embolization, occlusion, or bleeding, or to visualize tumor vascularity. The Seldinger technique is the preferred approach. An appropriately shaped catheter is introduced, usually at the femoral artery site, and advanced into the orifice of the desired artery. The radiographer observes the following steps:

- Accomplish each of these selective studies initially with the patient in the supine position for single-plane frontal projections.
- Direct the central ray perpendicular to the film.
- Usually, obtain a preliminary radiograph to establish optimum exposure and positioning.
- If necessary, use oblique projections for improved visualization or to avoid superimposition of vessels.
- Obtain radiographs for all abdominal visceral studies during suspended expiration.

The following are various types of selective abdominal visceral arteriograms.

Celiac arteriogram

The celiac artery normally arises from the aorta at the level of T12 and carries blood to the stomach, liver, spleen, and pancreas.

- For the angiographic examination, center the patient to the film.
- Direct the central ray to L1 (Fig. 26-21).
- Make the exposures. Representative injection and film programs are 10 ml/sec for 40 ml total volume and two films per second for 5 seconds followed by one film per second for 5 seconds.

Hepatic arteriogram

The common hepatic artery branches from the right side of the celiac artery and supplies circulation to the liver, stomach, duodenum and pancreas.

- Position the patient to place the upper and right margins of the liver at the respective margins of the film (Fig. 26-22).
- Make the exposures. Representative injection and film programs are 8 ml/sec for 40 ml total volume and two films per second for 5 seconds followed by one film per second for 5 seconds.

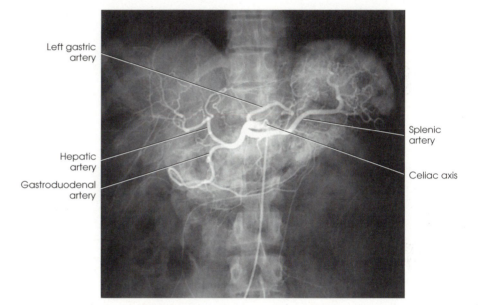

Fig. 26-21. Selective AP celiac arteriogram.

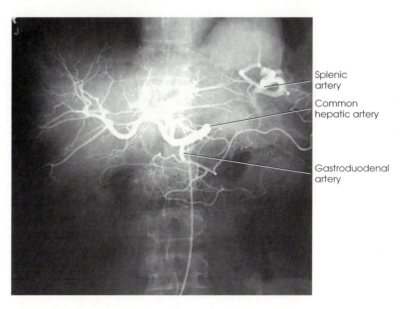

Fig. 26-22. Superselective hepatic arteriogram with overflow into splenic artery.

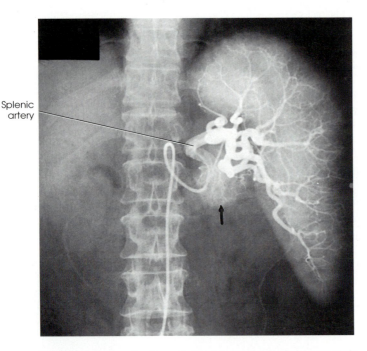

Fig. 26-23. Superselective splenic arteriogram with moderately enlarged spleen. *Arrow,* tail of pancreas.

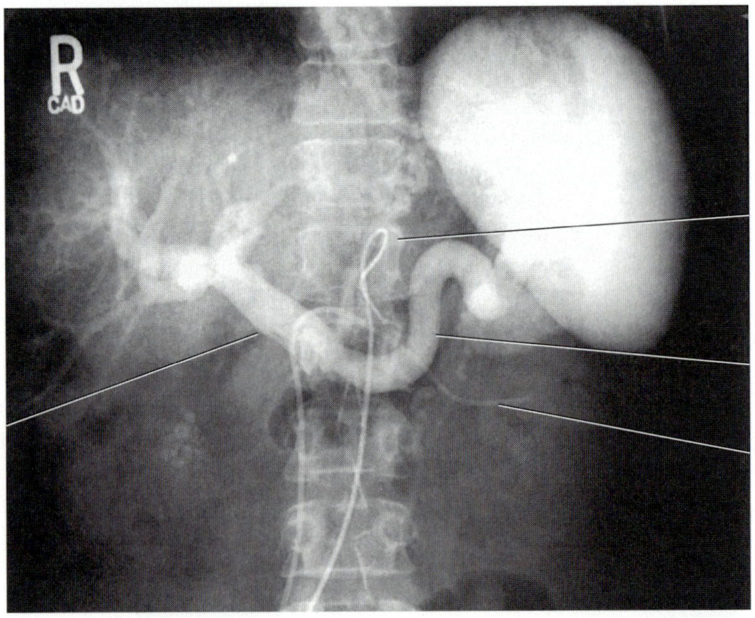

Fig. 26-24. Late-phase splenic arteriogram demonstrating portal system.

Splenic artery

Splenic artery catheter

Splenic vein

Portal vein

Catheter in left renal vein

R
CAD

Splenic arteriogram

The splenic artery branches from the left side of the celiac artery and supplies blood to the spleen and pancreas.

- Position the patient to place the left and upper margins of the spleen at the respective margins of the film (Figs. 26-23 and 26-24).
- Extend the length of the filming sequence, which will often allow adequate visualization of the portal system on the later radiographs. Splenic artery injection is, in fact, the common method of demonstrating the portal venous system.
- For demonstration of the portal vein, center the patient to the film.
- Make the exposures. Representative injection and film programs for a standard splenic arteriogram are 8 ml/sec for 40 ml total volume and two films per second for 5 seconds followed by one film per second for 5 seconds. Representative programs for portal vein visualization are 8 ml/sec for 80 ml total volume and one film per second for 20 seconds.

Superior mesenteric arteriogram

The superior mesenteric artery (SMA) supplies blood to the small intestine and the ascending and transverse colon. It arises at about the level of L1 and descends to L5-S1.

- To demonstrate the SMA, center the patient to the midline of the film.
- Direct the central ray to the level of L3 (Fig. 26-25).
- Make the exposures. Representative injection and filming programs are 8 ml/sec for 40 ml total volume and two films per second for 5 seconds followed by one film per second for 5 seconds.
- When attempting to visualize bleeding sites, conduct the filming at one film per second for 18 seconds.
- Use an increased injection volume and an extended filming sequence to optimize visualization of the mesenteric and portal veins.

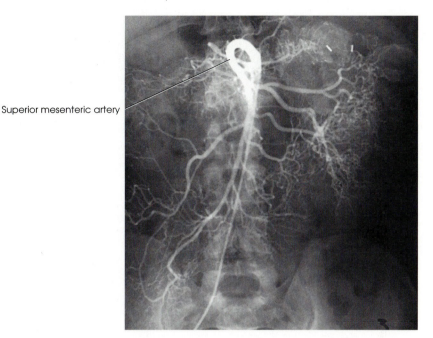

Superior mesenteric artery

Fig. 26-25. Selective superior mesenteric arteriogram.

Inferior mesenteric arteriogram

The inferior mesenteric artery (IMA) supplies blood to the splenic flexure, the descending colon, and the rectosigmoid area. It arises from the left side of the aorta at about the level of L3 and descends into the pelvis.

- To best visualize the IMA, use a 15-degree RAO or LPO position that places the descending colon and rectum at the left and inferior margins of the film (Fig. 26-26).
- Make the exposures. A representative injection program is 3 ml/sec for 15 ml total volume. Filming is the same as that performed for the SMA.

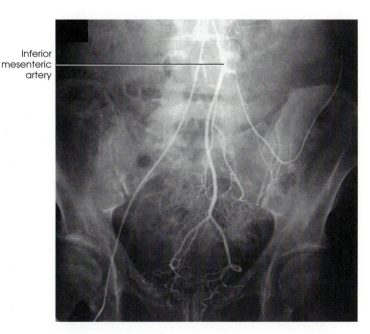

Inferior mesenteric artery

Fig. 26-26. Selective inferior mesenteric arteriogram.

Abdominal visceral arteriography

533

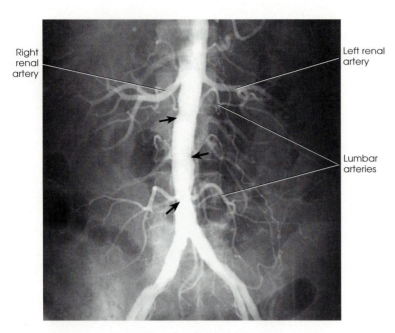

Right renal artery

Left renal artery

Lumbar arteries

Fig. 26-27. Renal flush arteriogram showing atherosclerotic changes in the aorta *(arrows)*.

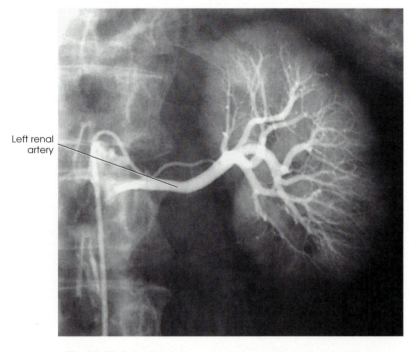

Left renal artery

Fig. 26-28. Selective left renal arteriogram in early arterial phase.

Renal arteriogram

The renal arteries arise from the right and left side of the aorta between L1 and L2 and supply blood to the respective kidneys.

- Check the patient's intravenous urogram or renal flush arteriogram for the exact size and location of the kidneys before performing this selective study. This step enables the radiographer to collimate precisely to the kidney being studied and ensures exact centering of the patient and central ray.
- For a right renal arteriogram, position the patient so that the central ray enters at the level of L2 midway between the center of the spine and the patient's right side.
- For a selective left renal arteriogram, position the patient so that the central ray usually enters at the level of L1 and midway between the center of the spine and the patient's left side (Figs. 26-27 and 26-28).
- Make the exposures. A renal flush arteriogram may be accomplished by injecting 25 ml/sec for 40 ml total volume through a multiple side hole catheter positioned in the aorta at the level of the renal arteries. A representative selective injection is 8 ml/sec for 12 ml total volume. Filming for both methods of injections is commonly three to six films per second for 2 to 3 seconds followed by nephrogram films, perhaps only one or two, made between 5 and 10 seconds after the beginning of the injection.

• • •

Other arteries branching from the aorta may be selectively studied to demonstrate the anatomy and possible pathologic condition. The positioning for these procedures depends on the area to be studied and on the surrounding structures.

Central Venography

Blood in veins flows proximally. Injection into a central venous structure may not opacify the peripheral veins that *anastomose* to it. However, the position of peripheral veins can be indirectly documented by the filling defect from unopacified blood in the opacified central vein. The radiographer observes the following guidelines:

- Place the patient in the supine position for either a single-plane AP or PA projection or biplane projections.
- Obtain lateral projections at increased SID, if possible, to reduce magnification, and move the patient's arms out of the field of view.
- Remember that collimation to the long axis of the vena cava will improve image quality but may prevent visualization of peripheral or *collateral* veins.

Superior vena cavogram

A superior vena cavogram is performed primarily to rule out the existence of thrombus or the occlusion of the superior vena cava. Injection may be made through a needle or angiographic catheter introduced into a vein in an antecubital fossa, although superior opacification results from injection through a catheter positioned in the axillary or subclavian vein. Radiographs should include the opacified subclavian vein, the upper central chest including the superior vena cava, and the right atrium (Fig. 26-29). The injection program depends mostly on whether a needle, angiographic catheter, or regular catheter is used. A representative program for a catheter injection is 10 to 15 ml/sec for 30 to 50 ml total volume. Radiographs are produced in both planes, if desired, at a rate of one or two films per second for 5 to 10 seconds and are made at the end of suspended inspiration.

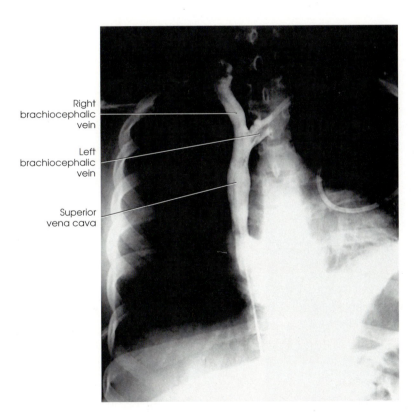

Right brachiocephalic vein

Left brachiocephalic vein

Superior vena cava

Fig. 26-29. AP superior vena cava.

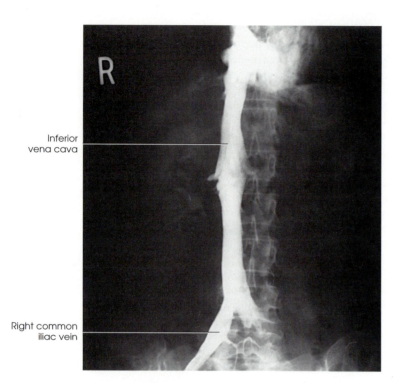

Inferior
vena cava

Right common
iliac vein

Fig. 26-30. AP inferior vena cava.

Inferior vena cavogram

An inferior vena cavogram is performed primarily to rule out the existence of thrombus or the occlusion of the inferior vena cava. Injection is usually made through a multiple side hole catheter inserted through the femoral vein and positioned in the common iliac vein or the inferior aspect of the inferior vena cava. Radiographs may need to include the opacified vasculature from the catheter tip to the right atrium (Figs. 26-30 and 26-31). Representative injection and film programs are 25 ml/sec for 50 ml total volume and two films per second for 4 to 8 seconds in both planes. Filming begins at the end of suspended expiration.

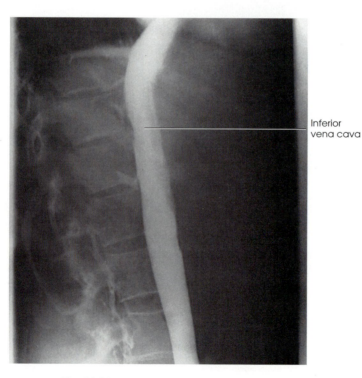

Inferior
vena cava

Fig. 26-31. Lateral inferior vena cava.

Selective Visceral Venography

The visceral veins are often visualized by extending the filming program of the corresponding visceral artery injection. For example, the veins that drain the small bowel are normally visualized by extending the filming program of a superior mesenteric arteriogram. Portal venography can be performed by injecting the portal vein directly from a percutaneous anterior abdominal wall approach, but it is usually accomplished by late-phase filming of a splenic artery injection. Some visceral veins are catheterized, however, for optimum visualization, blood sampling, or blood pressure measurements obtained through the catheter.

Hepatic venogram

A hepatic venogram is usually performed to rule out stenosis or thrombosis of the hepatic veins. The hepatic veins are also catheterized to obtain pressure measurements from the liver interior. The hepatic veins carry blood from the liver to the inferior vena cava. (The portal vein carries nutrient-rich blood from the other organs of digestion to the liver.) The hepatic veins are most easily catheterized from an upper limb vein approach, but a femoral vein approach may also be used.

- Place the patient in the supine position for AP or PA projections that include the liver tissue and the extreme upper inferior vena cava (Fig. 26-32).
- Make the exposures. Representative injection and film programs are 10 ml/sec for 30 ml total volume and one film per second for 8 seconds.
- Make films at the end of suspended expiration.

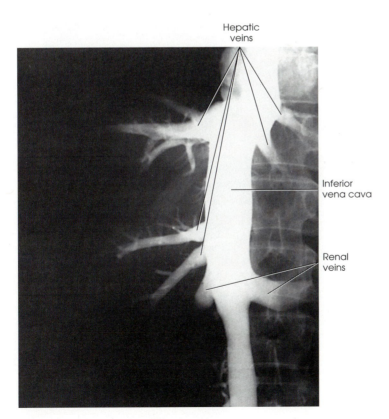

Fig. 26-32. Hepatic vein visualization from inferior vena caval injection overflow.

Renal venogram

A renal venogram is usually performed to rule out thrombosis of the renal vein. The renal vein is also catheterized for blood sampling, usually to measure the production of renin, an enzyme produced by the kidney when it lacks adequate blood supply. The renal vein is most easily catheterized from an upper limb vein approach, but a femoral vein approach may also be used.

- Place the patient in the supine position for a single-plane AP or PA projection.
- Center the selected kidney to the film, and collimate the field to include the kidney and area of the inferior vena cava (Fig. 26-33).
- Make the exposures. Representative injection and filming programs are 8 ml/sec for 16 ml total volume and two films per second for 4 seconds.
- Make films at the end of suspended expiration.

Left renal veins

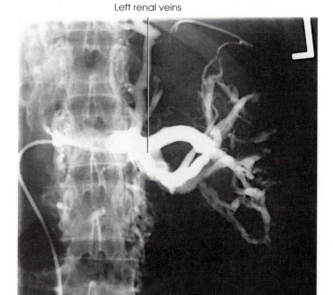

Fig. 26-33. Selective left renal venogram, AP projection.

Circulatory system

Peripheral Angiography
Upper limb arteriograms

Upper limb (extremity) arteriograms are most often performed to evaluate traumatic injury or an arteriovenous shunt created for renal dialysis. They are usually obtained by using the Seldinger technique to introduce a catheter, usually at a femoral artery site, and positioning it for selective injection into the subclavian artery. The contrast medium may also be injected at a more distal site through a catheter or needle. The area to be radiographed may therefore be just a hand or other selected part of the arm, or it may include the entire upper limb and thorax. The equipment available and the condition of the patient control the filming procedure. The recommended projection is a true AP with the arm extended and the hand supinated. Hand arteriograms may be obtained in the supine or prone arm position (Figs. 26-34 and 26-35). The injection and filming programs depend on the equipment used. Injection varies from around 3 or 4 ml/sec through a large needle positioned distally to around 10 ml/sec through a proximally positioned catheter. Filming using a long film cassette changer may be performed with 1- or 2-second delays between exposures. A representative program for a rapid film changer may be two films per second for 5 seconds followed by one film per second for 5 seconds.

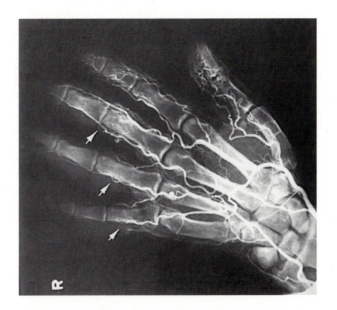

Fig. 26-34. Right hand arteriogram (2:1 magnification), showing severe arterio-occlusive disease *(arrows)* affecting digits after cold-temperature injury.

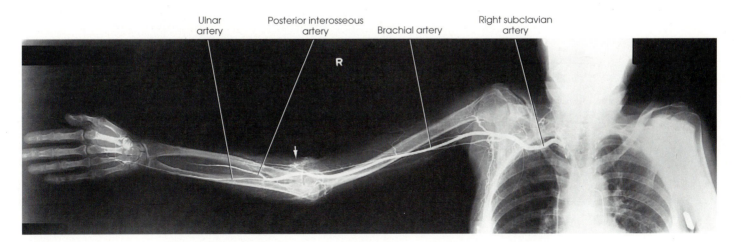

Fig. 26-35. Right upper limb arteriogram showing iatrogenic occlusion of radial artery *(arrow).*

Upper limb venograms

Upper limb (extremity) venograms are most often performed to look for thrombosis. The contrast medium is injected through a needle or catheter into a superficial vein at the elbow or wrist. The radiographs should cover the vasculature from the wrist or elbow to the superior vena cava. The patient position selected may be determined by fluoroscopy, or the patient may be positioned for an AP projection with the hand supinated. The projection and filming sequence depend on the location of the injection site and the limitations and condition of the patient and equipment (Fig. 26-36). If the injection and filling of veins are observed with a fluoroscopic spot film device, radiographs can be exposed as the vessels opacify. If a Bucky tray or film changer is used, a series of films with a delay of a few seconds between exposures is normally obtained. Injections may be made by hand, or an automatic injector may be set to deliver a total of 40 to 80 ml at a rate of 1 to 4 ml/sec, depending on whether a needle or catheter is used. If the study is performed with the patient supine, tourniquets positioned proximal to the wrist and elbow are required to force the contrast medium into the deep veins.

Cephalic vein   Basilic vein   Subclavian vein

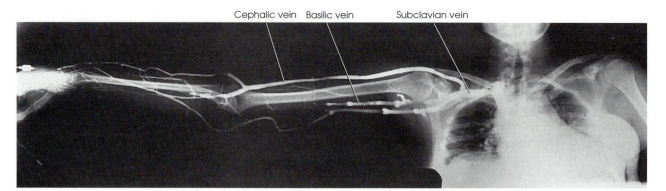

Fig. 26-36. Normal right upper limb venogram.

Aortofemoral arteriograms

Aortofemoral arteriograms are usually performed to determine if atherosclerotic disease is the cause of *claudication*. A catheter is usually introduced into a femoral artery using the Seldinger technique. The catheter tip is positioned superior to the aortic bifurcation so that bilateral arteriograms are simultaneously obtained. When only one leg is to be examined, the catheter tip is placed below the bifurcation, or the contrast medium is injected through a needle placed in the femoral artery. The radiographer then observes the following guidelines:

- For a bilateral examination, place the patient in the supine position for single-plane AP projections and center the patient to the midline of the film changer to include the area from the renal arteries to the ankles.
- Place the patient in the prone position for a translumbar catheterization if needed.
- For either patient position, internally rotate the legs 30 degrees.
- For best results, use a cassette changer with 120 cm long film.
- If the cassette changer is not available, have the radiographs obtain overlap to ensure coverage of all vasculature. Such overlapping radiographs can be produced automatically by specialized moving tables.
- Make exposures of the opacified lower abdominal aorta and aortic bifurcation with the patient in suspended expiration.

Film programs will vary and are set based on the predicted rate of flow through the long arterial course of the lower limb. Flow through normal arteries may take as little as 10 seconds, whereas flow through severely diseased arteries may take 30 seconds or more. A representative injection program designed to create a long bolus of contrast medium is 13 ml/sec for 80 ml total volume (Fig. 26-37).

Examinations of a specific area of the leg (e.g., popliteal fossa or foot) are occasionally performed. For these procedures the preferred injection site is usually the femoral artery. AP, lateral, or both projections may be obtained with the patient centered to the designated area.

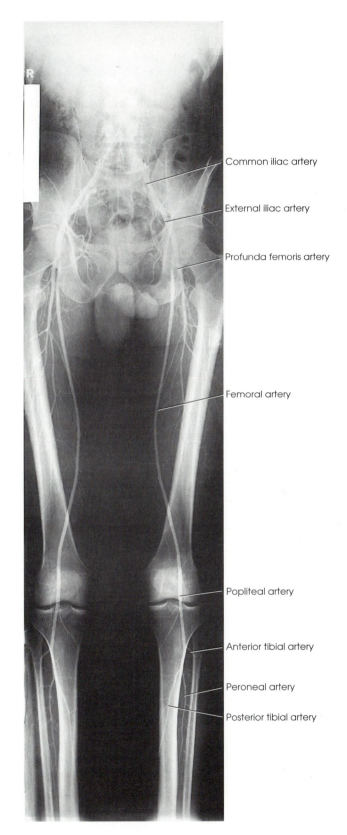

Fig. 26-37. Normal aortofemoral arteriogram in late arterial phase.

Common iliac artery

External iliac artery

Profunda femoris artery

Femoral artery

Popliteal artery

Anterior tibial artery

Peroneal artery

Posterior tibial artery

Peripheral angiography

541

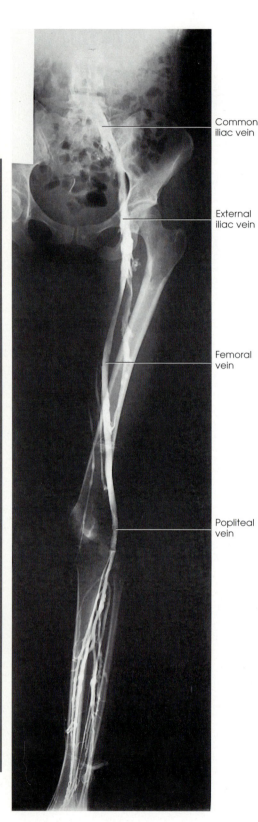

Common
iliac vein

External
iliac vein

Femoral
vein

Popliteal
vein

Fig. 26-38. Normal left lower limb venogram.

Lower limb venograms

Lower limb (extremity) venograms are common and are usually performed to rule out thrombosis of the deep veins of the leg. These venograms are usually obtained by making an injection through a needle placed directly into a superficial vein in the foot. The radiographer then observes the following guidelines:

- Obtain radiographs with the patient on a tilt table in a semi-upright position at a minimum angle of 45 degrees if possible.
- Begin filming at the ankle and proceed superiorly to include the inferior vena cava as the injection continues.
- Exact positioning is often determined with fluoroscopic aid; without fluoroscopy, usually obtain AP projections with the leg internally rotated 30 degrees to include the entire area of interest (Fig. 26-38).
- Perform lateral projections if needed.
- If filming is performed with the patient supine, apply tourniquets just proximal to the ankle and knee to force filling of the deep veins in the leg.
- Usually, expose serial radiographs obtained with a Bucky tray or film changer 5 to 10 seconds apart. Injections may be made by hand, or an automatic injector may be set to deliver 1 or 2 ml/sec for a total of 50 to 100 ml.

• • •

In all angiographic procedures, precise methods must be followed, and the sequence of filming and injection must be determined in consultation with the physician. As in all surgical procedures, great care must be exercised to ensure that sterile techniques are strictly maintained. Precise positioning of the patient is also essential so that the desired body part will be adequately demonstrated. It is imperative that careful and complete cooperation be maintained among the physician, the radiographer, and the patient to obtain radiographs with the maximum amount of diagnostic information.

Angiography in the Future

Visceral and peripheral angiography is a dynamic profession that challenges angiographers to keep abreast with new techniques and equipment. New diagnostic modalities that reduce or eliminate irradiation may be developed that will possibly replace some current angiographic procedures. Some diagnostic information, however, can be obtained only through conventional angiographic methods. Angiography will, therefore, continue to examine vasculature and, through therapeutic procedures, provide beneficial treatment to the body.

Cerebral angiography is the term used to denote radiologic examinations of the blood vessels of the brain by means of injecting the vessels with a radiopaque contrast medium. The procedure was introduced by Egas Moniz[1] in 1927. It is performed to investigate intracranial *aneurysms* or other vascular *lesions* and to demonstrate tumor masses, which are shown by displacement of the normal cerebrovascular pattern or by the tumor's circulation.

The brain is supplied by four trunk vessels: the right and left common carotid arteries, which supply the anterior circulation, and the right and left vertebral arteries, which supply the posterior circulation. These paired arteries branch from the arch of the aorta and ascend through the neck, as shown in Fig. 26-39.

The left common carotid artery originates directly from the aortic arch. The right common carotid artery arises with the right subclavian artery about 1½ inches (3.7 cm) higher at the *bifurcation* of the brachiocephalic artery (Fig. 26-40). The left subclavian artery originates di-

[1]Egas Moniz AC: L'encéphalographie artérielle, son importance dans la localisation des tumeurs cérébrales, Rev Neurol 2:72-90, 1927.

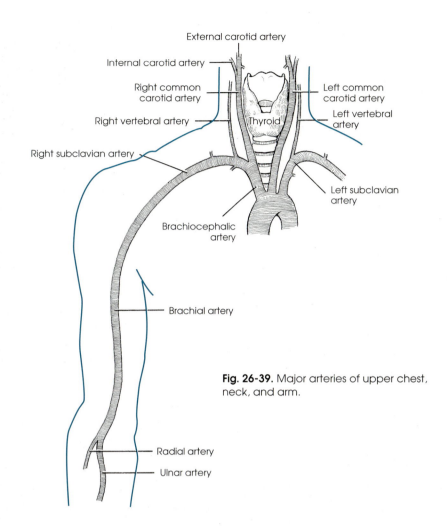

Fig. 26-39. Major arteries of upper chest, neck, and arm.

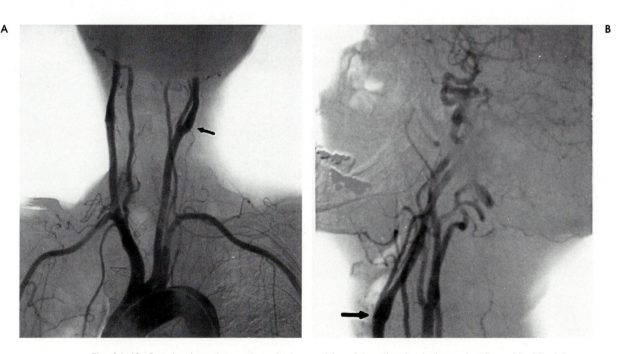

Fig. 26-40. Cerebral angiography, photographic subtraction technique. **A,** AP and **B,** AP oblique (RPO position) of aortic arch demonstrating excellent visualization of extracranial carotid and vertebral arteries. Normal left common carotid bifurcation *(arrows)*.

Cerebral angiography

543

rectly from the arch of the aorta. The vertebral arteries arise from the subclavian arteries. *Anomalies* in the origin of these vessels are common.

Each common carotid artery passes superiorly and somewhat laterally alongside the trachea and larynx to the level of C4, where each divides into internal and external carotid arteries. The latter vessel contributes to the supply of the *meninges* but not to that of the intracerebral circulation. The internal carotid artery enters the cranium through the carotid foramen of the temporal bone and then bifurcates into the anterior and middle cerebral arteries. They, in turn, branch and rebranch to supply the anterior circulation of the respective hemisphere of the brain (Fig. 26-41).

The vertebral arteries ascend through the cervical transverse foramina and then pass medially to enter the cranium through the foramen magnum. The verte-

bral arteries unite to form the basilar artery, which, after a short superior course along the posterior surface of the dorsum sellae, bifurcates into the right and left posterior cerebral arteries. The blood supply to the posterior fossa (cerebellum) originates from the vertebral and basilar arteries (Fig. 26-42).

The anterior and posterior cerebral arteries are connected by communicating arteries at the level of the midbrain to form the circulus arteriosus, commonly known as the circle of Willis. The anterior communicating artery forms an anastomosis between the anterior cerebral arteries. The right and left posterior communicating arteries each form an anastomosis between the internal carotid artery and the posterior cerebral artery on their side of the cerebral circulation.

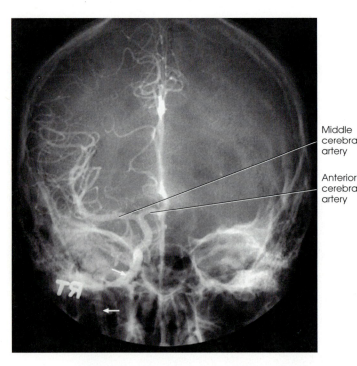

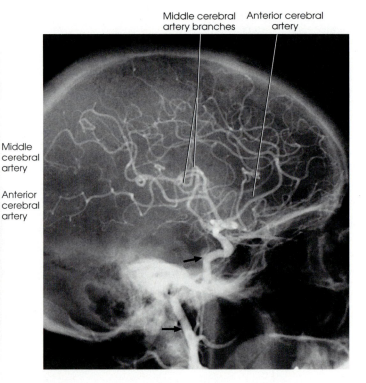

Middle cerebral artery branches

Anterior cerebral artery

Middle cerebral artery

Anterior cerebral artery

Fig. 26-41. Carotid arteriograms showing internal carotid artery *(arrows)* and anterior cerebral blood circulation.

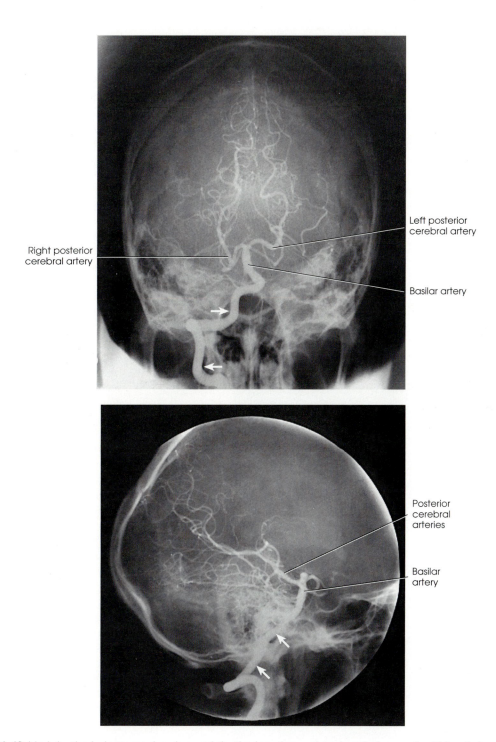

Right posterior
cerebral artery

Left posterior
cerebral artery

Basilar artery

Posterior
cerebral
arteries

Basilar
artery

Fig. 26-42. Vertebral arteriograms showing vertebral artery *(arrows)* and posterior cerebral blood circulation.

TECHNIQUE

Cerebral angiography should be performed only in facilities equipped to produce studies of high technical quality with minimum risk to the patient. The ability to obtain rapid-sequence biplane radiographs with automatic injection represents the minimum standard. This equipment is available in all major medical centers and in most large community hospitals.

Access to the carotid, vertebral, and cerebral vessels is almost universally accomplished by catheterization from the femoral artery (Fig. 26-43). If this route is blocked by previous surgical procedures such as aortofemoral bypass grafting or intrinsic atherosclerotic disease, catheterization from a brachial or axillary artery approach is frequently employed. The entire intracerebral circulation can also be visualized by direct puncture and injection of the left common carotid artery and a right retrograde brachial artery injection. This technique is associated with a higher complication rate and significantly more discomfort to the patient. Selective catheterization techniques also allow the study of internal and external carotid circulations separately, which is useful in delineating the blood supply of some forms of cerebral tumors and vascular malformations.

The final position of the catheter depends on the information sought from the angiographic study. When atherosclerotic disease of the extracranial carotid, subclavian, and vertebral arteries is being evaluated, an injection of the aortic arch with filming of the extracranial portion of these vessels is an appropriate way to begin. Selective studies depend on fluoroscopic positioning of an appropriate catheter in a stable but *nonocclusive* position in the proximal segment of the carotid or vertebral artery of interest.

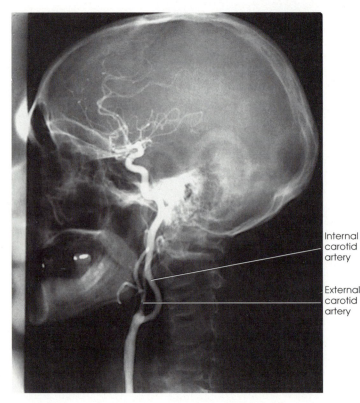

Fig. 26-43. Lateral intracranial and extracranial carotid arteriogram with catheter in right common carotid artery orifice by way of femoral artery catheterization.

Internal carotid artery

External carotid artery

CIRCULATION TIME AND FILMING PROGRAM

According to the estimation of Egas Moniz,[1] only 3 seconds is the usual time required for the blood to circulate from the internal carotid artery to the jugular vein, the circulation time being slightly prolonged by the injected contrast solution. Greitz,[2] who measured the cerebral circulation time as "the time between the points of maximum concentration [of contrast medium] in the carotid siphon and in the parietal veins," found a normal mean value of 4.13 seconds. Thus time is a highly important factor in cerebral angiography.

Certain pathologic conditions significantly alter the cerebral circulation time. *Arteriovenous malformations* shorten the transit time, and increased intracranial pressure or arterial spasm may cause a considerable delay.

A standard radiographic program should include a radiograph taken before the arrival of contrast material to serve as a subtraction mask (see discussion of the photographic subtraction technique at the end of this chapter) and rapid-sequence films at one and one-half to three films per second in the AP and lateral projections during the early, or arterial, phase (first 1½ to 2½ seconds) (Fig. 26-44). After the arterial phase, filming may be slowed to one film per second for the capillary, or parenchymal, phase (Fig. 26-45) and maintained at one film per second or every other second for the venous phase (Fig. 26-46) of the angiogram. The entire program should cover 7 to 10 seconds depending on the preference of the angiographer. The filming program must be tailored to demonstrate the suspected pathologic condition.

Injection rates and volumes through the catheter are coupled with the filming program, usually by automatic means. Injections at rates of 5 to 9 ml/sec for 1 to 2 seconds are most often employed in the cerebral vessels, with variations dependent on vessel size and the patient's circulatory status.

[1]Egas Moniz AC: L'angiographie cérébrale, Paris, 1934, Masson & Cie.
[2]Greitz T: A radiologic study of the brain circulation by rapid serial angiography of the carotid artery, Acta Radiol Suppl 140, 1956.

Fig. 26-44 . Right lateral arteriogram showing arterial phase of circulation.

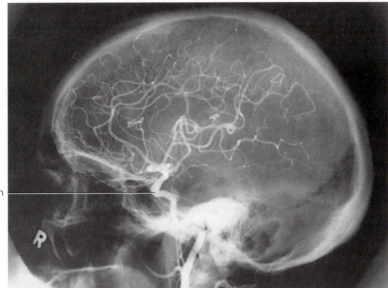

Carotid siphon

Fig. 26-45. Capillary phase of carotid circulation.

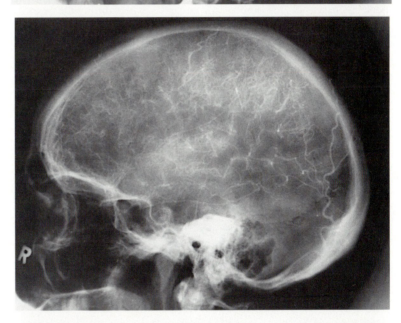

Fig. 26-46. Venous phase of circulation.

(Courtesy Dr. John A. Goree.)

Cerebral veins

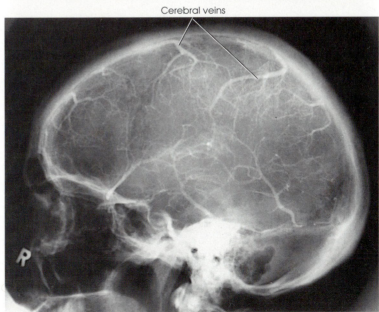

EQUIPMENT

Rapid-sequence biplane imaging using either film or DSA with electronically coupled automatic injection is used almost universally in cerebral angiography. Special training and experience are necessary to use this sophisticated and expensive equipment. The operational and filming capabilities of cerebral angiographic units are diverse and vary considerably according to the manufacturer. However, routine maintenance of all equipment is essential to ensure reliable performance. Careful attention to maintenance and other details by technical and professional staff members is necessary to prevent unnecessary delay in completing studies and inconvenient downtime.

Collimating to the area of the head and neck is essential for improving image quality in the nonmagnified study. The standard tube collimator may be used for this purpose, or lead cutout diaphragms may be additionally positioned on the collimator. These diaphragms may have openings in the shape of a circle or a "keyhole." Keyhole diaphragm openings are rounded in the area of the cranium and taper inward in the area of the neck. The frontal and lateral keyhole diaphragms are each designed to resemble the shape of the head and neck in their respective images.

PREPARATION OF PATIENT

Other than withholding the preceding meal, preliminary preparation of the patient depends on his or her condition and is accordingly determined by the radiologist and the referring physician. Whenever possible, adult patients are examined under local anesthesia in conjunction with sedation. Adequate sedation minimizes the intensity of the burning pain felt along the course of the injected vessel and in the areas supplied by it during the rapid injections of the iodinated medium. The sedative has the further advantage of lessening the possibility of a reaction resulting in reflex movement during initial arterial filming at or before the end of each injection. It is imperative that the conscious patient receive a careful explanation of what to expect during the examination and what is expected of him or her. This explanation is essential for the successful completion of the examination.

PREPARATION OF EXAMINING ROOM

It cannot be said too often that radiographic examining rooms and every item in them should be as scrupulously clean as any other room used for medical purposes. The room should be fully prepared, with every item needed or likely to be needed on hand before the patient is admitted. Cleanliness and advance preparation are of vital importance in examinations that must be carried out under aseptic conditions. The radiographer should observe the following guidelines in preparing the room:

- Check the radiographic machine and all working parts of the equipment, and adjust the controls for the exposure technique to be employed.
- Place identification markers and all accessories in a convenient location.
- Have compression and restraining bands ready for application.
- Adapt immobilization of the head (by suitable strapping) to the type of equipment employed.
- Make arrangements for immediate processing of the films as the examination proceeds.

The sterile and nonsterile items required for the introduction of the contrast medium vary according to the method of injection. The supplies specified by the radiologist for each procedure should be listed in the angiographic procedure book. Sterile trays or packs, set up to specifications, can usually be obtained from the central sterile-supply room. Otherwise, it is the responsibility of a qualified member of the technologic staff to prepare them. Extra sterile supplies should always be on hand in case of an accident. Preparation of the room includes having life-supporting emergency equipment immediately available.

RADIATION PROTECTION

As in all radiographic examinations, the patient is protected by filtration totaling not less than 2.5 mm of aluminum, by sharp restriction of the beam of radiation to the area being examined, and by avoidance of repeat exposures. In angiography each repeated exposure necessitates a repeated injection of the iodinated compound. For this reason, only skilled and specifically trained radiographers should be assigned to take part in these examinations.

Angiography suites should be designed to allow observation of the patient at all times as well as to provide adequate protection to the physician and radiology personnel. These goals are usually accomplished with leaded glass observation windows.

POSITION OF PATIENT

In positioning the patient, the following steps are observed:
- Place the patient in the supine position for the entire examination, as required by all cerebral angiographic injection methods.
- Regardless of whether the patient is awake, place suitable supports under points of strain—the small of the back, the knees, and the ankles—and cover the patient according to room temperature.
- Apply wrist restraints and compression bands across the body as indicated by the patient's condition.
- When the catheter is in place, there is little danger of unseating it during positioning; however, exercise care to prevent excessive patient motion, especially with extremely selective studies.

POSITION OF HEAD

The centering and angulation of the central ray required for the demonstration of the anterior circulation differ from that required for the demonstration of the posterior circulation, but the same head position is used for the basic AP and lateral projections of both regions. The following steps are observed:
- For the initial right-angle studies, center the head to both the AP and lateral image receptors.
- Then adjust the head to place its median sagittal plane exactly perpendicular to the headrest and consequently exactly parallel with the laterally placed film changer.
- Place the infraorbitomeatal line perpendicular to the horizontal plane when positioning is accomplished manually.
- Base the central ray angulation for caudally inclined AP and AP oblique projections from the vertically placed infraorbitomeatal line, or adjust the central ray so that it is parallel to the floor of the anterior fossa, as indicated by a line extending from the supraorbital margin to a point 2 cm superior to the external acoustic (auditory) meatus.

Head positioning is presented in this chapter as if the image receptors were fixed in the horizontal and vertical planes. This necessitates the use of facial landmarks for precise positioning of the head in relationship to the central ray to achieve certain projections. In some angiographic suites, however, fluoroscopy can be used to determine the final position of the head and the angulation of the central ray required to achieve the desired image.

The literature on cerebral angiography contains numerous position variations concerning the degree of central ray angulation, the base from which it should be angled or the line that it should parallel, and the degree of part rotation for oblique studies. The most frequently employed images, and reasonably standard specifications for obtaining them, have been selected for inclusion in this chapter.

The number of radiographs required for satisfactory delineation of a lesion depends on the nature and location of the lesion. Oblique projections and/or variations in central ray angulation are taken to separate the vessels that overlap in the basic positions and to evaluate any existing abnormality.

Aortic Arch Angiogram (for Cranial Vessels)

An aortic arch angiogram is most commonly performed to visualize atherosclerotic or occlusive disease of the extracranial carotid, vertebral, and subclavian arteries. A multiple side hole catheter is positioned in the arch of the aorta so that the subsequent injection fills all of the vessels simultaneously.

For best results, simultaneous biplane oblique projections are produced so that superimposition of vessels is minimized.

The following steps are observed:

- Place the patient in an RPO position on the tabletop, with the median sagittal plane of the head either perpendicular to the AP film changer or in an RPO position. This patient position opens the aortic arch for the AP oblique projection and frees the carotid and vertebral arteries from superimposition for the lateral oblique projection.
- Raise the patient's chin to superimpose the inferior margin of the mandible onto the occiput so that as much of the neck as possible is exposed in the frontal radiograph.
- Move the patient's shoulders inferiorly so that they are removed as much as possible from the lateral image.
- Use offset biplane film changers for this procedure if possible.
- Position the lateral film changer approximately 15 cm superior to the AP changer so that the lateral projection exposes the head and neck while the AP projection exposes the neck and upper chest.
- For the AP projection, direct the central ray perpendicular to the center of the film to enter the patient at a level 3 cm superior to the sternal angle.
- Direct the central ray for the lateral projection perpendicular to the midline of the vertically oriented grid and to usually enter the patient a few centimeters inferior to the angle of the mandible.
- Collimate the lateral field in the anteroposterior aspect (see Fig. 26-40).

A representative injection program for an aortic arch examination is 30 to 35 ml/sec for a total volume of 60 to 70 ml. A representative film program is two to three films per second in each plane for 4 seconds. Because subtraction films are frequently produced from aortic arch angiograms, it is important that the initial films are exposed before the injection begins. An alternative film program exposes one film in each plane, pauses 1 second as the injection begins, and then continues with two to three films per second for 3 seconds.

Anterior Circulation

LATERAL PROJECTION

- Center the patient's head to the vertically placed film.
- Extend the head enough to place the infraorbitomeatal line perpendicular to the horizontal.
- Adjust the head to place the median sagittal plane vertically and thereby parallel with the plane of the film.
- Adapt immobilization to the type of equipment being employed.
- Perform lateral projections of the anterior, or carotid, circulation with the central ray directed horizontal to a point slightly cranial to the auricle and midway between the forehead and the occiput. This centering allows for variation (Figs. 26-47 to 26-49).

For assistance in identifying the cerebral vessels in these and the following radiographs, see Fig. 26-72 at the end of this section of this chapter.

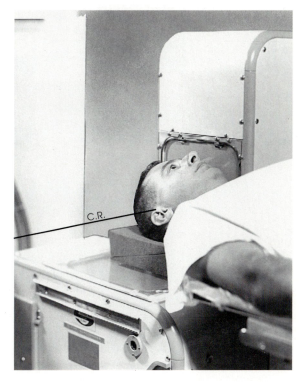

Fig. 26-47. Cerebral angiogram, lateral projection.

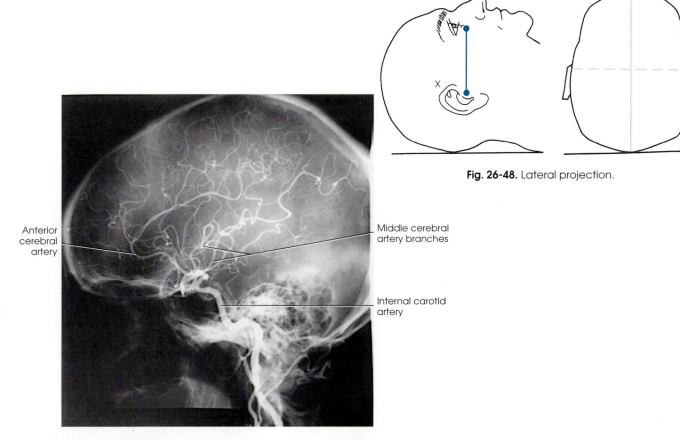

Fig. 26-48. Lateral projection.

Anterior cerebral artery

Middle cerebral artery branches

Internal carotid artery

Fig. 26-49. Cerebral angiogram. Lateral projection demonstrating anterior circulation.

(Courtesy Joyce Torzewski, R.T.)

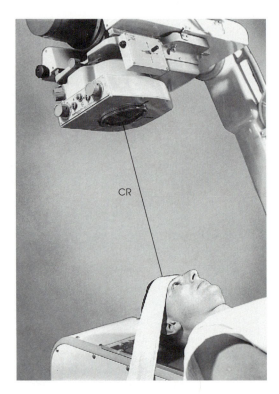

Fig. 26-50. Carotid angiogram, AP axial (supraorbital) projection.

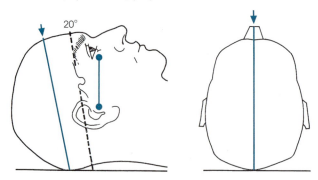

Fig. 26-51. AP axial (supraorbital).

Anterior Circulation
AP AXIAL PROJECTION (SUPRAORBITAL)

- Adjust the head so that its median sagittal plane is centered over and perpendicular to the midline of the grid and so that it is extended enough to place the infraorbitomeatal line vertically.
- Immobilize the head.
- To achieve the goal in this radiograph, superimpose the supraorbital margins on the superior margin of the petrous ridges so that the vessels are projected above the floor of the anterior cranial fossa.
- Obtain this result in a majority of patients by directing the central ray 20 degrees caudal along a line passing 2 cm superior to and parallel with a line extending from the supraorbital margin to a point 2 cm superior to the external acoustic meatus; the latter line coincides with the floor of the anterior fossa (Figs. 26-50 to 26-52).

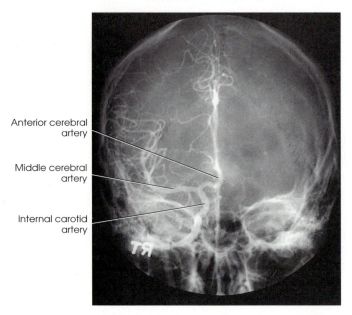

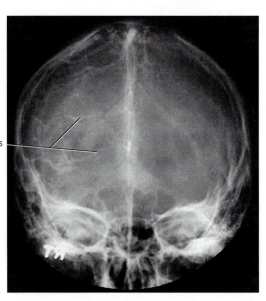

Fig. 26-52. Serial carotid angiograms, AP axial (supraorbital) projection. *Left,* arterial and, *right* venous phases of circulation.

Anterior Circulation

AP AXIAL OBLIQUE PROJECTION (SUPRAORBITAL)

- For demonstration of the region of the anterior communicating artery, maintain the preceding head position, except rotate the head approximately 30 degrees away from the injected side.
- Direct the central ray 20 degrees caudal (Figs. 26-53 and 26-54).

AP AXIAL PROJECTION (TRANSORBITAL)

The AP axial (transorbital) projection demonstrates the middle cerebral artery and its main branches within the orbit.

- Adjust the head for the basic AP projection.

- Direct the central ray through the midorbits at an average angle of 20 degrees cephalad; it should coincide with a line passing through the center of the orbit and a point about 2 cm superior to the auricle of the ear (Figs. 26-55 and 26-56).

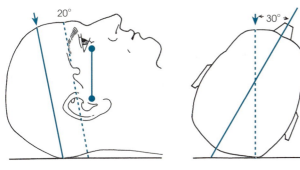

Fig. 26-53. AP axial oblique (supraorbital) projection.

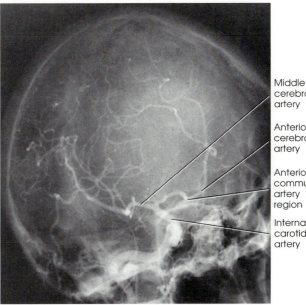

Fig. 26-54. Carotid arteriogram. AP axial oblique (supraorbital) projection.

(Courtesy Dr. John A. Goree.)

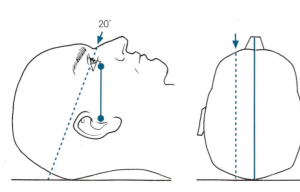

Fig. 26-55. AP axial (transorbital) projection.

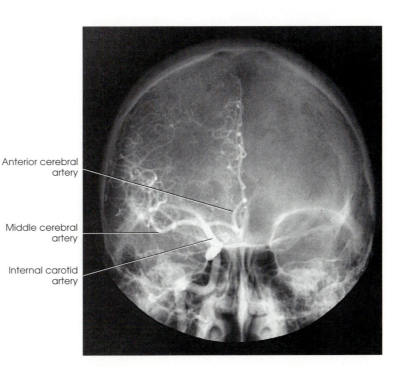

Fig. 26-56. Carotid arteriogram. AP axial (transorbital) projection.

Anterior Circulation

AP AXIAL OBLIQUE PROJECTION (TRANSORBITAL)

The oblique transorbital projection demonstrates the internal carotid bifurcation and the anterior communicating and middle cerebral arteries within the orbital shadow.

- From the position for the basic AP transorbital, rotate the head approximately 30 degrees away from the injected side.
- Angle the central ray 20 degrees cephalad and center it to the midorbit of the uppermost side (Figs. 26-57 and 26-58).

AP AXIAL AND AP OBLIQUE PROJECTIONS

AP axial and/or AP axial oblique projections are used in carotid angiography, when indicated, for further evaluation of vessel displacement or of aneurysms.

For an AP axial projection, the following steps are observed:

- Adjust the head in the basic position.
- Direct the central ray to the region approximately 1½ in (4 cm) superior to the glabella at an average angle of 30 degrees caudad; it exits at the level of the external acoustic meatus (Figs. 26-59 to 26-61).

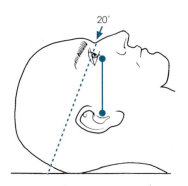

Fig. 26-57. AP axial oblique (transorbital) projection.

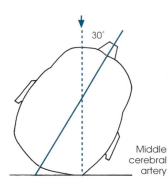

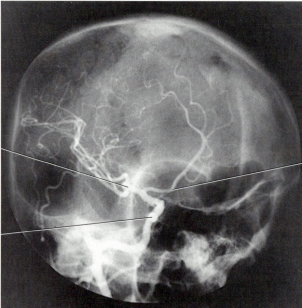

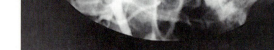

Fig. 26-58. Carotid angiogram: AP axial oblique (transorbital) projection.

(Courtesy Dr. John A. Goree.)

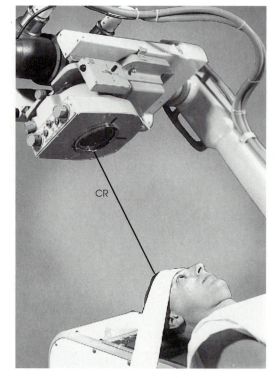

Fig. 26-59. AP axial projection.

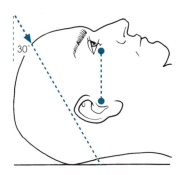

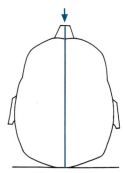

Fig. 26-60. AP axial projection.

For an AP axial oblique projection, the following steps are observed:
- Rotate the head 35 to 45 degrees away from the injected side.
- Angle the central ray 30 degrees caudad (Figs. 26-62 and 26-63).

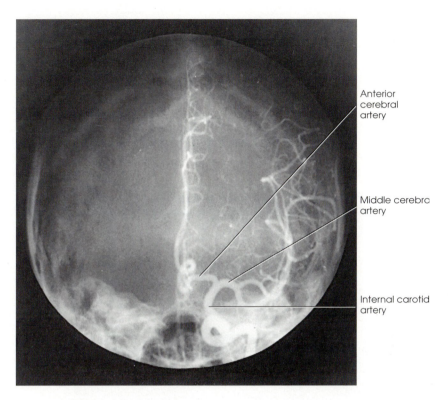

Fig. 26-61. Carotid angiogram: AP axial projection.

Anterior cerebral artery

Middle cerebra artery

Internal carotid artery

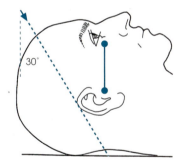

Fig. 26-62. AP axial oblique projection.

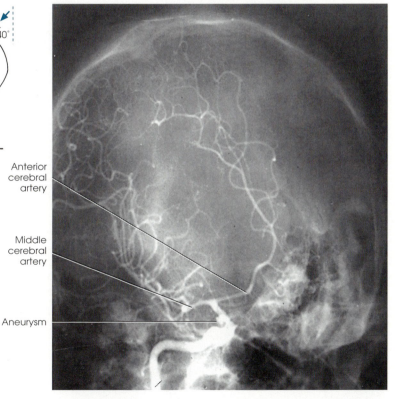

Anterior cerebral artery

Middle cerebral artery

Aneurysm

Fig. 26-63. Carotid angiogram: AP axial oblique projection showing small internal carotid artery aneurysm at posterior communicating junction.

(Courtesy Dr. John A. Goree.)

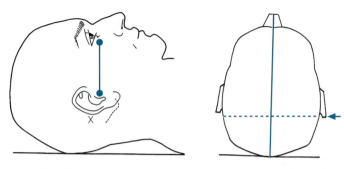

Fig. 26-64. Lateral projection for posterior circulation.

Posterior Circulation
LATERAL PROJECTION

- Center the patient's head to the vertically placed film.
- Extend it enough to place the infraorbitomeatal line perpendicular to the horizontal plane and then adjust it to place the median sagittal plane vertical and thereby parallel with the plane of the film.
- Rigidly immobilize the head.
- Perform lateral projections of the posterior, or vertebral, circulation with the central ray directed horizontal to the mastoid process at a point about 1 cm superior to and 2 cm posterior to the external acoustic meatus.
- Restrict the exposure field to the middle and posterior fossae for lateral studies of the posterior circulation, the inclusion of the entire skull being neither necessary nor, from the standpoint of optimum technique, desirable (Figs. 26-64 to 26-67).

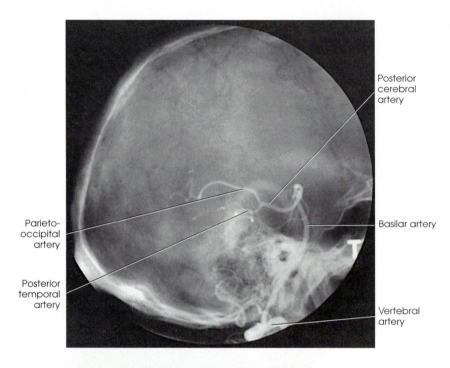

Posterior cerebral artery

Basilar artery

Parieto-occipital artery

Posterior temporal artery

Vertebral artery

Fig. 26-65. Cerebral angiogram. Lateral projection in early arterial phase showing vertebral artery and posterior vascular structures.

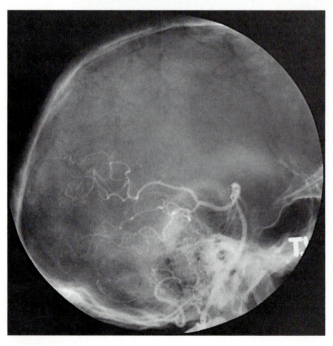

Fig. 26-66. Cerebral angiogram. Lateral projection in arterial phase.

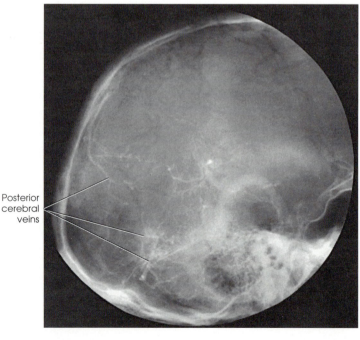

Posterior cerebral veins

Fig. 26-67. Cerebral angiogram, lateral projection in venous phase. Contrast medium for above serial angiograms was introduced by percutaneous retrograde injection into left brachial artery.

Posterior Circulation

AP AXIAL PROJECTION

- Adjust the head so that its median sagittal plane is centered over, and is perpendicular to, the midline of the grid, and extend the head enough so that the infraorbitomeatal line is vertical.
- Immobilize the head.
- Direct the central ray to the region approximately 1½ in (4 cm) superior to the glabella at an angle of 30 to 35 degrees caudad; it exits at the level of the external acoustic meatuses. For this projection the supraorbital margins are positioned approximately 2 cm below the superior margins of the petrous ridges (Figs. 26-68 and 26-69).

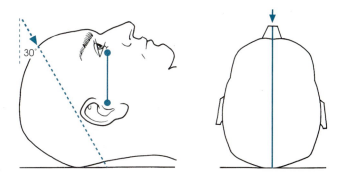

Fig. 26-68. AP axial projection for posterior circulation.

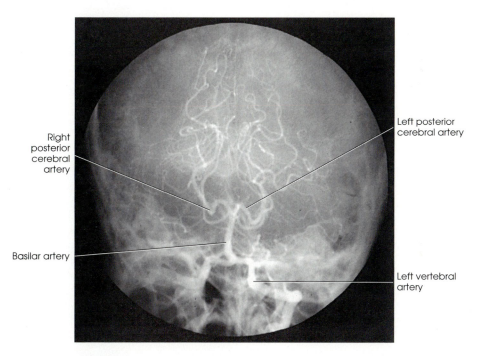

Right posterior cerebral artery

Left posterior cerebral artery

Basilar artery

Left vertebral artery

Fig. 26-69. AP axial projection; arterial phase of posterior circulation.

(Courtesy Dr. John A. Goree.)

Posterior Circulation
SUBMENTOVERTICAL PROJECTION

A modified submentovertical projection (SMV) is sometimes employed in the investigation of the posterior circulation. It is also used for the anterior circulation when a middle fossa lesion is suspected.

The success of this projection depends on the patient's ability to hyperextend the neck and maintain this hyperextension for the time required for a filming sequence. This body position may not be possible for elderly patients with cervical degenerative arthritis (Figs. 26-70 and 26-71). Fig. 26-72 shows the intracerebral circulation.

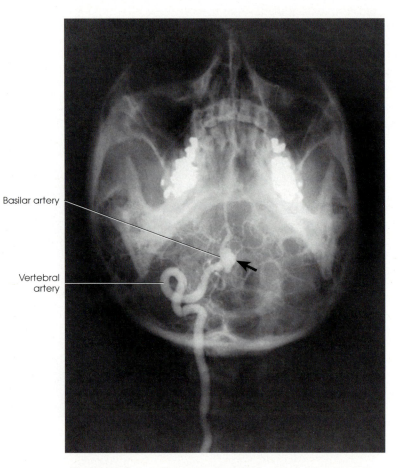

Basilar artery

Vertebral artery

Fig. 26-71. Transaxillary selective right submentovertical vertebral arteriogram showing excellent opacification of right vertebral artery and aneurysm *(arrow)* of vertebrobasilar junction.

(Courtesy Dr. K.Y. Chynn.)

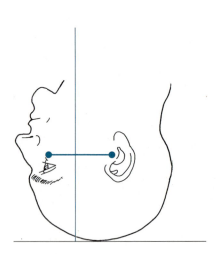

Fig. 26-70. Submentovertical projection.

A CHART OF THE INTRACEREBRAL CIRCULATION

Second Edition

BERTEN C. BEAN, M.D.
Department of Radiology, Buffalo General Hospital
Buffalo, New York

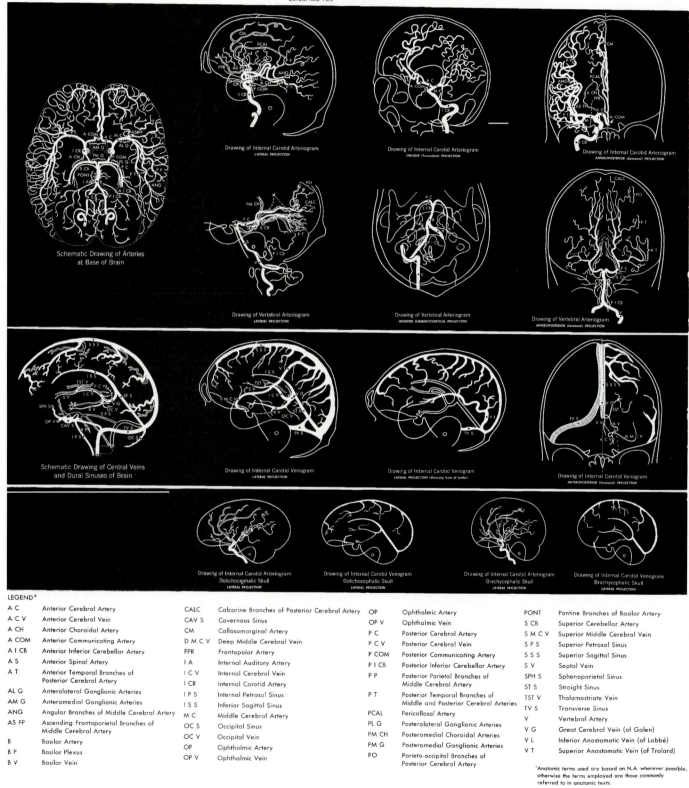

Schematic Drawing of Arteries at Base of Brain

Drawing of Internal Carotid Arteriogram — *LATERAL PROJECTION*

Drawing of Internal Carotid Arteriogram — *OBLIQUE (Transorbital) PROJECTION*

Drawing of Internal Carotid Arteriogram — *ANTEROPOSTERIOR (Semiaxial) PROJECTION*

Drawing of Vertebral Arteriogram — *LATERAL PROJECTION*

Drawing of Vertebral Arteriogram — *MODIFIED SUBMENTOVERTICAL PROJECTION*

Drawing of Vertebral Arteriogram — *ANTEROPOSTERIOR (Semiaxial) PROJECTION*

Schematic Drawing of Central Veins and Dural Sinuses of Brain

Drawing of Internal Carotid Venogram — *LATERAL PROJECTION*

Drawing of Internal Carotid Venogram — *LATERAL PROJECTION (Showing Vein of Labbé)*

Drawing of Internal Carotid Venogram — *ANTEROPOSTERIOR (Semiaxial) PROJECTION*

Drawing of Internal Carotid Arteriogram — Dolichocephalic Skull — *LATERAL PROJECTION*

Drawing of Internal Carotid Venogram — Dolichocephalic Skull — *LATERAL PROJECTION*

Drawing of Internal Carotid Arteriogram — Brachycephalic Skull — *LATERAL PROJECTION*

Drawing of Internal Carotid Venogram — Brachycephalic Skull — *LATERAL PROJECTION*

LEGEND*

A C	Anterior Cerebral Artery
A C V	Anterior Cerebral Vein
A CH	Anterior Choroidal Artery
A COM	Anterior Communicating Artery
A I CB	Anterior Inferior Cerebellar Artery
A S	Anterior Spinal Artery
A T	Anterior Temporal Branches of Posterior Cerebral Artery
AL G	Anterolateral Ganglionic Arteries
AM G	Anteromedial Ganglionic Arteries
ANG	Angular Branches of Middle Cerebral Artery
AS FP	Ascending Frontoparietal Branches of Middle Cerebral Artery
B	Basilar Artery
B P	Basilar Plexus
B V	Basilar Vein
CALC	Calcarine Branches of Posterior Cerebral Artery
CAV S	Cavernous Sinus
CM	Callosomarginal Artery
D M C V	Deep Middle Cerebral Vein
FPR	Frontopolar Artery
I A	Internal Auditory Artery
I C V	Internal Cerebral Vein
I CR	Internal Carotid Artery
I P S	Internal Petrosal Sinus
I S S	Inferior Sagittal Sinus
M C	Middle Cerebral Artery
OC S	Occipital Sinus
OC V	Occipital Vein
OP	Ophthalmic Artery
OP V	Ophthalmic Vein

OP	Ophthalmic Artery
OP V	Ophthalmic Vein
P C	Posterior Cerebral Artery
P C V	Posterior Cerebral Vein
P COM	Posterior Communicating Artery
P I CB	Posterior Inferior Cerebellar Artery
P P	Posterior Parietal Branches of Middle Cerebral Artery
P T	Posterior Temporal Branches of Middle and Posterior Cerebral Arteries
PCAL	Pericallosal Artery
PL G	Posterolateral Ganglionic Arteries
PM CH	Posteromedial Choroidal Arteries
PM G	Posteromedial Ganglionic Arteries
PO	Parieto-occipital Branches of Posterior Cerebral Artery

PONT	Pontine Branches of Basilar Artery
S CB	Superior Cerebellar Artery
S M C V	Superior Middle Cerebral Vein
S P S	Superior Petrosal Sinus
S S S	Superior Sagittal Sinus
S V	Septal Vein
SPH S	Sphenoparietal Sinus
ST S	Straight Sinus
TST V	Thalamostriate Vein
TV S	Transverse Sinus
V	Vertebral Artery
V G	Great Cerebral Vein (of Galen)
V L	Inferior Anastomotic Vein (of Labbé)
V T	Superior Anastomotic Vein (of Trolard)

*Anatomic terms used are based on N.A. wherever possible; otherwise the terms employed are those commonly referred to in anatomic texts.

Fig. 26-72. Intracerebral circulation.

Interventional radiology is a process that intervenes, or interferes, with the course of a disease process or other medical condition. It has a therapeutic, rather than diagnostic, purpose. Since its conception in the early 1960s, the realm of interventional radiology has become so vast and sophisticated that periodicals struggle to keep abreast of the rapidly advancing specialty.

Interventional radiology allows the angiographer to assume an important role in the management and reduction of disease in many patients. In most cases the interventional procedure has helped reduce the length of a patient's stay in the hospital and helped some patients avoid surgery, lowering medical costs for those patients.

All interventional radiologic procedures must include two integral aspects. The first aspect is the interventional or medical side of the procedure in which the highly skilled radiologist uses needles, catheters, and special medical devices (e.g., occluding coils, guide wires) to produce an improvement in the process of the patient. The second aspect involves using fluoroscopy and radiography for guiding and documenting the progress of the steps taken during the first process. The radiographer, specially trained in the angiographic and interventional laboratory, has a very important role in assisting the angiographer in the interventional procedures.

In the succeeding pages, the interventional procedures more frequently performed are described. The selected bibliography at the end of this chapter provides a listing of resources containing more detailed information.

Circulatory system

Percutaneous Transluminal Angioplasty

Percutaneous transluminal angioplasty (PTA) is a therapeutic radiologic procedure designed to dilate or reopen stenotic or occluded areas within a vessel using a catheter introduced by the Seldinger technique. PTA was first described by Dotter and Judkins[1] in 1964 using a coaxial catheter method. The first step in this method is passing a wire guide through the narrowed area of a vessel. Then a smaller catheter is passed over the wire guide through the *stenosis* to begin the dilation process. Finally, a larger catheter is passed over the smaller catheter positioned through the stenosis to cause further dilation (Fig. 26-73). Although this method can achieve dilation of stenoses, it has the significant disadvantage of creating an arteriotomy as large as the dilating catheters.

In 1974 Gruntzig and Hopff[2] introduced the double-lumen balloon-tipped catheter. One lumen allows the passage of a wire guide and fluids through the catheter. The other lumen communicates with a balloon at the distal end of the catheter that, when inflated, expands to a size much larger than the catheter. These catheters are available in sizes ranging from 4.5 to 9 Fr. with attached balloons varying in length and expanding to diameters of 2 to 20 mm or more (Fig. 26-74).

Fig. 26-75 illustrates the process of balloon angioplasty. Of course, the stenosis is initially identified on a previously conducted angiogram. The balloon diameter used for a procedure is often the measured diameter of the normal artery adjacent to the stenosis. The angioplasty procedure is often conducted at the same time through the same catheterization site as the initial

[1]Dotter CT and Judkins MP: Transluminal treatment of arteriosclerotic obstruction: description of a new technique and preliminary report of its application, Circulation 30:654-670, 1964.

[2]Gruntzig A and Hopff H: Perkutane rekanalisation chronischer arterieller Verschlusse mit einem neuen dilatationskatheter; modifikation der Dotter-Technik, Deutsch Med Wochenschr 99:2502-2511, 1974.

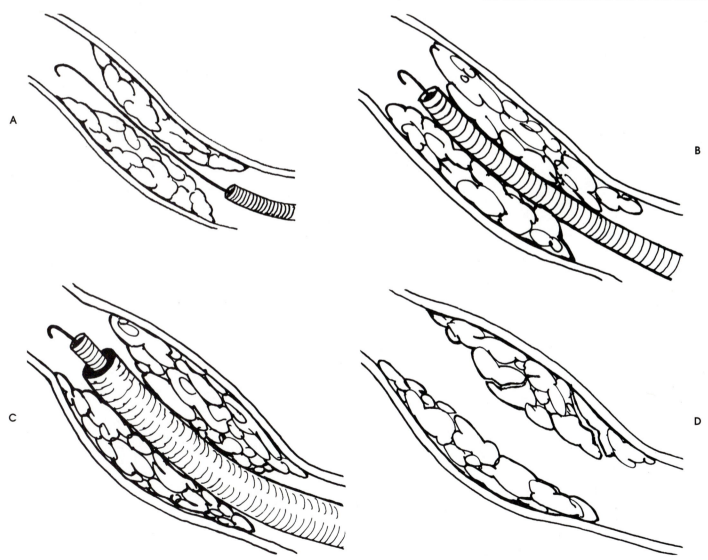

Fig. 26-73. Coaxial angioplasty of atherosclerotic stenosis. **A,** Wire guide advanced through stenosis. **B,** Small catheter advanced through stenosis. **C,** Large catheter advanced through stenosis. **D,** Postangioplasty stenotic area.

(Illustrated by Stephen G. Moon, M.S., and David R. Schumick, B.S.)

diagnostic examination. After the wire guide is positioned across the stenosis, the angiographic catheter is removed over the wire guide and the balloon-tipped catheter is introduced and directed by the wire guide through the stenosis. The balloon is usually inflated with a diluted contrast medium mixture for 15 to 45 seconds, depending on the degree of stenosis and the particular vessel being treated. The balloon is then deflated and repositioned or withdrawn from the lesion. Contrast medium can then be injected through the angioplasty catheter for a repeat angiogram. Success of the angioplasty procedure may be additionally determined by comparing transcatheter blood pressure measurements from a location distal and a location proximal to the lesion site. Nearly equal pressures indicate a reopened stenosis.

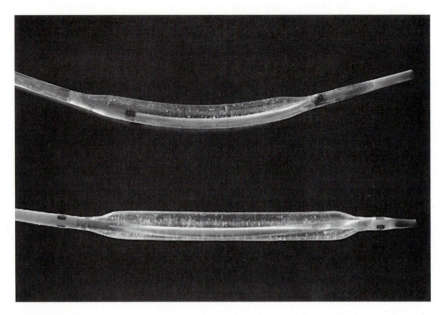

Fig. 26-74. Magnified view of balloon angioplasty catheter deflated *(above)* and inflated *(below)*.

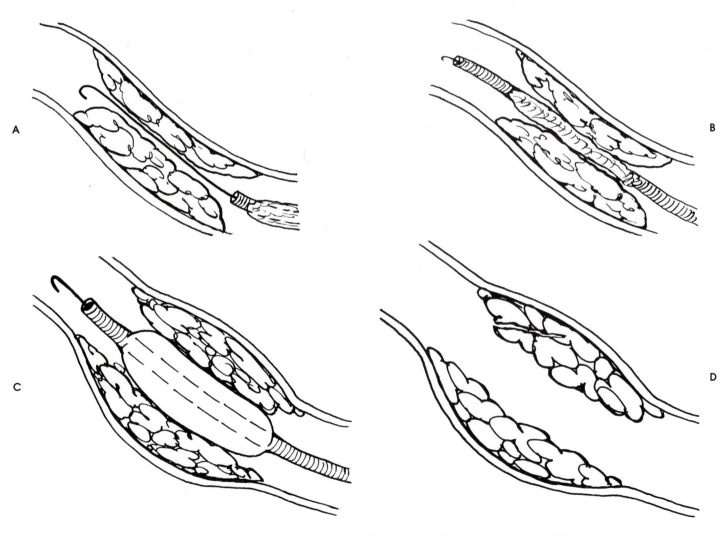

Fig. 26-75. Balloon angioplasty of atherosclerotic stenosis. **A,** Wire guide advanced through stenosis. **B,** Balloon across stenosis. **C,** Balloon inflated. **D,** Postangioplasty stenotic area.

(Illustrated by Stephen G. Moon, M.S., and David R. Schumick, B.S.)

Transluminal angioplasty can be performed in virtually any vessel that can be reached percutaneously with a catheter. It is most commonly performed in the renal, iliac, and femoral arteries, and the procedure is primarily used for therapy within an artery (Figs. 26-76 and 26-77). In 1978, however, Molnar and Stockum[1] described the use of balloon angioplasty for dilation of strictures within the biliary system (Fig. 26-78). Balloon angioplasty is also conducted in venous structures and in the ureteral and gastrointestinal tracts.

Balloon angioplasty has been used successfully to manage various diseases that cause arterial narrowing. The most common form of arterial stenosis treated by transluminal angioplasty is caused by atherosclerosis. Dotter and Judkins speculated that this atheromatous mass was soft and inelastic and therefore could be compressed against the artery wall. The success of coaxial and balloon method angioplasty was initially attributed to enlargement of the arterial lumen because of compression of the atherosclerotic plaque. Later research showed, however, that the plaque does not compress. If plaque surrounds the inner diameter of the artery, it cracks at its thinnest portion as the lumen

---

[1]Molnar W and Stockum AE: Transhepatic dilatation of choledochoenterostomy strictures, Radiology 129:59, 1978.

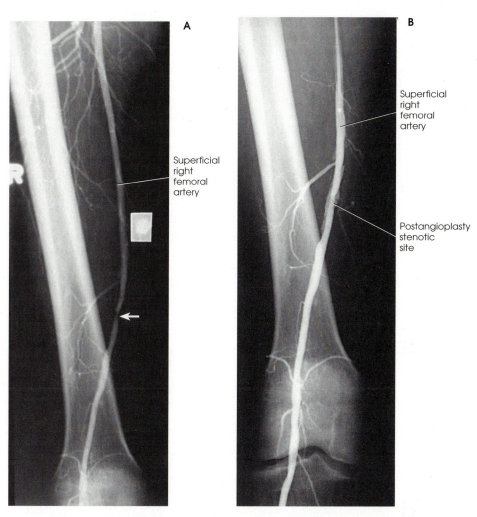

Superficial right femoral artery

Superficial right femoral artery

Postangioplasty stenotic site

Fig. 26-76. Femoral arteriogram: **A,** stenosis *(arrow)* and, **B,** postangioplasty femoral arteriogram.

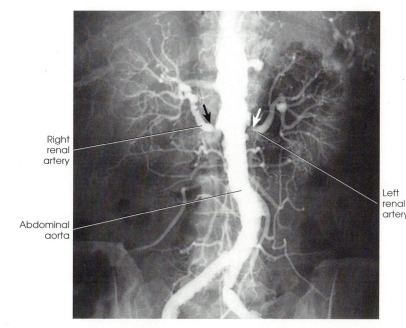
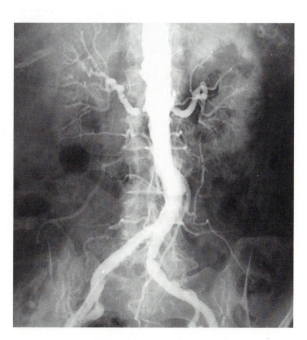

Right renal artery

Abdominal aorta

Left renal artery

Fig. 26-77. A, Renal flush angiogram showing bilateral renal artery stenosis *(arrows)* and **B,** angiogram showing improved postangioplasty left renal artery.

is expanded. Continued expansion cracks the arterial wall's inner layer, the intima, then stretches and tears the middle layer, the media, and finally stretches the outer layer, the adventitia. The arterial lumen is increased by permanently enlarging the artery's outer diameter. Restenosis, when it occurs, is usually caused by deposits of new plaque, not arterial wall collapse.

In addition to balloon angioplasty, other angioplasty technologies treat atherosclerotic disease. Some of these technologies involve the use of lasers. In laser-tipped angioplasty, laser energy is directed through a special catheter and pulsed at the atheromatous mass to vaporize it. It leaves a smooth, carbonized surface up to 5 mm in diameter, which is somewhat larger than the catheter tip. In thermal angioplasty a laser-heated probe is advanced through an atheroma to recanalize the vessel lumen. It also creates a smoother surface than balloon angioplasty, resulting in less restenosis at the lesion site. Sometimes, a balloon angioplasty procedure follows lumen recanalization to further expand the vessel lumen.

Percutaneous atherectomy is an angioplasty technology that removes an atheroma by cutting it. Atherectomy catheters are of two types, rotational and directional. A rotational catheter system has a blunt cam at the distal tip of the catheter that rotates at speeds up to 100,000 rpm. A fluid mixture is infused through the catheter as the cam rotates, creating a radial fluid spray. Together, the rotating cam and fluid spray cut and recirculate atherosclerotic material until it is micropulverized, while sparing normal tissue. A balloon angioplasty procedure frequently follows lumen restoration by this method. A directional atherectomy catheter system has, at its distal end, a cylindrically shaped chamber called the housing with an opening along one side called the housing window. Opposite the housing window is a balloon that, when inflated, presses the atheromatous mass into the window. A round, rotating cutter is then advanced through the housing to cut the atheroma, which is collected in the distal housing chamber. The balloon is then deflated, and the housing window is rotated 90 degrees in the vessel. The procedure is repeated until the atheroma has been removed circumferentially from the vessel lumen.

A final possibility for percutaneous treatment of vessel stenoses is the placement of vascular stents. A vascular stent is a wire or plastic cylinder that is introduced through a catheter system and positioned across a stenosis to keep the narrowed area spread apart. These devices permanently remain in the vessel (Fig. 26-79).

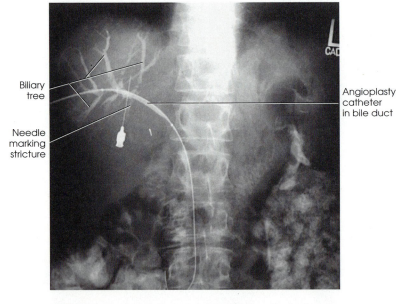

Biliary tree

Needle marking stricture

Angioplasty catheter in bile duct

Fig. 26-78. Radiograph showing balloon catheter in common bile duct.

The success of PTA in the management of atherosclerosis has made it a significant alternative to surgical procedures as a treatment for this disease. PTA is not indicated in all cases, however. Long segments of occlusion, for example, may be best treated by surgery. PTA has a lower risk than surgery but is not risk-free. Generally, patients must be able to tolerate the surgical procedure that may be required to repair vessel damage that could be caused by PTA. Unsuccessful attempts of transluminal angioplasty procedures rarely prevent, or complicate, any necessary subsequent surgery. In selected cases the procedure is effective and almost painless and can be repeated as often as necessary with no apparent increase in risk to the patient. The recovery time is often no longer than the time required to stabilize the arteriotomy site, usually a matter of hours, and general anesthesia is normally not required. Therefore the length of the hospital stay and the cost to the patient are reduced.

Although most PTA procedures occur in the radiology angiographic laboratory, angioplasty involving the arteries of the heart is generally performed in a more specialized laboratory. Percutaneous transluminal coronary angioplasty (PTCA) takes place in the cardiac catheterization laboratory because of the possibility of potentially serious cardiac complications. (See Chapter 31 for further information on PTCA.)

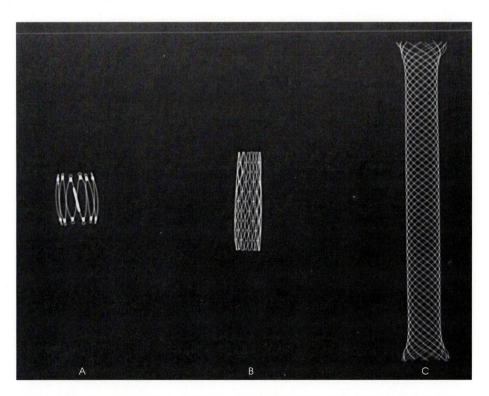

Fig. 26-79. Vascular stents. **A,** Gianturco-Rosch Biliary Z-stent; **B,** Palmaz; **C,** Wallstent.

Transcatheter Embolization

Transcatheter embolization was first discovered by Nusbaum and Baum[1] in 1963 when they found that active bleeding in various areas of the body could be demonstrated with angiography. *Extravasated blood*, when mixed with injected contrast media, appears as a collection of small "pools" at the bleeding site. They later discovered that this bleeding could be adequately managed through angiographic procedures.

Transcatheter embolization involves the therapeutic introduction of various substances to occlude or drastically reduce the blood flow within a vessel. The three main purposes for embolization are (1) to stop active bleeding sites, (2) to end blood flow to diseased or malformed areas (e.g., tumors or arteriovenous malformations), and (3) to stop or reduce blood flow to a particular area of the body before surgery.

Patient condition and the situation must be considered when choosing an embolizing agent. The radiologist in consultation with the attending physician will usually identify the appropriate agent to be used. Embolizing agents must be administered with care to ensure that they flow to the predetermined vessel. Once given, *they cannot be retrieved and their effects are irreversible*. Many types of embolizing agents exist, and their use depends on whether the occlusion is to be temporary or permanent. Table 26-1 lists some of the most widely used agents.

[1]Nusbaum M and Baum S: Radiographic demonstration of unknown sites of gastrointestinal bleeding, Surg Forum 14:374-375, 1963.

Table 26-1. Embolization agents

Permanent	Temporary
Ivalon (polyvinyl alcohol)	Gelfoam
Silicone beads	Microfibrillar collagen (Avitene)
Gianturco stainless steel coils	Vasoconstrictors (vasopressin, Pitressin)
Detachable balloons	

When the occlusion is to be temporary, for example, in gastrointestinal bleeding, occlusion need be sustained only until adequate *hemostasis* occurs. Gelfoam, which is a spongelike substance that can be formed into large or small *pledgets*, may be used and injected into the vessel. After each Gelfoam injection, however, contrast medium injections should follow to check the progress of the occlusion. After satisfactory embolization occurs, the Gelfoam will remain intact for a number of days.

Vasoconstricting drugs can be used to temporarily reduce blood flow. Although vasoconstrictors, such as vasopressin (Pitressin), do not function as emboli, they drastically constrict the vessels, which results in hemostasis.

When permanent occlusion is desired, as in trauma to the pelvis that causes hemorrhage or when vascular tumors are supplied by large vessels, the Gianturco stainless steel coil is most widely used for occlusion. This coil (Fig. 26-80) is simply a looped segment of guide wire with dacron fibers attached that functions to produce *thrombogenesis*. These coils are initially straight and are easily introduced into a catheter that has been placed into the desired vessel. The coil is then pushed out of the catheter tip with a wire guide. The coil assumes its looping shape immediately as it enters the bloodstream. It is important that the catheter tip be specifically placed in the vessel so the coil will "spring" into precisely the desired area. Numerous coils can be "stacked" as needed to occlude the vessel.

An indication for this type of embolization is shown in the arteriogram in Fig. 26-81 where a large vascular tumor is demonstrated in the upper and middle portions of the right kidney. A significant reduction of surgical bleeding was noted in a subsequent *nephrectomy* because of the embolization therapy (Fig. 26-82).

Transcatheter embolization has also been used in the cerebral vasculature of the brain. *Arteriovenous malformations* within the cerebral vasculature can be managed with the use of silicone beads or tissue adhesives. Very small catheters (2 or 3 Fr.) are passed through a larger catheter that is positioned in the internal carotid artery. The smaller catheter is then manipulated into the appropriate cerebral vessel and the embolic material injected through it until sufficient embolization occurs.

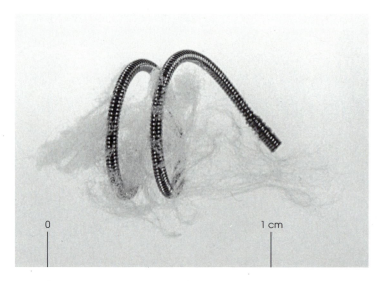

Fig. 26-80. Gianturco stainless steel occluding coil (magnified).

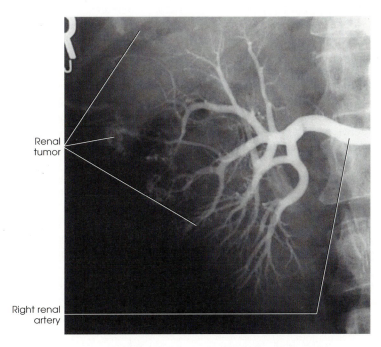

Renal
tumor

Right renal
artery

Fig. 26-81. Selective right renal arteriogram.

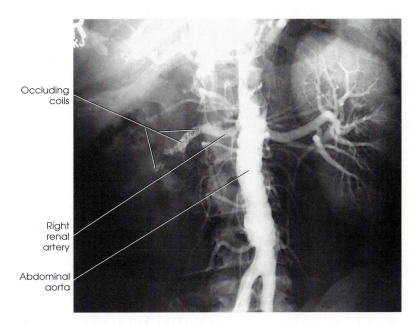

Occluding
coils

Right
renal
artery

Abdominal
aorta

Fig. 26-82. Postembolization renal flush angiogram on same patient as in Fig. 26-81.

Percutaneous Nephrostomy Tube Placement and Related Procedures

Nephrostomy tube drainage is indicated in the patient who has some type of ureteral or bladder blockage that causes *hydronephrosis*. If urine cannot be eliminated from the kidney, renal failure with necrosis to the kidney will occur.

A nephrostomy tube is a catheter that has multiple side holes at the distal end through which urine can enter. The urine will drain into a bag connected to the proximal end of the catheter outside the patient's body. These catheters range in size from 8 to 24 Fr. and are usually about 30 cm in length. Nephrostomy tubes are also placed in patients with kidney stones to facilitate subsequent passage of ultrasonic lithotripsy catheters through the tract from the flank to the renal pelvis created by the nephrostomy tube.

The renal pelvis must be opacified to provide a target for percutaneous nephrostomy tube placement. A percutaneous nephrostogram may be performed to accomplish this. For this procedure the patient is positioned prone or in an anterior oblique position on the tabletop. The patient's back and posterolateral aspect of the affected side are prepared and surgically draped. Following the administration of a local anesthetic, a 7-inch thin-wall cannula needle is passed through the back under fluoroscopic control and the cannula is removed. The needle is examined for drainage of urine. When urine returns through the needle, the needle is injected with contrast medium to opacify the renal pelvis.

A particular calyx of the opacified renal pelvis is often selected as the target for the nephrostomy tube placement. Following administration of a local anesthetic, a 7-inch cannula needle is inserted through the posterolateral aspect of the back and directed toward the renal pelvis. A fluoroscopic C arm offers a distinct advantage for this process. The C arm can be obliqued to match the angle between the needle insertion site and the target. The needle can then be advanced directly toward the target visualized on the fluoroscopic monitor. The C arm is then obliqued 90 degrees from this angle to see if the needle tip has reached the renal pelvis or calyx. When the needle tip has entered the desired target, a wire guide is passed through the needle into the renal pelvis and is then maneuvered into the proximal ureter for additional support. The needle is then removed, the tract dilated, and the drainage catheter is passed over the wire guide and into the renal pelvis. The pigtail end of the catheter must be placed well within the renal pelvis and not outside the kidney itself or in the proximal ureter (Figs. 26-83 and 26-84). The catheter's position is maintained by attaching it to a fixation disk or other device that is then sutured or taped to the body wall. A dressing is applied over the entry site. Either the fixation device or the dressing must prevent the catheter from becoming kinked, which would prevent drainage out through the catheter. Periodic antegrade nephrostograms may be performed by injecting the drainage catheter to evaluate anatomy and the functionality of the catheter.

Nephrostomy tubes may be placed for temporary or permanent external drainage of urine. Nephrostomy tubes that are left in place for a long time need to be exchanged periodically for new ones. A wire guide is inserted through the existing catheter, and the catheter is removed, leaving the wire guide in place. A new nephrostomy tube is then passed over the wire guide and positioned in the renal

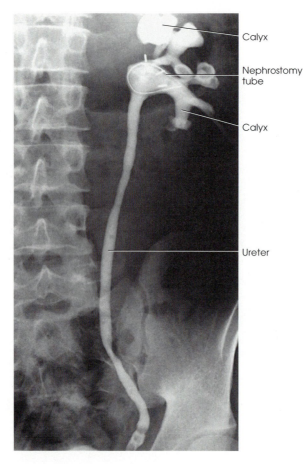

Fig. 26-83. Nephrostogram through Coop Loop drainage tube.

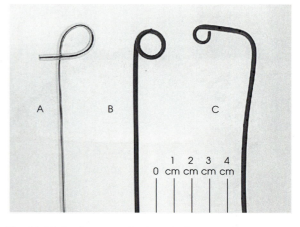

Fig. 26-84. Drainage catheters: **A,** Coop Loop nephrostomy catheter; **B,** Vance nephrostomy catheter; and, **C,** Ring biliary drainage catheter.

pelvis. Nephrostomy tubes can be permanently removed by simply pulling them out. The tract from the body wall to the renal pelvis usually closes in a day or so without complication.

In addition to nephrostomy tube placement, other *uroradiologic* procedures occur in the angiographic and interventional laboratory. *Percutaneous nephrolithotomy* offers the patient an alternative to surgical removal of kidney stones. Only stones that are relatively small can be removed by this method. Large stones may require surgery or ultrasonic lithotripsy for removal. The percutaneous nephrolithotomy procedure begins like a nephrostomy tube placement. After a wire is passed into the renal pelvis and ureter, a large tract is formed by using dilators or a balloon-tipped catheter. Then a sheath large enough to facilitate removal of the stone is placed between the renal pelvis and body wall. A stone basket or other retrieval catheter is introduced through the tract and manipulated to grasp the stone (Figs. 26-85 and 26-86). The stone is removed by withdrawing the retrieval catheter as it grasps the stone. The sheath is then also withdrawn, and a nephrostomy tube is placed in the renal pelvis to drain urine and any blood resulting from trauma from the procedure. The nephrostomy tube is eventually removed.

Angioplasty of stenoses in the ureteral system, renal cyst puncture with drainage, and percutaneous antegrade ureteral stent placement are additional procedures. A ureteral stent is a double-ended pigtail catheter that is passed into the ureter and remains inside the body, with one end placed into the renal pelvis and the other into the bladder (Fig. 26-87). This catheter is used when a constriction of the ureter or ureterovesicular junction is present, blocking the drainage of urine from the renal pelvis. The stent has multiple side holes at both pigtail ends that allow urine to drain into one end and exit the other end. The stent provides an internal passageway for urine across the area of blockage. Usually a nephrostomy tube is initially placed to provide access to the renal pelvis and to allow a tract to form in the body. At a later time a wire guide is passed through the nephrostomy tube and down the ureter into the bladder. The nephrostomy tube is removed and the stent is inserted over the wire guide using a catheter-like pusher. Usually a nephrostomy tube is replaced to provide external drainage until it is known that the stent is providing internal drainage. These stents can usually be removed through the urethra by a cystoscopic procedure.

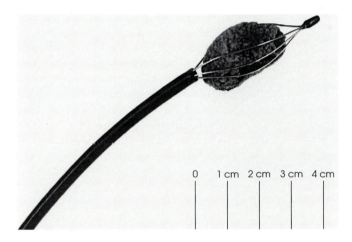

Fig. 26-85. Retrieval catheter and basket with large renal stone.

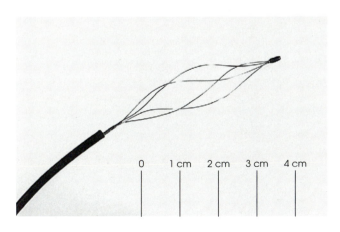

Fig. 26-86. Retrieval catheter with stone basket extended.

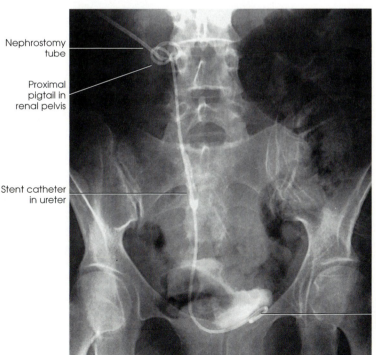

Nephrostomy tube

Proximal pigtail in renal pelvis

Stent catheter in ureter

Distal pigtail in bladder

Fig. 26-87. Postplacement radiograph of ureteral stent.

Inferior Vena Caval Filter Placement

As discussed earlier in this chapter, pulmonary angiography primarily evaluates embolic disease of the lungs. A pulmonary embolus is usually a blood clot, but it does not form in the lungs. Instead, it commonly forms as a *thrombus*, usually in the deep veins of the leg (Fig. 26-88). When such a thrombus becomes dislodged and migrates, it is called an *embolus*. An embolus originating in the leg may migrate through the inferior vena cava and right side of the heart and finally lodge in the pulmonary arteries. A filter can be percutaneously placed in the inferior vena cava to trap such an embolus.

The idea of interrupting the pathway of an embolus is not a new one. Surgical interruption of the common femoral vein was first described in 1784, and surgical interruption of the inferior vena cava was described in 1868. These procedures and the partial surgical interruption procedures that evolved from them had a high rate of complication, not only from the surgical process but also from inadequate venous drainage from the lower limbs. Catheterization technology led to the development of detachable balloons for occluding the inferior vena cava, but that procedure also resulted in complications from inadequate venous flow from the lower limbs. The first true filter designed to trap emboli while maintaining vena caval *patency* was introduced in 1967 by Mobin-Uddin. It consisted of six metal struts joined at one end to form a conical shape which was then covered by a perforated plastic canopy. The plastic canopy proved to be too occlusive, however, and the Mobin-Uddin filter is no longer in use. Because of its striking resemblance to an open umbrella, vena caval filters of all types were for many years referred to as "umbrella filters."

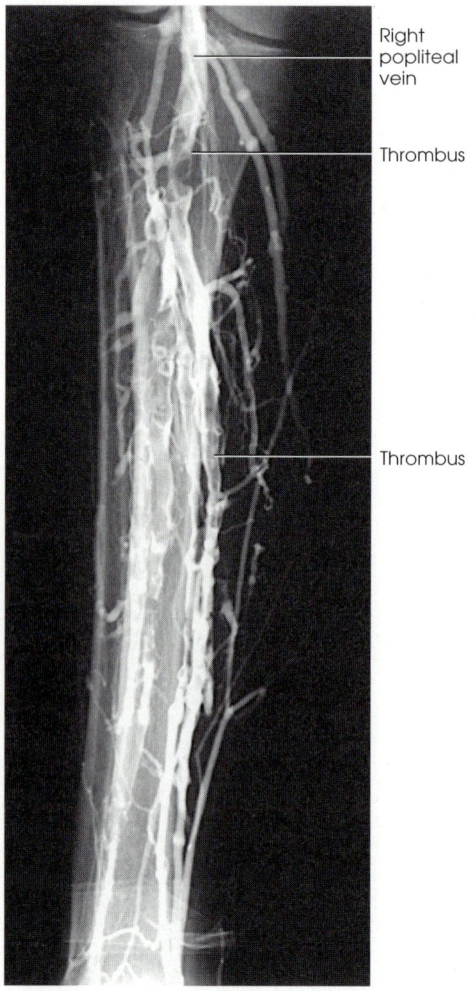

Right popliteal vein

Thrombus

Thrombus

Fig. 26-88. Lower limb venogram.

Lower limb vein thrombosis is not necessarily an indication for inferior vena caval filter placement. Normally, blood-thinning medications are administered to treat deep vein thrombosis. When such anticoagulant therapy is contraindicated because of hemorrhaging or the risk of hemorrhaging, filter placement may be indicated. The filter placement itself has associated risks. They include thrombosis of the vein through which the filter is introduced and caval thrombosis, but these risks are normally not life-threatening after the placement of a filter. It is important to note that inferior vena caval filter placement is not a treatment for deep venous thrombosis of the leg but a therapy intended to reduce the chance of pulmonary embolism.

Inferior vena caval filters are available in a variety of forms. All of these filters are initially compact inside an introducer catheter device and assume their functional shape as they are released (Fig. 26-89). The introducers are passed through sheaths ranging in size from 9 to 29 Fr.

The filters are made of inert metals and most are designed for permanent placement. The Kimray-Greenfield filter is composed of six wire struts joined at the apex to form a conical shape. Each strut has a hook on its end that engages the wall of the vena cava. The Titanium Greenfield filter is a modification of the Kimray-Greenfield which is introduced through a smaller venotomy. The Vena Tech filter also consists of six metal struts forming a cone, but each strut ends with a side rail that is parallel to the wall of the vena cava. The side rails have barbs to hold the filter in place. The Gianturco-Roehm Bird's Nest filter consists of a bundle of fine wire anchored on each end by a V-shaped hook wire strut. The Simon Nitinol filter is composed of wire that has thermal memory. This allows the device, which is very compact in its introducer, to achieve a completely different shape when placed in the body temperature environment of the vena cava. Inferiorly it has six wire struts forming a cone, and superiorly it has seven overlapping loops of wire for additional clot-trapping capability. Some filters are designed for temporary placement. They have a hook on the bottom that allows them to be grasped by a catheter snare device and removed percutaneously. Another temporary filter remains attached to its introducer catheter, which is used to retrieve it. Some temporary filters must be removed within approximately 10 days or they will become permanently attached to the vena cava endothelium. Other filter designs are in use in other countries. Inferior vena caval filter development continues, and new designs will certainly become available.

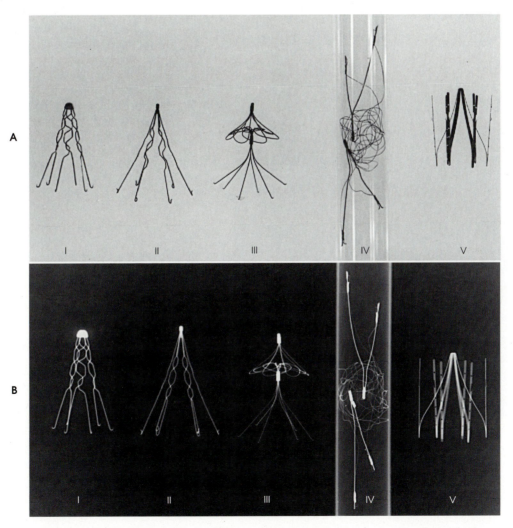

Fig. 26-89. Vena cava filters. **I,** Kimray-Greenfield; **II,** Titanium Greenfield; **III,** Simon Nitinol; **IV,** Gianturco-Roehm Bird's Nest; **V,** Vena Tech. **A,** Photographic, and **B,** radiographic images.

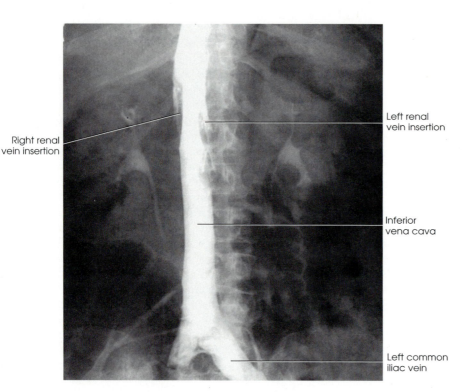

Right renal
vein insertion

Left renal
vein insertion

Inferior
vena cava

Left common
iliac vein

Fig. 26-90. Inferior vena cavogram.

The filters are percutaneously inserted through a femoral, jugular, or antecubital vein, usually for placement in the inferior vena cava just inferior to the renal veins. Placement inferior to the renal veins is important to avoid risking renal vein thrombosis, which could result if the vena cava is occluded superior to the level of the renal veins by a large thrombus in a filter. An inferior vena cavogram is performed using the Seldinger technique, usually from the right femoral vein approach because it provides the straightest course into the inferior vena cava. The inferior vena cavogram defines the anatomy including the level of the renal veins, determines the diameter of the vena cava, and rules out the presence of a thrombus (Fig. 26-90). A filter insertion from the jugular or antecubital approach may be indicated if a thrombus is present in the inferior vena cava. The diameter of the vena cava may influence the choice of filter, because each filter has a maximum diameter. The filter insertion site is dilated to accommodate the filter introducer. The filter remains sheathed until it reaches the desired level and is released from its introducer by the angiographer. The introducing system is then removed and external compression is applied to the venotomy site until hemorrhage ceases. A post-placement plain radiograph is obtained to document the location of the filter (Fig. 26-91).

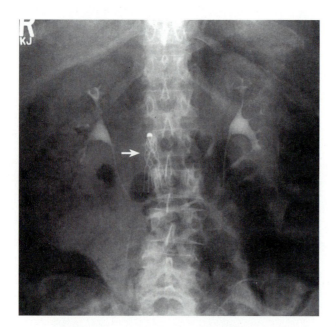

Fig. 26-91. Postplacement radiograph showing filter in place *(arrow)*.

Transjugular Intrahepatic Portosystemic Shunt

The portal circulation drains blood from the digestive organs to the liver. The blood passes through the liver tissue and is returned to the inferior vena cava via the hepatic veins. Disease processes can increase the resistance of blood flow through the liver. This elevates the portal circulation's blood pressure—a condition known as portal hypertension—and causes blood to flow instead through *collateral* veins to return to the systemic circulation. The *varices* that eventually result can be life-threatening if they bleed. The creation of a portosystemic shunt can decrease portal hypertension and the associated risk of variceal bleeding by allowing the portal venous circulation to bypass its normal course through the liver tissue. The percutaneous intervention for creating an artificial low pressure pathway between the portal and hepatic veins is called a transjugular intrahepatic portosystemic shunt (TIPS).

Portography and hepatic venography are usually performed prior to a TIPS procedure to delineate anatomy and confirm *patency* of these vessels. Ultrasound may be used for this purpose. Transcatheter blood pressure measurements may also be obtained to confirm the existence of a pressure gradient between the portal and hepatic veins. An intravascular marker placed in the portal vein through a needle guided by CT may act as a target during the TIPS procedure.

To accommodate all of the catheter and needle manipulations during the TIPS procedure, a long sheath is passed from a right internal jugular venous puncture site to the middle or right hepatic vein. An hepatic venogram may be performed at this time. A special long needle is passed into the hepatic vein and advanced through the liver tissue into the portal vein. The needle is exchanged for a balloon-tipped angioplasty catheter, and the tract through the liver tissue is dilated. An angiographic catheter may be passed through the tract and advanced into the splenic vein for a splenoportal venogram. An intravascular stent is positioned across the tract to maintain its patency (Fig. 26-92). The tract and stent may be further enlarged with balloon-tipped catheters until the desired reduction in pressure gradient between the portal and hepatic veins is achieved. The sheath is then removed from the internal jugular vein and external pressure is applied until hemostasis at the venotomy occurs.

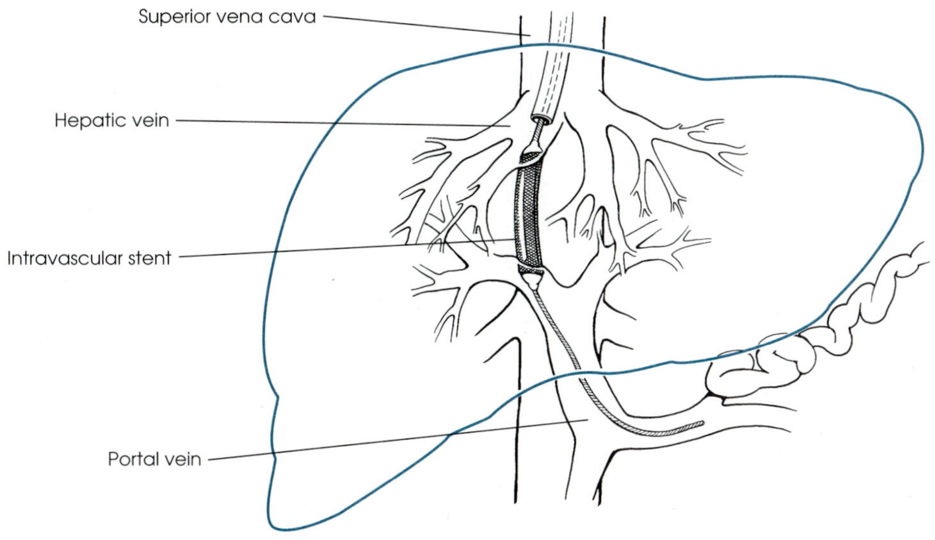

Other Procedures

When an arteriogram demonstrates thrombosis, the procedure may be continued for thrombolytic therapy. Blood clot–dissolving medications can be infused through an angiographic catheter positioned against the thrombus. Special infusion catheters that have side holes may be manipulated directly into the clot. Periodic repeat arteriograms evaluate the progress of lysis (dissolution). The catheter may need to be advanced under fluoroscopic control to keep it against or in the clot as lysis progresses.

Catheters can also be used to percutaneously remove foreign bodies, such as catheter fragments, from vasculature. A variety of snares are available for this purpose. The snare catheter is introduced using the Seldinger technique and manipulated under fluoroscopic control to grasp the foreign body. Then the snare and foreign body are withdrawn as a unit.

Interventional radiologic procedures are also performed in the biliary system and include biliary drainage and biliary stone removal. For more information, see the section on the biliary tract in Chapter 16, Volume 2 of this atlas.

Interventional Radiology: Present and Future

Interventional procedures bring therapeutic capabilities into the hands of the radiologist. Procedures that are done initially for diagnosis can be extended, using the same basic techniques, to perform therapeutic processes. New equipment is continually becoming available to improve techniques and broaden the scope of percutaneous intervention. Although use of the catheter for angiographic diagnosis may wane, its ability to provide therapy percutaneously ensures a future for angiography.

Fig. 26-92. Intravascular stent placement in a TIPS procedure.

Lymphography is a general term applied to radiologic examinations of the lymph vessels and nodes (Figs. 26-93 and 26-94) after they have been opacified by an injected iodinated contrast medium. The study of the lymph vessels, which may be called *lymphangiography,* is carried out within the first hour after injection of the contrast material. The study of the lymph nodes, which may be called *lymphadenography,* is made 24 hours after injection of the contrast medium. The lymph vessels empty the contrast agent within a few hours. The nodes normally retain the contrast substance for 3 to 4 weeks. Abnormal nodes may retain the medium for several months, so that delayed lymphadenograms may be made, as indicated, without further injection.

PURPOSE

The primary indication for lymphography is to assess the clinical extent of lymphomas. Lymphography may also be indicated in patients in whom there is clinical evidence of obstruction or other impairment of the lymphatic system.

CONTRAST MEDIA

Lymphography is currently performed with the use of an iodinated oil contrast medium and by the direct-injection technique developed by Kinmonth, Harper, and Taylor.[1] A water-soluble, iodinated contrast medium may be used to delineate the lymphatic vessels and nodes of the limbs, but these agents are miscible with lymph and undergo dilution, and they diffuse out through the lymphatic walls so rapidly that they cannot be used to study the proximal lymphatics.

The oily contrast medium currently employed is ethiodized oil (Ethiodol). This agent affords opacification of the lymphatic vessels for several hours after the injection. The lymph nodes are outlined on the studies of the vessels, but their internal structure does not become optimally opacified until about 24 hours later.

[1]Kinmonth JB, Harper RAK, and Taylor GW: Lymphangiography by radiologic methods, J Fac Radiologists 6:217-223, 1955.

DYE SUBSTANCE

Ordinarily the peripheral lymphatic vessels cannot be easily identified because of their small size and lack of color. For identification of the lymphatic vessels on the dorsum of the feet and hands, a blue dye that is selectively absorbed by the lymphatics is injected subcutaneously into the first and second interdigital web spaces about 15 minutes before the examination. The dyes frequently used for this purpose are 11% patent blue violet and 4% sky blue.

Following patent blue violet injection, the patient's urine and skin will be tinted blue. This condition disappears within a few hours.

PRECAUTIONS

As in any procedure involving injection of foreign materials, untoward reactions must be anticipated. The patient must be observed closely, and appropriate medications and resuscitation equipment must be nearby.

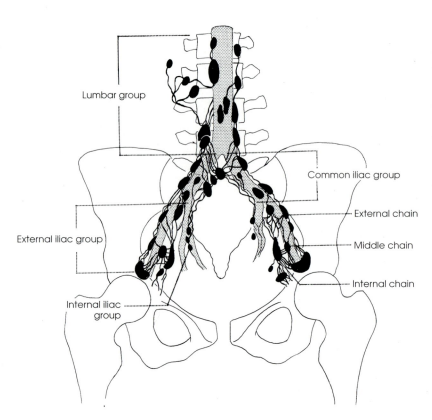

Fig. 26-93. Iliopelvic-aortic lymphatic system (after Cuneo and Marcille). Anterior projection.

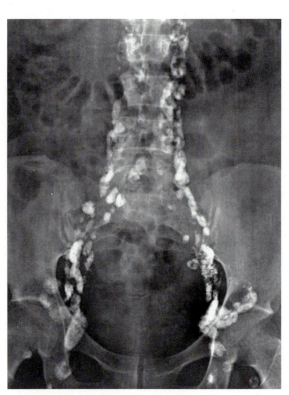

Fig. 26-94. AP projection of iliopelvic-abdominoaortic lymph nodes.

INJECTION SITES

Lymphography is limited to easily accessible injection sites—the lymphatics of the feet and of the hands. Most examinations are performed by injection of the lymphatics of the feet. This injection route provides visualization of the lymphatic structures of the lower limb, the groin, the iliopelvic-abdominoaortic region, and the thoracic duct. Injection of the lymphatics of the hands provides visualization of the upper limb and of the axillary, infraclavicular, and supraclavicular regions.

FILMING PROCEDURE

Radiographs are made within the first hour after completion of the injection for the demonstration of the lymph vessels (Fig. 26-95). A second series of radiographs, which may include tomographic studies, is made 24 hours later to demonstrate the lymph nodes.

The exposure factors employed for lymphographic studies are the same as those used for bone studies of the respective region.

Tomography and magnification radiography are other techniques sometimes required to obtain better delineation of the opacified lymph nodes.

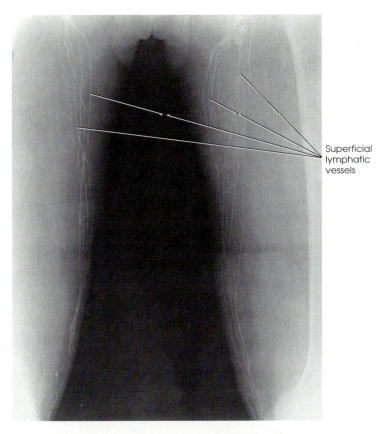

Superficial lymphatic vessels

Fig. 26-95. Superficial lymphatics of thigh taken 10 minutes after completion of dorsal pedal lymphatic injection.

Lymphatic Injection of Feet

Preceding the examination, the following steps are observed:

- Thoroughly wash the patient's feet.
- Shave the areas about the sites of injection and incision.
- Place the patient in the supine position for the injection procedure and keep the patient in that position until the lymphangiographic studies have been completed. The injection need not be made in a radiographic examining room; it may be carried out in an operating room, and the patient may be on a padded stretcher, ready for conveyance to the radiology department.
- Surgically cleanse and drape both feet.

The blue dye is injected subcutaneously into the first and second interdigital web spaces of each foot to stain the lymph for identification of the lymphatic vessels. The dye may be mixed with a local anesthetic to minimize the pain of the injections.

About 15 minutes after the injection of the blue dye, a local anesthetic (1% lidocaine) is injected subcutaneously in an amount sufficient to distend the tissues overlying the body of the first metatarsal, which is the site of cutdown for exposure and cannulation of the lymphatic vessel. A small (2 cm) longitudinal incision is made over the body of the first metatarsal immediately lateral to the extensor tendon of the great toe. (Some physicians advocate a transverse incision at this site.) The dye-filled lymphatic vessel is seen as a fine blue vessel in the subcutaneous tissue. The vessel is dissected free of surrounding tissue and is then cannulated with a 27- or 30-gauge needle connected to polyethylene tubing. The needle is tied securely in the vessel, and the tubing is connected to the syringe containing the contrast medium. An automatic injection device is used. A total of 6 ml of the contrast medium is slowly injected into each lower limb over a period of 30 minutes.

Confirmation that the injection is intralymphatic and not intravenous may be determined fluoroscopically or radiographically. After completion of the injection, the needle is removed, the overlying skin incision closed with interrupted silk sutures, and a dressing applied. The lymphatic vessel is not ligated or disturbed in any way. The patient, still in the supine position, is prepared for filming (Fig. 26-96).

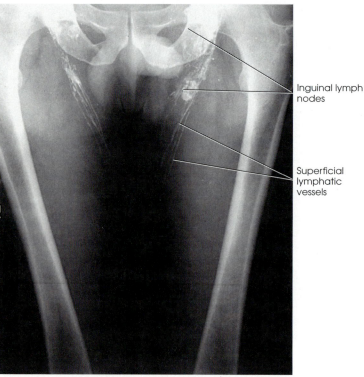

Inguinal lymph nodes

Superficial lymphatic vessels

Fig. 26-96. Lymphangiogram. Delayed radiograph of same patient as in Fig. 26-95. Superficial lymphatic vessels of thigh are opacified, and contrast medium is in superficial inguinal lymph node group.

ILIOPELVIC-ABDOMINOAORTIC REGION

- Take three radiographs, AP and 30-degree right and left AP oblique images, for each of the two iliopelvic-abdominoaortic studies. The lymphangiograms are taken within the first hour after injection of the contrast medium (Figs. 26-97 and 26-98). These radiographs show the contrast medium within the lymph vessels that run concurrently with the femoral and iliac arteries, veins, and nerves, as well as the lymph vessels in the paraspinal areas. After the contrast medium has concentrated in the lymph nodes 24 hours later, lymphadenograms are taken (Fig. 26-99).
- Record all radiographs on 14 × 17 inch (35 × 43 cm) films positioned to include the lower border of the ischium.
- Direct the central ray vertically and centered at the level of the crests of the ilia.

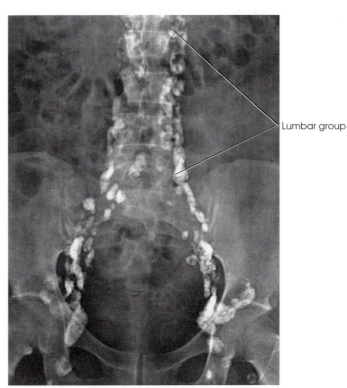

Lumbar group

Fig. 26-97. Normal AP lymphangiogram.

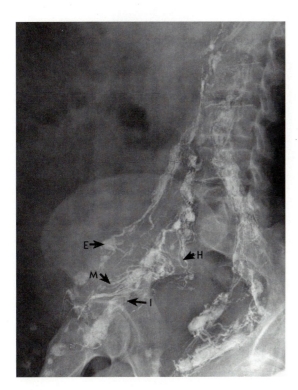

Fig. 26-98. Lymphangiogram of iliopelvic-aortic region. Right AP oblique position showing external chain, *E,* middle chain, *M,* and internal chain, *I,* of external and common iliac groups. *H,* Internal iliac group.

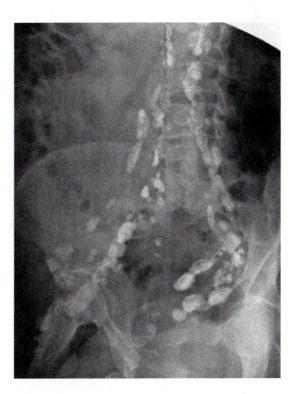

Fig. 26-99. Lymphadenogram 24 hours later of same patient as in Figs. 26-97 and 26-98.

THORACIC DUCT

- Obtain two radiographs, AP and left lateral projections, for each of two serial studies of the thoracic duct. The contrast medium remains in the thoracic duct for less than an hour after completion of the injection; thus the studies must be timed accordingly (Fig. 26-100).

- Make the exposures on 14 × 17 inch (35 × 43 cm) films that are adjusted to place the upper margin of the film 2 inches (5 cm) above the supraclavicular region.

- Direct the central ray perpendicularly to the midpoint of the film.

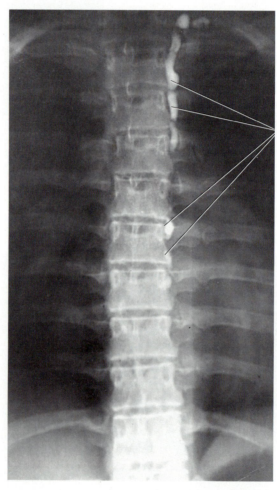

Thoracic duct

Fig. 26-100. AP projection showing opacification of superior portion of thoracic duct. Segmented appearance is caused by valves in lymph vessels.

LOWER LIMB

- Take three AP projections, centered respectively at the level of the midtibias, the level of the midfemora, and for the groin at the level of the symphysis pubis, for the demonstration of the lymphatic vessels. Radiographs are taken for the demonstration of the lymph nodes of the lower limbs 24 hours later.
- Make the exposures on 14 × 17 inch (35 × 43 cm) films.
- Direct the central ray vertically (Figs. 26-101 and 26-102).

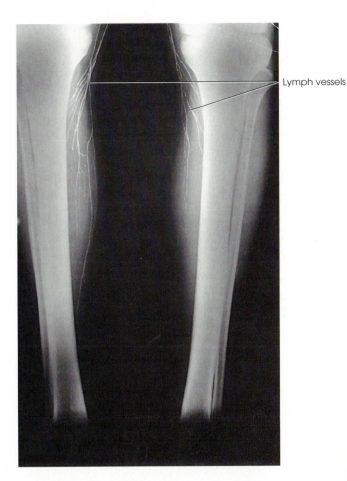

Lymph vessels

Fig. 26-101. Lymphangiogram of legs 10 minutes after injection.

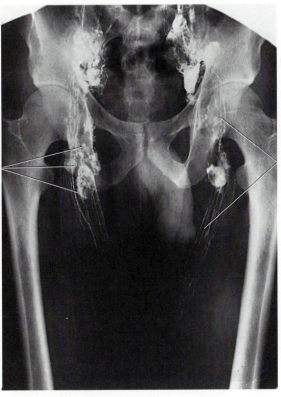

Inguinal lymph nodes

Lymph vessels

Fig. 26-102. Lymphangiogram of inguinal region and upper thighs.

Lymphography

579

Lymphatic Injection of Hands

The general procedure for lymphatic injection of the hands is the same as for the feet. Blue dye is injected into the dorsal surface of the first and second interdigital web spaces. A longitudinal skin incision is made on the dorsum of the hand, parallel to and on the ulnar side of the tendon of the musculus extensor pollicis longus over the base of the first or second metacarpal. A 30-gauge needle is used for cannulation. Four milliliters of the contrast medium is injected. This quantity is sufficient to visualize the lymphatics of the upper limb and the lymph nodes of the axilla.

UPPER LIMB

- Take AP and lateral projections on 14 × 17 inch (35 × 43 cm) films for the lymphangiograms and the later lymphadenograms of the arm and forearm.
- Place the films diagonally to include the greatest length of the limb.
- Direct the central ray vertical and center it to the elbow (Fig. 26-103).

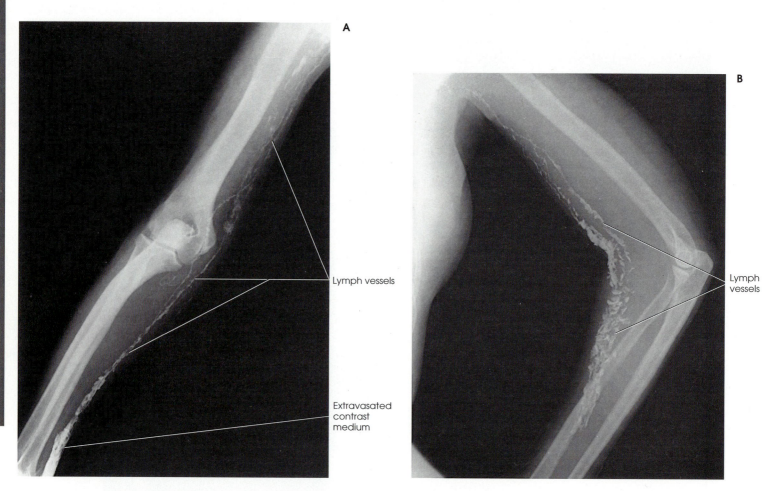

Lymph vessels

Extravasated contrast medium

Lymph vessels

Fig. 26-103. Lymphangiograms. **A,** AP and **B,** lateral of upper limb, showing fluting of vessels and extravasation of contrast medium.

AXILLA

- Take AP and 45-degree AP oblique projections for each series of studies of the axilla.
- Perform these studies on 11 × 14 inch (30 × 35 cm) films that are adjusted to include the supraclavicular region.
- Direct the central ray vertical and center it to the region of the coracoid process (Fig. 26-104).

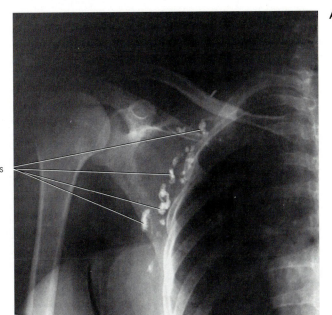

A

Axillary lymph nodes

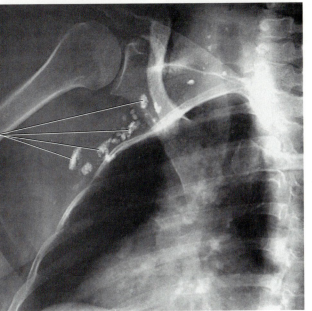

B

Axillary lymph nodes

Fig. 26-104. Lymphadenograms. **A,** AP and, **B,** oblique axilla.

DONALD L. SUCHER*

Photographic subtraction, introduced by Ziedses des Plantes,[1] is a technique by which bone structure images are subtracted, or canceled out, from a film of the bones plus opacified vessels, leaving an unobscured image of the vessels. The technique can be applied in all forms of angiography, wherever the vessels are superimposed in bone structures.

With the increasing popularity of digital subtraction angiography (see Chapter 35), the use of photographic subtraction has decreased in many institutions. However, photographic subtraction remains relatively widely used and, in some cases, is increasing in popularity. One such area of increasing frequency occurs in evaluation of joint replacements (see discussion of contrast arthrography, Chapter 12, Volume 1, of this atlas).

[1]Ziedses des Plantes BG: Subtraktion: eine roentgenographische Methode zur separaten Abbildung bestimmter Teile des Objekts, Fortschr Roentgenstr 52:69-79, 1935.
*Visual Presentation Specialist, Department of Radiology, Children's Hospital, 300 Longwood Avenue Boston, MA 02114.

The purpose of subtraction in angiography and other specialized procedures is to fully define all vessels containing contrast material and at the same time eliminate the confusing overlying bone images. Following are a few terms that pertain to the subtraction technique:

registration Matching of one image over another so that bony landmarks are precisely superimposed. When so arranged, films are taped together to prevent slippage. Composites discussed herein may involve two or more films.

reversal film (also called a **positive mask** or **diapositive**) Reverse-tone duplicate of radiographic image, showing black changed to white and white to black. This positive transparency is obtained by exposing single-emulsion film through traditional radiographic film.

zero, or base, film (also called the **control film**) This film must show bone structures only, and there must be no patient motion whatever between it and subsequent contrast studies. For these reasons, zero film is exposed just before contrast medium is injected into vessels.

EQUIPMENT AND MATERIALS

Items needed for subtraction include the following:

1. A contact printer similar to the one illustrated in Fig. 26-105. Several units are available that can also be used to duplicate radiographs.
2. Radiographic processing facilities.
3. A horizontally oriented illuminator for registration of images.
4. Films:
   a. Subtraction mask film for making the reversal masks.
   b. Subtraction print film for making photographic prints of the final subtracted image.

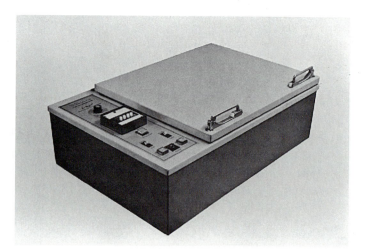

Fig. 26-105. Contact printer such as that used during exposure steps in producing subtraction prints.

Circulatory system

First-Order Subtraction

The simplest method of photographic subtraction is called first-order subtraction (Fig. 26-106) and consists of obtaining a positive mask, or reversal, of the first film (zero film) of the angiographic series (the one that does not contain contrast material). When the reversal mask is superimposed over a film in the series that contains contrast material, the positive and negative images of the bones tend to cancel each other out, and only the vessels can be seen. The vessels are not canceled out because they were present on only one film—the one containing the contrast material. A contact printer makes a print of this combination of films.

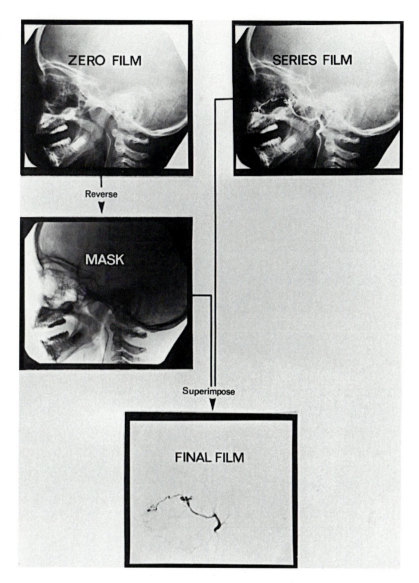

Fig. 26-106. First-order subtraction process.

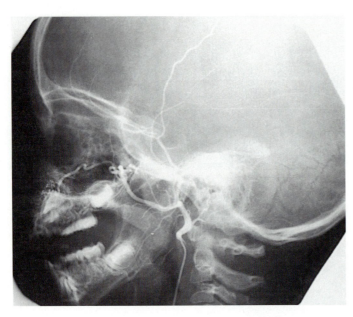

Fig. 26-107. Angiographic series radiograph.

FIRST-ORDER SUBTRACTION PROCEDURE

- In a darkroom, place the nonemulsion side of the sheet of subtraction mask film in contact with the zero film and expose it for approximately 5 seconds* to light. When processed, this becomes the mask.

On a light box, carefully register the mask over the selected series film (Fig. 26-107), and tape the two securely together.

In the darkroom, place the mask-series film combination in contact with the emulsion side of a sheet of subtraction print film, which is then exposed for approximately 5 seconds* to light. This produces the final subtraction image (Fig. 26-108).

---

*Time will vary according to equipment and material used.

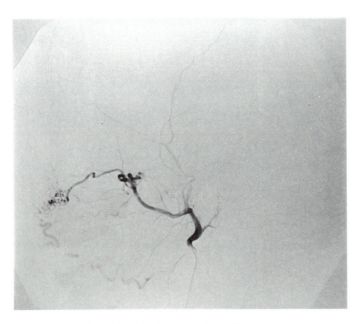

Fig. 26-108. First-order subtraction print.

Second-Order Subtraction

The reversal of the zero film obtained in the first-order subtraction is usually not the exact reversal of the density of the selected angiographic film; thus the subtraction result is imperfect. The imperfection can be corrected with what is called second-order subtraction. This process involves producing another film, called a secondary or correction mask, which compensates for the slight differences. Hanafee and Shinno[1] led the way toward this improved subtraction method. Their method of second-order subtraction consists of superimposing the zero film on its own reversal mask. The additional print that results from the transmission of light through the two films, which in theory would be the exact opposite of each other, produces a faint radiographic image that corrects for the small "photographic mistake" between the first two. The reversal of the zero film, the correction film, and the film containing contrast material are carefully registered; this combination is then exposed to obtain the final subtraction print.

A further advancement toward the goal of complete subtraction was published by Sucher and Strand[2] in 1974. This second-order subtraction modification is called composite-mask subtraction or white-over-white technique. When correctly applied, this technique approaches almost total elimination of both bony structure and soft tissue, leaving a display of the vessels in high-contrast reproduction (Fig. 26-109).

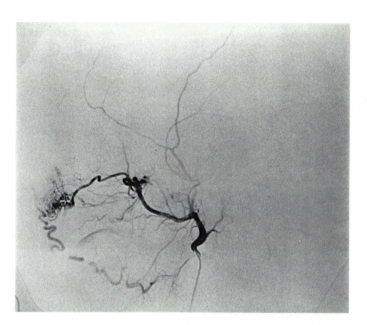

Fig. 26-109. Composite-mask, white-over-white technique. Bone has been completely removed, allowing improved visualization of vessels.

[1]Hanafee W and Shinno JM: Second-order subtraction with simultaneous bilateral carotid, internal carotid injections, Radiology 86:334-341, 1966.
[2]Sucher DL and Strand RD: Composite mask subtraction, white over white technique, Radiology 113:470-472, 1974.

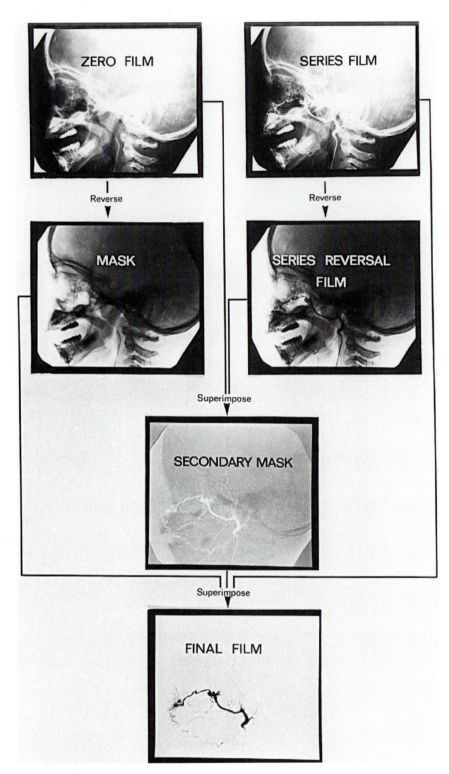

Fig. 26-110. Composite-mask subtraction process.

COMPOSITE-MASK SUBTRACTION PROCEDURE

The following steps are illustrated in Fig. 26-110.

- In a darkroom, place the nonemulsion side of a sheet of subtraction mask film in contact with the zero film and expose it for approximately 5 seconds* to light. When processed this becomes the mask.
- In a darkroom, place the emulsion side of a sheet of subtraction mask film in contact with the selected angiographic series film, which is then exposed to light. This process produces the series reversal film.
- On a light box, carefully register the series reversal film with the zero film, and tape the two securely together.
- In a darkroom, place the zero–series reversal film combination in contact with the emulsion side of a sheet of subtraction mask film and expose it for approximately 20 seconds* to light. This process produces the secondary mask.
- On a light box, carefully register the series film and the mask, and tape the two securely together. To this composite carefully register and tape the secondary mask.
- In a darkroom, place the series film—mask—secondary mask combination in contact with the emulsion side of a sheet of subtraction print film and expose it for approximately 35 seconds* to light. The final subtraction image is thus produced.

*Time will vary according to equipment and material used.

A comparison of second-order subtraction with composite-mask subtraction shows the steps to be almost identical. The only procedural difference is that in second-order subtraction the secondary mask is made by registering the zero film and the zero reversal mask. In composite-mask subtraction, the zero film and the angiographic series reversal film are superimposed to produce the secondary mask. Although the procedures are similar, the composite-mask subtraction technique is recommended when increased resolution is required.

In recent years marked advancement has been made by the production of films specifically designed for subtraction. In addition to the advantage of 90-second processing, these films often allow subtractions of adequate or even excellent quality to be made with the single-order subtraction technique. Composite-mask subtraction is recommended only when small structures require increased definition for visualization or when illustrations of high quality are needed for publications.

Definition of Terms

anastomose Join.

aneurysm A sac formed by local enlargement of a weakened artery wall.

angiography The radiographic study of vessels.

anomaly A variation from the normal pattern.

aortic dissection Tear in the inner lining of the aortic wall that allows blood to enter and track along the muscular coat.

arteriography The radiologic examination of arteries after the injection of a radiopaque contrast medium.

arteriovenous malformation An abnormal anastomosis or communication between an artery and a vein.

atherosclerosis Condition in which fibrous and fatty deposits on the luminal wall of an artery may cause obstruction of the vessel.

bifurcation The place where a structure divides into two branches.

biplane Two x-ray exposure planes 90 degrees from another; usually frontal and lateral.

cinefluorography Same as cineradiography; the making of a motion picture record of successive images on a fluoroscopic screen.

claudication Cramping of the leg muscles after physical exertion because of a chronically inadequate blood supply.

collateral Secondary or accessory.

embolus Foreign material, often thrombus, that detaches and moves freely in the bloodstream.

extravasation The escape of fluid from a vessel into the surrounding tissue.

film changer Device that transports films into and out of the exposure field for serial imaging.

hematoma A local swelling filled with effused blood.

hemostasis Stopping of blood flow or hemorrhage.

hydronephrosis Distention of the pelvis and calices of the kidney with urine caused by ureteral obstruction.

iatrogenic Caused by a therapeutic or diagnostic procedure.

lesion An injury or other damaging change to an organ or tissue.

lymphadenography Radiographic study of the lymph nodes.

lymphangiography Radiographic study of the lymph vessels.

lymphography Radiographic evaluation of the lymphatic channels and lymph nodes.

meninges The three membranes that envelop the brain and spinal cord.

nephrectomy Surgical removal of the kidney.

nephrostomy Surgical opening into the kidney's collecting system.

nonocclusive Being not completely closed or shut; allowing blood flow.

patency The state of being open or unobstructed.

percutaneous Effected or introduced through the skin.

percutaneous nephrolithotomy A uroradiologic procedure performed to extract stones from within the kidney or proximal ureter.

percutaneous transluminal angioplasty Surgical correction of a vessel from within the vessel using catheter technology.

pledget A small piece of material used as a dressing or plug.

stenosis Constriction or narrowing of a passage or an orifice.

thrombogenesis The formation of a blood clot.

thrombosis Formation or existence of a blood clot.

thrombus A blood clot obstructing a blood vessel or cavity of the heart.

uroradiology The radiologic and interventional study of the urinary tract.

varices Irregularly swollen veins.

venography The radiologic study of veins after the injection of radiopaque contrast medium.

SELECTED BIBLIOGRAPHY

Abrams HL: Abrams angiography: vascular and interventional radiology, ed 3, Boston, 1983, Little, Brown & Co.

Abrams HL: Angiography, ed 3, Boston, 1983, Little, Brown & Co.Athanasoulis CA et al: Interventional radiology, Philadelphia, 1982, WB Saunders.

Abramson AF and Mitty HA: Update on interventional treatment of urinary obstruction, Urol Radiol 14:234-236, 1992.

Bierman HR et al: Intra-arterial catheterization of viscera in man, Am J Roentgenol Radium Ther Nucl Med 66:555-568, 1951.

Bull JWD: History of neuroradiology, the presidential address delivered at the British Institute of Radiology, Oct 20, 1960, Br J Radiol 34:69-84, 1961.

Chase NE and Kricheff II: Cerebral angiography in the evaluation of patients with cerebrovascular disease, Radiol Clin North Am 4:131-144, 1966.

Chopp M et al: Clinical dosimetry during cerebral arteriography, Neuroradiology 20(2):79-81, 1980.

Clouse ME and Wallace S: Lymphatic imaging—lymphography, computed tomography and scintigraphy, ed 2, Baltimore, 1985, Williams & Wilkins.

Cromwell LD, Kerber CW, and Vermeere WR: A wedge filter for craniocervical angiography, AJR 129(6):1125-1127, 1977.

Doi K et al: X-ray imaging of blood vessels to the brain by use of magnification stereoscopic technique, Adv Neurol 30:175-189, 1981.

Dotter CT and Judkins MP: Transluminal treatment of arteriosclerotic obstruction: description of a new technique and preliminary report of its application, Circulation 30:654-70, 1964.

Dreesen RG and Becker GJ: Effects of streptokinase in thrombolytic therapy: a radiology research project, Radiol Technol 58:211-214, 1987.

Ferrucci JT et al: Interventional radiology of the abdomen, ed 2, Baltimore, 1985, Williams & Wilkins.

Fisher HW: Viscosity, solubility, and toxicity in the choice of an angiographic contrast medium, Angiography 16:759-766, 1965.

Fitz CR and Harwood-Nash DC: Neonatal radiology; special procedure techniques in infants, Radiol Clin North Am 13:(2):181-198, 1975.

Fu WR: Angiography of trauma, Springfield, Ill, 1972, Charles C Thomas, Publisher.

Greitz T: A radiologic study of the brain circulation by rapid serial angiography of the carotid artery, Acta Radiol, suppl 140, 1956.

Gruntzig A and Hopff H: Perkutane rekanalisation chronischer arterieller Verschlusse mit einem neuen dilatationskatheter; modifikation der Dotter-Technik, Deutsch Med Wochenschr 99:2502-2511, 1974.

Hacker H: Detail angiography—direct x-ray enlargement in serial angiography, Electromedica 38:346-349, 1970.

Hinck VC and Dotter CT: Appraisal of current techniques for cerebral angiography, Am J Roentgenol Radium Ther Nucl Med 107:626-630, 1969.

Hoppe JO and Archer S: X-ray contrast media for cardiovascular angiography, Angiology 11:244-254, 1960.

Johnsrude IS et al: A practical approach to angiography, ed 2, Boston, 1987, Little, Brown & Co.

Judkins MP et al: Lumen following safety J-guide for catheterization of tortuous vessels, Radiology 88:1127-1130, 1967.

Kadir S: Diagnostic angiography, Philadelphia, 1986, WB Saunders.

Katzen BT: Interventional diagnostic and therapeutic procedures, New York, 1980, Springer-Verlag New York.

Kerber C et al: Selective cerebral angiography through the axillary artery, Neuroradiology 10(3):131-135, 1975.

Lammer J and Karnel F: Percutaneous transluminal laser angioplasty with contact probes, Radiology 168(3):733-737, 1988.

Lang EK: Transcatheter embolization of pelvic vessels for control of intractable hemorrhage, Radiology 140:331-339, 1981.

Langes EK et al: Catheter atherectomy: functional results in peripheral arterial disease, Angiology 40(9):830-834, 1989.

Lin JP: Techniques of cerebral angiography, Radiol Clin North Am 12(2):223-240, 1974.

Mani RL: A new double-curve catheter for selective femoro-cerebral angiography, Radiology 94:607-611, 1980.

Mani RL and Gross RC: Keyhole cone device for lateral magnification cerebral angiography, Am J Radiol 129(1):165-166, 1977.

Miller K: Advantages of a low-osmolality ionic contrast medium in intra-arterial applications, Radiol Technol 59:43-48, 1987.

Mills CS and Van Aman ME: Modified technique for percutaneous transfemoral pulmonary angiography, Cardiovasc Interven Radiol 9:52-53, 1986.

Molnar W and Stockum AE: Transhepatic dilatation of choledochoenterostomy strictures, Radiology 129:59, 1978.

Morris JL and Wylie I: Cerebral angiotomography, Radiology 120(1):105-109, 1976.

Newman GE et al: Peripheral artery atherectomy: description of technique and report of initial results, Radiology 169(3):677-680, 1988.

Newton TH: The axillary artery approach to arteriography of the aorta and its branches, Am J Roentgenol Radium Ther Nucl Med 89:275-283, 1963.

Newton TH and Potts DG: Radiology of the skull and brain—angiography, vol 2, book 1, Great Neck, 1986, Medibooks.

Numaguchi Y, Hoffman JC Jr, and Sones PJ Jr: Femoral percutaneous catheterization in infants and small children for cerebral angiography, Radiology 116(2):451, 1975.

Osborn AG: Introduction to cerebral angiography, New York, 1980, Harper & Row, Publishers.

Pais SO: Diagnostic and therapeutic angiography in the trauma patient, Semin Roentgenol 27:211-232, 1992.

Rakofsky M: Quantified analysis of a carotid angiogram, Neuroradiology 20(2):53-71, 1980.

Ramsey RG: Neuroradiology, ed 2, Philadelphia, 1987, WB Saunders.

Reuter SR et al: Gastrointestinal angiography, ed 3, Philadelphia, 1986, WB Saunders.

Ring EJ and McLean GK: Interventional radiology: principals and techniques, Boston, 1981, Little, Brown & Co.

Roehm JOF et al: The bird's nest inferior vena cava filter: progress report, Radiology 168:745-749, 1988.

Rose BS, Simon DC, Hess ML, and Van Aman ME: Percutaneous transfemoral placement of the Kimray-Greenfield vena cava filter, Radiology 165:373-376, 1987.

Seldinger SI: Catheter replacement of the needle in percutaneous arteriography, Acta Radiol 39:368-376, 1953.

Shimizu H, Sato O, and Kobayashi M: A new method of autotomography with cerebral angiography (angioautotomography), Neuroradiology 9(4):203-208, 1975.

Smith DC and Tidwell J: Adjustable sliding aluminum wedge filter: device for angiographic enhancement, Radiol Technol 49(4):459-471, 1978.

Smith GA et al: Experimental evaluation of cerebral angiography, J Neurosurg 8:556-563, 1951.

Smith GR and Loop JW: A simple method of femorocerebral catheterization, Radiology 118(3):733-734, 1976.

Snopek AM: Fundamentals of special radiographic procedures, Philadelphia, 1984, WB Saunders.

Staton R: Lymphography, Radiol Technol 55:233-238, 1984.

Takahashi M: Magnification factor, position, and true size of an object in stereoscopic magnification radiography, Radiology 142(1):215-217, 1982.

Takahashi M and Ozawa Y: Stereoscopic magnification angiography using a twin focal-spot x-ray tube, Radiology 142(3):791-792, 1982.

Takahashi M et al: Serial cerebral angiography in stereoscopic magnification, AJR 126(6):1211-1216, 1976.

Thorn A and Voight K: Rotational cerebral angiography: procedure and value, Am J Neuroradiol 4(3):289-291, 1983.

Tortorici MR: Fundamentals of angiography, St Louis, 1982, Mosby.

Von Sonnenberg E and Mueller PR: Practical interventional radiology, Philadelphia, 1989, WB Saunders.

Whitley JE and Whitley NO: Angiography: techniques and procedures, St Louis, 1971, Warren H Green.

Wilkens RA and Viamonte M, editors: Interventional radiology, Boston, 1982, Blackwell Scientific Publications.

Wood EH, Taveras JM, and Tenner MS: The brain and eye—an atlas of tumor radiology, St Louis, 1975, Mosby.

Anatomic terms used are based on *Nomina Anatomica* wherever possible; otherwise terms employed are those usually referred to in anatomic texts. From Bean BC: A chart of the intracerebral circulation, ed 2, Med Radiogr Photogr 34:25, 1958; courtesy Dr Berton C Bean and Eastman Kodak Co.

Chapter 27

SECTIONAL ANATOMY FOR RADIOGRAPHERS

TERRI BRUCKNER

Cranial region
Thoracic region
Abdominopelvic region

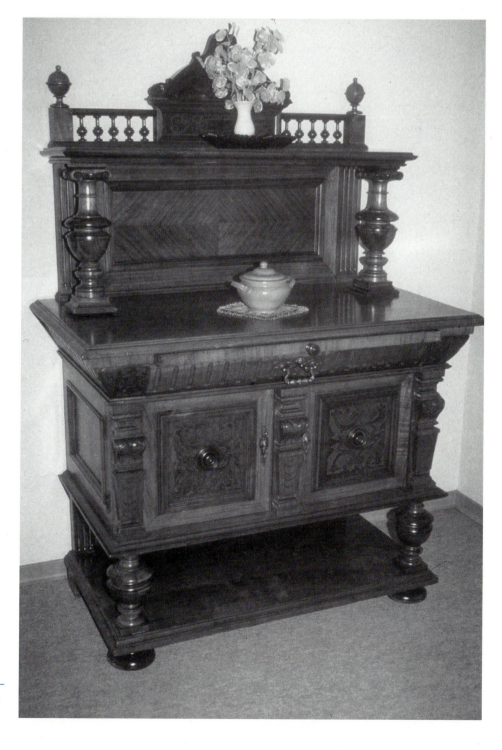

A buffet on display in the birthplace of Dr. Roentgen.

An understanding of the relationships between organ and skeletal structures is essential for the identification and localization of specific anatomic structures when using computed imaging modalities. The trend in the development of new imaging methods is toward sectional reconstruction, whether using x-ray, magnetic resonance, or diagnostic medical sonography. The purpose of this chapter is to provide the radiographer who possesses a background in general anatomy with an orientation to sectional anatomy and to correlate such with structures demonstrated on images from the various imaging modalities.

The cadaver sections were selected as being representative of major organ structures for each of the body regions and are *depicted from the inferior surface*. The major anatomic structures normally seen when using current imaging modalities have been labeled. For each cadaver section presented, representative images have been included to provide an orientation to anatomic structures normally seen using the available imaging modalities. It must be understood that the cadaver sections and diagnostic images will not match exactly; therefore, some structures will be seen on only one of the illustrations for each body region.

When axial images are viewed, it is useful to imagine that one is standing at the patient's feet and looking toward the head. With this orientation, the patient's right side will be to the viewer's left and vice versa. The anterior aspect of the patient is usually at the top of the image, and the posterior is at the bottom. All relational terms in the following discussion refer to the body in normal anatomic position.

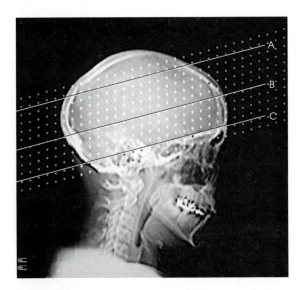

Fig. 27-1. CT localizer or scout image of skull.

Cranial Region

The computed tomography (CT) localizer, or scout, image (Fig. 27-1) represents a lateral image of the cranium. CT imaging for the cranium may be performed with the gantry parallel to or angled 15 to 20 degrees to the orbitomeatal line (OML). Magnetic resonance (MR) imaging of the cranium generally results in images parallel to the orbitomeatal or infra-orbitomeatal plane. For further details on patient positioning, see the chapters describing computed tomography (Chapter 33) and magnetic resonance imaging (Chapter 36). Because the imaging planes may be different for the cadaver sections and the CT and MR images, some variation will exist in the anatomical structures visualized on corresponding illustrations in this section.

Three identifying lines represent the approximate levels for each of the labeled cadaver sections and images for this region. The cranial cadaver section seen in Fig. 27-2 is sectioned through the frontal and parietal bones. The cortex, or outer layer of gray matter, is clearly differentiated from the deeper white matter (myelinated fibers). The numerous gyri (convolutions) and sulci (fissures) are demonstrated. The cerebral hemispheres are separated by the longitudinal fissure. Invaginated in this fissure is a fold of dura mater, the falx cerebri. The superior sagittal sinus is a venous drainage system that runs through the superior margin of the falx and is closely related to the contour of the superior skull margin. In cross section, the anterior and posterior aspects of this sinus can be seen in the midline deep to the bony plates. Two of the five cerebral lobes are seen (frontal and parietal). The division between these lobes is the central sulcus. The corona radiata is a tract of white matter that connects all parts of the cerebral hemisphere to the internal capsule.

The corresponding CT image demonstrates the structures discussed above (Fig. 27-3). The superior sagittal sinus appears white because of the introduction of contrast medium.

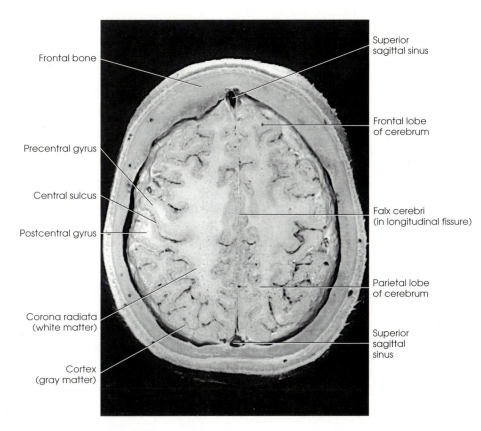

Fig. 27-2. Cadaver section corresponding to level A in Fig. 27-1.

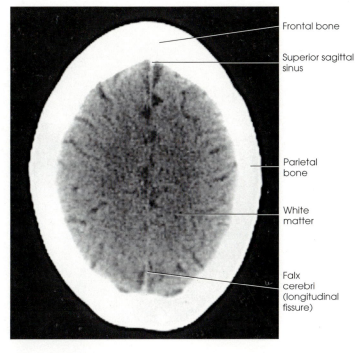

Fig. 27-3. Computed tomography (CT) image representing the anatomic structures located at level A in Fig. 27-1.

(Courtesy Theresa Spotts, R.T.)

591

The axial section through the midcranial region demonstrates the primary structures of the cerebral hemispheres (Fig. 27-4). The falx cerebri is shown within the longitudinal fissure with the superior sagittal sinus in the anterior and posterior margins. The hemispheres are joined by a tract of white (myelinated) fibers known as the corpus callosum. The anterior portion of the corpus callosum is the genu, and the posterior portion is the splenium. In this section, the frontal, temporal, and occipital lobes are visualized along with the insula (fifth lobe or island of Reil), which is deep to the temporal lobe at the lateral sulcus (lateral fissure of Sylvius). At this level, the anterior and posterior horns (cornu) of the lateral ventricles are seen. The membranous layer between the anterior horns is the septum pellucidum. Within each posterior horn is the choroid plexus, a capillary network for the formation of cerebrospinal fluid. Deep to the cortex, much of the cerebrum is composed of tracts of white matter. Several areas of gray matter are found deep within the white matter. These areas of gray matter relay and coordinate informa-tion and are known collectively as the basal nuclei (ganglia) or cerebral nuclei. The major components of the basal nuclei (ganglia) are the caudate nucleus, the claustrum, the lentiform nucleus (composed of the putamen and the globus pallidus), and the amygdaloid body. The lentiform nucleus is separated from the caudate nucleus and the thalamus by a tract of white matter known as the internal capsule. The caudate nucleus is located lateral to each anterior horn of the lateral ventricles. The midline third ventricle is visualized at this level. The thalamus, which serves as a central relay station for sensory impulses to the cerebral cortex, is located surrounding the third ventricle. Between the third ventricle and the splenium of the corpus callosum is the pineal body. This is an important anatomic landmark because of its tendency to calcify in adults. Branches of the anterior cerebral arteries are found in the longitudinal fissure, just anterior to the genu of the corpus callosum. Branches of the middle cerebral arteries are found in the lateral fissures.

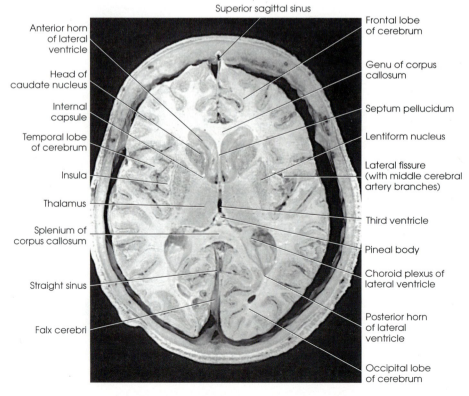

Fig. 27-4. Cadaver section corresponding to level B in Fig. 27-1.

Fig. 27-5 is an MR image that corresponds to the cadaver section discussed previously. In this T1-weighted image, bone cortex appears black because of a lack of signal return. The high content of fat in the marrow cavity will appear white on these images. Cerebrospinal fluid within the ventricles appears dark. Note the differentiation between gray and white matter structures.

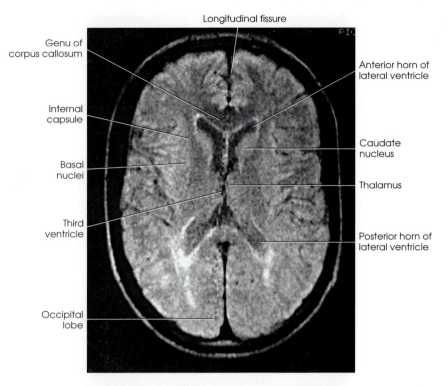

Fig. 27-5. Magnetic resonance (MR) image representing the structures located at level B in Fig. 27-1.

(Courtesy Picker International.)

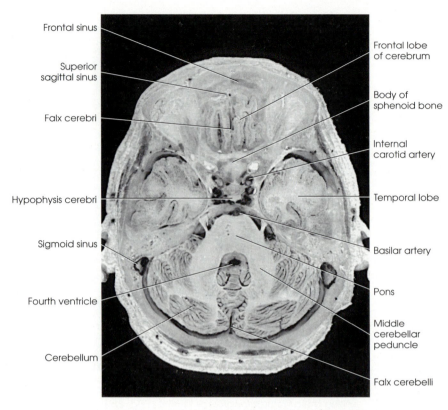

Frontal sinus

Superior
sagittal sinus

Falx cerebri

Hypophysis cerebri

Sigmoid sinus

Fourth ventricle

Cerebellum

Frontal lobe
of cerebrum

Body of
sphenoid bone

Internal
carotid artery

Temporal lobe

Basilar artery

Pons

Middle
cerebellar
peduncle

Falx cerebelli

Fig. 27-6. Cadaver section corresponding to level C in Fig. 27-1.

The cross section through the base of the cranium demonstrates the inferior portions of the cerebrum, the brainstem, the cerebellum, and the associated major skeletal structures (Fig. 27-6). The frontal sinuses and the inferiormost portions of the frontal lobes are seen in the anterior skull, along with the supraorbital fat. The temporal lobes are found in the middle cranial fossa between the lesser wings of the sphenoid bone and the pars petrosa of the temporal bone. The hypophysis cerebri (pituitary gland) is located in the hypophyseal fossa of the sella turcica, formed by the body of the sphenoid bone. The internal carotid arteries lie lateral to the sella turcica between the anterior clinoid processes and the hypophysis cerebri (pituitary gland). Posterior to the sphenoid bone is the pons, a portion of the brain that relays impulses between the medulla oblongata and the cerebrum. Extending laterally and dorsally from the pons are the middle cerebellar peduncles, which transmit impulses between the pons and the cerebellum. The basilar artery lies in the midline directly anterior to the pons. The major portion of the posterior fossa is occupied by the cerebellum.

The cerebellum functions as a reflex center for coordinating skeletal muscle movements. The cerebellum is divided into two hemispheres that are joined by the midline vermis. A fold of dura mater, the falx cerebelli, is found between the cerebellar hemispheres. The fourth ventricle is seen between the pons and the cerebellum. Posterior to the cerebellum, the transverse dural venous sinuses pass laterally in the margin of the tentorium cerebelli. As the transverse sinuses reach the pars petrosae, they change direction and are now called the sigmoid sinuses. The sigmoid sinuses ultimately exit the cranium via the jugular foramina, at which point they are known as the internal jugular veins.

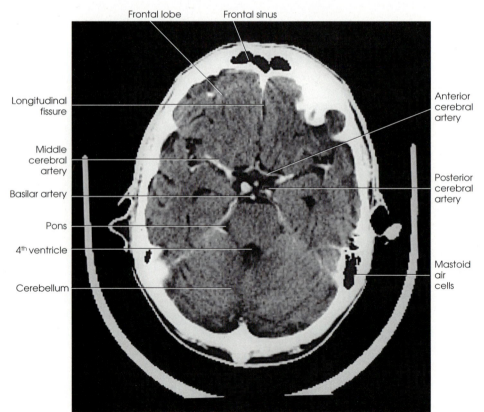

Frontal lobe   Frontal sinus

Longitudinal
fissure

Middle
cerebral
artery

Basilar artery

Pons

4th ventricle

Cerebellum

Anterior
cerebral
artery

Posterior
cerebral
artery

Mastoid
air
cells

Fig. 27-7. CT image representing the anatomic structures located at level C in Fig. 27-1.

Fig. 27-7 is a CT scan through the region of the circulus arteriosus (circle of Willis), the pons, and the cerebellum. Contrast medium makes the vascular structures visible on this image. The circulus arteriosus encircles the optic chiasm and the stalk of the hypophysis cerebri (pituitary gland). It is the anastomosis of the anterior and posterior blood supply to the brain. The main vessels that comprise the circulus arteriosus are the anterior cerebral arteries, the anterior communicating arteries, the posterior cerebral arteries, and the posterior communicating arteries. The anterior and middle cerebral arteries are branches of the internal carotid artery; the posterior cerebral arteries are branches of the basilar artery, which is seen in the CT image directly anterior to the pons.

Fig. 27-8 is an MR image through the orbits and posterior fossa. (Note the difference in orientation to the orbitomeatal plane between this MR image and the preceding cadaver and CT images.) The optic nerves can be seen extending posteriorly from the eyeballs toward the optic chiasm. The ethmoidal air cells and sphenoidal sinuses are both visualized at this level. Posterior and lateral to the sphenoidal sinuses are the internal carotid arteries in the carotid canal. Posterior to the sphenoidal sinuses is the clivus, the junction of the dorsum sellae and the basilar portion of the occipital bone. Associated with the posterior clivus are the basilar artery and the pons. The black areas of signal void lateral to the pons are the dense bony pars petrosae. The tragi and auricles of the ears are seen lateral to the petrous regions.

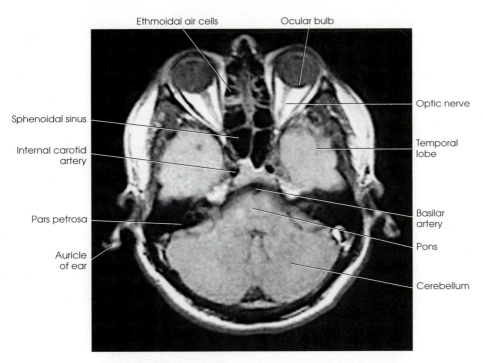

Fig. 27-8. MR image representing the anatomic structures located at level C in Fig. 27-1.

(Courtesy Picker International.)

The cadaver section in Fig. 27-9 is through the third cervical vertebra. At this level the hyoid bone (which serves as an attachment for the muscles of the tongue) is visualized. The submandibular (salivary) gland is found lateral to the hyoid at this level. Immediately posterior to the submandibular glands are the internal and external carotid arteries. These arteries are enclosed in the carotid sheath along with the internal jugular vein and vagus nerve. The vertebral arteries can be seen in the neck within the transverse foramina of the cervical vertebrae. The sternocleidomastoid muscles, which attach to the mastoid processes and the sternum and clavicle, are visualized lateral to the internal jugular veins.

Anterior to the vertebra is the laryngeal portion of the pharynx. The epiglottic cartilage is in the anterior pharynx.

Fig. 27-10 is a CT image through the hyoid bone. This image is slightly inferior to the cadaver section and demonstrates the symphysis of the mandible anterior to the hyoid (with the suprahyoid muscles between). Deep to the hyoid bone is the epiglottic cartilage. The internal jugular vein and common carotid arteries are well visualized because of contrast media enhancement for this particular scan.

The next cadaver section and CT image correspond to the body of the sixth cervical vertebra (Figs. 27-11 and 27-12). The thyroid cartilage (Adam's apple) is seen surrounding the larynx and vocal cords. The cricoid cartilage is seen posterior to the vocal cords, and the terminal laryngopharynx is posterior to the cricoid cartilage. The thyroid gland has an H-shaped configuration with two lateral lobes connected by a horizontal portion (isthmus). The lobes of the thyroid gland are found on the posterolateral aspects of the thyroid cartilage (and in lower sections lateral to the trachea) and appear highlighted on CT scans because of normal iodine content. At this level the common carotid artery, internal jugular vein, and vagus nerve are on each side of the pharynx enclosed within the carotid sheath. The vagus nerve is not seen on these images. The vertebral arteries are noted again within the transverse foramina of C6. The sternocleidomastoid muscles lie anterior to the internal jugular veins and lateral to the thyroid cartilage at this level. The large posterior muscle masses lateral to the vertebral column are the trapezius muscles.

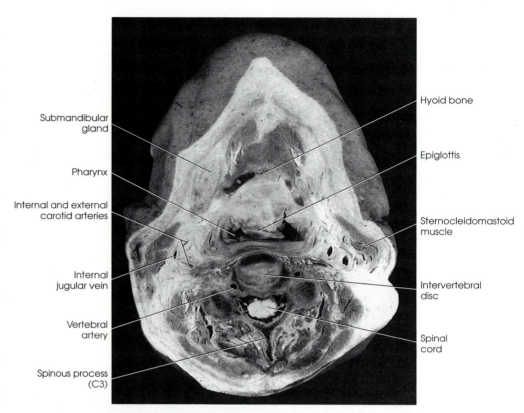

Fig. 27-9. Axial cadaver section through the third cervical vertebra.

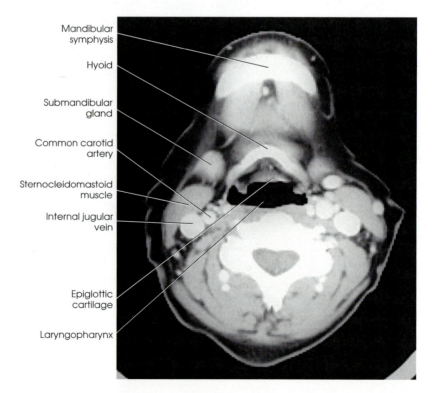

Fig. 27-10. CT image through the fourth cervical vertebra corresponding to Fig. 27-9.

(Courtesy Lyn VanDervort, R.T.)

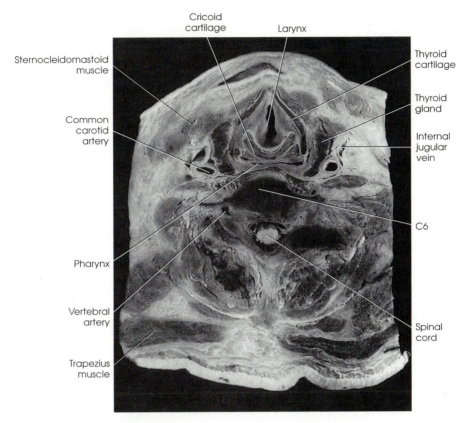

Fig. 27-11. Cadaver section through the sixth cervical vertebra.

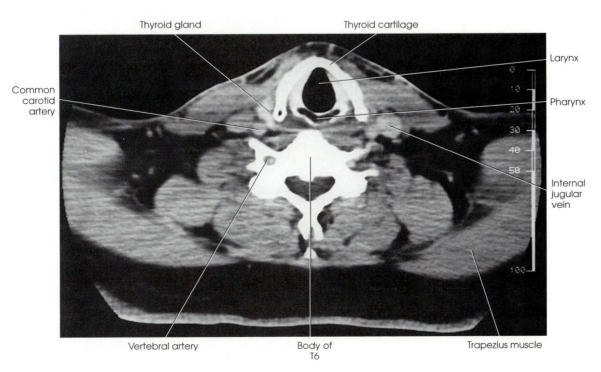

Fig. 27-12. CT image through the sixth cervical vertebra corresponding to Fig. 27-11.

(Courtesy Angelique Jacopin, R.T.)

It is increasingly common to find images in sagittal, coronal, and oblique planes. CT scanners have the capability to image in the axial and coronal planes and reconstruct the information in alternate planes. MR, on the other hand, is capable of direct axial, sagittal, oblique, and coronal imaging. Representative images have been selected in the sagittal and coronal planes to help interpret the anatomy demonstrated.

Fig. 27-13 is a midline sagittal MR image of the cranium. The relationship between the cerebral hemisphere, cerebellum, and brainstem is demonstrated. In this image the frontal, parietal, and occipital lobes of the cerebrum are seen and correspond to the cranial bones. The corpus callosum is a white matter tract that connects the hemispheres and is found at the inferior aspect of the parietal lobe. Cerebrospinal fluid appears dark on this T1-weighted image, making it relatively easy to trace the ventricular system. The anterior horn of the lateral ventricle is inferior to the genu of the corpus callosum. The midline third ventricle receives cerebrospinal fluid by way of the intraventricular foramen (of Monro) and is not optimally visualized in this image. Cerebrospinal fluid drains from the third ventricle via the cerebral aqueduct (of Sylvius), which can be found within the midbrain (between the corpora quadrigemina and the cerebral peduncles). The fourth ventricle is also a midline structure and is situated between the pons and the cerebellum. The large air-filled sphenoidal sinus is located anterior to the pons. Superior to this, the hypophysis cerebri (pituitary gland) rests within hypophyseal fossa formed by the sella turcica. Directly superior to the hypophysis cerebri is the optic chiasm.

Several vascular structures are well demonstrated in this image. The basilar artery appears between the clivus and the pons. The great cerebral vein (of Galen) is posterior to the splenium of the corpus callosum. Between the cerebrum and the cerebellum, the straight sinus (one of the dural venous sinuses) is noted within the tentorium cerebelli.

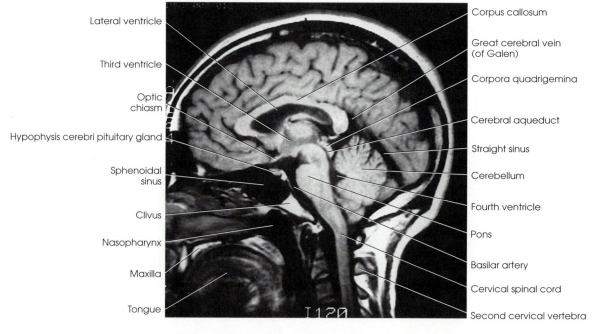

Lateral ventricle

Third ventricle

Optic chiasm

Hypophysis cerebri pituitary gland

Sphenoidal sinus

Clivus

Nasopharynx

Maxilla

Tongue

Corpus callosum

Great cerebral vein (of Galen)

Corpora quadrigemina

Cerebral aqueduct

Straight sinus

Cerebellum

Fourth ventricle

Pons

Basilar artery

Cervical spinal cord

Second cervical vertebra

Fig. 27-13. Sagittal MR image through the median sagittal plane.

A CT localizer, or scout, image is included as a reference for the next three coronal images (Fig. 27-14). Fig. 27-15 is a coronal MR image through the anterior horns of the lateral ventricles and the pharyngeal structures. The anterior portions of the cerebral hemispheres are joined by the corpus callosum, which is immediately superior to the lateral ventricles. The membrane between the anterior horns (of the lateral ventricles) is the septum pellucidum. On the lateral aspect of each cerebral hemisphere is the lateral fissure (of Sylvius), which divides the frontal lobe from the temporal lobe. The insula (insular lobe) lies deep to this fissure. Structures of the basal nuclei can again be identified. The caudate nucleus is seen lateral to the anterior horns. Inferolateral to the caudate nucleus are the putamen and globus pallidus (labeled basal nuclei). The anterior portion of the third ventricle is found in the midline inferior to the lateral ventricles. Inferior to the third ventricle are the optic chiasm and the hypophysis cerebri (pituitary gland). The superior and inferior sagittal sinuses occupy the margins of the falx cerebri in the longitudinal fissure between the hemispheres of the cerebrum. The internal carotid arteries occupy the cavernous sinus along with several cranial nerves and are found lateral to the hypophysis cerebri (pituitary gland) and sella turcica. Branches of the middle cerebral arteries occupy the lateral fissures of the cerebrum. Several air-filled structures are seen on this image, and they are (from superior to inferior) the sphenoidal sinus, nasopharynx, and oropharynx. This image also demonstrates the rami of the mandible along with the masseter and pterygoid muscles. The submandibular (salivary) glands are found deep to the gonions (angles) of the mandible.

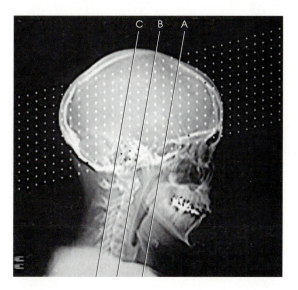

Fig. 27-14. CT localizer or scout image of the skull.

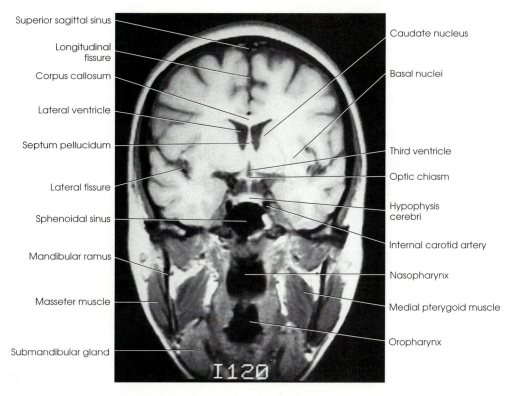

Fig. 27-15. Coronal MR image corresponding to level A in Fig. 27-14.

Superior sagittal sinus
Longitudinal fissure
Corpus callosum
Lateral ventricle
Septum pellucidum
Lateral fissure
Sphenoidal sinus
Mandibular ramus
Masseter muscle
Submandibular gland

Caudate nucleus
Basal nuclei
Third ventricle
Optic chiasm
Hypophysis cerebri
Internal carotid artery
Nasopharynx
Medial pterygoid muscle
Oropharynx

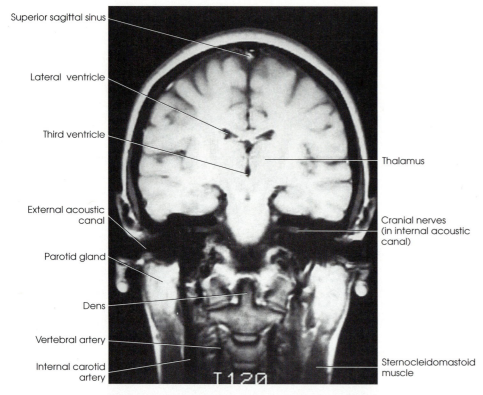

Superior sagittal sinus

Lateral ventricle

Third ventricle

Thalamus

External acoustic canal

Cranial nerves (in internal acoustic canal)

Parotid gland

Dens

Vertebral artery

Internal carotid artery

Sternocleidomastoid muscle

T120

Fig. 27-16. Coronal MR image corresponding to level B in Fig. 27-14.

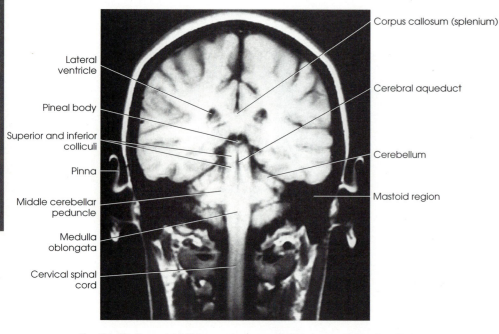

Lateral ventricle

Corpus callosum (splenium)

Pineal body

Cerebral aqueduct

Superior and inferior colliculi

Pinna

Cerebellum

Middle cerebellar peduncle

Mastoid region

Medulla oblongata

Cervical spinal cord

Fig. 27-17. Coronal MR image corresponding to level C in Fig. 27-14.

Fig. 27-16 is a coronal MR image through the bodies of the lateral ventricles, the brainstem, and the bodies of the cervical vertebrae. The third ventricle is well demonstrated and bordered laterally by the thalamus. The cartilaginous structures of the external ear surround the external acoustic (auditory) meatus and canal. The dark region (low signal return) medial to the external acoustic canal corresponds to the petrous portion of the temporal bone. Within this region the seventh and eighth (facial and vestibulocochlear) cranial nerves are found in the internal acoustic canal. The first three cervical vertebrae are detailed in this section with the dens (odontoid process) of the axis (C2) seen between the lateral masses of the atlas (C1). The vertebral arteries are demonstrated within the transverse foramina, lateral to the bodies of cervical vertebrae. The internal carotid arteries are found more laterally in the neck between the sternocleidomastoid muscles and the cervical spine. The large whitish masses inferior to the external acoustic canals are the parotid (salivary) glands.

Fig. 27-17 shows a coronal MR image through the lateral ventricles, brainstem, and spinal cord. The splenium of the corpus callosum is found between the lateral ventricles. Inferior to the splenium is the midline pineal body. The cerebral aqueduct (of Sylvius) is also a midline structure found within the midbrain. On either side of the cerebral aqueduct are the superior and inferior colliculi (corpora quadrigemina), which are associated with visual and auditory reflexes. Two large white matter tracts are seen extending laterally, inferior to the colliculi. These are the middle cerebellar peduncles, which conduct impulses between the pons and the cerebellum. Portions of the cerebellum are visualized superior and inferior to the middle cerebellar peduncles. The medulla oblongata is the most inferior segment of the brainstem and is continuous with the spinal cord as it passes through the foramen magnum. The large dark areas (signal void) lateral to the cerebellum correspond to the bony mastoid portions of the temporal bone.

Thoracic Region

The CT localizer, or scout, image represents an AP projection of the thoracic region with three identifying lines (Fig. 27-18). These lines demonstrate the approximate three levels for each of the labeled cadaver sections for this region.

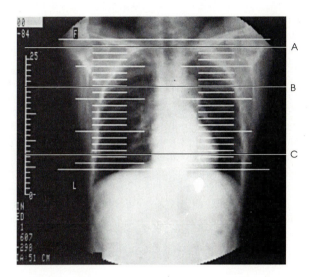

Fig. 27-18. CT localizer or scout image of thorax.

Figs. 27-19 and 27-20 represent a cadaver section and CT image at the level of T2 and demonstrate the relationship between the vertebral column, esophagus, and trachea. The inferior portion of the thyroid gland, which extends from C6 to T1, is positioned lateral to the trachea. The vertebral arteries are positioned lateral to the vertebral column, and the common carotid arteries are found lateral to the trachea. At this level the internal jugular veins are anterior to the carotid arteries. The apices of the lungs are visualized along with the first two ribs, the glenohumeral joint, and the sternal extremity of the clavicle. The trapezius, pectoral, and deltoid muscles are clearly seen. The muscles of the rotator cuff (supraspinatus, infraspinatus, subscapularis, and teres minor) stabilize the glenohumeral joint. At this level the supraspinatus, which lies superior to the scapular spine, is visualized on the cadaver section.

The CT scan at this level is slightly more inferior than the cadaver image. The five major vessels of the superior thorax are visualized posterior to the manubrium.

The right and left brachiocephalic veins are formed by the junction of the subclavian veins and the internal jugular veins. These will unite and form the superior vena cava at a more inferior level. The three branches of the aortic arch are also visualized on this image. From the patient's right to left they are the brachiocephalic artery, the left common carotid artery, and the left subclavian artery. The brachiocephalic artery gives rise to the right subclavian and right common carotid arteries, which are both seen in more superior sections of the thorax.

Figs. 27-21 and 27-22 represent a cadaver section and CT image at the level of T5 and demonstrate the great vessels superior to the heart. (The heart is normally positioned between T7 and T11, with the majority of the organ lying to the left of the midline.) The ascending aorta is found anteriorly in the midline; the descending aorta is related to the left anterolateral surface of the vertebral bodies. (This relationship between descending aorta and vertebral column is continuous through the thorax and abdomen.) The superior vena cava is located to the right of the ascending aorta, and the pulmonary trunk is located to the left of the ascending aorta at this level. The pulmonary trunk originates from the right ventricle of the heart and divides into the right and left pulmonary arteries, which carry deoxygenated blood to the lungs. In these figures the right and left pulmonary arteries are seen at the hilum of each lung. The azygos vein, which drains the thoracic and posterior abdominal walls, is positioned anterior and to the right of the vertebral column from its origination near the diaphragm until it arches anteriorly over the root of the right lung and empties into the superior vena cava at the level of T4 or T5. At the T5 vertebral level the trachea divides into the left and right primary bronchi. The thoracic duct, one of the major channels for lymphatic drainage, generally originates at the twelfth thoracic vertebra and ascends the thorax in the posterior mediastinum between the aorta and the azygos vein. The duct ultimately empties into the venous blood system at the junction of the left subclavian and internal jugular veins.

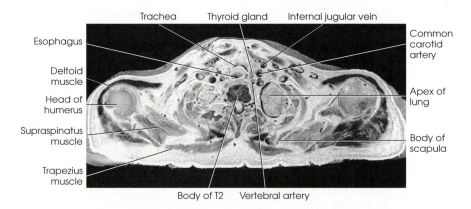

Fig. 27-19. Cadaver section corresponding to level A of Fig. 27-18 at the second thoracic vertebra.

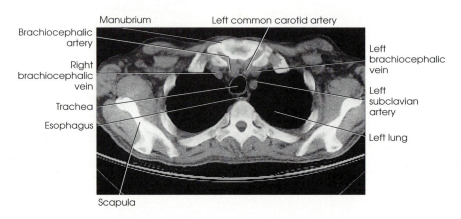

Fig. 27-20. CT image corresponding to Fig. 27-19.

(Courtesy Theresa Spotts, R.T.)

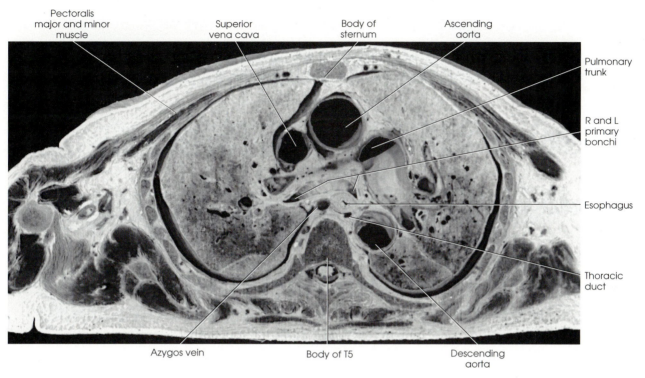

Pectoralis major and minor muscle

Superior vena cava

Body of sternum

Ascending aorta

Pulmonary trunk

R and L primary bonchi

Esophagus

Thoracic duct

Azygos vein

Body of T5

Descending aorta

Fig. 27-21. Cadaver section corresponding to level B of Fig. 27-18 at the fifth thoracic vertebra.

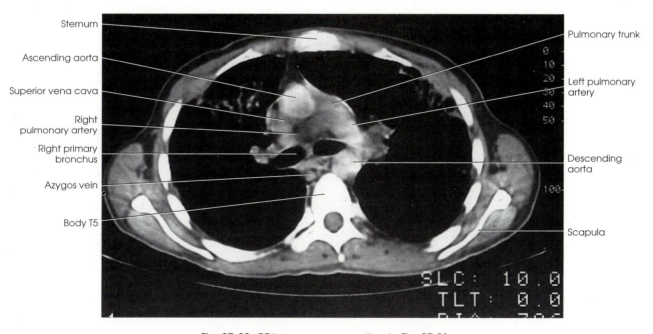

Sternum

Ascending aorta

Superior vena cava

Right pulmonary artery

Right primary bronchus

Azygos vein

Body T5

Pulmonary trunk

Left pulmonary artery

Descending aorta

Scapula

SLC: 10.0
TLT: 0.0

Fig. 27-22. CT image corresponding to Fig. 27-21.

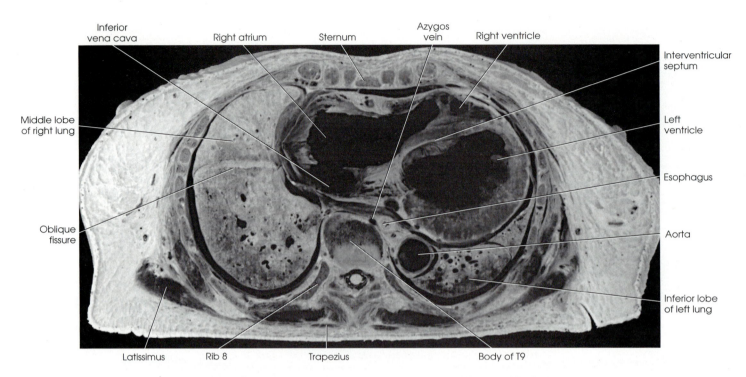

Fig. 27-23. Cadaver section corresponding to level C in Fig. 27-18 at the ninth thoracic vertebra.

Labels (clockwise from top left): Inferior vena cava — Right atrium — Sternum — Azygos vein — Right ventricle — Interventricular septum — Left ventricle — Esophagus — Aorta — Inferior lobe of left lung — Body of T9 — Trapezius — Rib 8 — Latissimus — Oblique fissure — Middle lobe of right lung

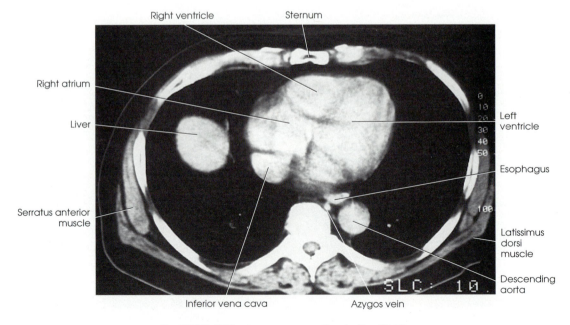

Fig. 27-24. CT image corresponding to Fig. 27-23.

Labels: Right ventricle — Sternum — Right atrium — Liver — Serratus anterior muscle — Inferior vena cava — Azygos vein — Left ventricle — Esophagus — Latissimus dorsi muscle — Descending aorta

SLC: 10

The cadaver section and CT image depicted in Figs. 27-23 and 27-24 demonstrate the lungs and the midsection of the heart. Generally, when the heart is imaged in cross section, the left atrium will be the most superior structure encountered, and the pulmonary veins will be seen emptying into it (not seen on these illustrations). The right atrium will be seen lying the farthest toward the right side of the body, anterior and somewhat inferior to the left atrium. The inferior vena cava may be seen at this level as it enters the right atrium. The right ventricle lies to the left of the right atrium and anterior to the more muscular left ventricle. The interventricular septum can be seen between the ventricles.

The lungs are divided into superior and inferior lobes by the diagonally oriented oblique fissure. The superior lobes lie superior and anterior to the inferior lobes. The superior lobe of the right lung is further divided by the horizontal fissure, with the lower portion termed the middle lobe. The left lung has no horizontal fissure. The inferior and anterior portion of the left lung (corresponding to the right middle lobe) is termed the lingula.

Muscular structures that can be seen at this level include the trapezius, latissimus dorsi, and serratus anterior muscles. The esophagus is normally seen anterior and slightly to the left of the vertebral column at this level as it veers toward the esophageal hiatus of the diaphragm. Fig. 27-24 demonstrates the superior portion of the liver bulging against the base of the right lung. The descending aorta normally lies along the left anterolateral surface of the vertebral column, and the azygos vein is normally on the right anterolateral surface. The azygos vein, esophagus, and aorta are abnormally displaced to the left in Figs. 27-33 and 27-24 due to patient pathology.

Fig. 27-25 presents a sagittal MR image through the midline structures of the neck and upper thorax. The air-filled pharynx and trachea are easily identified. The cartilaginous flap within the laryngeal portion of the pharynx is the epiglottis. Spinal structures are well seen in this image, and the relationship between the intervertebral disks and the spinal cord is clearly depicted. The major blood vessels of the superior thorax are seen posterior to the manubrium. The most anterior of these vessels is the left brachiocephalic vein, which ultimately unites with the right bra-chiocephalic vein to form the superior vena cava. Posterior to the brachiocephalic vein is a portion of the aortic arch with the origin of the brachiocephalic artery. Inferior to the arch is the right pulmonary artery.

The coronal MR image in Fig. 27-26 is slightly posterior to the median coronal plane and also demonstrates structures of the neck and superior thorax. The distal cervical and superior thoracic vertebrae can be identified. On the patient's left side, note the humeral head, clavicle, acromion process, and acromioclavicular joint. The tracheal bifurcation is seen on this image. The aortic arch and left pulmonary artery are found in close proximity to the left main bronchus. From the superior aspect of the arch extends the left subclavian artery. The heart and lungs are not ideally imaged in this scan because of motion artifacts. (See Chapter 36 on magnetic resonance imaging for methods to overcome this problem.)

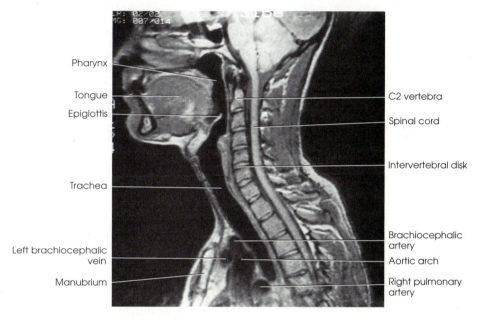

Fig. 27-25. Midline sagittal MR image through the neck and upper thorax.

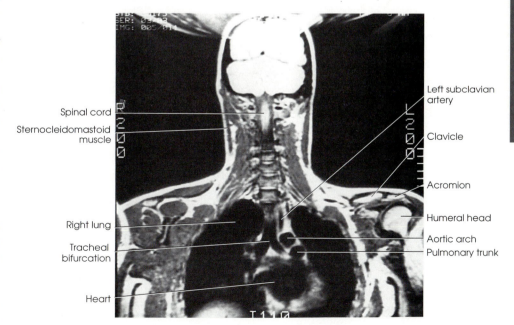

Fig. 27-26. Magnetic resonance image of the neck and thorax through the median coronal plane.

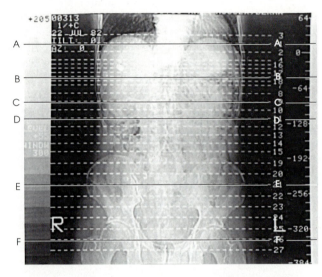

Fig. 27-27. CT localizer or scout image of the abdominopelvic region.

Abdominopelvic Region

Fig. 27-27 is a CT localizer, or scout, image representing an AP projection of the abdominopelvic region. It has six identifying lines demonstrating the levels for each of the labeled cadaver sections and images for this region.

Figs. 27-28 and 27-29 represent structures seen at the T10-11 levels (corresponding to level A in the localizer image, Fig. 27-27). The cadaver section (Fig. 27-28) demonstrates the right hemidiaphragm surrounding the superior portion of the liver and the left hemidiaphragm in its entirety. (The multiple white spots in this patient's liver are pathologic.) The pericardial fat at the apex of the heart is seen to the left of the liver. The esophagus, posterior to the liver, has migrated toward the patient's left as it nears its entrance into the stomach. The aorta is in its normal position, anterior and slightly left of the vertebral body. The inferior vena cava (IVC) appears embedded within the liver. Hepatic veins are draining into the IVC at this level. The CT scan (Fig. 27-29) is at a slightly more inferior level. The lower lobes of both lungs are seen. The right hemidiaphragm surrounds the superior portion of the liver. The spleen and contrast-filled stomach are seen on the patient's left side surrounded by the left hemidiaphragm and the lower lobe of the left lung. The esophagus still appears in the midline. The IVC is difficult to see in this image because of its proximity to the isodense liver tissue.

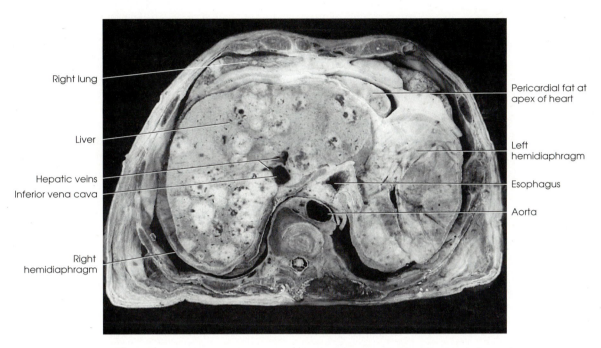

Right lung

Liver

Hepatic veins

Inferior vena cava

Right
hemidiaphragm

Pericardial fat at
apex of heart

Left
hemidiaphragm

Esophagus

Aorta

Fig. 27-28. Cadaver section corresponding to level A in Fig. 27-27 at the tenth thoracic
vertebra.

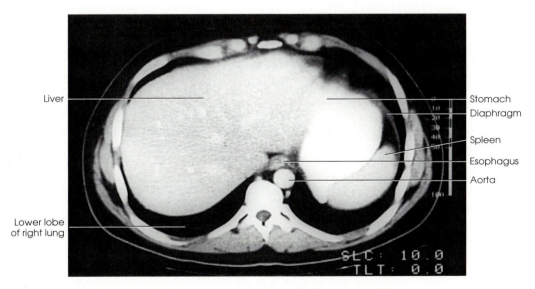

Liver

Lower lobe
of right lung

Stomach
Diaphragm

Spleen

Esophagus

Aorta

Fig. 27-29. CT image corresponding to Fig. 27-28.

The cadaver section and CT image at the level of T12 demonstrate the relationship between the liver, stomach, and spleen (Figs. 27-30 and 27-31). The cardiac portion of the stomach is located at approximately the level of T11 in the anterior aspect of the left upper quadrant, and the pyloric portion normally lies anterior to L2. The spleen, located between the levels of T12 and L1, is in the posterolateral aspect of the left upper quadrant posterior to the fundus of the stomach. The liver is generally found between T11 and L3 and occupies the entire right upper quadrant. The right lobe of the liver has two small subdivisions, the caudate and quadrate lobes, which are bounded by the gall bladder, the ligamentum teres, and the IVC. The left lobe of liver stretches across the midline and into the left upper quadrant. The suprarenal (adrenal) glands are normally located superior to the kidney. The right suprarenal gland is found at this level between the liver and the right diaphragmatic crus. The abdominal aorta is positioned anterior and to the left of the vertebral column with the celiac trunk projecting anteriorly. The three branches of the celiac trunk (hepatic, splenic, left gastric arteries) supply the liver, spleen, pancreas, and stomach with oxygen-rich blood. The splenic artery runs a very tortuous course and normally cannot be visualized in its entirety in axial sections. The IVC can be seen in its normal position anterior and to the right of the vertebral column. Branches of the portal vein are seen within the liver. The muscles of the abdomen are located between the lower rib cage and the crests of the ilia. This group of muscles includes the external oblique, internal oblique, and transverse abdominal muscles. The two rectus abdominis muscles are located on the anterior aspect of the abdomen on either side of the midline and extend from the symphysis pubis to the xiphoid process. The psoas muscles originate from the body of the twelfth thoracic vertebra and the transverse processes of the lumbar vertebrae and descend the abdomen lateral to the vertebral bodies. The quadratus lumborum muscles are located posterolateral to the psoas muscles through the abdomen.

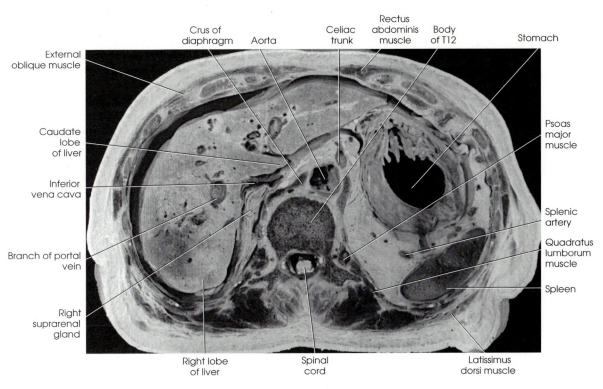

Fig. 27-30. Cadaver section corresponding to level B of Fig. 27-27 at the twelfth thoracic vertebra.

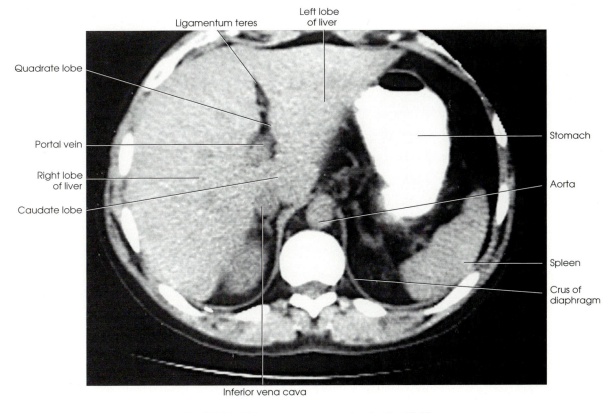

Fig. 27-31. CT image corresponding to Fig. 27-30.

The cadaver section and CT image at the level of the second lumbar vertebra demonstrate the inferior aspect of the liver with the porta hepatis (Figs. 27-32 and 27-33). At the porta hepatis the vasculature of the liver can be seen in its normal configuration, with the hepatic duct lying anterior to the hepatic artery and the portal vein lying posterior to the hepatic artery. The superior pole of the left kidney is visualized along with the pylorus of the stomach. The pancreas lies essentially in a horizontal plane posterior to the stomach and liver. The head of the pancreas is near the liver and surrounded by the duodenum (C-loop). The tail of the pancreas is slightly superior to the head and is located near the hilum of the spleen. The transverse colon arches posteriorly, then inferiorly, near the spleen at the left colic (splenic) flexure, which is seen on the CT scan at this level. Posterior to the left lobe of the liver and the neck of the pancreas, the junction of the splenic vein and the superior mesenteric vein is visualized. This junction is the origin for the portal vein. The superior mesenteric artery lies anterior and to the left of the aorta and can be seen originating from the aorta in the CT scan. The IVC is seen as the left renal vein empties into it. Lateral to the vertebral body are the psoas muscles. The quadratus lumborum muscles are seen between the psoas muscles and the transverse processes of the lumbar vertebrae. The spinal cord normally terminates at the level of the first lumbar vertebra. Inferior to L1, the spinal nerves (cauda equina) are seen within the spinal canal.

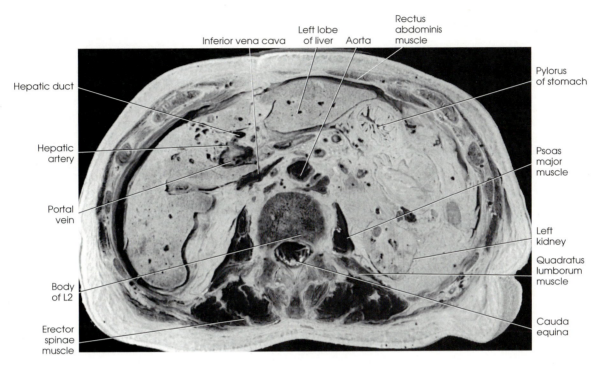

Inferior vena cava

Left lobe of liver

Aorta

Rectus abdominis muscle

Hepatic duct

Pylorus of stomach

Hepatic artery

Psoas major muscle

Portal vein

Left kidney

Quadratus lumborum muscle

Body of L2

Erector spinae muscle

Cauda equina

Fig. 27-32. Cadaver section corresponding to level C of Fig. 27-27 at the second lumbar vertebra.

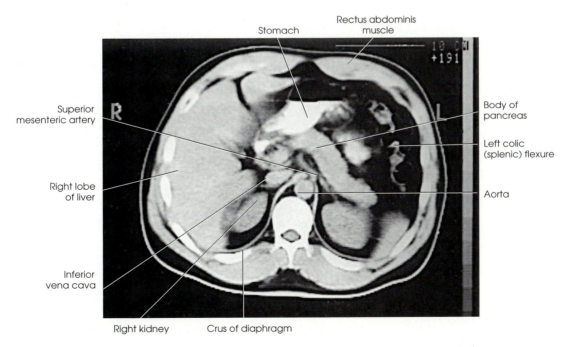

Stomach

Rectus abdominis muscle

Superior mesenteric artery

Body of pancreas

Right lobe of liver

Left colic (splenic) flexure

Aorta

Inferior vena cava

Right kidney

Crus of diaphragm

Fig. 27-33. CT image corresponding to Fig. 27-32. Note the crus (tendinous origin) of the diaphragm surrounding the aorta.

Figs. 27-34 and 27-35 represent the level of the intervertebral disk between L2 and L3. At this level the gall bladder is seen lying against the inferior aspect of the liver. The pylorus of the stomach and the first, or horizontal, portion (bulb) of the duodenum are anterior in the abdomen. The descending colon is seen in the left posterior and lateral aspect of the abdomen. The ascending colon is seen in Fig. 27-34 lateral to the right kidney as it makes its anterior turn toward the transverse colon (hepatic flexure). This level demonstrates the hilum of each kidney and the head, neck, and body of the pancreas (across the midline). The IVC is seen behind the head of the pancreas with the right renal vein emptying into it. The superior mesenteric vessels and aorta are located posterior to the body of the pancreas.

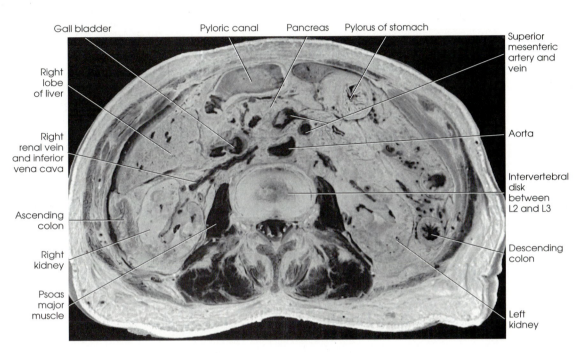

Gall bladder   Pyloric canal   Pancreas   Pylorus of stomach

Superior mesenteric artery and vein

Right lobe of liver

Right renal vein and inferior vena cava

Aorta

Intervertebral disk between L2 and L3

Ascending colon

Right kidney

Descending colon

Psoas major muscle

Left kidney

Fig. 27-34. Cadaver section corresponding to level D of Fig. 27-27 at the interspace between the second and third lumbar vertebrae.

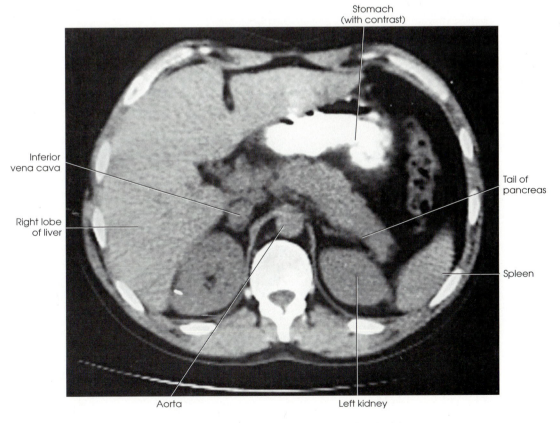

Stomach (with contrast)

Inferior vena cava

Right lobe of liver

Tail of pancreas

Spleen

Aorta   Left kidney

Fig. 27-35. CT image corresponding to Fig. 27-34.

The cadaver section and CT image seen in Figs. 27-36 and 27-37 are at the midsacral level and demonstrate the wing (ala) of the ilium, the anterior superior iliac spine (ASIS), and the sacroiliac (SI) joints. At the posterolateral aspect of the ilium the three gluteal muscles are visualized. The iliacus muscle is seen lining the internal aspect of the iliac wings near the psoas muscles. The cecum is found at the right anterior aspect of the pelvic cavity and the descending colon at the left lateral aspect. Multiple loops of small intestine are found throughout this level in the images. The abdominal aorta bifurcates at the fourth lumbar vertebra into the common iliac arteries. Each common iliac artery divides at the level of the ASIS into internal and external iliac arteries. The internal iliac arteries tend to be located in the posterior pelvis and branch to feed the pelvic structures. The external iliac vessels will be found progressively anterior in succeeding inferior sections to become the femoral vessels at the superior aspect of the thigh. The internal and external iliac veins unite inferior to the ASIS to form the common iliac veins, and the IVC is formed anterior to the fifth lumbar vertebra by the junction of the common iliac veins. The common iliac veins are positioned at the anterior aspects of the sacrum with the internal and external iliac arteries lateral to the veins in these images. Through the abdomen and at this level the ureters are located along the anterior aspect of the psoas muscles and can be seen filled with contrast in the CT image (Fig. 27-37). In the female pelvis, the ovaries are normally located laterally in the pelvis near the anterior superior iliac spines.

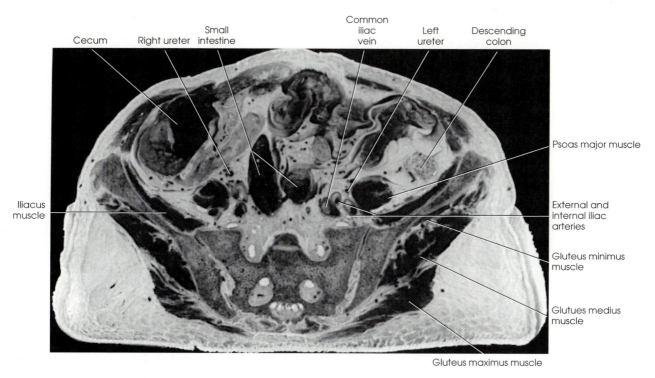

Cecum — Right ureter — Small intestine — Common iliac vein — Left ureter — Descending colon

Iliacus muscle

Psoas major muscle

External and internal iliac arteries

Gluteus minimus muscle

Glutues medius muscle

Gluteus maximus muscle

Fig. 27-36. Cadaver section corresponding to level E of Fig. 27-27 at the anterior superior iliac spine (ASIS).

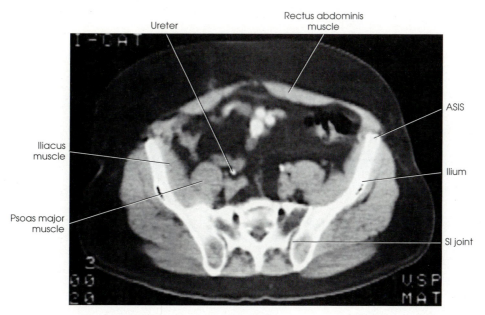

Ureter — Rectus abdominis muscle

Iliacus muscle

Psoas major muscle

ASIS

Ilium

SI joint

Fig. 27-37. CT image corresponding to Fig. 27-36.

(Courtesy Tom Meridith, R.T.)

The cadaver section and CT image seen in Figs. 27-38 and 27-39 are at a level just superior to the symphysis pubis. The ischial spines, acetabula, femoral heads, and greater trochanters are visualized. The relationship between the rectum, vagina, wall of the bladder, and superior aperture of the urethra is demonstrated from posterior to anterior in the pelvic region. The external iliac vessels are now known as the femoral vessels, with the name change occurring at the inguinal ligament, which is found between the symphysis pubis and the ASIS. The iliopsoas muscles (formed by the junction of the psoas and iliacus muscles) are found anterior to the femoral heads; the obturator internus muscle, with its characteristic right-angle bend, is found medial to the acetabulum.

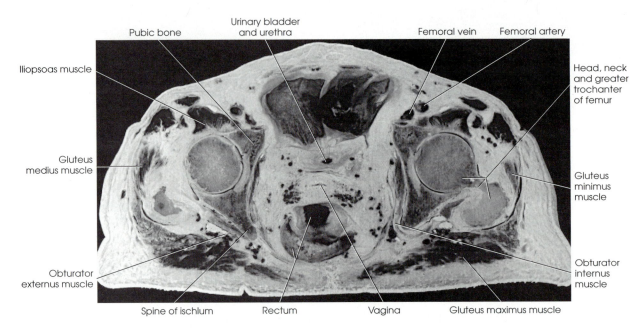

Fig. 27-38. Cadaver section corresponding to level F of Fig. 27-27 at the coccyx (female).

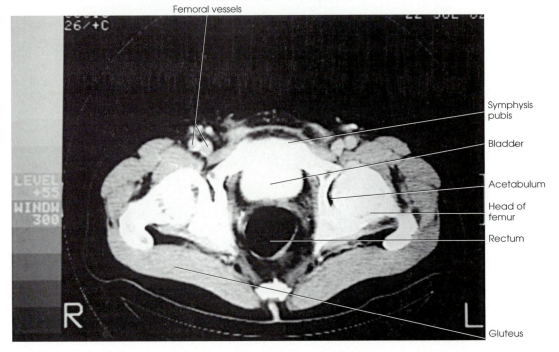

Fig. 27-39. CT image corresponding to Fig. 27-38.

Figs. 27-40 and 27-41 are of a male pelvic cadaver section and a corresponding MR image. These figures highlight structures of the male reproductive system. At this level the relationship between the rectum, prostate gland, and symphysis pubis is noted. The prostatic portion of the urethra is seen within the prostate. Posterior to the prostate are the prostatic venous plexus and the ductus deferens. The spermatic cord contains the ductus deferens and the testicular vessels, and it is found superficial and lateral to the symphysis pubis.

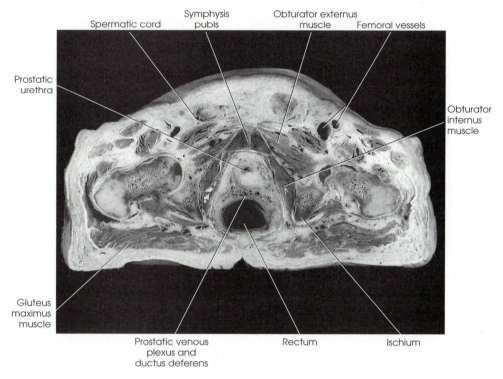

Fig. 27-40. Cadaver section corresponding to level F of Fig. 27-27 at the coccyx (male).

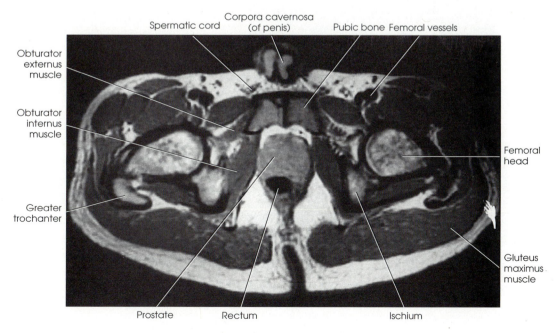

Fig. 27-41. MR image corresponding to Fig. 27-40.

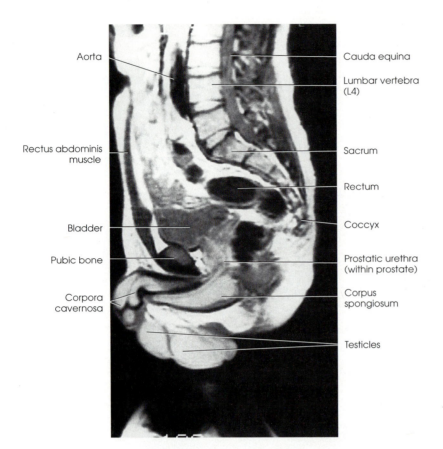

Aorta

Cauda equina

Lumbar vertebra (L4)

Rectus abdominis muscle

Sacrum

Rectum

Bladder

Coccyx

Pubic bone

Prostatic urethra (within prostate)

Corpora cavernosa

Corpus spongiosum

Testicles

Fig. 27-42. MR image of the abdominopelvic region at the median sagittal plane.

Fig. 27-42 is a sagittal MR image of the structures of the abdomen and pelvis near the midline. The third, fourth, and fifth lumbar vertebrae, the sacrum, and the coccyx are visualized. The cauda equina is seen descending the spinal canal. Anterior to the vertebral bodies is the distal portion of the abdominal aorta. At the level of the fourth lumbar vertebra, the aorta bifurcates to form the right and left common iliac arteries. The large areas of signal void anterior to the sacrum represent the rectum. The bladder is anterior to the rectum and superior to the prostate. The urethra appears faintly, traversing the prostate. The corpus spongiosum and corpora cavernosa of the penis are inferior and anterior to the symphysis pubis. The right and left testes are seen inferior to the penile structures. The rectus abdominis muscle extends superiorly from the pubis in the anterior abdominal wall.

A coronal MR image through the femoral heads and greater trochanter is found in Fig. 27-43. The femoral heads are demonstrated within the acetabula. The crests of the ilia are visualized with their associated musculature. The internal surface of the iliac bone is lined by the iliacus muscle. In this image the psoas muscles are seen joining the iliacus muscles to form the iliopsoas muscles. (Iliopsoas muscles are visualized on more anterior sections of the pelvis.) Gluteus medius and minimus muscles are found external to the iliac bones. The bladder and prostate are seen within the pelvic cavity. Superior to the bladder is a portion of the sigmoid colon. The right ductus deferens is found lateral to the neck of the bladder. Between the rami of the pubic bones are the corpus spongiosum and the corpora cavernosa. The scrotum is seen inferior to the penis and between the gracilis muscles of the thighs.

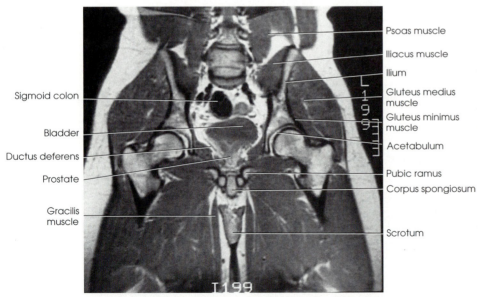

Sigmoid colon

Psoas muscle

Iliacus muscle

Ilium

Gluteus medius muscle

Gluteus minimus muscle

Bladder

Ductus deferens

Acetabulum

Prostate

Pubic ramus

Corpus spongiosum

Gracilis muscle

Scrotum

Fig. 27-43. MR image of the abdominopelvic region at the midcoronal plane.

SELECTED BIBLIOGRAPHY

Bo WJ et al: Basic atlas of cross-sectional anatomy, ed 2, Philadelphia, 1990, WB Saunders.

Cahill DR: Atlas of human cross-sectional anatomy, Philadelphia, 1984, Lea & Febiger.

Carter BL et al: Cross-sectional anatomy: computed tomography and ultrasound correlation, Englewood Cliffs, NJ, 1977, Appleton-Century-Crofts.

Chiu L, Lipcamon J, and Yiu-Chiu V: Clinical computed tomography, Rockville, Md, 1986, Aspen Publishers.

Christoforidis A: Atlas of axial, sagittal, and coronal anatomy, Philadelphia, 1988, WB Saunders.

Elster A, Goldman A, and Handel S: Magnetic resonance imaging, Philadelphia, 1987, JB Lippincott.

Hagen-Ansert S: The anatomy workbook, Philadelphia, 1986, JB Lippincott.

Hayran M et al: Evaluation of the temporal bone by anatomic sections and computed tomography, Surgical & Radiologic Anatomy 14:169-173, 1992.

Karssemeijer N et al: Recognition of organs in CT-image sequences: a model guided approach, Comput Biomed Res 21:434-448, 1988.

Keiffer S and Heitzman E: An atlas of cross-sectional anatomy, Hagerstown, Md, 1979, Harper & Row.

Koritke J and Sick H: Atlas of sectional human anatomy, Germany, 1988, Urban & Schwarzenberg.

Ledley RS, Huang HK, and Mazziotta JC: Cross-sectional anatomy: an atlas for computerized tomography, Baltimore, 1977, Williams & Wilkins.

Metrewelli C: Practical abdominal ultrasound, St Louis, 1978, Mosby.

Novelline R and Squire L: Living anatomy: a working atlas using computed tomography, magnetic resonance and angiography images, St Louis, 1986, Mosby.

Peterson R: A cross-sectional approach to anatomy, St Louis, 1978, Mosby.

Taylor K: Atlas of gray scale ultrasonography, New York, 1978, Churchill Livingstone.

Wagner M and Lawson TL: Segmental anatomy, New York, 1982, Macmillan Publishing Co.

Wicke L: Atlas of radiologic anatomy, ed 4, Baltimore, 1987, Urban & Schwarzenberg.

Selected bibliography

BIBLIOGRAPHY

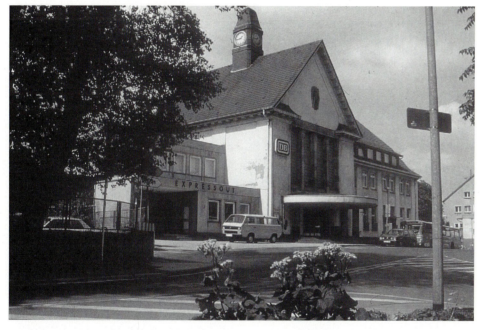

The train station in Lennep, Germany.

PALATE, PHARYNX, LARYNX

For bibliographic citations before 1964, please see the fifth edition of this atlas. For citations from 1964 through 1974, see the sixth or seventh edition.

1975   Samuel E: Xerography or conventional radiography for laryngeal examination? Can J Otolaryngol 4:59-63, 1975.

Tegtmeyer CJ et al: The value of tantalum powder as a contrast medium in laryngography, Can J Otolaryngol 4:81-85, 1975.

1976   Hemmingsson A and Löfroth PO: Xeroradiography and conventional radiography in examination of the larynx, Acta Radiol [Diagn] 17:723-732, 1976.

1977   Rossato RG and Wrightson P: Dionosil swallow: a test of laryngeal protection, Surg Neurol 7:24, 1977.

1978   Archer CR et al: Computer tomography of the larynx, J Comput Assist Tomogr 2:404-411, 1978.

Momose KJ and Macmillan AS Jr: Roentgenologic investigations of the larynx and trachea, Radiol Clin North Am 16:321-341, 1978.

Ting YM, Curran J and Maklad N: Xeroradiography of the larynx, Australas Radiol 22:39-41, 1978.

Weber AL et al: Cartilaginous tumors of the larynx and trachea, Radiol Clin North Am 16:261-267, 1978.

1979   Bergman AB, Neiman HL and Warpeha RL: Computed tomography of the larynx, Laryngoscope 89:812-817, 1979.

Mancuso AA and Hanafee WN: A comparative evaluation of computed tomography and laryngography, Radiology 133:131-138, 1979.

1980   La Rossa D et al: Video-radiography of the velopharyngeal portal using the Towne's view, J Maxillofac Surg 8:203-205, 1980.

Mancuso AA, Tamakawa Y and Hanafee WN: CT of the fixed vocal cord, AJR 135:7529-7534, 1980.

Mancuso AA et al: Computed tomography of the nasopharynx: normal and variants of normal, Radiology 137:113-121, 1980.

Noscoe NJ: Xerotomography of the larynx—an aid to radiotherapy planning, Radiography 46:199-205, 1980.

Parsons CA et al: The role of computed tomography in tumours of the larynx, Clin Radiol 31:529-533, 1980.

1981   Archer CR et al: Staging of carcinoma of the larynx: comparative accuracy of CT and laryngography, AJR 136:571-575, 1981.

Bowen A et al: Radiologic imaging in otorhinolaryngology, Pediatr Clin North Am 28:905-939, 1981.

Dunbar JS and Kramer SS: Radiology of trauma to the pediatric larynx, Ear Nose Throat J 60:356-365, 1981.

Friedman WH et al: Computed tomography vs. laryngography: a comparison of relative diagnostic value, Otolaryngol Head Neck Surg 89:579-586, 1981.

Gamsu G, Mark AS and Webb WR: Computed tomography of the normal larynx during quiet breathing and phonation, J Comput Assist Tomogr 5:353-360, 1980.

Gamsu G et al: CT in carcinoma of the larynx and pyriform sinus: value of phonation scans, AJR 136:577-584, 1981.

Gregor RT and Michaels L: Computed tomography of the larynx: a clinical and pathologic study, Head Neck Surg 3:284-296, 1981.

Jeans WD, Fernando DC and Maw AR: How should adenoidal enlargement be measured? a radiological study based on interobserver agreement, Clin Radiol 32:337-340, 1981.

Julian WL, Noscoe NJ and Berry RJ: Xeroradiographic tomography of the larynx, Clin Radiol 32:577-583, 1981.

Sagel SS et al: High resolution computed tomography in the staging of carcinoma of the larynx, Laryngoscope 91:292-300, 1981.

Weiss C and Blackley F: Feasibility of using computerized tomography in diagnosing nasopharyngeal closure, J Commun Disord 14:43-50, 1981.

1982   Curtis DJ: Laryngeal dynamics, CRC Crit Rev Diagn Imaging 18:29-80, 1982.

Ekberg O and Sigurjonsson SV: Movement of the epiglottis during deglutition: a cineradiographic study, Gastrointest Radiol 7:101-107, 1982.

Feuerbach S, Gullotta U and Schmeisser KJ: Computed tomography of pharyngo-laryngeal carcinoma, Eur J Radiol 2:105-108, 1982.

Kassel EE, Noyek AM and Cooper PW: High resolution computerized tomography in otorhinolaryngology, J Otolaryngol 11:297-306, 1982.

Mafee MF: Dynamic CT and its application to otolaryngology—head and neck surgery, J Otolaryngol 11:207-318, 1982.

Martinez CR et al: Computed tomography of the neck, Ann Otol Rhinol Laryngol [Suppl] 99:1-31, 1982.

Noscoe NJ: High definition radiographic analysis of voice and its disorders, Radiography 48:147-150, 1982.

Noyek AM, Shulman HS and Steinhardt MI: Contemporary laryngeal radiology—a clinical perspective, J Otolaryngol 11:178-185, 1982.

Schneider G, Sager WD and Lepuschutz H: Multidirectional tomography and high resolution CT in lesions of the paranasal sinuses and the pharyngeal cavity, Acta Radiol [Diagn] (Stockh) 23:63-69, 1982.

Shulman HS, Noyek AM and Steinhardt MI: CT of the larynx, J Otolaryngol 11:395-406, 1982.

Silverman PM et al: High-resolution multiplanar CT images of the larynx, Invest Radiol 17:634-637, 1982.

Silverman PM et al: Work in progress: high-resolution, thin-section computed tomography of the larynx, Radiology 145:723-725, 1982.

1983   Bohlman ME et al: CT demonstration of pharyngeal narrowing in adult obstructive sleep apnea, AJR 140:543-548, 1983.

Brown BM et al: Digital subtraction laryngography, Radiology 147:655-657, 1983.

Curtis DJ and Sepulveda GU: Epiglottic motion: video recording of muscular dysfunction, Radiology 148:473-477, 1983.

Deeb ZE: Plain roentgenography in the evaluation of unilateral vocal cord mobility, Am J Otolaryngol 4:92-100, 1983.

Glazer HS et al: Computed tomography of laryngoceles, AJR 140:549-552, 1983.

Mafee MF et al: Computed tomography of the larynx: correlation with anatomic and pathologic studies in cases of laryngeal carcinoma, Radiology 147:123-128, 1983.

Noscoe NJ et al: Examination of vocal fold movement by ultra-short pulse x radiography, Br J Radiol 56:641-645, 1983.

Silverman PM, Johnson GA and Korobkin M: High-resolution sagittal and coronal reformatted CT images of the larynx, AJR 140:819-822, 1983.

Silverman PM and Korobkin M: High-resolution computed tomography of the normal larynx, AJR 140:875-879, 1983.

Silverman PM, Korobkin M and Rauch RF: Digital radiographic localization for CT scanning of the larynx, AJR 141:1329-1330, 1983.

Suratt PM et al: Fluoroscopic and computed tomographic features of the pharyngeal airway in obstructive sleep apnea, Am Rev Respir Dis 127:487-492, 1983.

Unger JM and Chintepalli KN: Computed tomography of the parapharyngeal space, J Comput Assist Tomogr 7:605-609, 1983.

1984   Apter AJ, Levine MS and Glick SN: Carcinomas of the base of the tongue: diagnosis using double-contrast radiography of the pharynx, Radiology 151:123-126, 1984.

Cohn ER et al: Barium sulphate coating of the nasopharynx in lateral view videofluoroscopy, Cleft Palate J 21:7-17, 1984.

Horowitz BL, Woodson GE and Bryan RN: CT of laryngeal tumors, Radiol Clin North Am 22:265-279, 1984.

Kaffe I et al: The greater palatine foramen in periapical radiographs imaged with the bisecting angle technique, Dentomaxillofac Radiol 13:117-124, 1984.

Mafee MF: CT of the normal larynx, Radiol Clin North Am 22:251-264, 1984.

Silver AJ, Sane P and Hilal SK: CT of the nasopharyngeal region: normal and pathologic anatomy, Radiol Clin North Am 22:161-176, 1984.

Weber A: Radiology of the larynx, Otolaryngol Clin North Am 17:13-28, 1984.

1985   Cooper C et al: Ultrasound evaluation of the normal fetal upper airway and esophagus, J Ultrasound Med 4:343-346, 1985.

Ekberg O and Nylander G: Double-contrast examination of the pharynx, Gastrointest Radiol 10:263-271, 1985.

Jones B, Kramer SS and Donner MW: Dynamic imaging of the pharynx, Gastrointest Radiol 10:213-224, 1985.

Swartz JD et al: High resolution computed tomography. III. The larynx and hypopharynx, Head Neck 7:231-242, 1985.

1986 Ekberg O: Posture of the head and pharyngeal swallowing, Acta Radiol [Diagn] (Stockh) 27:691-696, 1986.

Khoo FY et al: The normal nasopharyngogram, AJR 147:145-148, 1986.

Singh AP et al: Computerized axial tomography of the nose, paranasal sinuses, nasopharynx and pterygoid regions, J Laryngol Otol 100:907-914, 1986.

Unger JM: Computed tomography of the parapharyngeal space, CRC Crit Rev Diagn Imaging 26:265-290, 1986.

1987 Moon JB and Smith WL: Application of cine computed tomography to the assessment of velopharyngeal form and function, Cleft Palate J 24:226-232, 1987.

Rubesin SE, Jones B and Donner MW: Contrast pharyngography: the importance of phonation, AJR 148:269-272, 1987.

Rubesin SE, Jones B and Donner MW: Radiology of the adult soft palate, Dysphagia 2:8-17, 1987.

Rubesin SE et al: Lines of the pharynx, Radiographics 7:217-237, 1987.

1988 Birch Iensen M, Borgstrom PS and Ekberg O: Cineradiography in closed and open pharyngeal swallow, Acta Radiol 29:407-410, 1988.

Carter BL and Runge VS: Imaging modalities for the study of the paranasal sinuses and nasopharynx, Otolaryngol Clin North Am 21:395-420, 1988.

Parker AJ, Bingham BJ and Osborne JE: The swallowed foreign body: is it in the nasopharynx? Postgrad Med J 64:201-203, 1988.

Penning L: Radioanatomy of upper airways in flexion and retroflexion of the neck, Neuroradiology 30:17-21, 1988.

Rubesin SE and Glick SN: The tailored double-contrast pharyngogram, CRC Crit Rev Diagn Imaging 28:133-179, 1988.

Rubesin SE et al: Contrast examination of the soft palate with cross sectional correlation, Radiographics 8:641-665, 1988.

Zinreich SJ et al: Three-dimensional CT for cranial facial and laryngeal surgery, Laryngoscope 98:1212-1219, 1988.

1989 Braun IF: MRI of the nasopharynx, Radiol Clin North Am 27:315-330, 1989.

Cross RR, Shapiro MD and Som PM: MRI of the parapharyngeal space, Radiol Clin North Am 27:353-378, 1989.

Curtin HD: Imaging of the larynx: current concepts, Radiology 173:1-11, 1989.

Kassel EE, Keller MA and Kucharczyk W: MRI of the floor of the mouth, tongue and orohypopharynx, Radiol Clin North Am 27:331-351, 1989.

Stutley J, Cooke J and Parsons C: Normal CT anatomy of the tongue, floor of mouth and oropharynx, Clin Radiol 40:248-253, 1989.

Teresi LM, Lufkin RB and Hanafee WN: Magnetic resonance imaging of the larynx, Radiol Clin North Am 27:393-406, 1989.

Towler CR and Young SW: Magnetic resonance imaging of the larynx, Magn Reson Q 5:228-241, 1989.

1990 Halvorsen RA Jr: The pharynx and esophagus, Curr Opin Radiol 2:385-393, 1990.

Hoffman EA and Gefter WB: Multimodality imaging of the upper airway: MRI, MR spectroscopy, and ultrafast X-ray CT, Prog Clin Biol Res 345:291-301, 1990.

Jabour BA, Lufkin RB and Hanafee WN: Magnetic resonance imaging of the larynx, Top Magn Reson Imaging 2:60-68, 1990.

Lanzieri CF and Bangert B: Magnetic resonance imaging of the nasopharynx, Top Magn Reson Imaging 2:39-47, 1990.

Lenz M: Oropharynx and oral cavity, Curr Opin Radiol 2:128-139, 1990.

McKenna KM et al: Magnetic resonance imaging of the tongue and oropharynx, Top Magn Reson Imaging 2:49-59, 1990.

Rothrock SG, Pignatiello GA and Howard RM: Radiologic diagnosis of epiglottitis: objective criteria for all ages, Ann Emerg Med 19:978-982, 1990.

1991 Halvorsen RA Jr: Imaging of the pharynx and the esophagus, Curr Opin Radiol 3:397-406, 1991.

Lenz M and Kersting-Sommerhoff B: Imaging of the oropharynx and oral cavity, Curr Opin Radiol 3:67-75, 1991.

Rubesin SE and Laufer I: Pictorial review: principles of double-contrast pharyngography, Dysphagia 6:170-178, 1991.

Takasugi JE and Godwin JD: The airway, Semin Roentgenol 26:175-190, 1991.

Taylor AJ, Dodds WJ and Stewart ET: Pharynx: value of oblique projections for radiographic examination, Radiology 178:59-61, 1991.

1993 Muller-Miny H, Eisele DW and Jones B: Dynamic radiographic imaging following total laryngectomy, Head Neck 15:342-347, 1993.

TRACHEA AND THYMUS

For bibliographic citations before 1964, please see the fifth edition of this atlas. For citations from 1964 through 1974, see the sixth or seventh edition.

1976 Galvin PG and Devlin HB: Outpatient thyrography: its value in the diagnosis of thyroid and mediastinal lesions, Proc R Soc Med 69:848-851, 1976.

1979 Aita JF: Body computerized tomography and the thymus, Arch Neurol 36:20-21, 1979.

1980 Kormano M and Yrjana J: The posterior tracheal band: correlation between computed tomography and chest radiography, Radiology 136:689-694, 1980.

Sone S et al: Normal anatomy of thymus and anterior mediastinum by pneumomediastinography, AJR 134:81-89, 1980.

1981 Quattromani FL et al: Fascial relationship of the thymus: radiologic-pathologic correlation in neonatal pneumomediastinum, AJR 137:1209-1211, 1981.

1982 Baron RL et al: Computed tomography of the normal thymus, Radiology 142:121-125, 1982.

Gamsu G and Webb WR: Computed tomography of the trachea: normal and abnormal, AJR 139:321-326, 1982.

Haskin PH and Goodman LR: Normal tracheal bifurcation angle: a reassessment, AJR 139:879-882, 1982.

Heiberg E et al: Normal thymus: CT characteristics in subjects under age 20, AJR 138:491-494, 1982.

1983 Gamsu G and Webb WR: Computed tomography of the trachea and mainstem bronchi, Semin Roentgenol 18:51-60, 1983.

Griscom NT: Cross-sectional shape of the child's trachea by computed tomography, AJR 140:1103-1106, 1983.

1984 Breatnach E, Abbott GC and Fraser RG: Dimensions of the normal human trachea, AJR 142:903-906, 1984.

Day DL and Gedgaudas E: Symposium on Nonpulmonary Aspects in Chest Radiology: the thymus, Radiol Clin North Am 22:519-538, 1984.

1985 Simerman LP et al: The Montgomery tracheal cannula: radiological assessment, J Can Assoc Radiol 36:49-51, 1985.

Westra D and Verbeeten B Jr: Some anatomical variants and pitfalls in computed tomography of the trachea and mainstem bronchi. II. Compression or anatomical variants? Diagn Imaging 54:285-297, 1985.

1987 Harris GJ et al: Standard biplane roentgenography is highly sensitive in documenting mediastinal masses, Ann Thorac Surg 44:238-241, 1987.

1988 Ellis K, Austin JH and Jaretzki A III: Radiologic detection of thymoma in patients with myasthenia gravis, AJR 151:873-881, 1988.

Geelhoed GW: Tracheomalacia from compressing goiter: management after thyroidectomy, Surgery 104:1100-1108, 1988.

Laks Y and Barzilay Z: Foreign body aspiration in childhood, Pediatr Emerg Care 4:102-106, 1988.

Penning L: Radioanatomy of upper airways in flexion and retroflexion of the neck, Neuroradiology 30:17-21, 1988.

1989 Williams MP: Problems in radiology: CT assessment of the thymus, Clin Radiol 40:113-114, 1989.

1990 Riebel T and Wartner R: Use of non-ionic contrast media for tracheobronchography in neonates and young infants, Eur J Radiol 11:120-124, 1990.

1991 Dawlatly EE, al-Arfaj AL and al-Azizi MA: Paediatric foreign bodies: the lessons of failure and near misses, J Laryngol Otol 105:755-759, 1991.

Szmigielski W et al: Powdered diatrizoic acid for radiography of the respiratory tract. I. Experimental investigation, Acta Radiol 32:415-420, 1991.

Szmigielski W et al: Powdered diatrizoic acid for radiography of the respiratory tract. II. Clinical application, Acta Radiol 32:467-473, 1991.

Takasugi JE and Godwin JD: The airway, Semin Roentgenol 26:175-190, 1991.

1992 Boothroyd AE et al: The magnetic resonance appearances of the normal thymus in children, Clin Radiol 45:378-381, 1992.

Davis SD and Umlas SL: Radiology of congenital abnormalities of the chest, Curr Opin Radiol 4:25-35, 1992.

Manninen MP et al: Diagnosis of tracheal carcinoma at chest radiography, Acta Radiol 33:546-547, 1992.

1993 Dennie CJ and Coblentz CL: The trachea: normal anatomic features, imaging and causes of displacement, Can Assoc Radiol J 44:81-89, 1993.

THYROID GLAND

For bibliographic citations before 1964, please see the fifth edition of this atlas. For citations from 1964 through 1974, see the sixth or seventh edition.

1976 Galvin PG and Devlin HB: Outpatient thyrography: its value in the diagnosis of thyroid and mediastinal lesions, Proc R Soc Med 69:848-851, 1976.

Mojab K and Ghosh BC: Thyroid angiography, Am J Surg 132:620-622, 1976.

1977 Wolf BS: Visualization of the thyroid gland with computed tomography, Radiology 123:368, 1977.

1978 Weber AL et al: Cartilaginous tumors of the larynx and trachea, Radiol Clin North Am 16:261-267, 1978.

1980 Binder RE et al: Diagnosis of posterior mediastinal goiter by computed tomography, J Comput Assist Tomogr 4:550-552, 1980.

Leopold GR: Ultrasonography of superficially located structures, Radiol Clin North Am 18:161-173, 1980.

Ram MD and Griffen WO: Thyroidography as a technique for localization of parathyroid adenomas, Am Surg 46:50-54, 1980.

1981 Komolafe F: Radiological patterns and significance of thyroid calcification, Clin Radiol 32:571-575, 1981.

Mahboubi S, Tenore A and Kirkpatrick JA: Diagnosis of ectopic thyroid: value of pretracheal soft-tissue measurements, AJR 137:717-719, 1981.

Som PM et al: Some CT findings in occult thyroid disease, J Comput Assist Tomogr 5:516-518, 1981.

1982 Glazer GM, Axel L and Moss AA: CT diagnosis of mediastinal thyroid, AJR 138:495-498, 1982.

Komolafe F: Cervical spine changes in goiters, Clin Radiol 33:25-29, 1982.

Martinez CR et al: Computed tomography of the neck, Ann Otol Rhinol Laryngol [Suppl] 99:1-31, 1982.

Popmihailova H and Yaneva R: Xeroradiography—a method for exploring the thyroid gland pathology, Endocrinologie 20:113-121, 1982.

Reede DL, Whelan MA and Bergeron RT: Computed tomography of the infrahyoid neck. I. Normal anatomy, Radiology 145:389-395, 1982.

1983 Bashist B, Ellis K and Gold RP: Computed tomography of intrathoracic goiters, AJR 140:455-460, 1983.

Becker TS et al: Electron radiography in the evaluation of solitary nodules in the thyroid gland, AJR 140:398-399, 1983.

Iida Y et al: Thyroid CT number and its relationship to iodine concentration, Radiology 147:793-795, 1983.

Noyek AM et al: Thyroid tumor imaging, Arch Otolaryngol 109:205-224, 1983.

1984 Silverman PM et al: Computed tomography in the evaluation of thyroid disease, AJR 142:897-902, 1984.

1985 Goblyos P et al: Liquid crystal thermography of the thyroid, Eur J Radiol 5:291-294, 1985.

1987 Beckers C: Trends in thyroid imaging, Horm Res 26:28-32, 1987.

Ott RJ et al: Measurement of radiation dose to the thyroid using positron emission tomography, Br J Radiol 60:245-251, 1987.

1988 Chen JJ et al: Single photon emission computed tomography of the thyroid, J Clin Endocrinol Metab 66:1240-1246, 1988.

Geelhoed GW: Tracheomalacia from compressing goiter: management after thyroidectomy, Surgery 104:1100-1108, 1988.

Higgins CB and Auffermann W: MR imaging of thyroid and parathyroid glands: a review of current status, AJR 151:1095-1106, 1988.

1989 Smith ML and Wraight EP: Oblique views in thyroid imaging, Clin Radiol 40:505-507, 1989.

Van Middlesworth L: Effects of radiation on the thyroid gland, Adv Intern Med 34:265-284, 1989.

1990 Gross MD and Shapiro B: Scintigraphic imaging of the thyroid, parathyroid, and adrenal glands, Curr Opin Radiol 2:851-859, 1990.

1991 Imanishi Y et al: Measurement of thyroid iodine by CT, J Comput Assist Tomogr 15:287-290, 1991.

Schneider K: Sonographic imaging of the thyroid in children, Prog Pediatr Surg 26:1-14, 1991.

DIAPHRAGM

For bibliographic citations before 1964, please see the fifth edition of this atlas. For citations from 1964 through 1974, see the sixth or seventh edition.

1975 Ramachandran S, Warakaulle MB and Vinayagamurthy V: The diaphragm in chest radiology, Med J Aust 1:680-682, 1975.

1979 Bein ME: Plain film diaphragm view as an adjunct to full lung tomography, AJR 133:217-220, 1979.

Gelfand DW and Ott DJ: Areae gastricae traversing the esophageal hiatus: a sign of hiatus hernia, Gastrointest Radiol 4:127-129, 1979.

1980 Govoni AF and Whalen JP: The respiratory diaphragm and the gastroesophageal hiatus: anatomo-radiological considerations, ROEFO 132:15-20, 1980.

1983 Naidich DP et al: Computed tomography of the diaphragm: normal anatomy and variant, J Comput Assist Tomogr 7:633-640, 1983.

Naidich DP et al: Computed tomography of the diaphragm: peridiaphragmatic fluid localization, J Comput Assist Tomogr 7:641-649, 1983.

Stewart ME et al: Radiology of the diaphragm as two muscles, Invest Radiol 18:155-159, 1983.

1986 Gale ME: Anterior diaphragm: variations in the CT appearance, Radiology 161:635-639, 1986.

1989 Tarver RD et al: Imaging the diaphragm and its disorders, J Thorac Imaging 4:1-18, 1989.

Verschakelen JA et al: Sonographic appearance of the diaphragm: a cadaver study, JCU 17:222-227, 1989.

1990 Heitzman ER: Kerley Pergamon lecture: The diaphragm. Radiologic correlations with anatomy and pathology, Clin Radiol 42:15-19, 1990.

1992 Graham NJ and Muller NL: The diaphragm, Can Assoc Radiol J 43:250-257, 1992.

1993 Saifuddin A and Arthur RJ: Congenital diaphragmatic hernia—a review of pre- and postoperative chest radiology, Clin Radiol 47:104-110, 1993.

ABDOMEN

For bibliographic citations before 1964, please see the fifth edition of this atlas. For citations from 1964 through 1974, see the sixth or seventh edition.

1975 Bookstein JJ and Walter JF: The role of abdominal radiography in hypertension secondary to renal or adrenal disease, Med Clin North Am 59:169-200, 1975.

Love L: Radiology of abdominal trauma, JAMA 231:1377-1380, 1975.

1976 Lee PW: The plain x-ray in the acute abdomen: a surgeon's evaluation, Br J Surg 63:763-766, 1976.

1977 Bryk D: Radiological evaluation of small bowel activity in the acute abdomen, CRC Crit Rev Diagn Imaging 10:99-128, 1977.

Seibert JJ and Parvey LS: The telltale triangle: use of the supine cross table lateral radiograph of the abdomen in early detection of pneumoperitoneum, Pediatr Radiol 5:209-210, 1977.

1978 Stanley J: Current status of computed tomography in the abdomen, J Belge Radiol 61:345-347, 1978.

1979 Churchill RJ et al: CT imaging of the abdomen: methodology and normal anatomy, Radiol Clin North Am 17:13-24, 1979.

Sheedy PF et al: Computed tomography of the abdominal organs, Adv Intern Med 24:455-479, 1979.

Symposium on abdominal imaging, Radiol Clin North Am 17:1-168, 1979.

Thorpe JA: The plain abdominal radiograph in acute appendicitis, Ann R Coll Surg Engl 61:45-47, 1979.

1980 de Lacey et al: Rationalizing abdominal radiography in the accident and emergency department, Clin Radiol 31:453-455, 1980.

Lawson TL et al: Abdominal computed radiography: evaluation of low-contrast lesions, Invest Radiol 15:215-219, 1980.

Oon CL: A method of localizing the plane of CT scans of the abdomen, J Comput Assist Tomogr 4:268-277, 1980.

Robbins AH et al: Further observations on the medical efficacy of computed tomography of the chest and abdomen, Radiology 137:719-725, 1980.

Roub LW et al: Early clinical experience with direct peritoneal enhancement for abdominal computed tomography, Comput Tomogr 4:217-224, 1980.

1981 Burgener FA and Hamlin DJ: Contrast enhancement in abdominal CT: bolus vs infusion, AJR 137:351-358, 1981.

Federle MP et al: Evaluation of abdominal trauma by computed tomography, Radiology 138:637-644, 1981.

Han SY, Shin MS and Tishler JM: Plain film findings of hydropneumoperitoneum, AJR 136:1195-1197, 1981.

Morin ME: Contrast enhancement of the soft tissues of the abdomen, CRC Crit Rev Diagn Imaging 15:237-271, 1981.

1982 Cherian MJ et al: Prone films of abdomen—a diagnostic tool in intestinal obstruction, Australas Radiol 26:255-260, 1982.

Eisenberg RL et al: Evaluation of plain abdominal radiographs in the diagnosis of abdominal pain, Ann Intern Med 97:257-261, 1982.

Kleinhaus U, Goldsher D and Kaftori JK: Computed tomographic diagnosis of abdominal abscesses, Radiologe 22:230-234, 1982.

McCook TA, Ravin CE and Rice RP: Abdominal radiography in the emergency department: a prospective analysis, Ann Emerg Med 11:7-8, 1982.

1983 Acin F et al: Anatomy of the upper abdomen: computerized tomography, Morphol Med 3:165-171, 1983.

Jones TK, Walsh JW, and Maull KI: Diagnostic imaging in blunt trauma of the abdomen, Surg Gynecol Obstet 157:389-398, 1983.

Kormano M et al: Dynamic contrast enhancement of the upper abdomen: effect of contrast medium and body weight, Invest Radiol 18:364-367, 1983.

1984 Chambers SE and Best JJ: A comparison of dilute barium and dilute water-soluble contrast, Clin Radiol 35:463-464, 1984.

Gyll C: Horizontal versus vertical, or lying down is better, Br J Radiol 57:191-193, 1984.

1985 Fodor J III et al: Indications for the use of high kVp in the plain film examination of the abdomen, Radiol Technol 57:159-161, 1985.

1986 Ball DS et al: Contrast medium precipitation during abdominal CT, Radiology 158:258-260, 1986.

Greene CS: Indications for plain abdominal radiography in the emergency department, Ann Emerg Med 15:257-260, 1986.

Mirvis SE et al: Plain film evaluation of patients with abdominal pain: are three radiographs necessary? AJR 147:501-503, 1986.

1987 Baldwin JE et al: Image quality of abdominal computed tomography in the elderly, Age Aging 16:261-264, 1987.

Bury R: Radiological investigations of the abdomen and digestive tract, Practitioner 231:693-698, 1987.

Feuerstein IM and Margulis AR: Semierect computed tomography of the abdomen using the Imatron ultrafast CT scanner, J Comput Assist Tomogr 11:1107-1108, 1987.

Piper KJ: Reappraisal of the erect abdominal radiograph, Radiography 53:19-21, 1987.

Raptopoulos V et al: Fat-density oral contrast agent for abdominal CT, Radiology 164:653-656, 1987.

Van Dyke JA, Holley HC and Anderson SD: Review of iliopsoas anatomy and pathology, Radiographics 7:53-84, 1987.

Yeh HC: Adrenal gland and nonrenal retroperitoneum, Urol Radiol 9:127-140, 1987.

1988 Baumgartner RN et al: Abdominal composition quantified by computed tomography, Am J Clin Nutr 48:936-945, 1988.

Belli AM and Williams MP: Graft versus host disease: findings on plain abdominal radiography, Clin Radiol 39:262-264, 1988.

Campbell JP and Gunn AA: Plain abdominal radiographs and acute abdominal pain, Br J Surg 75:554-556, 1988.

Curati WL and Greco A: Magnetic resonance imaging of the abdomen—1988, Br J Hosp Med 40:121-123, 1988.

Jeffrey RB Jr et al: Radiologic imaging of AIDS, Curr Probl Diagn Radiol 17:73-117, 1988.

Lee JK: Magnetic resonance imaging of the retroperitoneum, Urol Radiol 10:48-51, 1988.

Platt JF and Glazer GM: IV contrast material for abdominal CT: comparison of three methods, AJR 151:275-277, 1988.

Sundram SR: Direct coronal imaging of the abdomen and pelvis, Radiography 54:86-92, 1988.

Thoeni RF and Filson RG: Abdominal and pelvic CT: use of oral metoclopramide to enhance bowel opacification, Radiology 169:391-393, 1988.

Wood ML, Runge VM and Henkelman RM: Overcoming motion in abdominal MR imaging, AJR 150:513-522, 1988.

1989 Anonymous: MRI in the abdomen and pelvis, Semin Ultrasound CT MR 10:1-77, 1989.

Collins JD et al: Anatomy of the abdomen, back, and pelvis as displayed by magnetic resonance imaging. I. J Natl Med Assoc 81:680-684, 1989.

Collins JD et al: Anatomy of the abdomen, back, and pelvis as displayed by magnetic resonance imaging. II. J Natl Med Assoc 81:809-813, 1989.

Collins JD et al: Anatomy of the abdomen, back, and pelvis as displayed by magnetic resonance imaging. III. J Natl Med Assoc 81:857-861, 1989.

Hall-Craggs MA: Interventional abdominal ultrasound: recent advances, Br J Hosp Med 42:176-182, 1989.

Harris TM and Cohen MD: Abdominal magnetic resonance imaging, Pediatr Radiol 20:10-19, 1989.

Kaufman RA: Technical aspects of abdominal CT in infants and children, AJR 153:549-554, 1989.

Lewis BD and James EM: Current applications of duplex and color Doppler ultrasound imaging: abdomen, Mayo Clinic Proc 64:1158-1169, 1989.

van Waes PF, Feldberg MA and Barth P: Comparison of Telebrix Gastro and Gastrografin in abdominal computed tomography, Eur J Radiol 9:179-181, 1989.

1990 Barker CS and Lindsell DR: Ultrasound of the palpable abdominal mass, Clin Radiol 41:98-99, 1990.

Charnley RM and Hardcastle JD: Intraoperative abdominal ultrasound, Gut 31:368-369, 1990.

Gross GW, Ehrlich SM and Wang Y: Diagnostic quality of portable abdominal radiographs in neonates with necrotizing enterocolitis: digitized vs nondigitized images, AJR 154:779-783, 1990.

Hamm B, Laniado S and Saini S: Contrast-enhanced magnetic resonance imaging of the abdomen and pelvis, Magn Reson Q 6:108-135, 1990.

Jelinek GA and Banham ND: Reducing the use of plain abdominal radiographs in an emergency department, Arch Emerg Med 7:241-245, 1990.

Mueller PR and vanSonnenberg E: Interventional radiology in the chest and abdomen, N Engl J Med 322:1364-1374, 1990.

Niemi P et al: Superparamagnetic particles as gastrointestinal contrast agent in magnetic resonance imaging of lower abdomen, Acta Radiol 31:409-411, 1990.

Vogel HJ, Schipper J and Hermans J: Abdominal ultrasonography: improved image quality with the combined use of a diet and laxatives, JCU 18:627-630, 1990.

1991 Bach DB: Telebrix: a better-tasting oral contrast agent for abdominal computed tomography, Can Assoc Radiol J 42:98-101, 1991.

Caron KH: Magnetic resonance imaging of the pediatric abdomen, Semin Ultrasound CT MR 12:448-474, 1991.

Daya D and McCaughey WT: Pathology of the peritoneum: a review of selected topics, Semin Diagn Pathol 8:277-289, 1991.

Kressel HY: Insights of an abdominal imager: what do we need for MRI enhancement? Magn Reson Med 22:314-318, 1991.

Mutgi A, Williams JW and Nettleman M: Renal colic: utility of the plain abdominal roentgenogram, Arch Intern Med 151: 1589-1592, 1991.

Plewa MC: Emergency abdominal radiography, Emerg Med Clin North Am 9:827-852, 1991.

Shirkhoda A: Diagnostic pitfalls in abdominal CT, Radiographics 11:969-1002, 1991.

1992 Hamed MM et al: Dynamic MR imaging of the abdomen with gadopentetate dimeglumine: normal enhancement patterns of the liver, spleen, stomach, and pancreas, AJR 158:303-307, 1992.

Hamm B: Contrast materials for cross-sectional imaging of the abdomen, Curr Opin Radiol 4:93-104, 1992.

Merritt CR: Doppler color imaging: abdomen, Clin Diagn Ultrasound 27:141-194, 1992.

Rothrock SG, Green SM and Hummel CB: Plain abdominal radiography in the detection of major disease in children: a prospective analysis, Ann Emerg Med 21:1423-1429, 1992.

1993 Stark DD, Fahlvik AK and Klaveness J: Abdominal imaging, J Magn Reson Imaging 3:285-295, 1993.

Weill FS, Rohmer P and Parizet C: Work in progress CAVUS: transcaval ultrasonography of abdominal organs, preliminary results, J Ultrasound Med 12:91-95, 1993.

PERITONEUM

For bibliographic citations before 1964, please see the fifth edition of this atlas. For citations from 1964 through 1974, see the sixth or seventh edition.

1979 Dunnick NR et al: Intraperitoneal contrast infusion for assessment of intraperitoneal fluid dynamics, AJR 133:221-223, 1979.

1980 Roub LW et al: Early experience with direct peritoneal enhancement for abdominal computed tomography, Comput Tomogr 4:217-224, 1980.

1981 Jeffrey RB, Federle MP and Goodman PC: Computed tomography of the lesser peritoneal sac, Radiology 141:117-122, 1981.

Love L et al: Computed tomography of extraperitoneal sacs, AJR 136:781-789, 1981.

1982 Oliphant M and Berne BS: Computed tomography of the subperitoneal space: demonstration of direct spread of intraabdominal disease, J Comput Assist Tomogr 6:1127-1137, 1982.

1984 Gullmo A, Broome A and Smedberg S: Herniography, Surg Clin North Am 64:229-244, 1984.

1987 Qibi NM: New technique of blind peritoneal biopsy, BMJ 295:638, 1987.

1991 Daly BD, Guthrie JA and Couse NF: Pneumoperitoneum without peritonitis, Postgrad Med J 67:999-1003, 1991.

Daya D and McCaughey WT: Pathology of the peritoneum: a review of selected topics, Semin Diagn Pathol 8:277-289, 1991.

Levine MS et al: Diagnosis of pneumoperitoneum on supine abdominal radiographs, AJR 156:731-735, 1991.

1992 Stapakis JC and Thickman D: Diagnosis of pneumoperitoneum: abdominal CT vs. upright chest film, J Comput Assist Tomogr 16:713-716, 1992.

1993 Hindley A and Cole H: Use of peritoneal insufflation to displace the small bowel during pelvic and abdominal radiotherapy in carcinoma of the cervix, Br J Radiol 66: 67-73, 1993.

RETROPERITONEAL PNEUMOGRAPHY

For bibliographic citations before 1964, please see the fifth edition of this atlas. For citations from 1964 through 1974, see the sixth or seventh edition.

1979 Korobkin M, Callen PW and fisch AE: Computed tomography of the pelvis and retroperitoneum, Radiol Clin North Am 17:301-319, 1979.

1980 Sones PJ: Computed tomography of the retroperitoneum, Appl Radiol 9:40-50, 1980.

1981 Kuhns LR: Computed tomography of the retroperitoneum in children, Radiol Clin North Am 19:495-501, 1981.

1982 Seigel MJ et al: Clinical utility of CT in pediatric retroperitoneal disease: 5 years experience, AJR 138:1011-1017, 1982.

1983 Engel IA et al: Large posterior abdominal masses: computed tomography localization, Radiology 149:203-209, 1983.

1987 Munechika H et al: Computed tomography of retroperitoneal cystic lymphangiomas, J Comput Assist Tomogr 11:116-119, 1987.

Yeh HC: Adrenal gland and nonrenal retroperitoneum, Urol Radiol 9:127-140, 1987.

1988 de Lange EE, Black WC and Mills SE: Radiologic features of retroperitoneal cystic hamartoma, Gastrointest Radiol 13:266-270, 1988.

Goldman SM, Davidson AJ and Neal J: Retroperitoneal and pelvic hemangiopericytomas: clinical, radiologic, and pathologic correlation, Radiology 168:13-17, 1988.

Kaibara N et al: A comparison of pelvic retroperitoneal pneumography and computed tomography in the assessment of extramural invasion of rectal carcinoma, Jpn J Surg 18:675-680, 1988.

UPPER ABDOMINAL ORGANS (LIVER, SPLEEN, PANCREAS)
Liver

For bibliographic citations before 1964, please see the fifth edition of this atlas. For citations from 1964 through 1974, see the sixth or seventh edition.

1977 Levitt RG et al: Accuracy of computed tomography of the liver and biliary tract, Radiology 124:123-128, 1977.

Stephens DH et al: Computed tomography of the liver, AJR 128:579-590, 1977.

1978 Claesson G et al: Roentgen stereophotogrammetry for evaluation of liver volume and shape, Acta Radiol Diagn 19:423-432, 1978.

Progress in clinical radiology: diagnostic imaging of the liver and bile ducts, Invest Radiol 13:265-278, 1978.

Schapiro RL and Chiu LC: Computed tomography of the liver: a review, CT 2:331-341, 1978.

1979 Cynn WS et al: Infusion hepatotomography for evaluation of obstructive jaundice, AJR 132:187-190, 1979.

1980 Gelfand DW: Anatomy of the liver, Radiol Clin North Am 18:187-194, 1980.

Kreel L: Computed tomography of the liver and gallbladder, J R Coll Physicians Lond 14:81-90, 1980.

Vermess M et al: Clinical trials with a new intravenous liposoluble contrast material for computed tomography of the liver and spleen, Radiology 137:217-222, 1980.

Wegener OH, Mutzel W and Souchon R: Contrast media for computer tomography of the liver, Acta Radiol 21:239-247, 1980.

Yeh HS and Rabinowitz JG: Ultrasonography and computed tomography of the liver, Radiol Clin North Am 18:321-338, 1980.

1981 Dixon AK et al: The use of the right decubitus position in computed tomography of the liver and pancreas, Clin Radiol 32:113-116, 1981.

1983 Aisen AM et al: Hepatic imaging: positron emission tomography, digital angiography, and nuclear magnetic resonance imaging, Hepatology 3:1024-1030, 1983.

Foley WD et al: Contrast enhancement technique for dynamic hepatic computed tomographic scanning, Radiology 147:797-803, 1983.

Feeny PC and Marks WM: Computed tomographic arteriography of the liver, Radiology 148:193-197, 1983.

Sexton CC and Zeman RK: Correlation of computed tomography, sonography, and gross anatomy of the liver, AJR 141:711-718, 1983.

Standertskjold-Nordenstam CG, Somer K and Kivisaari L: Lobar liver anatomy: definition by CT, Eur J Radiol 3:234-235, 1983.

1985 Perkerson RB Jr et al: CT densities in delayed iodine hepatic scanning, Radiology 155:445-446, 1985.

1986 Gattoni F et al: Intra-arterial digital angiography of the liver: comparison with conventional angiography, Rays 11:91-96, 1986.

Weinreb JC et al: Imaging the pediatric liver: MRI and CT, AJR 147:785-790, 1986.

1987 Champetier J et al: Magnetic resonance imaging of the liver by frontal (coronal) sections, Surg Radiol Anat 9:107-121, 1987.

Valleix D et al: Ultrasonographic anatomy of the liver, Surg Radiol Anat 9:123-134, 1987.

1988 Feeny PC: Hepatic CT: state of the art, Radiology 168:319-323, 1988.

Glazer GM: MR imaging of the liver, kidneys, and adrenal glands, Radiology 166:303-312, 1988.

Kashiwagi T et al: Three-dimensional demonstration of liver and spleen by a computer, Acta Radiol 29:27-31, 1988.

Sigel B et al: Intraoperative ultrasound of the liver and pancreas, Adv Surg 21:213-244, 1988.

Zeman RK et al: CT of the liver: a survey of the prevailing methods for administration of contrast material, AJR 150:107-109, 1988.

1989 Adam A: Percutaneous techniques in the liver and biliary system: recent advances, Br J Hosp Med 42:102-110, 1989.

Cho YD, Yum HY and Park YH: Hepatocellular carcinoma with skeletal metastasis: management with intraarterial radioactive iodine, J Belge Radiol 72:267-271, 1989.

Clouse ME: Current diagnostic imaging modalities of the liver, Surg Clin North Am 69:193-234, 1989.

Foley WD: Dynamic hepatic CT scanning, AJR 152:272-274, 1989.

Foley WD: Dynamic hepatic CT, Radiology 170:617-622, 1989.

Galli G, Salvatori M and Valenza V: Hepatobiliary scintigraphy, Rays 14:57-63, 1989.

Itoh K and Stark DD: Imaging of the liver, Curr Opin Radiol 1:71-75, 1989.

Nelson RC et al: Contrast-enhanced CT of the liver and spleen: comparison of ionic and nonionic contrast agents, AJR 153:973-976, 1989.

Weissleder R and Stark DD: Magnetic resonance imaging of the liver, Magn Reson Q 5:97-121, 1989.

1990 Anonymous: Interventional radiology of the liver. I. Cardiovasc Intervent Radiol 13:133-207, 1990.

Kim EE and Podoloff DA: Radionuclide studies of the liver and hepatobiliary system, Curr Opin Radiol 2:844-850, 1990.

Thoeni RF: Imaging of the liver, Curr Opin Radiol 2:413-425, 1990.

Vassiliades VC and Bernardino ME: Magnetic resonance imaging of the liver, Top Magn Reson Imaging 2:1-16, 1990.

1991 Cox IH, Foley WD and Hoffmann RG: Right window for dynamic hepatic CT, Radiology 181:18-21, 1991.

Grossman SJ and Joyce JM: Hepatobiliary imaging, Emerg Med Clin North Am 9:853-874, 1991.

Kavanagh G, McNulty J and fielding JF: Complications of liver biopsy: the incidence of pneumothorax and role of post biopsy chest x-ray, Ir J Med Sci 160:387-388, 1991.

Lim KO et al: Hepatobiliary MR imaging: first human experience with MnDPDP, Radiology 178:79-82, 1991.

Nelson RC: Techniques for computed tomography of the liver, Radiol Clin North Am 29:1199-1212, 1991.

Soyer P and Roche A: Three-dimensional imaging of the liver, Acta Radiol 32:432-435, 1991.

Stark DD: Physiological principles for the design of hepatic contrast agents, Magn Reson Med 22:324-8, 1991.

Walkey MM: Dynamic hepatic CT: how many years will it take 'til we learn? Radiology 181:17-18, 1991.

Watson A and Kalff V: Hepatobiliary imaging, Curr Opin Radiol 3:851-858, 1991.

1992 Ditchfield MR, Gibson RN and Fairlie N: Liver CT: a practical approach to dynamic contrast enhancement, Australas Radiol 36:210-213, 1992.

Finn JP, Clarke MP and Goldmann A: MR angiography of the liver, Semin Ultrasound CT MR 13:367-376, 1992.

Longmaid HE et al: Noninvasive liver imaging: new techniques and practical strategies, Semin Ultrasound CT MR 13:377-398, 1992.

Marchal G and Baert AL: Dynamic CT of the liver, Radiologe 32:211-216, 1992.

Paulson EK et al: CT arterial portography: causes of technical failure and variable liver enhancement, AJR 159:745-749, 1992.

Schuhmann-Giampieri G et al: Preclinical evaluation of Gd-EOB-DTPA as a contrast agent in MR imaging of the hepatobiliary system, Radiology 183:59-64, 1992.

Van Heertum RL et al: Hepatic SPECT imaging in the detection and clinical assessment of hepatocellular disease, Clin Nucl Med 17:948-953, 1992.

1993 Bluemke DA and fishman EK: Spiral CT of the liver, AJR 160:787-792, 1993.

Chambers TP et al: Hepatic CT enhancement: a method to demonstrate reproducibility, Radiology 188:627-631, 1993.

Dodd GD and Baron RL: Investigation of contrast enhancement in CT of the liver: the need for improved methods, AJR 160:643-645, 1993.

Miles KA, Hayball MP and Dixon AK: Functional images of hepatic perfusion obtained with dynamic CT, Radiology 188:405-411, 1993.

Mitchell DG: Hepatic imaging: techniques and unique applications of magnetic resonance imaging, Magn Reson Q 9:84-112, 1993.

Schuhmann-Giampieri G: Liver contrast media for magnetic resonance imaging: interrelations between pharmacokinetics and imaging, Invest Radiol 28:753-761, 1993.

Soyer P, Lacheheb D and Levesque M: CT arterial portography of the abdomen: effect of injecting papaverine into the mesenteric artery on hepatic contrast enhancement, AJR 160:1213-1215, 1993.

Spleen

For bibliographic citations before 1964, please see the fifth edition of this atlas. For citations from 1964 through 1974, see the sixth or seventh edition.

1980 Piekerski J et al: Computed tomography of the spleen, Radiology 135:683-689, 1980.

Vermess M et al: Clinical trials with a new intravenous liposoluble contrast material for computed tomography of the liver and spleen, Radiology 137:217-222, 1980.

1981 Glazer GM et al: Dynamic CT of the normal spleen, AJR 137:343-346, 1981.

1986 Quinn SF et al: Interventional radiology in the spleen, Radiology 161:289-291, 1986.

1988 Kurtz AB: The spleen, Clin Diagn Ultrasound 23:139-164, 1988.

Kashiwagi T et al: Three-dimensional demonstration of liver and spleen by a computer, Acta Radiol 29:27-31, 1988.

Pugh P, Brenner M and Milne EN: Splenic size on routine chest films in AIDS: diagnostic and prognostic significance, J Thorac Imaging 3:40-51, 1988.

1989 Nelson RC et al: Contrast-enhanced CT of the liver and spleen: comparison of ionic and nonionic contrast agents, AJR 153:973-976, 1989.

1990 Rummeny EJ: Imaging of the spleen, Curr Opin Radiol 2:426-433, 1990.

1991 Mirowitz SA et al: Dynamic gadolinium-enhanced MR imaging of the spleen: normal enhancement patterns and evaluation of splenic lesions, Radiology 179:681-686, 1991.

Pancreas

For bibliographic citations before 1964, please see the fifth edition of this atlas. For citations from 1964 through 1974, see the sixth or seventh edition.

1978 Crade M, Taylor KJ and Rosenfeld AT: Water distention of the gut in the evaluation of the pancreas by ultrasound, AJR 131:348-349, 1978.

1980 Karp W et al: Angiography and ultrasound examination in the evaluation of pancreatic lesions, Acta Radiol 21:169-176, 1980.

Simeone JF, Witterberg J and Ferrucci JT: Modern concepts of imaging of the pancreas, Invest Radiol 15:6-18, 1980.

1981 Dixon AK et al: The use of the right decubitus position in computed tomography of the liver and pancreas, Clin Radiol 32:113-116, 1981.

Stuck KJ and Kuhna LR: Improved visualization of the pancreatic tail after maximum distension of the stomach, J Comput Assist Tomogr 5:509-512, 1981.

1982 Kivisaari L, Makela P and Aarimaa M: Pancreatic mobility: an important factor in pancreatic computed tomography, J Comput Assist Tomogr 6:854-856, 1982.

Kolmannskog F et al: Computed tomography and ultrasound of the normal pancreas, Acta Radiol 23:443-451, 1982.

Levitt RG et al: Computed tomography of the pancreas: 3-second scanning versus 18-second scanning, J Comput Assist Tomogr 6:259-267, 1982.

1983 Creed L et al: Fluoroscopically guided percutaneous pancreatography, Gastrointest Radiol 8:147-148, 1983.

1984 Frick MP et al: Pancreas imaging by computed tomography after endoscopic retrograde pancreatography, Radiology 150:191-194, 1984.

Jaffe MH et al: Endoscopic retrograde computed tomography of the pancreas, J Comput Assist Tomogr 8:63-66, 1984.

Stark DD et al: Magnetic resonance and CT of the normal and diseased pancreas: a comparative study, Radiology 150:153-162, 1984.

1985 Clark LR et al: Enhanced pancreatic CT imaging utilizing a geometric magnification, Invest Radiol 20:531-538, 1985.

Lavelle MI et al: Demonstration of pancreatic parenchyma by digital subtraction techniques during endoscopic retrograde cholangiopancreatography, Clin Radiol 36:405-407, 1985.

Noble PN: Computed tomography of the pancreas, Radiography 51:205-210, 1985.

Op den Orth JO: Tubeless hypotonic duodenography with water: a simple aid in sonography of the pancreatic head, Radiology 154:826, 1985.

1986 Brady PG: Endoscopic retrograde cholangiopancreatography: its role in diagnosis and therapy of pancreatitis, Postgrad Med 79:253-6, 259-61, 1986.

1987 Allendorph M et al: Endoscopic retrograde cholangiopancreatography in children, J Pediatr 110:206-211, 1987.

Lees WR and Heron CW: US-guided percutaneous pancreatography: experience in 75 patients, Radiology 165:809-813, 1987.

Marta MR: Endoscopic retrograde cholangiopancreatography: its role in diagnosis and treatment, Focus Crit Care 14:62-63, 1987.

Muranaka T et al: CT retrograde pancreatography using an indwelling balloon catheter, Radiat Med 5:42-47, 1987.

Op den Orth JO: Sonography of the pancreatic head aided by water and glucagon, Radiographics 7:85-100, 1987.

Vogelzang RL and Gore RM: Bolus-rapid infusion of contrast medium: simplified technique for optimal computed tomography pancreatography without use of dynamic scanning, J Comput Assist Tomogr 11:1-3, 1987.

1988 Freeny PC: Radiology of the pancreas: two decades of progress in imaging and intervention, AJR 150:975-981, 1988.

Goldberg BB: The pancreas, Clin Diagn Ultrasound 23:165-193, 1988.

McCune WS: ERCP—the first twenty years, Gastrointest Endosc 34:277-278, 1988.

Raptopoulos V et al: CT of the pancreas with a fat-density oral contrast regimen, AJR 150:1303-1306, 1988.

Yuh WT et al: Pancreatic transplant imaging, Radiology 167:679-683, 1988.

1989 Ghazi A and Washington M: Endoscopic retrograde cholangiopancreatography, endoscopic sphincterotomy, and biliary drainage, Surg Clin North Am 69:1249-1274, 1989.

Hansell DT et al: endoscopic sphincterotomy for bile duct stones in patients with intact gallbladders, Br J Surg 76:856-858, 1989.

Hayward SR et al: Emergent endoscopic retrograde cholangiopancreatography: a highly specific test for acute pancreatic trauma, Arch Surg 124:745-746, 1989.

Kerzel W et al: Extracorporeal piezoelectric shockwave lithotripsy of multiple pancreatic duct stones under ultrasonographic control, Endoscopy 21:229-231, 1989.

Kozarek RA et al: Endoscopic placement of pancreatic stents and drains in the management of pancreatitis, Ann Surg 209:261-266, 1989.

Lindstrom E and Ihse I: Computed tomography findings in pancreas divisum, Acta Radiol 30:609-613, 1989.

London NJ et al: Contrast-enhanced abdominal computed tomography scanning and prediction of severity of acute pancreatitis: a prospective study, Br J Surg 76:268-272, 1989.

Smith FW et al: low-field (0.08 T) magnetic resonance imaging of the pancreas: comparison with computed tomography and ultrasound, Br J Radiol 62:796-802, 1989.

Ueda D: Sonographic measurement of the pancreas in children, JCU 17:417-423, 1989.

Vecchioli A et al: Duodenal endoscopic approach: ERCP, Rays 14:27-35, 1989.

Whittwell AE et al: Blunt pancreatic trauma: prospective evaluation of early endoscopic retrograde pancreatography, South Med J 82:586-591, 1989.

Yuh WT et al: Application of magnetic resonance imaging in pancreas transplant, Diabetes 38 (Suppl 1):27-29, 1989.

Yuh WT et al: Pancreatic transplants: evaluation with MR imaging, Radiology 170:171-177, 1989.

1990 Banerjee AK, Grainger SL and Thompson RP: Trial of low versus high osmolar contrast media in endoscopic retrograde cholangiopancreatography, Br J Clin Pract 44:445-447, 1990.

Feretis CB et al: Evaluation of a new catheter (ER-PT) suitable for both diagnostic ERCP and endoscopic papillotomy, Gastrointest Endosc 36:598-599, 1990.

Freeny PC: Radiology of the pancreas, Curr Opin Radiol 2:452-461, 1990.

Martin DF and Tweedle DE: Retroperitoneal perforation during ERCP and endoscopic sphincterotomy: cases, clinical features and management, Endoscopy 22:174-175, 1990.

Murayama S et al: MR imaging of pancreas in cystic fibrosis, Pediatr Radiol 20:536-539, 1990.

Seto H et al: Pancreas divisum: CT and ERCP findings, Radiat Med 8:20-21, 1990.

1991 Barkin JS et al: A comparative study of contrast agents for endoscopic retrograde pancreatography, Am J Gastroenterol 86:1437-1441, 1991.

Gulliver DJ, Cotton PB and Baillei J: Anatomic variants and artifacts in ERCP interpretation, AJR 156:975-980, 1991.

Herman TE and Siegel MJ: CT of the pancreas in children AJR 157:375-379, 1991.

Kubo S et al: Assessment of pancreatic blood flow with positron emission tomography and oxygen-15 water, Ann Nucl Med 5:133-138, 1991.

Oi I: Technical guidance of endoscopic pancreatocholangiography, Int J Pancreatol 9:1-6, 1991.

Rogalla CJ: Pancreatic duct calculi: treatment by pulsed dye laser, AORN J 53:1506-1517, 1991.

Tart RP et al: Enteric MRI contrast agents: comparative study of five potential agents in humans, Magn Reson Imaging 9:559-568, 1991.

Tham RT et al: Cystic fibrosis: MR imaging of the pancreas, Radiology 179:183-186, 1991.

1992 Dupuy DE, Costello P and Ecker CP: spiral CT of the pancreas, Radiology 183:815-818, 1992.

Fishman EK et al: Spiral CT of the pancreas with multiplanar display, AJR 159:1209-1215, 1992.

Mitchell DG et al: Pancreatic disease: findings on state-of-the-art MR images, AJR 159:533-538, 1992.

Nakamura H et al: Pancreatic angiography using balloon catheter occlusion and a vasoconstrictor, Radiat Med 10:48-49, 1992.

Shimizu S et al: Diagnostic ERCP, Endoscopy 24:95-99, 1992.

Taylor AJ et al: filling defects in the pancreatic duct on endoscopic retrograde pancreatography, AJR 159:1203-1208, 1992.

Vitale GC: Interventional endoscopic retrograde cholangiopancreatography: state of the art. I. J R Coll Surg Edinb 37:289-297, 1992.

Vitale GC: Interventional endoscopic retrograde cholangiopancreatography: state of the art. II. J R Coll Surg Edinb 37:357-368, 1992.

Yasuda K et al: Clinical application of ultrasonic probes in the biliary and pancreatic duct, Endoscopy 24 (Suppl 1):370-375, 1992.

1993 Brambs HJ and Claussen CD: Pancreatic and ampullary carcinoma: ultrasound, computed tomography, magnetic resonance imaging and angiography, Endoscopy 25:58-68, 1993.

Cushing GL et al: Intraluminal ultrasonography during ERCP with high-frequency ultrasound catheters, Gastrointest Endosc 39:432-435, 1993.

Shirai Z et al: The usefulness of endoscopic retrograde cholangiopancreatography in infants and small children, Am J Gastroenterol 88:536-541, 1993.

Thornton J and Axon A: Towards safer endoscopic retrograde cholangiopancreatography, Gut 34:721-724, 1993.

PANCREATOGRAPHY BY SURGICAL METHODS

For bibliographic citations before 1964, please see the fifth edition of this atlas. For citations from 1964 through 1974, see the sixth or seventh edition.

1975 Clouse ME, Gregg JA and Sedgwick CE: Angiography vs. pancreatography in diagnosis of carcinoma of the pancreas, Radiology 114:605-610, 1975.

Leach RE, Riley JC and Davis WD Jr: Endoscopic retrograde choledochopancreatography, South Med J 68:49-51, 1975.

Schmarsow R and Peters PE: The pancreatographic effect during pharmacoangiography of the pancreas, Acta Radiol [Diagn] 16:73-80, 1975.

1977 Falkenstein DB et al: Influence of endoscopic manipulation and patient position on cholangiographic interpretation in endoscopic retrograde cholangiopancreatography, Radiology 122:836-838, 1977.

Smulewicz JJ et al: Pancreatography: follow-up, N Y State J Med 77:41-44, 1977.

Wilkins RA and Hatfield A: Cholangiopancreatography and pancreatic cytology in carcinoma of the pancreas, AJR 128:747-749, 1977.

1978 Nelson EW: Accuracy and consistency of pancreatography, Am J Surg 136:740-743, 1978.

Sage MR and Perrett LV: Computerized tomography of pancreas, Australas Radiol 22:145-150, 1978.

1979 Burrell MI et al: Diagnostic imaging procedures in acute pancreatitis: comparison of ultrasound, intravenous cholangiography, and oral cholecystography, JAMA 242:342-343, 1979.

Frank ED: Computed tomography of the pancreas: a new roentgenographic examination, Radiol Technol 50:403-409, 1979.

Reuben A and Cotton PB: Endoscopic retrograde cholangiopancreatography in carcinoma of the pancreas, Surg Gynecol Obstet 148:179-184, 1979.

1980 Cotton PB et al: Gray-scale ultrasonography and endoscopic pancreatography in pancreatic diagnosis, Radiology 134:453-459, 1980.

1981 Arndt RD et al: Iodipamide-enhanced computed tomography of the pancreas, Radiology 139:491-493, 1981.

Blustein PK et al: Endoscopic retrograde cholangiopancreatography in pancreatitis in children and adolescents, Pediatrics 68:387-393, 1981.

1982 Hamilton I et al: Metrizamide as contrast medium in endoscopic retrograde cholangiopancreatography, Clin Radiol 33:293-295, 1982.

1983 Cooper MJ and Williamson RCN: The value of operative pancreatography, Br J Surg 70:577-580, 1983.

Creed L et al: Fluoroscopically guided percutaneous pancreatography, Gastrointest Radiol 8:147-148, 1983.

Matter D, Spinelli G and Warter P: Ultrasonically guided percutaneous pancreatography, JCU 11:401-404, 1983.

1988 Sigel B et al: Intraoperative ultrasound of the liver and pancreas, Adv Surg 21:213-244, 1988.

1992 Printz H et al: Intraoperative ultrasonography in surgery for chronic pancreatitis, Int J Pancreatol 12:233-237, 1992.

1993 Cotton PB: Endoscopic retrograde cholangiopancreatography and laparoscopic cholecystectomy, Am J Surg 165:474-478, 1993.

BILIARY TRACT (CHOLEGRAPHY BY ORAL AND INTRAVENOUS METHODS)

For bibliographic citations before 1964, please see the fifth edition of this atlas. For citations from 1964 through 1974, see the sixth or seventh edition.

1975 Cohen WN and Freeman JB: Development and evaluation of use of cholecystokinin in the diagnosis of a calculous gallbladder disease, Can J Surg 18:571-577, 1975.

Fuchs WA and Preisig R: Prolonged drip-infusion cholangiography, Br J Radiol 48:539-544, 1975.

Laufer I and Gledhill L: The value of the fatty meal in oral cholecystography, Radiology 114:525-527, 1975.

Parks MP: Radiological concepts of cholecystokinin cholecystography, Radiol Technol 46:335-342, 1975.

Scholz FJ, Johnston DO and Wise RE: Intravenous cholangiography: optimum dosage and methodology, Radiology 114:413-518, 1975.

1976 Herzog RJ and Nelson JA: The role of cholecystokinin in radiographic opacification of the gallbladder, Invest Radiol 11:440-447, 1976.

Leopold GR et al: Gray scale ultrasonic cholecystography: a comparison with conventional radiographic techniques, Radiology 121:445-448, 1976.

1977 Bartrum RJ Jr, Crow HC and Foote SR: Ultrasonic and radiographic cholecystography, N Engl J Med 296:538-541, 1977.

Behan M et al: The concentration maximum concept in intravenous cholangiography, Br J Radiol 50:551-554, 1977.

Dodds WJ and Stewart ET: Upright spot filming of the gallbladder using pneumatic compression, AJR 128:334-335, 1977.

1978 Holden WS and Jones G: Limitations of the cholecystogram, Clin Radiol 29:651-655, 1978.

Imhof H and Doi K: Applications of radiographic magnification technique with an ultra-high speed rare-earth screen/film system to oral cholecystography, Radiology 129:173-178, 1978.

Loeb PM et al: The effect of fasting on gallbladder opacification during oral cholecystography: a controlled study in normal volunteers, Radiology 126:395-401, 1978.

Neschis M, King MC and Murphy RA: Cholecystokinin cholecystography in the diagnosis of acalculous extrahepatic biliary tract disorders, Am J Gastroenterol 70:593-599, 1978.

1979 Anderson JF: Value of plain radiographs prior to oral cholecystography, Radiology 133:309-310, 1979.

Evans AF and Whitehouse GH: The effect of glucagon on infusion cholangiography, Clin Radiol 30:499-506, 1979.

Mehta MH, Hynes DM and Osuszek A: Flow-chart for sequential cholecystography, J Can Assoc Radiol 30:23-25, 1979.

Wetzner SM, Vincent ME and Robbins AH: Ceruletide-assisted cholecystography: a clinical assessment, Radiology 131:23-26, 1979.

1980 Detwiler RP et al: Ultrasonography and oral cholecystography: a comparison of their use in the diagnosis of gallbladder disease, Arch Surg 115:1096-1098, 1980.

Goodman MW et al: Is intravenous cholangiography still useful? Gastroenterology 79:642-645, 1980.

Hamilton B and Hurley GD: Some aspects of radiography in oral cholecystography, Radiology 46:197, 1980.

Hoeffel JC et al: Oral cholecystography: is the fatty meal always necessary? Radiologe 20:24-27, 1980.

Krook PM et al: Comparison of real-time cholecystosonography and oral cholecystography, Radiology 135:145-148, 1980.

1981 Brenner RJ et al: The oblique bending view of oral cholecystography, Radiology 138:733-734, 1981.

Miller RE et al: Grid selection for oral cholecystography, Radiology 139:234-235, 1981.

Simeone JF and Ferrucci JT: New trends in gallbladder imaging, JAMA 246:380-383, 1981.

1982 Atkinson GO Jr and Gay BB Jr: Choledochal cysts in children: radiologic features, South Med J 75:1215-1221, 1982.

Levy MD: Preoperative diagnosis of gallbladder disease, Compr Ther 8:40-43, 1982.

Pretorius DH, Gosink BB and Olson LK: CT of the opacified biliary tract: use of calcium ipodate, AJR 138:1073-1075, 1982.

Thompson WM et al: Gallbladder density and iodine concentration in humans during oral cholecystography: a comparison of iopanoic and iopronic acid, Invest Radiol 17:621-628, 1982.

1983 Berk RN, Leopold GR and Fordtran JS: Imaging of the gallbladder, Adv Intern Med 28:387-408, 1983.

Greenberg M, Rubin JM and Greenberg BM: Appearance of the gallbladder and biliary tree by CT cholangiography, J Comput Assist Tomogr 7:788-794, 1983.

Krebs CA and Carson J: Gallbladder examinations: a comparison between sonography and radiography, Radiol Technol 54:181-188, 1983.

McConnell CA, Whitehouse GH and Evans AF: Gallbladder contraction and bile duct opacification in oral cholecystography—a comparison of different methods, Br J Radiol 56:371-376, 1983.

Okuda K and Tsuchiya Y: Ultrasound anatomy of the biliary system, Clin Gastroenterol 12:49-63, 1983.

1984 Andrews RC and Hawkins IF: The Hawkins needle-guide system for percutaneous catheterization. I. AJR 142:1191-1195, 1984.

Cockrell CH and Cho SR: Upright tomographic oral cholecystography, Radiology 151:797, 1984.

Culp WC: Buoyancy of gallstones in varying concentrations of contrast, AJR 143:79-81, 1984.

Gollock JM: The single cannula method, Surg Gynecol Obstet 158:87-88, 1984.

Lehmann AL: Brief ties with a vascular tourniquet, Surg Gynecol Obstet 158:500-501, 1984.

Niederau C, Sonnenberg A and Mueller J: Comparison of the extrahepatic bile duct size measured by ultrasound, Gastroenterology 87:615-621, 1984.

1986 Parulekar SG: Evaluation of the prone view for cholecystosonography, J Ultrasound Med 5:617-624, 1986.

Thompson WM: The optimal radiographic technique for operative and T-tube cholangiography, CRC Crit Rev Diagn Imaging 26:107-176, 1986.

vanSonnenberg E et al: Diagnostic and therapeutic percutaneous gallbladder procedures, Radiology 160:23-26, 1986.

1987 Widmann WD et al: An improved double-lumen biliary catheter for cholangiography, Am J Surg 154:317-319, 1987.

1988 Kane RA: The biliary system, Clin Diagn Ultrasound 23:75-137, 1988.

1989 Das AK et al: Percutaneous transhepatic ultrasonic cholelithotripsy, Arch Surg 124:747-748, 1989.

Galli G, Salvatori M and Valenza V: Hepatobiliary scintigraphy, Rays 14:57-63, 1989.

Goldberg HI: Imaging of the biliary system, Curr Opin Radiol 1:76-80, 1989.

Irving HC: Studying the gall bladder, BMJ 298:977-978, 1989.

Teplick SK: Diagnostic and therapeutic interventional gallbladder procedures, AJR 152:913-916, 1989.

vanSonnenberg E et al: Interventional radiology in the gallbladder, Radiographics 9:39-49, 1989.

1990 Burhenne HJ: The history of interventional radiology of the biliary tract, Radiol Clin North Am 28:1139-1144, 1990.

Goldberg HI: Biliary tract, Curr Opin Radiol 2:434-440, 1990.

Kim EE and Podoloff DA: Radionuclide studies of the liver and hepatobiliary system, Curr Opin Radiol 2:844-850, 1990.

Lette J et al: Standing views to differentiate gallbladder or bile leak from duodenal activity on cholescintigrams, Clin Nucl Med 15:231-236, 1990.

Liddell RM et al: Normal intrahepatic bile ducts: CT depiction, Radiology 176:633-635, 1990.

Wong K et al: Nonvisualized gallbladder on oral cholecystography: implications for lithotripsy, Gastrointest Radiol 15:126-128, 1990.

1991 Burrell MI et al: The biliary tract: imaging for the 1990s, AJR 157:223-233, 1991.

Cohen SM and Kurtz AB: Biliary sonography, Radiol Clin North Am 29:1171-1198, 1991.

Grossman SJ and Joyce JM: Hepatobiliary imaging, Emerg Med Clin North Am 9:853-874, 1991.

Haller JO: Sonography of the biliary tract in infants and children, AJR 157:1051-1058, 1991.

Lim KO et al: Hepatobiliary MR imaging: first human experience with MnDPDP, Radiology 178:79-82, 1991.

Meilstrup JW, Hopper KD and Thieme GA: Imaging of gallbladder variants, AJR 157:1205-1208, 1991.

Stott MA et al: Ultrasound of the common bile duct in patients undergoing cholecystectomy, JCU 19:73-76, 1991.

Watson A and Kalff V: Hepatobiliary imaging, Curr Opin Radiol 3:851-858, 1991.

Zeman RK and Garra BS: Gall bladder imaging: the state of the art, Gastroenterol Clin North Am 20:127-156, 1991.

1992 Brakel K et al: Accuracy of ultrasound and oral cholecystography in assessing the number and size of gallstones: implications for non-surgical therapy, Br J Radiol 65:779-783, 1992.

Girard MJ et al: Wallstent metallic biliary endoprosthesis: MR imaging characteristics, Radiology 184:874-876, 1992.

Schuhmann-Giampieri G et al: Preclinical evaluation of Gd-EOB-DTPA as a contrast agent in MR imaging of the hepatobiliary system, Radiology 183:59-64, 1992.

Yasuda K et al: Clinical application of ultrasonic probes in the biliary and pancreatic duct, Endoscopy 24 (Suppl 1):370-375, 1992.

1993 Heaton KW et al: An explanation for gallstones in normal-weight women: slow intestinal transit, Lancet 341:8-10, 1993.

BILIARY DUCTS (CHOLANGIOGRAPHY BY SURGICAL METHODS)

For bibliographic citations before 1964, please see the fifth edition of this atlas. For citations from 1964 through 1974, see the sixth or seventh edition.

1975 Leach RE, Riley JC and Davis WD Jr: Endoscopic retrograde choledochopancreatography, South Med J 68:49-54, 1975.

Redeker AG et al: Percutaneous transhepatic cholangiography: an improved technique, JAMA 231:386-387, 1975.

1976 Buonocore E: Transhepatic percutaneous cholangiography, Radiol Clin North Am 14:527-542, 1976.

Menuck L and Amberg J: The bile ducts, Radiol Clin North Am 14:499-525, 1976.

Morin ME, Baker DA and Marsan RE: Demonstration of dilated biliary ducts by total-body opacification: differentiation of surgical from nonsurgical jaundice, Radiology 121:307-309, 1976.

1977 Blackstone MO and Blum AL: Endoscopic retrograde cholangiography, Am J Dig Dis 22:474-475, 1977.

Borge J: Operative cholangiography: new cholangiogram catheter clamp and improved technique, Arch Surg 112:340-342, 1977.

Falkenstein DB et al: Influence of endoscopic manipulation and patient position on cholangiographic interpretation in endoscopic retrograde cholangiopancreatography, Radiology 122:836-838, 1977.

1978 Berci G et al: Modern operative fluorocholangiography: utopia or overlooked entity? Gastrointest Radiol 3:401-406, 1978.

Berci G et al: Operative fluoroscopy and cholangiography: the use of modern radiologic technics during surgery, Am J Surg 135:32-35, 1978.

Chatterji B, Majumdar P and Mukherjee S: Percutaneous transhepatic cholangiography, J Indian Med Assoc 70:130-133, 1978.

Goldberg HI et al: Capability of CT body scanning and ultrasonography to demonstrate the status of the biliary ductal system in patients with jaundice, Radiology 129:731-737, 1978.

Hopton D: Common bile duct perfusion combined with operative cholangiography, Br J Surg 65:852-854, 1978.

Siegel JH: ERCP update: diagnostic and therapeutic applications, Gastrointest Radiol 3:311-318, 1978.

1979 Elyaderani M and Gabriele OF: Percutaneous cholecystostomy and cholangiography in patients with obstructive jaundice, Radiology 130:601-602, 1979.

Pedano NC: Operative cholangiography, JAOA 78:662-665, 1979.

1981 Rabinov KR: Operative cholangiography, Med Radiogr Photogr 57:18-20, 1981.

Shimizu H et al: The diagnostic accuracy of computed tomography in obstructive biliary disease: a comparative evaluation with direct cholangiography, Radiology 138:411-416, 1981.

1982 Ajao OG: A simple technique of intraoperative cholangiography, Trop Doct 12:211-212, 1982.

1983 Cotton PB: Direct choledochography and related diagnostic methods, Clin Gastroenterol 12:101-107, 1983.

Kelly TR and fink JA: A new inflatable T-tube for completion cholangiography, Surg Gynecol Obstet 157:374-376, 1983.

Kumar SS and Looney CM: A simple method for operative cholangiography, Surg Gynecol Obstet 157:482-484, 1983.

Thompson WM et al: High kVp vs. low kVp for t-tube and operative cholangiography, Radiology 146:635-642, 1983.

1984 Connon JJ: Direct cholangiography: its diagnostic and therapeutic role, Can Med Assoc J 130:266-268, 1984.

Nichols DM and Burhenne HJ: Magnification in cholangiography, AJR 141:947-949, 1984.

Schwartz SA: A technique for operative cholangiography to evaluate failure, Surg Gynecol Obstet 158:589-590, 1984.

1985 Burchard KW et al: Standard T-tube cholangiogram: a safe method of cholangiography, RI Med J 68:405-407, 1985.

Case WG: Use of a snugging ligature for securing a cholangiogram catheter, Ann R Coll Surg Engl 67:19, 1985.

1986 Thompson WM: The optimal radiographic technique for operative and T-tube cholangiography, CRC Crit Rev Diagn Imaging 26:107-176, 1986.

vanSonnenberg E et al: Diagnostic and therapeutic percutaneous gallbladder procedures, Radiology 160:23-26, 1986.

1987 Allendorph M et al: Endoscopic retrograde cholangiopancreatography in children, J Pediatr 110:206-211, 1987.

Buckley AR et al: Intraoperative imaging of the biliary tree. Sonography vs. operative cholangiography, J Ultrasound Med 6:589-595, 1987.

Faulkner K et al: Fluoroscopic peroperative cholangiography: technique and associated, Br J Surg 74:753-754, 1987.

Marta MR: Endoscopic retrograde cholangiopancreatography: its role in diagnosis and treatment, Focus Crit Care 14:62-63, 1987.

Widmann WD et al: An improved double-lumen biliary catheter for cholangiography, Am J Surg 154:317-319, 1987.

1988 Gibson RN: Interventional radiology in the biliary tract, Br J Hosp Med 40:374-378, 1988.

Jacob ET and Bronsther B: A double ballooned inflatable and collapsible T-tube for selective, proximal or distal cholangiography, Surg Gynecol Obstet 166:84-86, 1988.

McCune WS: ERCP—the first twenty years, Gastrointest Endosc 34:277-278, 1988.

Motson RW et al: Digital subtraction cholangiography: a new technique for visualising the common bile duct during cholecystectomy, Ann R Coll Surg Engl 70:135-138, 1988.

1989 Adam A: Percutaneous techniques in the liver and biliary system: recent advances, Br J Hosp Med 42:102-110, 1989.

Ghazi A and Washington M: Endoscopic retrograde cholangiopancreatography, endoscopic sphincterotomy, and biliary drainage, Surg Clin North Am 69:1249-1274, 1989.

Hansell DT et al: Endoscopic sphincterotomy for bile duct stones in patients with intact gallbladders, Br J Surg 76:856-858, 1989.

vanSonnenberg E et al: Interventional radiology in the gallbladder, Radiographics 9:39-49, 1989.

Vecchioli A et al: Duodenal endoscopic approach: ERCP, Rays 14:27-35, 1989.

Vipond MN et al: Technique for operative cholangiography after endoscopic sphincterotomy, Br J Surg 76:571, 1989.

1990 al-Jurf A: A simplified technique to relax the sphincter of Oddi during intraoperative cholangiography, Surg Gynecol Obstet 170:163-164, 1990.

Banerjee AK, Grainger SL and Thompson RP: Trial of low versus high osmolar contrast media in endoscopic retrograde cholangiopancreatography, Br J Clin Pract 44:445-447, 1990.

Cwikiel W, Ivancev K and Lunderquist A: Interventional radiology of the biliary tract: metallic stents, Radiol Clin North Am 28:1203-1210, 1990.

Feretis CB et al: Evaluation of a new catheter (ER-PT) suitable for both diagnostic ERCP and endoscopic papillotomy, Gastrointest Endosc 36:598-599, 1990.

Martin DF and Tweedle DE: Retroperitoneal perforation during ERCP and endoscopic sphincterotomy: causes, clinical features and management, Endoscopy 22:174-175, 1990.

Phillips EH et al: The importance of intraoperative cholangiography during laparoscopic cholecystectomy, Am Surg 56:792-795, 1990.

Shively EH et al: Operative cholangiography, Am J Surg 159:380-384, 1990.

Yee AC and Ho CS: Percutaneous transhepatic biliary drainage: a review, CRC Crit Rev Diagn Imaging 30:247-279, 1990.

1991 Barkin JS et al: A comparative study of contrast agents for endoscopic retrograde pancreatography, Am J Gastroenterol 86:1437-1441, 1991.

Berlin RB and Berlin RB Jr: A closed system for intraoperative cystic duct cholangiography, Surg Gynecol Obstet 172:61-62, 1991.

Blatner ME et al: Cystic duct cholangiography during laparoscopic cholecystectomy, Arch Surg 126:646-649, 1991.

Pietrafitta JJ et al: Cholecystcholangiography during laparoscopic cholecystectomy: cholecystcholangiography or cystic duct cholangiography, J Laparoendosc Surg 1:197-206, 1991.

1992 Berci G: Biliary ductal anatomy and anomalies: the role of intraoperative cholangiography during laparoscopic cholecystectomy, Surg Clin North Am 72:1069-1075, 1992.

Bley WR and Ahmad I: Peroral radiographic placement of biliary stents, J Vasc Interv Radiol 3:375-377, 1992.

Cantwell DV: Routine cholangiography during laparoscopic cholecystectomy, Arch Surg 127:483-484, 1992.

Corder AP, Scott SD and Johnson CD: Place of routine operative cholangiography at cholecystectomy, Br J Surg 79:945-947, 1992.

Gillams A et al: Can cholangiography be safely abandoned in laparoscopic cholecystectomy, Ann R Coll Surg Engl 74:248-251, 1992.

Harvey MH, Cahill J and Wastell C: Laparoscopic cholangiography: a simple inexpensive technique using readily available materials, Br J Surg 79:1178-1179, 1992.

Kumar SS: Laparoscopic cholangiography: a new method and device, J Laparoendosc Surg 2:247-254, 1992.

Shimizu S et al: Diagnostic ERCP, Endoscopy 24:95-99, 1992.

Vitale GC: Interventional endoscopic retrograde cholangiopancreatography: state of the art. I. J R Coll Surg Edinb 37:289-297, 1992.

Vitale GC: Interventional endoscopic retrograde cholangiopancreatography: state of the art. II. J R Coll Surg Edinb 37:357-368, 1992.

1993 Carlson MA et al: Routine or selective intraoperative cholangiography in laparoscopic cholecystectomy, J Laparoendosc Surg 3:27-33, 1993.

Cotton PB: Endoscopic retrograde cholangiopancreatography and laparoscopic cholecystectomy, Am J Surg 165:474-478, 1993.

Kuster GG, Gilroy S and Graefen M: Intraoperative cholangiography for laparoscopic cholecystectomy, Surg Gynecol Obstet 176:411-417, 1993.

Phillips EH: Routine versus selective intraoperative cholangiography, Am J Surg 165:505-507, 1993.

Shirai Z et al: The usefulness of endoscopic retrograde cholangiopancreatography in infants and small children, Am J Gastroenterol 88:536-541, 1993.

Thornton J and Axon A: Towards safer endoscopic retrograde cholangiopancreatography, Gut 34:721-724, 1993.

ALIMENTARY TRACT
General

For bibliographic citations before 1964, please see the fifth edition of this atlas. For citations from 1964 through 1974, see the sixth or seventh edition.

1978 Kressel HY et al: Computed tomographic evaluation of disorders affecting the alimentary tract, Radiology 129:451-455, 1978.

1979 Eisenberg RI and Hedgcock MW: The ellipse sign: an aid in the diagnosis of acute ulcers, J Can Assoc Radiol 30:26-29, 1979.

1980 Anderson W et al: Barium sulfate preparations for use in double-contrast examination of the upper gastrointestinal tract, Br J Radiol 53:1150-1159, 1980.

Cohen M et al: The use of metrizamide (Amipaque) to visualize the gastrointestinal tract in children: a preliminary report, Clin Radiol 31:635-641, 1980.

1981 Ominsky SH and Margulis AR: Radiographic examination of the upper gastrointestinal tract: a survey of current techniques, Radiology 139:11-17, 1981.

1982 Foley MJ, Ghahremani GG and Rogers LF: Reappraisal of contrast media used to detect upper gastrointestinal perforations: comparison of ionic water-soluble media with barium sulfate, Radiology 144:231-237, 1982.

Freeman H and Redmond P: Double-contrast examination of the gastrointestinal tract: an overview for the radiologic technologist, Radiol Technol 53:555-559, 1982.

Lee KR: Computed tomography of the gastrointestinal tract, CRC Crit Rev Diagn Imaging 18:121-165, 1982.

1983 Op den Orth JO: Imaging techniques for detection and extent determination of cancer, Prog Clin Biol Res 132:363-364, 1983.

Ott DJ and Gelfand DW: Gastrointestinal contrast agents: indications, uses, and risks, JAMA 249:2380-2384, 1983.

Ratcliffe JF: The use of ioxaglate in the pediatric gastrointestinal tract: a report of 25 cases, Clin Radiol 34:579-583, 1983.

Rauch RF et al: Can ultrasound examination of the pancreas and gallbladder follow a barium UGI on the same day? Invest Radiol 18:523-525, 1983.

1984 Trenkner SW and Laufer I: Double-contrast examination. I. Oesophagus, stomach and duodenum, Clin Gastroenterol 13:41-73, 1984.

1985 de Lange EE and Shaffer HA Jr: Barium suspension formulation for use with the bubbly barium method, Radiology 154:825, 1985.

1986 Frigerio A et al: Bromide as a relaxant for the radiological examination, Curr Med Res Opin 10:319-325, 1986.

McKee MW and Jurgens RW Jr: Barium sulfate products for roentgenographic examination of the gastrointestinal tract, Am J Hosp Pharm 43:145-148, 1986.

1987 Bury R: Radiological investigations of the abdomen and digestive tract, Practitioner 231:693-698, 1987.

Kastan DJ, Ackerman LV and Feczko PJ: Digital gastrointestinal imaging: the effect of pixel size on detection of subtle mucosal abnormalities, Radiology 162:853-856, 1987.

Robbins JA et al: A modification of the modified barium swallow, Dysphagia 2:83-86, 1987.

Rothe AJ, Young JW and Keramati B: The value of glucagon in routine barium investigations of the gastrointestinal tract, Invest Radiol 22:786-791, 1987.

1988 Belli AM and Williams MP: Graft versus host disease: findings on plain abdominal radiography, Clin Radiol 39:262-264, 1988.

Levine MS et al: Double-contrast upper gastrointestinal examination: technique and interpretation, Radiology 168:593-602, 1988.

1989 Carroll BA: US of the gastrointestinal tract, Radiology 172:605-608, 1989.

Munro TG: Brief communication: a simple model for teaching double-contrast examinations of the gastrointestinal tract, Can Assoc Radiol J 40:162-163, 1989.

Op den Orth JO: Use of barium in evaluation of disorders of the upper gastrointestinal tract: current status, Radiology 173:601-608, 1989.

Raptopoulos V: Technical principles in CT evaluation of the gut, Radiol Clin North Am 27:631-651, 1989.

1990 Foulner D: A sweet solution to a contrast problem, Br J Radiol 63:219-220, 1990.

Jeffrey RB Jr: Imaging of the gastrointestinal tract in the acquired immunodeficiency syndrome, Curr Opin Radiol 2:467-471, 1990.

Mittal A, Saha MM and Pandey KK: Peroral pneumo colon—a double contrast technique to evaluate distal ileum and proximal colon, Australas Radiol 34:72-74, 1990.

1991 Calzado A et al: Estimation of doses to patients from "complex" conventional x-ray examinations, Br J Radiol 64:539-546, 1991.

Long BW, Rafert JA and Cory D: Percutaneous feeding tube method for use in children, Radiol Technol 62:274-278, 1991.

Mitchell DG et al: Comparison of Kaopectate with barium for negative and positive enteric contrast at MR imaging, Radiology 181:475-480, 1991.

Suleiman OH et al: Tissue doses in the upper gastrointestinal fluoroscopy examination, Radiology 178:653-658, 1991.

Tart RP et al: Enteric MRI contrast agents: comparative study of five potential agents in humans, Magn Reson Imaging 9:559-568, 1991.

Tilcock C et al: Polymeric gastrointestinal MR contrast agents, J Magn Reson Imaging 1:463-467, 1991.

1992 Balzarini L et al: Magnetic resonance imaging of the gastrointestinal tract: investigation of baby milk as a low cost contrast medium, Eur J Radiol 15:171-174, 1992.

Dangman BC, Leichtner AM and Teele RL: The antegrade colonogram: extending the small bowel follow-through for children suspected of having colonic disease, Pediatr Radiol 22:573-576, 1992.

Macis G et al: Digital gastrointestinal radiography, Rays 17:482-502, 1992.

Mirowitz SA and Susman N: Use of nutritional support formula as a gastrointestinal contrast agent for MRI, J Comput Assist Tomogr 16:908-915, 1992.

Moeller G et al: Comparison of L-hyoscyamine, glucagon, and placebo for air-contrast upper gastrointestinal series, Gastrointest Radiol 17:195-198, 1992.

Takahashi M et al: Gastrointestinal examinations with digital radiography, Radiographics 12:969-978, 1992.

Tytgat GN and Fockens P: Endoscopic ultrasonography, Scand J Gastroenterol Suppl 192:80-87, 1992.

1993 Chou CK et al: Retrograde air insufflation in MRI: a technical note, Abdom Imaging 18:211-214, 1993.

Mirowitz SA: Contrast enhancement of the gastrointestinal tract on MR images using intravenous gadolinium-DTPA, Abdom Imaging 18:215-219, 1993.

Patten RM et al: Positive bowel contrast agent for MR imaging of the abdomen: phase II and III clinical trials, Radiology 189:277-283, 1993.

Esophagus

For bibliographic citations before 1964, please see the fifth edition of this atlas. For citations from 1964 through 1974, see the sixth or seventh edition.

1975 James AE: Barium or Gastrografin: which contrast media for diagnosis of esophageal tears? Gastroenterology 68:1103-1113, 1975.

Skucas J: Routine air-contrast examination of the esophagus, Radiology 115:482-484, 1975.

1977 House AJ and Griffiths GJ: The significance of an air oesophagogram visualized on conventional chest radiographs, Clin Radiol 28:301-305, 1977.

Proto AV and Lane EJ: Air in the esophagus: a frequent radiographic finding, AJR 129:433-440, 1977.

1978 Robbins AH et al: Revised radiologic concepts of the Barrett esophagus, Gastrointest Radiol 3:377-381, 1978.

1979 Hall FM: Esophageal communication with mediastinal cysts: classification and incidence (letter), Radiology 130:262, 1979.

1981 Balfe DM et al: Routine air-contrast esophagography during upper gastrointestinal examination, Radiology 139:739-741, 1981.

Cassel DM et al: Double-contrast esophagrams: the prone technique, Radiology 139:737-739, 1981.

Daffner RH: Computed tomography of the esophagus, CRC Crit Rev Diagn Imaging 14:191-242, 1981.

Humphrey A and Holland WG: Unsuspected esophageal foreign bodies, J Can Assoc Radiol 32:17-20, 1981.

1982 Lee SW: Double-contrast esophagography, Radiology 145:198, 1982.

1983 Hada M et al: Double-contrast cervical esophagography: use of a specially designed cup to aid double-contrast cervical esophagography, Radiat Med 1:211-215, 1983.

Haney PJ: Infant apnea: findings on the barium esophagram, Radiology 148:425-427, 1983.

Ott DJ, Gelfand DW and Wu WC: Sensitivity of single-contrast radiology in esophageal disease: a study of 240 patients with endoscopically verified abnormality, Gastrointest Radiol 8:105-110, 1983.

1984 Halvorsen RA and Thompson WA: Computed tomography of the gastroesophageal junction, CRC Crit Rev Diagn Imaging 21:183-228, 1984.

Levine MS et al: The tube esophagram: a technique for obtaining a detailed double-contrast examination of the esophagus, AJR 142:293-298, 1984.

Ott DJ et al: Cold barium suspensions in the clinical evaluation of the esophagus, Gastrointest Radiol 9:193-196, 1984.

Thompson WM et al: Computed tomography of the gastroesophageal junction: value of the left lateral decubitus view, J Comput Assist Tomogr 8:346-349, 1984.

1985 Cayea PD and Seltzer SE: A new barium paste for computed tomography of the esophagus, J Comput Assist Tomogr 9:214-216, 1985.

Cooper C et al: Ultrasound evaluation of the normal fetal upper airway and esophagus, J Ultrasound Med 4:343-346, 1985.

Maglinte DD et al: Flow artifacts in double-contrast esophagography, Radiology 157: 535-536, 1985.

Quint LE, Glazer GM and Orringer MB: Esophageal imaging by MR and CT: study of normal anatomy and neoplasms, Radiology 156:727-731, 1985.

Rohrmann CA Jr and Acheson MB: Esophageal perforation during double-contrast esophagram, AJR 145:283-284, 1985.

Samuelsson L and Tylen U: Delineation of the normal esophagus at computed tomography, Acta Radiol [Diagn] 26:665-669, 1985.

1986 Tash RR, Weingarten M and Geller M: An alternative technique for double-contrast esophagography (technical note), AJR 147:266-267, 1986.

1987 Robbins et al: A modification of the modified barium swallow, Dysphagia 2:83-86, 1987.

Yoong PM: A simple technique for double-contrast oesophagrams, Br J Radiol 60: 1021-1022, 1987.

1988 Conces DJ Jr, Tarver RD and Lappas JC: The value of opacification of the esophagus by low density barium, J Comput Assist Tomogr 12:202-205, 1988.

David EF: Drinking cup for double-contrast esophagography, Radiology 168:564-565, 1988.

Hill JW and DeLuca SA: Achalasia, Am Fam Physician 37:201-203, 1988.

Levine MS et al: Double-contrast upper gastrointestinal examination: technique and interpretation, Radiology 168:593-602, 1988.

1989 Goenka MK et al: Tube esophagogram: a better radiological technique for evaluation of esophageal diseases, Indian J Gastroenterol 8:45-46, 1989.

1990 Halvorsen RA Jr: The pharynx and esophagus, Curr Opin Radiol 2:385-393, 1990.

Levine MS, Rubesin SE and Ott DJ: Update on esophageal radiology, AJR 155:933-941, 1990.

Nakamura H et al: Esophageal varices evaluated by endoscopic ultrasonography: observation of collateral circulation during non-shunting operations, Surg Endosc 4:69-74, 1990.

1991 Chevallier JM et al: The thoracic esophagus: sectional anatomy and radiosurgical applications, Surg Radiol Anat 13:313-321, 1991.

Dawlatly EE, al-Arfaj AL and al-Azizi MA: Paediatric foreign bodies: the lessons of failure and near misses, J Laryngol Otol 105:755-759, 1991.

Halvorsen RA Jr: Imaging of the pharynx and the esophagus, Curr Opin Radiol 3:397-406, 1991.

Safford RE, Blackshear JL and Kapples EJ: Clinical utility of transesophageal echocardiography, South Med J 84:611-618, 1991.

1992 Kirks DR: Fluoroscopic catheter removal of blunt esophageal foreign bodies: a pediatric radiologist's perspective, Pediatr Radiol 22:64-65, 1992.

Pavone P et al: Gadopentetate dimeglumine-barium paste for opacification of the esophageal lumen on MR images, AJR 159:762-764, 1992.

1993 Baron TH and Richter JE: The use of esophageal function tests, Adv Intern Med 38:361-386, 1993.

Stomach and duodenum

For bibliographic citations before 1964, please see the fifth edition of this atlas. For citations from 1964 through 1974, see the sixth or seventh edition.

1975 Gelfand DW: The double contrast upper gastrointestinal examination in the Japanese style, Am J Gastroenterol 63:216-220, 1975.

Laufer I: A simple method for routine double contrast study of the upper gastrointestinal tract, Radiology 117:513-518, 1975.

Miller RE: The air contrast stomach examination: an overview, Radiology 117:743-744, 1975.

1976 Allan S and Coates RH: The accuracy of the barium meal in the diagnosis of carcinoma of the stomach, Australas Radiol 20:236-238, 1976.

Laufer I: Assessment of the accuracy of double contrast gastroduodenal radiology, Gastroenterology 71:874-878, 1976.

1977 Gold RP et al: The preliminary double contrast examination of the postoperative stomach, Radiology 124:297-305, 1977.

Mohammed SH and Hegedüs V: Double contrast examination of the stomach: an improved technique, Acta Radiol [Diagn] 18:249-256, 1977.

1978 Gohel VK and Laufer I: Double-contrast examination of postoperative stomach, Radiology 129:601-607, 1978.

James WB: The double-contrast meal: new high density barium sulphate powders, Br J Radiol 51:1020-1022, 1978.

Mäkelä P, Rossi I and Kormano M: Effect of glucagon on the double contrast examination of the stomach and duodenum, ROEFO 129:418-420, 1978.

1979 Freeny PC: Double contrast gastrography of the fundus and cardia: normal landmarks and their pathologic changes, AJR 133: 481-487, 1979.

Gourtsoyiannis NC and Nolan DJ: Combined fine needle percutaneous transhepatic cholangiography and hypotonic duodenography in obstructive jaundice, Clin Radiol 30:507-512, 1979.

Lukes PJ et al: Clinical significance of duodenal diverticula and value of hypotonic duodenography, Acta Radiol [Diagn] 20: 93-99, 1979.

1980 Smith JE et al: Demonstration of duodenal ulcers using micronized vs. non-micronized barium preparations, J Natl Med Assoc 72:863-864, 1980.

Virkkunen P and Lounatmaa K: On the differences between the BaSO4 particles and additives in media for the double contrast examination of the stomach, ROEFO 133:542-545, 1980.

Virkkunen P and Retulainen M: Visualization of the area gastrica in double contrast examination, Gastrointest Radiol 5:325-329, 1980.

1981 Crymes JE: Foreign bodies in the stomach and duodenum, J Fla Med Assoc 68:30-36, 1981.

Gallina F and Piga V: The insufflated barium meal technique: a new approach to the radiological examination of the upper digestive tract, Radiology 139:742-743, 1981.

Koehler RE et al: Evaluation of three effervescent agents for double-contrast upper gastrointestinal radiography, Gastrointest Radiol 6:111-114, 1981.

Virkkunen P and Kreula J: Effervescent agents in the double contrast examination of the stomach, Acta Radiol 22:261-265, 1981.

1982 Ott DJ, Gelfand DW and Wu WC: Detection of gastric ulcer: comparison of single- and double-contrast examination, AJR 139:93-97, 1982.

1983 Fraser GM and Earnshaw PM: The double-contrast barium meal: a correlation with endoscopy, Clin Radiol 34:121-131, 1983.

Kinnunen J et al: Effect of sodium bicarbonate pretreatment on barium coating of mucosa during double-contrast barium meal, ROEFO 139:199-201, 1983.

Soini I et al: Double-contrast examination of the stomach: 100 mm fluorography vs full-size radiography, Radiology 148:627-631, 1983.

Ziedses des Plantes BG Jr, Falke TH and Tjon TLB: CT of the stomach and duodenum. I. anatomy and postoperative stomach, Eur J Radiol 3:51-56, 1983.

1988 Hill JW and DeLuca SA: Achalasia, Am Fam Physician 37:201-203, 1988.

1989 Ghazi A and Washington M: Endoscopic retrograde cholangiopancreatography, endoscopic sphincterotomy, and biliary drainage, Surg Clin North Am 69:1249-1274, 1989.

Hammerman AM, Mirowitz SA and Susman N: The gastric air-fluid sign: aid in CT assessment of gastric wall thickening, Gastrointest Radiol 14:109-112, 1989.

Munro TG: Brief communication: a simple model for teaching double-contrast examinations of the gastrointestinal tract, Can Assoc Radiol J 40:162-163, 1989.

Op den Orth JO: Use of barium in evaluation of disorders of the upper gastrointestinal tract: current status, Radiology 173:601-608, 1989.

Scatarige JC and DiSantis DJ: CT of the stomach and duodenum, Radiol Clin North Am 27:687-706, 1989.

Worlicek H, Dunz D and Engelhard K: Ultrasonic examination of the wall of the fluid-filled stomach, JCU 17:5-14, 1989.

1990 al-Jurf A: A simplified technique to relax the sphincter of Oddi during intraoperative cholangiography, Surg Gynecol Obstet 170:163-164, 1990.

de Lange EE, Shaffer HA Jr and Croft BY: Radiographic examination of the stomach and duodenum: comparison of single-, double- and biphasic-contrast methods, Eur J Radiol 10:167-174, 1990.

Joharjy IA, Mustafa MA and Zaidi AJ: Fluid-aided sonography of the stomach and duodenum in the diagnosis of peptic ulcer disease in adult patients, J Ultrasound Med 9:77-84, 1990.

Martin DF and Tweedle DE: Retroperitoneal perforation during ERCP and endoscopic sphincterotomy: causes, clinical features and management, Endoscopy 22:174-175, 1990.

Op den Orth JO: The stomach and duodenum, Curr Opin Radiol 2:394-399, 1990.

Pandolfo I et al: Tumors of the ampulla diagnosed by CT hypotonic duodenography, J Comput Assist Tomogr 14:199-200, 1990.

1991 Suleiman OH et al: Tissue doses in the upper gastrointestinal fluoroscopy examination, Radiology 178:653-658, 1991.

1992 Moeller G et al: Comparison of L-hyoscyamine, glucagon, and placebo for air-contrast upper gastrointestinal series, Gastrointest Radiol 17:195-198, 1992.

Small intestine

For bibliographic citations before 1964, please see the fifth edition of this atlas. For citations from 1964 through 1974, see the sixth or seventh edition.

1977 Bryk D: Radiological evaluation of small bowel activity in the acute abdomen, CRC Crit Rev Diagn Imaging 10:99-128, 1977.

1979 Miller RE and Sellink JL: Enteroclyisis—the small bowel enema: how to succeed and how to fail, Gastrointest Radiol 4:469-483, 1979.

1980 Brun B and Hegedus V: Radiography of the small intestine with large amounts of cold contrast medium, Acta Radiol 21:65-70, 1980.

Glick SN et al: Meconium ileus equivalent: treatment with Hypaque enema, Diagn Imaging 49:149-152, 1980.

Nolan DJ and Piris J: Crohn's disease of the small intestine: a comparative study of the radiological and pathological appearances, Clin Radiol 31:591-596, 1980.

Novak D: Acceleration of small intestine contrast study by ceruletide, Gastrointest Radiol 5:61-65, 1980.

Robbins AH, Wetzner SM and Landy MD: Ceruletide-assisted examination of the small bowel, AJR 134:343-347, 1980.

Vallance R: An evaluation of the small bowel enema based on an analysis of 350 consecutive examinations, Clin Radiol 31:227-232, 1980.

1981 Ominsky SH et al: Radiographic evaluation of the upper gastrointestinal tract: survey of current techniques, Radiology 139:11, 1981.

Violon D et al: Improved retrograde ileography with glucagon, AJR 136:833-834, 1981.

1982 Fisher JK: Angled view of the distal small bowel, Radiology 144:417-418, 1982.

1983 Antes G and Lissner J: Double-contrast small-bowel examination with barium and methylcellulose, Radiology 148:37-40, 1983.

Fraser GM and Preston PG: The small bowel barium follow-through enhanced with an oral effervescent agent, Clin Radiol 34:673-679, 1983.

Law RL: The small bowel enema, Radiography 49:91-95, 1983.

Ratcliffe JF: The small bowel enema in children: a description of a technique, Clin Radiol 34:287-289, 1983.

Schnyder PA and Candardjis G: CT detection of benign and malignant abnormalities of the small bowel, Eur J Radiol 3:33-38, 1983.

1985 Fitzgerald EJ et al: Pneumocolon as an aid to small-bowel studies, Clin Radiol 36:633-637, 1985.

Op den Orth JO: Tubeless hypotonic duodenography with water: a simple aid in sonography of the pancreatic head, Radiology 154:826, 1985.

1986 Bloom SM, Philipps E and Paul RE Jr: Optimal double-contrast visualization of the posteriorly directed duodenal bulb, Radiology 161:549-550, 1986.

Frigerio A et al: Cimetropium bromide as a relaxant for the radiological examination of the stomach and duodenum, Curr Med Res Opin 10:319-325, 1986.

Ghahremani GG: Radiology of Meckel's diverticulum, CRC Crit Rev Diagn Imaging 26:1-43, 1986.

Monsein LH et al: Retrograde ileography: value of glucagon, Radiology 161:558-559, 1986.

Morewood DJ and Whitehouse GH: A comparison of three methods for performing barium follow-through, Br J Radiol 59:971-973, 1986.

Stringer DA et al: Value of the peroral pneumocolon in children, AJR 146:763-766, 1986.

1987 Bach DB: Single-contrast examination of the duodenum following enteroclysis, Can Assoc Radiol J 38:224-226, 1987.

Finke M: Enteroclysis: double contrast examination of the small bowel, Radiol Technol 59:143-149, 1987.

Freson M and Kottler RE: Anti-reflux small bowel enema tube, J Belge Radiol 70:49-51, 1987.

Maglinte DD et al: Small bowel radiography: how, when, and why, Radiology 163:297-305, 1987.

Nolan DJ and Cadman PJ: The small bowel enema made easy, Clin Radiol 38:295-301, 1987.

Thoeni RF: Radiography of the small bowel and enteroclysis: a perspective, Invest Radiol 22:930-936, 1987.

White MM and Bartram CI: Technique and evaluation of the double contrast ileostomy enema, Clin Radiol 38:621-624, 1987.

1988 Aspestrand F et al: Radiological appearance of the ampulla of Vater, Radiologe 28:533-535, 1988.

Barloon TJ et al: Small bowel enteroclysis survey, Gastrointest Radiol 13:203-206, 1988.

Belli AM and Williams MP: Graft versus host disease: findings on plain abdominal radiography, Clin Radiol 39:262-264, 1988.

Carlson HC: Small intestine enema, AJR 150:510-511, 1988.

Fraser GM and Adam RD: Modifications to the gas-enhanced small bowel barium follow-through, Clin Radiol 39:537-541, 1988.

Genkins SM and Dunnick NR: Small-bowel disease: categorization by CT examination, Invest Radiol 23:410-412, 1988.

Goei R, Lamers RJ and Lamers JJ: Enteroclysis: improved performance using a flow inducer, Acta Radiol 29:665-668, 1988.

Kobayashi S: A method for double contrast radiography of the small intestine, J Belge Radiol 71:365-374, 1988.

Schatzki R: Small intestinal enema. By Richard Schatzki, 1942 [classic article]. AJR 150:499-507, 1988.

Silverman PM et al: Computed tomography of the ileocecal region, Comput Med Imaging Graph 12:293-303, 1988.

1989 Baath L et al: Small bowel barium examination in children: diagnostic accuracy and clinical value as evaluated from 331 enteroclysis and follow-through examinations, Acta Radiol 30:621-626, 1989.

Chippindale AJ and Desai S: Experience with the Merck small bowel enema tube, Clin Radiol 40:518-519, 1989.

Colborn GL et al: The duodenum. III. Pathology, Am Surg 55:469-473, 1989.

Desaga JF: Visualization of the mucosal villi on double-contrast barium studies, Gastrointest Radiol 14:25-30, 1989.

Gilchrist AM and Mills JO: Radiological examination of the small bowel, Ulster Med J 58:124-130, 1989.

Merine D, fishman EK and Jones B: CT of the small bowel and mesentery, Radiol Clin North Am 27:707-715, 1989.

Op den Orth JO: Use of barium in evaluation of disorders of the upper gastrointestinal tract: current status, Radiology 173:601-608, 1989.

Scatarige JC and DiSantis DJ: CT of the stomach and duodenum, Radiol Clin North Am 27:687-706, 1989.

Thoeni RF: Small bowel, Curr Opin Radiol 1:60-65, 1989.

1990 Lappas JC and Maglinte DD: Enteroclysis—a technique for examining the small bowel, CRC Crit Rev Diagn Imaging 30:183-217, 1990.

Lappas JC and Maglinte DD: Small-bowel imaging, Curr Opin Radiol 2:400-406, 1990.

Richards DG and Stevenson GW: Laxatives prior to small bowel follow-through: are they necessary for a rapid and good-quality examination? Gastrointest Radiol 15:66-68, 1990.

Thoeni RF: The loop-torque maneuver: a method to facilitate intubation for enteroclysis, Gastrointest Radiol 15:325-326, 1990.

1991 Lappas JC and Maglinte DD: Imaging of the small bowel, Curr Opin Radiol 3:414-421, 1991.

Thoeni RF and Gould RG: Enteroclysis and small bowel series: comparison of radiation dose and examination time, Radiology 178:659-662, 1991.

Zalev AH and McLennan MK: Double-contrast hypotonic duodenography after enteroclysis, Can Assoc Radiol J 42:141-143, 1991.

1992 Dangman BC, Leichtner AM and Teele RL: The antegrade colonogram: extending the small bowel follow-through for children suspected of having colonic disease, Pediatr Radiol 22:573-576, 1992.

Lappas JC: Small bowel imaging, Curr Opin Radiol 4:32-38, 1992.

1993 Dixon PM, Roulston ME and Nolan DJ: The small bowel enema: a ten year review, Clin Radiol 47:46-48, 1993.

Klein HM and Gunther RW: Double contrast small bowel follow-through with an acid-resistant effervescent agent, Invest Radiol 28:581-585, 1993.

Mirowitz SA: Contrast enhancement of the gastrointestinal tract on MR images using intravenous gadolinium-DTPA, Abdom Imaging 18:215-219, 1993.

Large intestine

For bibliographic citations before 1964, please see the fifth edition of this atlas. For citations from 1964 through 1974, see the sixth or seventh edition.

1975 Meeroff JC, Jorgens J and Isenberg JI: The effect of glucagon on barium-enema examination, Radiology 115:5-7, 1975.

Rogers CW: Method for double contrast study of the colon, Med Radiogr Photogr 51:30-42, 1975.

1976 Goldstein HM and Miller MH: Air contrast colon examination in patients with colostomies, AJR 127:607-610, 1976.

Klawon M: Improved cleansing for colonic radiography, Radiol Technol 48:121-124, 1976.

Thijn CJ: Diagnostic radiology of the colon and rectum: review of the European radiological literature, Radiol Clin 45:396-401, 1976.

1977 Bakran A et al: Whole gut irrigation: an inadequate preparation for double contrast barium enema examination, Gastroenterology 73:28-30, 1977.

Laufer I: Air contrast studies of the colon in inflammatory bowel disease, CRC Crit Rev Diagn Imaging 9:421-427, 1977.

1978 Cargill A and Hately W: Technical note: preparation of the colon prior to radiology—a comparison of the effectiveness of castor oil, Dulcodos and X-Prep liquid, Br J Radiol 51:910-912, 1978.

1979 Gerson DE et al: The barium enema: evidence for proper utilization, Radiology 130:297-301, 1979.

Sarashina H et al: A new device for barium-enema examination following colostomy, Radiology 133:241-242, 1979.

Slanger A: Comparative study of a standardized senna liquid and castor oil in preparing patients for radiographic examination of the colon, Dis Colon Rectum 22:356-359, 1979.

1980 Clayton RS: A clean colon in one hour, Appl Radiol 9:669-677, 1980.

Dodds WJ: Rectal balloon catheters and the barium enema exam, Gastrointest Radiol 5:227-284, 1980.

Johanson JG: Oral administration of Amipaque in obstruction of the colon, Gastrointest Radiol 5:273-276, 1980.

1981 Gutwein I, Baer J and Holt PR: The effect of a formula diet on preparation of the colon for barium enema examination: impact on health care and costs, Arch Intern Med 141:993-996, 1981.

Kendrick RG: A comparison of four methods of bowel preparation for barium enema, Clin Radiol 32:95-97, 1981.

Pochaczevsky R: Irrigation kit for barium enemas, Appl Radiol 10:54, 1981.

1982 Fork FT, Lindstrom C and Ekelund G: The double-contrast examination in inflammatory large bowel disease: a prospective clinical, radiographic, and pathologic study, ROEFO 137:685-692, 1982.

Miller RE and Maglinte DD: Barium pneumocolon: technologist-performed "7 pump" method, AJR 139:1230-1232, 1982.

1983 Bartram CI, Preston DM and Lennard-Jones JE: The "air enema" in acute colitis, Gastrointest Radiol 8:61-65, 1983.

Eisenberg RL, Meyers PC and May ST: Optimum overhead views in double-contrast barium enema examinations, AJR 140:505-506, 1983.

Feczko PJ et al: Compensation filtration for decubitus radiography during double-contrast barium enema examinations, Radiology 149:848-850, 1983.

Foord KD, Morcos SK and Ward P: A comparison of mannitol and magnesium citrate preparations for double-contrast barium enema, Clin Radiol 34:309-312, 1983.

Fork FT, Lindstrom C and Ekelund G: Double-contrast examination in carcinoma of the colon and rectum: a prospective clinical series, Acta Radiol 24:177-188, 1983.

Fork FT, Lindstrom C and Ekelund G: Reliability of routine double-contrast examination (DCE) of the large bowel in polyp detection: a prospective clinical study, Gastrointest Radiol 8:163-172, 1983.

Johnson CD et al: Barium enemas of carcinoma of the colon: sensitivity of double- and single-contrast studies, AJR 140:1143-1149, 1983.

Mendoza FM and Gough DC: The radiologic anatomy of the puborectalis muscle, J Pediatr Surg 18:172-173, 1983.

Narasimharao KL et al: Prone cross-table lateral view: an alternative to the invertogram in imperforate anus, AJR 140:227-229, 1983.

Stoddart PG and Virjee J: The role of decubitus films in double-contrast barium enemas, Clin Radiol 34:681-682, 1983.

1984 Bartram CI, Mootoosamy IM and Lim IK: Washout versus non-washout (Picolax) preparation for double-contrast, Clin Radiol 35:143-146, 1984.

Gottesman L et al: The use of water-soluble contrast enemas in the diagnosis of acute lower left quadrant peritonitis, Dis Colon Rectum 27:84-88, 1984.

Lu CC: A new, safe balloon enema tip, Radiology 150:835-836, 1984.

Maglinte DD and Miller RE: Salvaging the failed pneumocolon: a simple maneuver, AJR 142:719-720, 1984.

Mahieu P, Pringo J and Bodart P: Defecography. I. Description of a new procedure and results in normal patients, Gastrointest Radiol 9:247-251, 1984.

Mintz MC and Seltzer SE: Oral administration of contrast medium for rectal opacification in pelvic computed tomography, J Comput Assist Tomogr 8:73-74, 1984.

Waneck R et al: Lateral distant view for improved accuracy in locating rectal tumors, AJR 142:519-523, 1984.

1985 Mitchell DG et al: Gastrografin versus dilute barium for colonic CT examination, J Comput Assist Tomogr 9:451-453, 1985.

Scheurich JW et al: Preparation for barium enema: comparison of a commercial formula, South Med J 78:838-840, 1985.

1986 Harding JA et al: Appendiceal filling by double-contrast barium enema, Gastrointest Radiol 11:105-107, 1986.

Roe AM, Bartolo DC and Mortensen NJ: Techniques in evacuation proctography in the diagnosis of intractable constipation and related disorders, J R Soc Med 79:331-333, 1986.

Schwab FJ et al: The barium enema scout film: cost effectiveness and clinical efficacy, Radiology 160:619-622, 1986.

Sprigg A et al: Compensation filtration in paediatric double-contrast barium enema, Clin Radiol 37:599-601, 1986.

1987 Feczko PJ and Halpert RD: Limiting overhead views in double-contrast colon examinations does not affect diagnostic accuracy, Gastrointest Radiol 12:175-177, 1987.

Fitzsimons P: A comparison of GoLYTELY and standard preparation for barium enema, J Can Assoc Radiol 38:109-112, 1987.

Gelfand DW, Ott DJ and Chen YM: Optimizing single- and double-contrast colon examinations, CRC Crit Rev Diagn Imaging 27:167-201, 1987.

Kastan DJ, Ackerman LV and Feczko PJ: Digital gastrointestinal imaging: the effect of pixel size on detection of subtle mucosal abnormalities, Radiology 162:853-856, 1987.

Olson DL et al: Efficacy of an intracassette filter for improved pneumocolon decubitus radiographs, AJR 148:547-549, 1987.

Smith C and Gardiner R: Efficacy of post-evacuation view after double-contrast barium enema, Gastrointest Radiol 12:268-270, 1987.

Thompson WM et al: Computed tomography of the rectum, Radiographics 7:773-807, 1987.

1988 Angelelli G and Macarini L: CT of the bowel: use of water to enhance depiction, Radiology 169:848-849, 1988.

Johnson JF: Pneumatosis in the descending colon: preliminary observations on the value of prone positioning, Pediatr Radiol 19:25-27, 1988.

Sato Y et al: Congenital anorectal anomalies: MR imaging, Radiology 168:157-162, 1988.

Stone EE and Conte FA: Glucagon-induced small bowel air reflux: degrading effects on double-contrast colon examination, Gastrointest Radiol 13:212-214, 1988.

1989 Boscaini M: Lower gastrointestinal endoultrasound, Surg Endosc 3:29-32, 1989.

Calandrino C: Barium enema procedure for the pediatric patient, Radiol Technol 60:209-213, 1989.

Campbell JB: Contrast media in intussusception, Pediatr Radiol 19:293-296, 1989.

Freimanis MG: Interval between cleansing enema and barium examination of the colon, Gastrointest Radiol 14:83-84, 1989.

Hirooka N et al: Sono-enterocolonography by oral water administration, JCU 17:585-589, 1989.

Johnson CD and Stephens DH: Computed tomography of the large bowel and appendix, Mayo Clin Proc 64:1276-1283, 1989.

Leighton DM and de Campo M: CT invertograms, Pediatr Radiol 19:176-178, 1989.

Munro TG: Brief communication: a simple model for teaching double-contrast examinations of the gastrointestinal tract, Can Assoc Radiol J 40:162-163, 1989.

Musk LC: Dynamic imaging of defaecation—the video proctogram, Radiogr Today 55:20-23, 1989.

Shorvon PJ et al: Defecography in normal volunteers: results and implications, Gut 30:1737-1749, 1989.

1990 Cooner WH: Reducing rectal injury from sonographically-guided transrectal needle biopsy of prostate: the "rule of finger," Urology 36:191-192, 1990.

Gelfand D: The colon, Curr Opin Radiol 2:407-412, 1990.

Gelfand DW and Ott DJ: Double-contrast enema: a simplified method for filling the colon, AJR 154:279-280, 1990.

Ginai AZ: Evacuation proctography (defecography): a new seat and method of examination, Clin Radiol 42:214-216, 1990.

Hughes T: A new positioning technique for barium enemas, Br J Radiol 63:723, 1990.

Marshall JB et al: Air-contrast barium enema studies after flexible proctosigmoidoscopy: randomized controlled clinical trial, Radiology 176:549-551, 1990.

Mittal A, Saha MM and Pandey KK: Peroral pneumo colon—a double contrast technique to evaluate distal ileum and proximal colon, Australas Radiol 34:72-74, 1990.

Rafert JA, Lappas JC and Wilkins W: Defecography: techniques for improved image quality, Radiol Technol 61:368-373, 1990.

Shiels WE II, Bisset GS III and Kirks DR: Simple device for air reduction of intussusception, Pediatr Radiol 20:472-474, 1990.

1991 Benson JT, Sumners JE and Pittman JS: Definition of normal female pelvic floor anatomy using ultrasonographic techniques, JCU 19:275-282, 1991.

Bradley MJ and Pilling D: The empty rectum on plain X-ray: does it have any significance in the neonate? Clin Radiol 43:265-267, 1991.

Gelfand DW, Chen MY and Ott DJ: Preparing the colon for the barium enema examination, Radiology 178:609-613, 1991.

Grosskreutz S et al: CT of the normal appendix, J Comput Assist Tomogr 15:575-577, 1991.

Kruyt RH et al: Normal anorectum: dynamic MR imaging anatomy, Radiology 179:159-163, 1991.

Ooms HW et al: Ultrasonography in the diagnosis of acute appendicitis, Br J Surg 78:315-318, 1991.

Stevens JK and Miller JI: Transrectal ultrasound: an aid to diagnosing prostate cancer, AORN J 53:1166-70, 1172-8, 1991.

Williams SM and Harned RK: Recognition and prevention of barium enema complications, Curr Probl Diagn Radiol 20:123-151, 1991.

1992 Bartram CI: Anal endosonography, Ann Gastroenterol Hepat (Paris) 28:185-189, 1992.

Bennett JD et al: Deep pelvic abscesses: transrectal drainage with radiologic guidance, Radiology 185:825-828, 1992.

Dangman BC, Leichtner AM and Teele RL: The antegrade colonogram: extending the small bowel follow-through for children suspected of having colonic disease, Pediatr Radiol 22:573-576, 1992.

Kruyt RH et al: Defecography and anorectal manometry, Eur J Radiol 15:166-170, 1992.

Mark DG, Rex DK and Lappas JC: Quality of air contrast barium enema performed the same day as incomplete colonoscopy with air insufflation, Gastrointest Endosc 38:693-695, 1992.

Papachrysostomou M et al: A method of computerised isotope dynamic proctography, Eur J Nucl Med 19:431-435, 1992.

Papachrysostomou M et al: Anal endosonography: which endoprobe? Br J Radiol 65:715-717, 1992.

Reading CC: Endorectal sonography, CRC Crit Rev Diagn Imaging 33:1-28, 1992.

Rioux M: Sonographic detection of the normal and abnormal appendix, AJR 158:773-778, 1992.

Smith DS et al: The role of abdominal x-rays in the diagnosis and management of intussusception, Pediatr Emerg Care 8:325-327, 1992.

Taccone A et al: New concepts in preoperative imaging of anorectal malformation: new concepts in imaging of ARM, Pediatr Radiol 22:196-199, 1992.

1993 Bray HJ and Mathieson JR: Quality of mucosal coating in double-contrast barium enema studies: comparison of two barium preparations, Can Assoc Radiol J 44:25-28, 1993.

Chou CK et al: Retrograde air insufflation in MRI: a technical note, Abdom Imaging 18:211-214, 1993.

Collier BD and Foley WD: Current imaging strategies for colorectal cancer, J Nucl Med 34:537-540, 1993.

Feuerbach S: Value of radiological techniques in the diagnosis and staging of colorectal carcinoma, Endoscopy 25:108-116, 1993.

Hageman MJ and Goei R: Cleansing enema prior to double-contrast barium enema examination: is it necessary? Radiology 187:109-112, 1993.

John H, Neff U and Kelemen M: Appendicitis diagnosis today: clinical and ultrasonic deductions, World J Surg 17:243-249, 1993.

Jorge JM et al: Cinedefecography and electromyography in the diagnosis of nonrelaxing puborectalis syndrome, Dis Colon Rectum 36:668-676, 1993.

Kaasbol MA, Hauge C and Nielsen MB: Case report: impaired rectal emptying caused by perineal herniation of the rectum: defaecographic demonstration using oblique projections, Br J Radiol 66:171-172, 1993.

Malone AJ Jr et al: Diagnosis of acute appendicitis: value of unenhanced CT, AJR 160:763-766, 1993.

Mirowitz SA: Contrast enhancement of the gastrointestinal tract on MR images using intravenous gadolinium-DTPA, Abdom Imaging 18:215-219, 1993.

Nielsen MB et al: Defecographic findings in patients with anal incontinence and constipation and their relation to rectal emptying, Dis Colon Rectum 36:806-809, 1993.

Papadaki PJ et al: A modified per os double-contrast examination of the colon in the elderly, ROFO 158:320-324, 1993.

Ramsden WH et al: Is the appendix where you think it is—and if not does it matter? Clin Radiol 47:100-103, 1993.

Steine S: Will it hurt, doctor? Factors predicting patients' experience of pain during double-contrast examination of the colon, BMJ 307:100, 1993.

Tham RT et al: Preparation of the colon for single- and double-contrast barium enema examination: a simplified method, Radiology 188:578-580, 1993.

Wald A et al: Scintigraphic studies of rectal emptying in patients with constipation and defecatory difficulty, Dig Dis Sci 38:353-358, 1993.

Walter DF et al: Colonic sonography: preliminary observations, Clin Radiol 47:200-204, 1993.

SINUS TRACTS AND FISTULAS

For bibliographic citations before 1964, please see the fifth edition of this atlas. For citations from 1964 through 1974, see the sixth or seventh edition.

1975 Weigen JF: A simple device for contrast injection of a cutaneous fistula, Radiology 116:733, 1975.

1976 Aragon GE and Eiseman B: Abdominal stab wounds: evaluation of sinography, J Trauma 16:792-797, 1976.

1977 Freidman PJ and Hellekant CA: Radiologic recognition of bronchopleural fistula, Radiology 124:289-295, 1977.

1979 Mikhael MA, Shackelford GD and Marchosky JA: Sinus tract injection: a technique for preoperative localization of cerebrospinal fluid fistula, Radiology 130:246-248, 1979.

1980 Aspestrand F: Demonstration of thoracic and abdominal fistulas by computed tomography, J Comput Assist Tomogr 4:536-537, 1980.

Sequeira FW and Smith WL: Seldinger sinography, Radiology 137:238-239, 1980.

1982 Frick MP et al: Evaluation of abdominal fistulas with computed body tomography, Comput Radiol 6:17-25, 1982.

1983 Elliot D and Tucker PE: The use of Silastic foam as an aid to sinography, Br J Radiol 56:128-130, 1983.

Hunter WN, Isenberg GW and Isenberg MS: Sinographic evaluation of fistulous lesions of the foot, J Foot Surg 22:97-99, 1983.

1984 Webb WR et al: Nuclear magnetic resonance of pulmonary arteriovenous fistula, J Comput Assist Tomogr 8:155-157, 1984.

1985 Johnson JF et al: Tracheoesophageal fistula: diagnosis with CT, Pediatr Radiol 15:134-135, 1985.

1986 Vaid YN and Shin MS: Computed tomography evaluation of tracheoesophageal fistula, J Comput Assist Tomogr 10:281-285, 1986.

1988 Chung JW et al: Computed tomography of cavernous sinus diseases, Neuroradiology 30:319-328, 1988.

Egund N and Pettersson H: Computed tomographic sinography in orthopedic radiology, Skeletal Radiol 17:96-100, 1988.

Hishikawa Y et al: Esophageal fistula: demonstration by CT, Radiat Med 6:115-116, 1988.

Narumi Y et al: Computed tomographic diagnosis of enterovesical fistulae: barium evacuation method, Gastrointest Radiol 13:233-236, 1988.

Rothman D and Dedick P: Vaginography for colovaginal fistula, N J Med 85:227-228, 1988.

Sundgren-Borgstrom P, Ekberg O and Lasson A: Radiology in cutaneous sinuses and fistulae, Radiologe 28:572-578, 1988.

Takahashi T et al: Localization of dural fistulas using metrizamide digital subtraction fluoroscopic cisternography, J Neurosurg 68:721-725, 1988.

1989 Koelbel G et al: Diagnosis of fistulae and sinus tracts in patients with Crohn disease: value of MR imaging, AJR 152:999-1003, 1989.

1992 Wittich GR: Radiologic treatment of abdominal abscesses with fistulous communications, Curr Opin Radiol 4:110-115, 1992.

1993 Outwater E and Schiebler ML: Pelvic fistulas: findings on MR images, AJR 160:327-330, 1993.

URINARY TRACT AND SUPRARENAL (ADRENAL) GLANDS

For bibliographic citations before 1964, please see the fifth edition of this atlas. For citations from 1964 through 1974, see the sixth or seventh edition.

1975 Elkin M: Radiology of the urinary tract: some consideration, Radiology 116:259-270, 1975.

Sane SM and Worshing RA Jr: Voiding cystourethrography: recent advances, Minn Med 58:148-153, 1975.

Sutton D: The radiological diagnosis of adrenal tumours, Br J Radiol 48:237-258, 1975.

1976 Lewis PJ et al: Routine intravenous urography in the investigation of hypertension, J Chronic Dis 29:785-791, 1976.

Pollack HM: Some limitations and pitfalls of excretory urography, J Urol 116:537-543, 1976.

1977 Feldman RA et al: Sensitive method for intraoperative roentgenograms, Urology 9:695-697, 1977.

Hall FM: Caudad angle view of the kidneys in excretory urography, Radiology 125:257, 1977.

Older RA: Radiologic approach to adrenal lesions, Urol Clin North Am 4:305-318, 1977.

Radhavaiah NV: Double contrast polycystography: new radiologic procedure, Urology 9:203-206, 1977.

1978 Harris RD et al: Value of computerized tomography in the evaluation of the kidney, Urology 12:729-732, 1978.

Hodgkinson CP: Metallic bead chain urethrocystography in preoperative and postoperative evaluation of gynecologic urologic problems, Clin Obstet Gynecol 21:725-735, 1978.

Karstaedt N et al: Computed tomography of the adrenal gland, Radiology 129:723-730, 1978.

Muir BB, Sinclair DJ and Duncan W: The role of radiology in the assessment of bladder cancer, Clin Radiol 29:479-485, 1978.

1979 Dixon GD, Brooks WH and Kunz A: Renal radiography with cephalad angulation and inspiration, Radiology 133:240-241, 1979.

Korobkin M et al: Computed tomography in the diagnosis of adrenal disease, AJR 132:231-238, 1979.

McCallum RW: The adult male urethra, normal anatomy, pathology, and method of urethrography, Radiol Clin North Am 17:227-244, 1979.

Newhouse JH and Pfister RC: The nephrogram, Radiol Clin North Am 17:213-226, 1979.

Thornbury JR: Perirenal anatomy: normal and abnormal, Radiol Clin North Am 17:321-331, 1979.

1980 Aadalen RJ et al: Exstrophy of the bladder: long-term results of bilateral posterior iliac osteotomies and two-stage anatomic repair, Clin Orthop 151:193-200, 1980.

Baert AL et al: Contrast enhancement by bolus technique in the CT examination of the kidney, Radiologe 20:279-287, 1980.

1981 Ala-Ketola L et al: Pre- and post-operative bead chain urethrocystography in female stress urinary incontinence, Acta Obstet Gynecol Scand 60:369-374, 1981.

Andresen J and Steenskov V: Radiologic and prognostic aspects of Wilms' tumors, Acta Radiol 22:353-358, 1981.

Bigongiari LR: The Seldinger approach to percutaneous nephrostomy and ureteral stent placement, Urol Radiol 2:141-145, 1981.

Elyaderani MK, Kalinowski D and Gabriele OF: Percutaneous nephrostomy by pigtail catheter in children, South Med J 74:421-423, 1981.

Hillman BJ et al: Recognition of bladder tumors by excretory urography, Radiology 138:319-323, 1981.

Sandler CM et al: Radiology of the bladder and urethra in blunt pelvic trauma, Radiol Clin North Am 19:195-211, 1981.

Saxton HM: Percutaneous nephrostomy—technique, Urol Radiol 2:131-139, 1981.

Simpson W, Cranage JD and Furness JA: Kidney size compared with vertebral height: importance of possible variations in normal values, Acta Radiol 22:321-324, 1981.

Wilson BC and Evill CA: Correlation of computed tomography and nephrography in quantitative comparison of urographic contrast agents, Radiology 140:127-134, 1981.

1982 Baert AL et al: Dynamic CT of the urogenital tract, Urol Radiol 4:69-83, 1982.

Dalla-Palma L and Rossi M: Advances in radiological anatomy of the kidney, Br J Radiol 55:404-412, 1982.

Jacobsen O and Andersen JT: Voiding cystourethrography with simultaneous pressureflow measurements: technique and findings in healthy elderly males, Acta Radiol [Diagn] (Stockh) 23:605-610, 1982.

Rubesin SE, Pollack HM and Banner MP: Simplified chain cystourethrography, Radiology 145:199-200, 1982.

Vela Navarrete R: Constant pressure flow-controlled antegrade pyelography, Eur Urol 8:265-268, 1982.

1983 Carroll PR and McAninch JW: Major bladder trauma: the accuracy of cystography, J Urol 130:887-888, 1983.

Leonidas JC et al: The one-film urogram in urinary tract infection in children, AJR 141:61-64, 1983.

McAlister WH and Griffith RC: Cystographic contrast media: clinical and experimental studies, AJR 141:997-1001, 1983.

Nepper-Rasmussen J, Nielsen PH and Kruse V: Pyeloureteral visualization using glucagon during intravenous urography, ROEFO 138:169-171, 1983.

Price RB et al: Biopsy of the right adrenal gland by the transhepatic approach, Radiology 148:566, 1983.

Roth D and Griffith DP: Operative renal radiography, Urology 21:60-61, 1983.

Thomsen HS: Pressures during retrograde pyelography, Acta Radiol [Diagn] (Stockh) 24:171-175, 1983.

Westby M, Ulmsten U and Asmussen M: Dynamic urethrocystography in women, Urol Int 38:329-336, 1983.

1984 Araki T and Murata Y: The VCU-pot: a new device for voiding cystourethrography, J Urol 132:266-267, 1984.

Gratale P: Advantages of table-top radiography in pediatric IVPs, Radiol Technol 55(3):34-37, 1984.

Gil Vernet JM and Culla A: Intraoperative three-dimensional radiography of the kidney (modified), J Urol 132:872-873, 1984.

Hillman BJ: Digital imaging of the kidney, Radiol Clin North Am 22:341-364, 1984.

Hu KN, Martz R and Vallandingham S: Use of the continuous-flush maneuver to prevent air bubbles on the urogram in a male patient: technical note, Urol Radiol 6:229, 1984.

Older RA et al: Diagnosis of adrenal disorders, Radiol Clin North Am 22:433-455, 1984.

Shafik A: Anal cystography: new technique of cystography, Urology 23:313-316, 1984.

Stephenson TF, Iyengar S and Rashid HA: Comparison of computerized tomography and excretory urography in detection and evaluation of renal masses, J Urol 131:11-13, 1984.

Thickman D et al: CT imaging of the unusually shaped bladder, J Comput Assist Tomogr 8:801-803, 1984.

Thompson WM et al: Iopamidol: new, nonionic contrast agent for excretory urography, AJR 142:329-332, 1984.

1985 Banner MP, Stein EJ and Pollack HM: Technical refinements in percutaneous nephroureterolithotomy, AJR 145:101-107, 1985.

Braun SD et al: Technique to facilitate percutaneous nephrostomy in non-obstructed kidneys, Cardiovasc Intervent Radiol 8:112-114, 1985.

Davies C et al: The radiological appearance of artificial urinary sphincters, Clin Radiol 36:95-99, 1985.

Davies P et al: The old and the new: a study of five contrast media for urography, Br J Radiol 58:593-597, 1985.

Jensen AR et al: Radiographic technique in the diagnosis of renal stones: a comparison of tomography and oblique projections, Eur J Radiol 5:125-126, 1985.

Krebs CA and Eisenberg RL: Ultrasound imaging of the adrenal glands, Radiol Technol 56:421-423, 1985.

Mendelson EB et al: Evaluation of the prone position in digital subtraction angiography, Cardiovasc Intervent Radiol 8:72-75, 1985.

Munro CJ: Computed tomography of the adrenal glands, Radiography 51:281-285, 1985.

Pahira JJ and Pollack HM: New self-developing film for intraoperative renal stone localization, Urology 25:418-424, 1985.

Sandler CM, Raval B and David CL: Computed tomography of the kidney, Urol Clin North Am 12:657-675, 1985.

Zollikofer CL et al: Antegrade pyelography, percutaneous nephrostomy and ureteral perfusion (Whitaker test) for the renal transplant recipient, ROEFO 142:193-200, 1985.

1986 Britton KE: Searching for the ideal kidney agent, Nucl Med Commun 7:145-147, 1986.

Kinnunen J: A 16-degree wedge pad for urography, Rontgenblatter 39:186-187, 1986.

Morewood DJ and Scally JK: An evaluation of the post-micturition radiograph following intravenous urography, Clin Radiol 37:499-500, 1986.

Newhouse JH: Image contrast and pulse sequences in urinary tract magnetic resonance imaging, Urol Radiol 8:120-126, 1986.

Uehara DT and Eisner RF: Indications for intravenous pyelography in trauma, Ann Emerg Med 15:266-269, 1986.

Uehara DT and Eisner RF: Indications for retrograde cystourethrography in trauma, Ann Emerg Med 15:270-272, 1986.

Westby M et al: Ovarian radiation dose during dynamic cystourethrography using videorecording and photofluorography, Acta Radiol [Diagn] (Stockh) 27:55-59, 1986.

Yoshioka S, Ochi K and Takeuchi M: Simple method for chain cystography, Urology 28:527-528, 1986.

Zeman RK et al: Computed tomography of renal masses: pitfalls and anatomic variants, Radiographics 6:351-372, 1986.

1987 Davies P et al: Comparison of two strengths of iohexol and iothalamate in urography, Urol Radiol 9:30-35, 1987.

Falke TH et al: Magnetic resonance imaging of the adrenal glands, Radiographics 7:343-370, 1987.

Imray TJ and Saigh JA: Importance of prone-position film during intravenous urography in detection of bladder tumors, Urology 29:228-230, 1987.

Kershaw A: Radionuclide imaging. 2. Renal studies in nuclear medicine, Radiography 53:244-248, 1987.

Lorentzen T, Dorph S and Hald T: Artificial urinary sphincters: radiographic evaluation, Acta Radiol 28:63-66, 1987.

Mawhinney RR and Gregson RH: Is ureteric compression still necessary? Clin Radiol 38:179-180, 1987.

Rhodes RA et al: Tomographic levels for intravenous urography: CT-determined guidelines, Radiology 163:673-675, 1987.

Roth D and Griffith DP: Operative renal radiography, Urology 135:12-13, 1987.

Sager EM et al: Contrast-enhanced computed tomography in carcinoma of the urinary bladder: the use of different injection methods, Acta Radiol 28:67-70, 1987.

Trewhella M et al: Dehydration, antidiuretic hormone and the intravenous urogram, Br J Radiol 60:445-447, 1987.

Yeh HC: Adrenal gland and nonrenal retroperitoneum, Urol Radiol 9:127-140, 1987.

1988 Egglin TK, Hahn PF and Stark DD: MRI of the adrenal glands, Semin Roentgenol 23:280-287, 1988.

Gattoni F et al: Digital subtraction angiography of the kidney, Br J Urol 62:214-218, 1988.

Glazer GM: MR imaging of the liver, kidneys, and adrenal glands, Radiology 166:303-312, 1988.

Katzberg RW: New and old contrast agents: physiology and nephrotoxicity, Urol Radiol 10:6-11, 1988.

Kumar R et al: Adrenal scintigraphy, Semin Roentgenol 23:243-249, 1988.

Mirk P et al: Sonography of normal lower ureters, JCU 16:635-642, 1988.

Mohammed SH: Suprapubic micturition cystourethrography, Acta Radiol 29:165-169, 1988.

Moulton JS: CT of the adrenal glands, Semin Roentgenol 23:288-303, 1988.

Penrose L: A new accessory for adult female voiding cystourethrograms, Radiol Technol 59:429-430, 1988.

Perri G et al: Digital subtraction radiography in voiding cystourethrography, Eur J Radiol 8:175-178, 1988.

Roberge Wade AP et al: The excretory urogram bowel preparation—is it necessary? J Urol 140:1473-1474, 1988.

Sfakianaki GN and Sfakianaki ED: Nuclear medicine in pediatric urology and nephrology, J Nucl Med 29:1287-1300, 1988.

Svetkey LP et al: Comparison of intravenous digital subtraction angiography and conventional arteriography in defining renal anatomy, Transplantation 45:56-58, 1988

Yeh HC: Ultrasonography of the adrenals, Semin Roentgenol 23:250-258, 1988.

1989   Ben Ami T, Rozin M and Hertz M: Imaging of children with urinary tract infection: a tailored approach, Clin Radiol 40:64-67, 1989.

Bretan PN Jr and Lorig R: Adrenal imaging: computed tomographic scanning and magnetic resonance imaging, Urol Clin North Am 16:505-513, 1989.

Dawson P: Contrast media for urography, Curr Opin Radiol 1:283-289, 1989.

Dedrick CG: Adrenal arteriography and venography, Urol Clin North Am 16:515-526, 1989.

Gordon D et al: Comparison of ultrasound and lateral chain urethrocystography in the determination of bladder neck descent, Am J Obstet Gynecol 160:182-185, 1989.

Gothlin JH: Is urethrocystography necessary? Curr Opin Radiol 1:293-296, 1989.

Keller MS: Renal Doppler sonography in infants and children, Radiology 172:603-604, 1989.

Marshall S, Pogany A and Anderson J: Technique for more rapid localization of distal ureteral obstruction, Urology 33:146-147, 1989.

Mushlin AI and Thornbury JR: Intravenous pyelography: the case against its routine use, Ann Intern Med 111:58-70, 1989.

Papanicolaou N, Pfister RC and Nocks BN: Percutaneous, large-bore, suprapubic cystostomy: technique and results, AJR 152:303-306, 1989.

Rickards D and Jones SN: Percutaneous interventional uroradiology, Br J Radiol 62:573-581, 1989.

Taylor A Jr and Halkar R: Radionuclide renal studies, Curr Opin Radiol 1:460-467, 1989.

Varpula M, Makinen J and Kiilholma P: Cough urethrocystography: the best radiological evaluation of female stress urinary incontinence? Eur J Radiol 9:191-194, 1989.

1990   Abdel-Dayem HM and Turoglu HT: Radionuclide renal studies, Curr Opin Radiol 2:834-843, 1990.

Beam C and Dunnick NR: Evaluation of iopamidol and diatrizoate in excretory urography: a double-blind clinical study, Invest Radiol 25:1255-1257, 1990.

Cervi PM et al: Digital radiography versus conventional radiography during excretory urography: our experience, Ann Radiol 33:321-328, 1990.

Dalla Palma L et al: Radiological anatomy of the kidney revisited, Br J Radiol 63:680-690, 1990.

Elkin M: Stages in the growth of uroradiology, Radiology 175:297-306, 1990.

Fanney DR, Casillas J and Murphy BJ: CT in the diagnosis of renal trauma, Radiographics 10:29-40, 1990.

Freeman LM: The radionuclide renal scan: past, present and future, Contrib Nephrol 79:87-98, 1990.

Hopper KD and Yakes WF: The posterior intercostal approach for percutaneous renal procedures: risk of puncturing the lung, spleen, and liver as determined by CT, AJR 154:115-117, 1990.

Klutke C et al: The anatomy of stress incontinence: magnetic resonance imaging of the female bladder neck and urethra, J Urol 143:563-566, 1990.

Lubat E and Weinreb JC: Magnetic resonance imaging of the kidneys and adrenals, Top Magn Reson Imaging 2:17-36, 1990.

Newhouse JH: MRI of the adrenal gland, Urol Radiol 12:1-6, 1990.

Rafal RB, Kosovsky PA and Markisz JA: Magnetic resonance imaging of the adrenal glands: a subject review, Clin Imaging 14:1-10, 1990.

Rasmussen F et al: Intravenous urography with a new non-ionic contrast media in a clinical phase III study: iopentol vs iohexol, Clin Radiol 41:37-41, 1990.

Redman JF: Female urologic diagnostic techniques, Urol Clin North Am 17:5-8, 1990.

1991   Bailey SR, Tyrrell PN and Hale M: A trial to assess the effectiveness of bowel preparation prior to intravenous urography, Clin Radiol 44:335-337, 1991.

Banerjee B and Brett I: Ultrasound diagnosis of horseshoe kidney, Br J Radiol 64:898-900, 1991.

Beierwaltes WH: Endocrine imaging: parathyroid, adrenal cortex and medulla, and other endocrine tumors. II. J Nucl Med 32:1627-1639, 1991.

Clorius JH and Irngartinger G: Renal studies in nuclear medicine, Curr Opin Radiol 3:828-839, 1991.

Debatin JF et al: Selective use of low-osmolar contrast media, Invest Radiol 26:17-21, 1991.

Frank JA et al: Functional MR of the kidney, Magn Reson Med 22:319-323, 1991.

Hjelm-Karlsson K: Dispelling the fear of the unknown. Effects of information to patients undergoing urography, Acta Radiol Suppl (Stockh) 375:7-29, 1991.

Hricak H et al: Female urethra: MR imaging, Radiology 178:527-535, 1991.

Hughes TH and Hine AL: The most advantageous timing of external ureteric compression during intravenous urography, Br J Radiol 64:314-317, 1991.

Kirshy DM et al: Autourethrography, Radiology 180:443-445, 1991.

McNicholas MM, Griffin JF and Cantwell DF: Ultrasound of the pelvis and renal tract combined with a plain film of abdomen in young women with urinary tract infection: can it replace intravenous urography? A prospective study, Br J Radiol 64:221-224, 1991.

Mutgi A, Williams JW and Nettleman M: Renal colic: utility of the plain abdominal roentgenogram, Arch Intern Med 151:1589-1592, 1991.

Osca JM et al: Unusual foreign bodies in the urethra and bladder, Br J Urol 68:510-512, 1991.

Rosenfield AT: Artifacts in urinary tract ultrasonography, Urol Radiol 12:228-232, 1991.

Todd AW et al: Plasma osmolality, iodine concentration and urographic images following high and low osmolar contrast media, Clin Radiol 43:331-336, 1991.

Vydareny KH et al: Diagnostic usefulness of post-void film in intravenous urogram, Urology 38:170-175, 1991.

Yamashita T and Ogawa A: Transperineal ultrasonic voiding cystourethrography using a newly devised chair, J Urol 146:819-823, 1991.

1992   Abramson AF and Mitty HA: Update on interventional treatment of urinary obstruction, Urol Radiol 14:234-236, 1992.

Archer RJ: Intrathoracic right kidney diagnosed by ultrasound, Australas Radiol 36:271-273, 1992.

Bagley DH, Liu JB and Goldberg BB: Use of endoluminal ultrasound of the ureter, Semin Urol 10:194-198, 1992.

Cameron HA et al: Investigation of selected patients with hypertension by the rapid-sequence intravenous urogram, Lancet 339:658-661, 1992.

Choyke PL: The urogram: are rumors of its death premature? Radiology 184:33-34, 1992.

Cleveland RH et al: Voiding cystourethrography in children: value of digital fluoroscopy in reducing radiation dose, AJR 158:137-142, 1992.

Danza FM et al: Digital genitourinary radiography, Rays 17:516-524, 1992.

Gavant ML, Ellis JV and Klesges LM: Maximizing opacification during excretory urography: effect of low-osmolarity contrast media, Can Assoc Radiol J 43:111-115, 1992.

Gavant ML and Siegle RL: Iodixanol in excretory urography: initial clinical experience with a nonionic, dimeric (ratio 6:1) contrast medium. Work in progress, Radiology 183:515-518, 1992.

Heyns CF and van Gelderen WF: Three-dimensional computed tomographic imaging of the pelvicaliceal system: analysis of factors influencing image quality, Eur Urol 22:298-302, 1992.

Jahn H and Muller Spath R: Ioversol in intravenous excretory urography: evaluation of radiographic quality, patient tolerance and safety in four clinical studies, Ann Radiol Paris 35:297-302, 1992.

Kim SH and Han MC: Reversed contrast-urine levels in urinary bladder: CT findings, Urol Radiol 13:249-252, 1992.

Loberant N: Emergency imaging of the urinary tract, Emerg Med Clin North Am 10:59-91, 1992.

Perri G et al: Digital subtraction radiography in pediatric cystourethrography, Child Nephrology & Urology 12:40-42, 1992.

Rickwood AM et al: Current imaging of childhood urinary infections: prospective survey, BMJ 304:663-665, 1992.

Shackelford GD, Kees-Folts D and Cole BR: Imaging the urinary tract, Clin Perinatol 19:85-119, 1992.

Sortland O et al: Iopentol in urography: a clinical comparison between iopentol and metrizoate including delayed reactions, Acta Radiol 33:368-373, 1992.

Stubbs DM: Emergency radiology of urinary tract injuries, Am J Emerg Med 10:242-250, 1992.

Thomsen HS and Dorph S: Interventional uroradiology today, Ann Med 24:167-169, 1992.

Thomsen HS, Vestergaard A and Dorph S: Quality of urography and renal clearance of ionic and nonionic contrast media, Invest Radiol 27:40-44, 1992.

Yoder IC and Papanicolaou N: Imaging the urethra in men and women, Urol Radiol 14:24-28, 1992.

Zoeller G et al: Digital radiography in urologic imaging: radiation dose reduction on urethrocystography, Urol Radiol 14:56-58, 1992.

1993 Chang TS, Bohm Velez M and Mendelson EB: Nongynecologic applications of transvaginal sonography, AJR 160:87-93, 1993.

Ditchfield MR and De Campo JF: Is the preliminary film necessary prior to the micturating cystourethrogram in children? Abdom Imaging 18:191-192, 1993.

Eschelman DJ and Sullivan KL: Exchange of an occluded nephroureteral stent by using a snare, Radiology 186:894-895, 1993.

Fultz PJ, Hampton WR and Totterman SM: Computed tomography of pyonephrosis, Abdom Imaging 18:82-87, 1993.

George CD et al: Bowel preparation before intravenous urography: is it necessary? Br J Radiol 66:17-19, 1993.

Rossleigh MA, Leighton DM and Farnsworth RH: Diuresis renography: the need for an additional view after gravity-assisted drainage, Clin Nucl Med 18:210-213, 1993.

Weese DL, Greenberg HM and Zimmern PE: Contrast media reactions during voiding cystourethrography or retrograde pyelography, Urology 41:81-84, 1993.

Zerin JM: Impact of contrast medium temperature on bladder capacity and cystographic diagnosis of vesicoureteral reflux in children, Radiology 187:161-164, 1993.

FEMALE REPRODUCTIVE SYSTEM
General

For bibliographic citations before 1964, please see the fifth edition of this atlas. For citations from 1964-1974, see the sixth or seventh edition.

1986 Haynor DR et al: Changing appearance of the normal uterus during the menstrual cycle: MR studies, Radiology 161:459-462, 1986.

1987 Carroll R and Gombergh R: Empty-bladder (hysterographic) view on US for evaluation of intrauterine devices. Work in progress, Radiology 163:822-823, 1987.

Granberg S and Wikland M: Comparison between endovaginal and transabdominal transducers for measuring ovarian volume, J Ultrasound Med 6:649-653, 1987.

Timor-Tritsch IE and Rottem S: Transvaginal ultrasonographic study of the fallopian tube, Obstet Gynecol 70:424-428, 1987.

1988 Birnholz J and Hrozencik D: Technical improvement for ultrasonic study of the endometrium, Int J Fertil 33:194-200, 1988.

Davison GB and Leeton J: A case of female infertility investigated by contrast-enhanced echo-gynecography, JCU 16:44-47, 1988.

Mintz MC and Grumbach K: Imaging of congenital uterine anomalies, Semin Ultrasound CT MR 9:167-174, 1988.

1989 Clark RL and Keefe B: Infertility: imaging of the female, Urol Radiol 11:233-237, 1989.

Jansen CA and van Os HC: Value and limitations of vaginal ultrasonography: a review, Hum Reprod 4:858-868, 1989.

McCarthy S: MR imaging of the uterus, Radiology 171:321-322, 1989.

Shapiro BS and DeCherney AH: Ultrasound and infertility, J Reprod Med 34:151-155, 1989.

1990 Winfield AC, Fleischer AC and Moore DE: Diagnostic imaging of fertility disorders, Curr Probl Diagn Radiol 19:1-38, 1990.

1991 Asztely M et al: Radiological study of changes in the pelvis in women following proctocolectomy, Int J Colorectal Dis 6:103-107, 1991.

Benson JT, Sumners JE and Pittman JS: Definition of normal female pelvic floor anatomy using ultrasonographic techniques, JCU 19:275-282, 1991.

Clewes J and Swallow J: The development of protocols for trans-vaginal sonography, Radiogr Today 57:19-22, 1991.

Hadar H et al: Air in vagina: indicator of intrapelvic pathology on CT, Acta Radiol 32:170-173, 1991.

Shatzkes DR, Haller JO and Velcek FT: Imaging of uterovaginal anomalies in the pediatric patient, Urol Radiol 13:58-66, 1991.

1992 Maroulis GB, Parsons AK and Yeko TR: Hydrogynecography: a new technique enables vaginal sonography to visualize pelvic adhesions and other pelvic structures, Fertil Steril 58:1073-1075, 1992.

Nasri MN: Transvaginal versus transrectal sonography in postmenopausal women, Br J Obstet Gynaecol 99:932-933, 1992.

Olson MC et al: MR imaging of the female pelvic region, Radiographics 12:445-465, 1992.

Schiller VL and Grant EG: Doppler ultrasonography of the pelvis, Radiol Clin North Am 30:735-742, 1992.

1993 Balen FG et al: Three-dimensional reconstruction of ultrasound images of the uterine cavity, Br J Radiol 66:588-591, 1993.

Chang TS, Bohm-Velez M and Mendelson EB: Nongynecologic applications of transvaginal sonography, AJR 160:87-93, 1993.

Hricak H: Current trends in MR imaging of the female pelvis, Radiographics 13:913-919, 1993.

Hricak H and Kim B: Contrast-enhanced MR imaging of the female pelvis, J Magn Reson Imaging 3:297-306, 1993.

Woodward PJ, Wagner BJ and Farley TE: MR imaging in the evaluation of female infertility, Radiographics 13:293-310, 1993.

Hysterosalpingography

For bibliographic citations before 1964, please see the fifth edition of this atlas. For citations from 1964 through 1974, see the sixth or seventh edition.

1975 Schwartz PE et al: Routine use of hysterosalpingography in endometrial carcinoma and postmenopausal bleeding, Obstet Gynecol 45:378-384, 1975.

1976 Lapido OA: Tests of tubal patency: comparison of laparoscopy and hysterosalpingography, Br Med J 2:1297-1298, 1976.

Mayall EM and Mayall GF: The radiology of the intrauterine contraceptive device, Clin Radiol 27:541-543, 1976.

1977 Markham GC, Bottomley JP and Ansell G: Dimer X in hysterosalpingography, Br J Radiol 50:101-104, 1977.

1978 Seppänen S, Lehtinen E and Holli H: Radiation dose in hysterosalpingography: modern 100 mm fluorography vs. fullscale radiography, Radiology 127:377-380, 1978.

1979 Cameron DD, Stirna MJ and Henry S: Hysterosalpingography using a Foley catheter, Radiology 131:542, 1979.

Horwitz RC et al: A radiological approach to infertility: hysterosalpingography, Br J Radiol 52:255-262, 1979.

Spring DB, Wilson RE and Arronet GH: Foley catheter hysterosalpingography: a simplified technique for investigating infertility, Radiology 131:543-544, 1979.

Stiris G and Andrew E: Hysterosalpingography with Amipaque, Radiology 130:795-796, 1979.

1980 Bateman BG, Nunley WC Jr and Kitchin JD III: Intravasation during hysterosalpingography using oilbase contrast media, Fertil Steril 34:439-443, 1980.

Kasby CB: Hysterosalpingography: an appraisal of current indications, Br J Radiol 53:279-282, 1980.

Spring DB and Boll DA: Prone hysterosalpingography, Radiology 136:235-236, 1980.

1981 Ekelund L and Karp W: Comparison between two radiographic contrast media for hysterosalpingography, Acta Obstet Gynecol Scand 60:393-394, 1981.

Kormano MJ, Goske MJ and Hamlin DJ: Attenuation and contrast enhancement of gynecologic organs and tumors in CT, Eur J Radiol 1:307-311, 1981.

Philipsen T and Hansen BB: Comparative study of hysterosalpingography and laparoscopy in infertile patients, Acta Obstet Gynecol Scand 60:149-151, 1981.

Yoder IC and Pfister RC: Angiodilator technique for hysterosalpingography in cervical os stenosis, Radiology 139:228-229, 1981.

1982 Montanari L, Bulgarelli C and Marra A: A comparison of hysterosalpingography and laparoscopy in the investigation of infertility, Clin Exp Obstet Gynecol 9:66-68, 1982.

Schutte HE: Comparative study: Endographine (diatrizoate), Vasurix polyvidone (acetrizoate), Dimer-x (iocarmate) and Hexabrix (ioxaglate) in hysterosalpingography, Diagn Imaging 51:277-283, 1982.

Totani R: The value of high-pressure hysterosalpingography with new cannula, Reproduction 6:167-177, 1982.

Winfield AC et al: Hysterosalpingography: comparison of Conray 60 and Sinografin, AJR 138:559, 1982.

1983 Cooper RA, Jabamoni R and Pieters CH: Fertility rate after hysterosalpingography with Sinografin, AJR 141:105-106, 1983.

Duff DE et al: Hysterosalpingography and laparoscopy: a comparative study, AJR 141:761-763, 1983.

Holst N, Abyholm T and Borgersen A: Hysterosalpingography in the evaluation of infertility, Acta Radiol [Diagn] 24:253-257, 1983.

Siegler AM: Hysterosalpingography, Fertil Steril 40:139-158, 1983.

Tolino A, Chiacchio G and Ciaramella F: Hysterosalpingography and laparoscopy in the study of infertile women, Clin Exp Obstet Gynecol 10:191-192, 1983.

1984 Austin RM et al: Catheter hysterosalpingography, Radiology 151:249, 1984.

Dan SJ and Goldstein MS: Fallopian tube occlusion with silicone: radiographic appearance, Radiology 151:603-605, 1984.

LaSala GB and Ghirardini G: Simple and practical technique for hysterosalpingography, Int J Fertil 29:33-34, 1984.

Richman TS et al: Fallopian tubal patency assessed by ultrasound following fluid injection. Work in progress, Radiology 152:507-510, 1984.

Snowden EU, Jarrett JC II and Dawood MY: Comparison of diagnostic accuracy of laparoscopy, hysteroscopy, and hysterosalpingography in evaluation of female infertility, Fertil Steril 41:709-713, 1984.

Winfield AC et al: Hexabrix as a contrast agent for hysterosalpingography, Radiology 152:232-233, 1984.

1985 Beyth Y, Navot D and Lax E: A simple improvement in the technique of hysterosalpingography achieving optimal imaging and avoiding possible complications, Fertil Steril 44:543-545, 1985.

1986 Alper MM et al: Quarrington. Pregnancy rates after hysterosalpingography with oil- and water-soluble contrast media, Obstet Gynecol 68:6-9, 1986.

el Kady AA et al: The value of x-ray with uterine sound in the diagnosis of IUDs with missing tails, Adv Contracept 2:161-167, 1986.

Kushner DC et al: Radiation dose reduction during hysterosalpingography: an application of scanning-beam digital radiography, Radiology 161:31-33, 1986.

La Sala GB et al: Simple and practical technique for hysterosalpingography: results obtained in 564 cases, Acta Eur Fertil 17:365-367, 1986.

1987 Bateman BG et al: Utility of the 24-hour delay hysterosalpingogram film, Fertil Steril 47:613-617, 1987.

Nielsen DT, Rasmussen F and Justesen P: A comparative study of hysterosalpingography and endoscopy/laparotomy in infertile patients, Eur J Radiol 7:260-262, 1987.

Nunley WC Jr et al: Intravasation during hysterosalpingography using oil-base contrast, Obstet Gynecol 70:309-312, 1987.

Rasmussen F, Justesen P and Tonner Nielsen D: Therapeutic value of hysterosalpingography with lipiodol ultra fluid, Acta Radiol 28:319-322, 1987.

Sholkoff SD: Balloon hysterosalpingography catheter, AJR 149:995-996, 1987.

1988 de Boer AD et al: Oil or aqueous contrast media for hysterosalpingography: a prospective, randomized, clinical study, Eur J Obstet Gynecol Reprod Biol 28:65-68, 1988.

Margolin FR: A new cannula for hysterosalpingography, AJR 151:729-730, 1988.

Wolf DM and Spataro RF: The current state of hysterosalpingography, Radiographics 8:1041-1058, 1988.

1989 Loy RA, Weinstein FG and Seibel MM: Hysterosalpingography in perspective: the predictive value of oil-soluble versus water-soluble contrast media, Fertil Steril 51:170-172, 1989.

Reshef E et al: Comparison between 1-hour and 24-hour follow-up radiographs in hysterosalpingography using oil based contrast media, Fertil Steril 52:753-755, 1989.

van der Weiden RM and van Zijl J: Radiation exposure of the ovaries during hysterosalpingography: is radionuclide hysterosalpingography justified? Br J Obstet Gynaecol 96:471-472, 1989.

1990 Thurmond AS and Rosch J: Fallopian tubes: improved technique for catheterization, Radiology 174:572-573, 1990.

Thurmond AS, Uchida BT and Rosch J: Device for hysterosalpingography and fallopian tube catheterization, Radiology 174:571-572, 1990.

1991 Brokensha C and Whitehouse G: A comparison between iotrolan, a non-ionic dimer, and a hyperosmolar contrast medium, Urografin, in hysterosalpingography, Br J Radiol 64:587-590, 1991.

Gurgan T et al: Radionuclide hysterosalpingography: a simple and potentially useful method of evaluating tubal patency, J Reprod Med 36:789-792, 1991.

Karasick S: Hysterosalpingography, Urol Radiol 13:67-73, 1991.

Lindequist S et al: Diagnostic quality and complications of hysterosalpingography: oil- versus water-soluble contrast media—a randomized prospective study, Radiology 179:69-74, 1991.

Meyerovitz MF: Hysterosalpingography and fallopian tube cannulation: use of a double-balloon introducing catheter, Radiology 181:901-902, 1991.

Peters AJ and Coulam CB: Hysterosalpingography with color Doppler ultrasonography, Am J Obstet Gynecol 164:1530-1532, 1991.

Rasmussen F et al: Therapeutic effect of hysterosalpingography: oil- versus water-soluble contrast media—a randomized prospective study, Radiology 179:75-78, 1991.

Schlief R and Deichert U: Hysterosalpingo-contrast sonography of the uterus and fallopian tubes: results of a clinical trial of a new contrast medium in 120 patients, Radiology 178:213-215, 1991.

Venezia R and Zangara C: Echohysterosalpingography: new diagnostic possibilities with S HU 450 Echovist, Acta Eur Fertil 22:279-282, 1991.

Yoder IC and Hall DA: Hysterosalpingography in the 1990s, AJR 157:675-683, 1991.

1992 Gleicher N et al: Standardization of hysterosalpingography and selective salpingography: a valuable adjunct to simple opacification studies, Fertil Steril 58:1136-1141, 1992.

Hofmann GE, Scott RT and Rosenwaks Z: Common technical errors in hysterosalpingography, Int J Fertil 37:41-43, 1992.

Krysiewicz S: Infertility in women: diagnostic evaluation with hysterosalpingography and other imaging techniques, AJR 159:253-261, 1992.

Maubon A et al: Fallopian tube recanalization by selective salpingography: an alternative to more invasive techniques? Hum Reprod 7:1425-1428, 1992.

Pellerito JS et al: Diagnosis of uterine anomalies: relative accuracy of MR imaging, endovaginal sonography, and hysterosalpingography, Radiology 183:795-800, 1992.

Rajah R, McHugo JM and Obhrai M: The role of hysterosalpingography in modern gynaecological practice, Br J Radiol 65:849-851, 1992.

Rouanet JP et al: Gynecologic interventional radiology, Acta Eur Fertil 23:69-77, 1992.

Yang KT et al: Radionuclide hysterosalpingography with technetium-99m-pertechnetate: application and radiation dose to the ovaries, J Nucl Med 33:282-286, 1992.

Yoder IC: Diagnosis of uterine anomalies: relative accuracy of MR imaging, endovaginal sonography, and hysterosalpingography, Radiology 185:343, 1992.

1993 Balen FG et al: Ultrasound contrast hysterosalpingography—evaluation as an outpatient procedure, Br J Radiol 66:592-599, 1993.

Brundin J et al: Developmental steps for radionuclide hysterosalpingography, Gynecol Obstet Invest 36:34-38, 1993.

Jacobson A and Uszler JM: A simplified technique for radionuclide hysterosalpingography, J Assist Reprod Gen 10:4-10, 1993.

Rosenwaks Z, Sultan KM and Davis OK: A novel technique for cervical cannulation during hysterosalpingography, Fertil Steril 59:1329-1330, 1993.

Tyrrell PN, McHugo JM and Hale M: Patients' perception of the hysterosalpingogram: the initial stages of the audit cycle, Br J Radiol 66:103-107, 1993.

Vaginography

For bibliographic citations before 1964, please see the fifth edition of this atlas. For citations from 1964 through 1974, see the sixth or seventh edition.

1982 Cooper RA: Vaginography: a presentation of new cases and subject review, Radiology 143:421-425, 1982.

1988 Hricak H, Chang YC and Thurnher S: Vagina: evaluation with MR imaging. I. Normal anatomy and congenital anomalies, Radiology 169:169-174, 1988.

Rothman D and Dedick P: Vaginography for colovaginal fistula, N J Med 85:227-228, 1988.

1991 Asztely M et al: Radiological study of changes in the pelvis in women following proctocolectomy, Int J Colorectal Dis 6:103-107, 1991.

Pelvic pneumography

For bibliographic citations before 1964, please see the fifth edition of this atlas. For citations from 1964 through 1974, see the sixth or seventh edition.

1976 Guistini FG: Pelvic pneumogynecography, W V Med J 72:197-204, 1976.

1981 Kolawole TM and Aimakhu VE: Pelvic pneumography in the investigation of patients with primary amenorrhoea, Diagn Imaging 50:20-28, 1981.

Fetography and placentography

For bibliographic citations before 1964, please see the fifth edition of this atlas. For citations from 1964 through 1974, see the sixth or seventh edition.

1976 Agüero O and Zighelboim I: Diagnostic radiology of fetal abnormalities, Int J Gynecol Obstet 14:314-319, 1976.

1977 Edelstone DI: Placental localization by ultrasound, Clin Obstet Gynecol 20:285-296, 1977.

Ogita S, Kamei T and Sugawa T: Estimation of fetal weight by fetography, Am J Obstet Gynecol 127:37-42, 1977.

1979 Panigel M, Leo FP and Donner MW: In vitro computed tomography of the human placenta, J Comput Assist Tomogr 3:181-183, 1979.

1980 Griscom NT and Driscoll SG: Radiography of stillborn fetuses and infants dying at birth, AJR 134:485-489, 1980.

Shiono PH, Chung CS and Myrianthopoulos NC: Preconception radiation, intrauterine diagnostic radiation, and childhood neoplasia, JNCI 65:681-686, 1980.

1981 Balsam D and Weiss RR: Amniography in prenatal diagnosis, Radiology 141:379-385, 1981.

1982 Hisley JC and Mangum C: Placental location in pregnancies following cesarean section, JCU 10:427-428, 1982.

Mossman KL and Hill LT: Radiation risks in pregnancy, Obstet Gynecol 60:237-242, 1982.

Schussman LC and Lutz LJ: Hazards and uses of prenatal diagnostic x-radiation, J Fam Pract 14:473-480, 1982.

Syed IB and Samols E: Medical x-ray exposure of the human embryo and fetus, Health Phys 42:61-64, 1982.

1983 Brent RL: The effects of embryonic and fetal exposure to x-ray, microwaves, and ultrasound, Clin Obstet Gynecol 26:484-510, 1983.

Jolley J: Antenatal screening for fetal abnormalities: experiences in a district general hospital, Radiography 49:157-159, 1983.

1986 Daw E: Amniography and fetography old diagnostic aids—new uses, Clin Exp Obstet Gynecol 13:10-11, 1986.

1993 Harris RD and Barth RA: Sonography of the gravid uterus and placenta: current concepts, AJR 160:455-465, 1993.

Pelvimetry

For bibliographic citations before 1964, please see the fifth edition of this atlas. For citations from 1964 through 1974, see the sixth or seventh edition.

1975 Klapholz H: A computerized aid to Ball pelvimetry, Am J Obstet Gynecol 121:1067-1070, 1975.

1976 Campbell JA: X-ray pelvimetry: useful procedure or medical nonsense? J Natl Med Assoc 68:514-520, 1976.

Johnson TH and Brown M: Twenty degree angle modification for pelvimetry, Radiol Technol 48:149-151, 1976.

Laurin S, Hegedüs V and Zurbriggen S: Pelvimetry in breech and cephalic presentation, Acta Radiol [Diagn] 17:856-860, 1976.

Zierolf EM and Kuhns LR: Carpenter's level aids true lateral radiograph during pelvimetry, J Can Assoc Radiol 27:286-287, 1976.

1978 Delise C and McCrann D: Pelvimetry and active management of labor, J Maine Med Assoc 69:321-323, 1978.

Walss-Rodriguez RJ and Keefer FJ: Assessment of X-ray pelvimetry in the management of labor, W V Med J 74:267-269, 1978.

1980 Fine EA, Bracken M and Berkowitz RL: An evaluation of the usefulness of x-ray pelvimetry: comparison of the Thoms and modified Ball methods with manual pelvimetry, Am J Obstet Gynecol 137:15-20, 1980.

Ohlsen H: Radiologic low-dose pelvimetry: indications and pelvimetry data, Acta Radiol 21:747-758, 1980.

Varner MW, Cruikshank DP and Laube DW: X-ray pelvimetry in clinical obstetrics, Obstet Gynecol 56:296-300, 1980.

1981 Jagani N et al: The predictability of labor outcome from a comparison of birth weight and x-ray pelvimetry, Am J Obstet Gynecol 139:507-511, 1981.

Laube DW, Varner MW and Cruikshank DP: A prospective evaluation of x-ray pelvimetry, JAMA 246:2187-2188, 1981.

1982 Arcarese JS and Morrison JL: The utilization of x-ray pelvimetry in the United States, Clin Obstet Gynecol 25:165-166, 1982.

Federle MP et al: Pelvimetry by digital radiography: a low-dose examination, Radiology 143:733-735, 1982.

Hernandez E et al: Roentgenographic pelvimetry in single vertex pregnancies, South Med J 75:439-442, 1982.

1983 Anderson JC, Chu WK and Dobry CA: Low radiation exposure pelvimetry by digital radiography, Nebr Med J 68:363-365, 1983.

Anderson N: X-ray pelvimetry: helpful or harmful? J Fam Pract 17:405-412, 1983.

1984 Lundh C et al: Radiographic pelvimetry—its use and possible radiation risk, Ups J Med Sci 89:135-146, 1984.

Suramo I et al: A low-dose CT pelvimetry, Br J Radiol 57:35-37, 1984.

1985 Adam P et al: Pelvimetry by digital radiography, Clin Radiol 36:327-330, 1985.

Claussen C et al: Pelvimetry by digital radiography and its dosimetry, J Perinat Med 13:287-292, 1985.

Mantero E, Cattaneo A and Costa S: The efficacy of X-ray pelvimetry, Rays 10:19-22, 1985.

Stark DD et al: Pelvimetry by magnetic resonance imaging, AJR 144:947-950, 1985.

1986 Brody AS et al: Artifacts seen during CT pelvimetry: implications for digital systems with scanning beams, Radiology 160:269-271, 1986.

Johnson GC: Pelvimetry revisited, AJR 147:409-411, 1986.

Kopelman JN et al: Computed tomographic pelvimetry in the evaluation of breech presentation, Obstet Gynecol 68:455-458, 1986.

Lenke RR and Shuman WP: Computed tomographic pelvimetry, J Reprod Med 31:958-960, 1986.

1987 Lao TT, Chin RK and Leung BF: Is x-ray pelvimetry useful in a trial of labour after caesarean section? Eur J Obstet Gynecol Reprod Biol 24:277-283, 1987.

Lotz H et al: Low dose pelvimetry with bi-plane digital radiography, Acta Radiol 28:577-580, 1987.

1988 al-Meshari AA: Routine lateral pelvimetry: a personal experience, Rays 13:43-48, 1988.

Dobson J and Nelson J: CT pelvimetry: replacing conventional with digital, Radiography 54:18-19, 1988.

1989 Moore MM and Shearer DR: Fetal dose estimates for CT pelvimetry, Radiology 171:265-267, 1989.

1991 al-Ahwani S et al: Magnetic resonance imaging of the female bony pelvis: MRI pelvimetry, J Belge Radiol 74:15-18, 1991.

Aronson D and Kier R: CT pelvimetry: the foveae are not an accurate landmark for the level of the ischial spines, AJR 156:527-530, 1991.

Gudgeon CW and Jarrett J: Pelvimetry—a squatter's view, Austral N Z J Obstet Gynaecol 31:221-222, 1991.

Nasrat H and Warda A: X-ray pelvimetry-reappraisal, Clin Exp Obstet Gynecol 18:27-33, 1991.

Raman S, Samuel D and Suresh K: A comparative study of X-ray pelvimetry and CT pelvimetry, Austral N Z J Obstet Gynaecol 31:217-220, 1991.

Smith RC and McCarthy S: Improving the accuracy of digital CT pelvimetry, J Comput Assist Tomogr 15:787-789, 1991.

Wiesen EJ et al: Improvement in CT pelvimetry, Radiology 178:259-262, 1991.

1992 Wade JP: Accuracy of pelvimetry measurements on CT scanners, Br J Radiol 65:261-263, 1992.

Wright AR, Cameron HM and Lind T: Magnetic resonance imaging pelvimetry: a useful adjunct in the management of the obese patient, Br J Obstet Gynaecol 99:852-853, 1992.

Wright AR et al: MR pelvimetry—a practical alternative, Acta Radiol 33:582-587, 1992.

1993 Morris CW, Heggie JC and Acton CM: Computed tomography pelvimetry: accuracy and radiation dose compared with conventional pelvimetry, Australas Radiol 37:186-191, 1993.

MALE REPRODUCTIVE SYSTEM

For bibliographic citations before 1964, please see the fifth edition of this atlas. For citations from 1964 through 1974, see the sixth or seventh edition.

1977 Gandhi MG: Testicular lymphography: a clinical study, J Urol 117:174, 1977.

Lein HH et al: Phlebography, urography, and lymphography in the diagnosis of metastases from testicular tumors, Acta Radiol. [Diagn] 18:177-185, 1977.

1978 Loveday BJ and Price JL: Soft tissue radiography of the testes, Clin Radiol 29:685-689, 1978.

1979 Meyer JJ et al: Transrectal seminal vesiculography, J Urol 121:129-130, 1979.

Raghavaiah NV: Prostatography, J Urol. 121:174-177, 1979.

Raghavaiah NV and Jordan WP Jr: Prostatic lymphography, J Urol 121:178-181, 1979.

1981 Comhaire F, Kunnen M and Nahoum C: Radiological anatomy of the internal spermatic vein(s) in 200 retrograde venograms, Int J Androl 4:379-387, 1981.

Kossoff J, Drane RJ, and Naimark A: Inflatable penile implant for impotence: radiologic evaluation, AJR 136:1109-1112, 1981.

Sharlip ID: Penile arteriography in impotence after pelvic trauma, J Urol 126:477-481, 1981.

1982 Bruhlmann W et al: Arteriography of the penis in secondary impotence, Urol Radiol 4:243-249, 1982.

Velcek D and Evans JA: Cavernosonography, Radiology 144:781-785, 1982.

1983 Frouws S, Reeders JW and Valcke AA: Corpus cavernosography, Diagn Imaging 52:145-153, 1983.

Puyua FA and Lewis RW: Corpus cavernosonography: pressure flow radiography, Invest Radiol 18:517-522, 1983.

Rajfer J et al: The use of computerized tomography scanning to localize the impalpable testis, J Urol 129:972-974, 1983.

1985 Al-Omari H, Girgis SM and Hanna AZ: Diagnostic value of vaso-seminal-vesiculography, Arch Androl 15:187-192, 1985.

Silverman PM, Dunnick NR and Ford KK: Computed tomography of the normal seminal vesicles, Comput Radiol 9:379-385, 1985.

1986 Fornage BD: Normal US anatomy of the prostate, Ultrasound Med Biol 12:1011-1021, 1986.

Gutman H, Golimbu M and Subramanyam BR: Diagnostic ultrasound of scrotum, Urology 27:72-75, 1986.

McClure RD and Hricak H: Scrotal ultrasound in the infertile man: detection of subclinical unilateral and bilateral varicoceles, J Urol 135:711-715, 1986.

1987 Fowler RC, Chennells PM and Ewing R: Scrotal ultrasonography: a clinical evaluation, Br J Radiol 60:649-654, 1987.

Martin B and Conte J: Ultrasonography of the acute scrotum, JCU 15:37-44, 1987.

McLeary RD: Future developments in ultrasonic imaging of the prostate, Prog Clin Biol Res 237:209-211, 1987.

Nagler HM and Thomas AJ Jr: Testicular biopsy and vasography in the evaluation of male infertility, Urol Clin North Am 14:167-176, 1987.

Resnick MI, Kursh ED and Bryan PJ: Magnetic resonance imaging of the prostate, Prog Clin Biol Res 243B:89-96, 1987.

Rockey KE and Cusack TJ: Ultrasound imaging of the scrotum: a pictorial guide to its varied capabilities, Postgrad Med 82:219-227, 1987.

1988 Amis ES Jr, Newhouse JH and Cronan JJ: Radiology of male periurethral structures, AJR 151:321-324, 1988.

Bookstein JJ: Penile angiography: the last angiographic frontier, AJR 150:47-54, 1988.

Chang Y and Hricak H: Magnetic resonance imaging of the prostate gland, Semin Ultrasound CT MR 9:343-351, 1988.

Demas BE: Computed tomography of the prostate gland, Semin Ultrasound CT MR 9:339-342, 1988.

Fritzsche PJ: MRI of the scrotum, Urol Radiol 10:52-57, 1988.

Hartnell GG: Radiological investigation of impotence, Br J Hosp Med 40:438-445, 1988.

Hartnell GG et al: Digital subtraction dynamic cavernosography, Br J Radiol 61:679-682, 1988.

Martin JF et al: Inflatable surface coil for MR imaging of the prostate, Radiology 167:268-270, 1988.

McClennan BL: Transrectal US of the prostate: is the technology leading the science? Radiology 168:571-575, 1988.

Rifkin MD: Prostate ultrasound, Semin Ultrasound CT MR 9:352-369, 1988.

Rosen MP, Walker TG and Greenfield AJ: Arteriography and radiology of impotence, Urol Radiol 10:136-143, 1988.

Thurnher S et al: Imaging the testis: comparison between MR imaging and US, Radiology 167:631-636, 1988.

1989 Benson CB, Doubilet PM and Richie JP: Sonography of the male genital tract, AJR 153:705-713, 1989.

Carter SS, Shinohara K and Lipshultz LI: Transrectal ultrasonography in disorders of the seminal vesicles and ejaculatory ducts, Urol Clin North Am 16:773-790, 1989.

King BF et al: Seminal vesicle imaging, Radiographics 9:653-676, 1989.

Patel PJ and Pareek SS: Scrotal ultrasound in male infertility, Eur Urol 16:423-425, 1989.

Rickards D: Imaging the prostate, Clin Radiol 40:335-336, 1989.

Rifkin MD: Prostate sonography: clinical indications and implications, Urol Radiol 11:238-240, 1989.

Satragno L, Martinoli C and Cittadini G: Magnetic resonance imaging of the penis: normal anatomy, Magn Reson Imaging 7:95-100, 1989.

1990 Rifkin MD, Dahnert W and Kurtz AB: State of the art: endorectal sonography of the prostate gland, AJR 154:691-700, 1990.

Schnall MD and Pollack HM: Magnetic resonance imaging of the prostate gland, Urol Radiol 12:109-114, 1990.

Schnall MD et al: Magnetic resonance imaging of the prostate, Magn Reson Q 6:1-16, 1990.

Winfield AC, Fleischer AC and Moore DE: Diagnostic imaging of fertility disorders, Curr Probl Diagn Radiol 19:1-38, 1990.

1991 Mattrey RF: Magnetic resonance imaging of the scrotum, Semin Ultrasound CT MR 12:95-108, 1991.

Pollack HM: Imaging of the prostate gland, Eur Urol 20 (Suppl 1):50-58, 1991.

Schultz-Lampel D et al: MRI for evaluation of scrotal pathology, Urol Res 19:289-292, 1991.

Secaf E et al: MR imaging of the seminal vesicles, AJR 156:989-994, 1991.

Stevens JK and Miller JI: Transrectal ultrasound: an aid to diagnosing prostate cancer, AORN J 53:1166-1170, 1991.

1992 Schnall MD et al: The seminal tract in patients with ejaculatory dysfunction: MR imaging with an endorectal surface coil, AJR 159:337-341, 1992.

1993 Hamper UM and Sheth S: Prostate ultrasonography, Semin Roentgenol 28:57-73, 1993.

Mirowitz SA, Brown JJ and Heiken JP: Evaluation of the prostate and prostatic carcinoma with gadolinium-enhanced endorectal coil MR imaging, Radiology 186:153-157, 1993.

Ramchandani P and Schnall MD: Magnetic resonance imaging of the prostate, Semin Roentgenol 28:74-82, 1993.

Richard WD et al: A method for three-dimensional prostate imaging using transrectal ultrasound, Comput Med Imaging Graph 17:73-79, 1993.

Schnall M: Magnetic resonance imaging of the scrotum, Semin Roentgenol 28:19-30, 1993.

SALIVARY GLANDS

For bibliographic citations before 1964, please see the fifth edition of this atlas. For citations from 1964 through 1974, see the sixth or seventh edition.

1977 Calcaterra TC et al: The value of sialography in the diagnosis of parotid tumors, Arch Otolaryngol 103:727-729, 1977.

Ferguson MM, Evans A and Mason WN: Continuous infusion pressure-monitored sialography, Int J Oral Surg 6:84-89, 1977.

1978 Azouz EM: The panoramic view in sialography, Radiology 127:267-268, 1978.

Kushner DC and Weber AL: Sialography of salivary gland tumors with fluoroscopy and tomography, AJR 130:941-944, 1978.

1979 Mancuso A, Rice D and Hanafee W: Computed tomography of the parotid gland during contrast sialography, Radiology 132:211-213, 1979.

1980 Som PM and Biller HF: The combined CT-sialogram, Radiology 135:387-390, 1980.

1981 Carter BL et al: Computed tomography and sialography. 1. Normal anatomy, J Comput Assist Tomogr 5:42-45, 1981.

Carter BL et al: Computed tomography and sialography. 2. Pathology, J Comput Assist Tomogr 5:46-53, 1981.

Cogan MI and Gill SP: Value of sialography and scintigraphy in diagnosis of salivary gland disorders, Int J Oral Surg (Suppl) 10:216-222, 1981.

Stone DN et al: Parotid CT sialography, Radiology 138:393-397, 1981.

1982 Bryan RN et al: Computed tomography of the major salivary glands, AJR 139:547-554, 1982.

Kassel EE: CT sialography. I. Introduction, technique, anatomy, and variants, J Otolaryngol 11(Suppl 12):1-10, 1982.

Massouh H and Dunscombe PB: Panoramic sialography: an alternative technique, Br J Radiol 55:735-739, 1982.

Sone S et al: CT of parotid tumors, AJNR 3:143-147, 1982.

1983 Bruneton JN et al: Indications for ultrasonography in parotid pathologies, ROEFO 138:22-24, 1983.

Conn IG, Wiesenfeld D and Ferguson MM: The anatomy of the facial nerve in relation to CT/sialography of the parotid gland, Br J Radiol 56:901-905, 1983.

Gullotta U and Schekatz A: Digital subtraction sialography, Eur J Radiol 3:339-340, 1983.

Wiesenfeld D, Ferguson MM and McMillan NC: Simultaneous computed tomography and sialography of the parotid and submandibular glands, Br J Oral Surg 21:268-276, 1983.

1984 Rabinov K, Kell T Jr and Gordon PH: CT of the salivary glands, Radiol Clin North Am 22:145-159, 1984.

Verhoeven JW: Choice of contrast medium in sialography, Oral Surg Oral Med Oral Pathol 57:323-337, 1984.

1985 Lightfoote JB, Friedenberg RM and Smolin MF: Digital subtraction ductography, AJR 144:635-638, 1985.

1987 Larsson SG, Lufkin RB and Hoover LA: Computed tomography of the submandibular salivary glands, Acta Radiol 28:693-696, 1987.

Moss EG: Sialography: a brief update, N J Med 84:39-41, 1987.

1988 Cooper RA, Tempany CM and Farrell B: Conventional and computed tomographic sialography in evaluating disorders of the parotid gland, Entechnology 20-35, 1988.

De Clerck LS et al: Ultrasonography and computer tomography of the salivary glands in the evaluation of Sjogren's syndrome: comparison with parotid sialography, J Rheumatol 15:1777-1781, 1988.

1989 Acton VJ: A helpful sialography technique, Australas Radiol 33:171-172, 1989.

Byrne MN et al: Preoperative assessment of parotid masses: a comparative evaluation of radiologic techniques to histopathologic diagnosis, Laryngoscope 99:284-292, 1989.

Gritzmann N: Sonography of the salivary glands, AJR 153:161-166, 1989.

March DE, Rao VM and Zwillenberg D: Computed tomography of salivary glands in Sjogren's syndrome, Arch Otolaryngol Head Neck Surg 115:105-106, 1989.

Rinast E, Gmelin E and Hollands Thorn B: Digital subtraction sialography, conventional sialography, high-resolution ultrasonography and computed tomography in the diagnosis of salivary gland diseases, Eur J Radiol 9:224-230, 1989.

Tabor EK and Curtin HD: MR of the salivary glands, Radiol Clin North Am 27:379-392, 1989.

Watson MG: Investigation of salivary gland disease, Ear Nose Throat J 68:84, 87-89, 93, 1989.

Yoshimura Y, Inoue Y and Odagawa T: Sonographic examination of sialolithiasis, J Oral Maxillofac Surg 47:907-912, 1989.

Zbaren P and Ducommun JC: Diagnosis of salivary gland disease using ultrasound and sialography: a comparison, Clin Otolaryngol 14:189-197, 1989.

1990 Nicholson DA: Contrast media in sialography: a comparison of Lipiodol Ultra Fluid and Urografin 290, Clin Radiol 42:423-426, 1990.

Pilbrow WJ et al: Salivary gland scintigraphy—a suitable substitute for sialography? Br J Radiol 63:190-196, 1990.

Pollei SR and Harnsberger HR: The radiologic evaluation of the parotid space, Semin Ultrasound CT MR 11:486-503, 1990.

Vogl TJ et al: Parotid gland: plain and gadolinium-enhanced MR imaging, Radiology 177:667-674, 1990.

1991 Akin I et al: Sialographic and ultrasonographic analyses of major salivary glands, Acta Otolaryngol Stockh 111:600-606, 1991.

Aslam MO et al: Technical report: wire guided sialography, Clin Radiol 44:350-351, 1991.

Bradley MJ, Ahuja A and Metreweli C: Sonographic evaluation of the parotid ducts: its use in tumour localization, Br J Radiol 64:1092-1095, 1991.

Corthouts B et al: Ultrasonography of the salivary glands in the evaluation of Sjogren's syndrome. Comparison with sialography, J Belge Radiol 74:189-192, 1991.

Herrmann A, Eckl M and Maier H: Parotid sialography with a new Zonarc program, Otolaryngol Head Neck Surg 104:421-424, 1991.

Ida M et al: Radiographic quality and patient discomfort in sialography: comparison of iohexol with iothalamate, Dentomaxillofac Radiol 20:81-86, 1991.

Kelly IM and Dick R: Technical report: interventional sialography: dormia basket removal of Wharton's duct calculus, Clin Radiol 43:205-206, 1991.

Larsson SG: Comparison of methods of imaging the salivary glands, Curr Opin Radiol 3:76-83, 1991.

Lewis MA et al: Clinical application of computerized continuous-infusion pressure-monitored sialography, Dentomaxillofac Radiol 20:68-72, 1991.

Luyk NH, Doyle T and Ferguson MM: Recent trends in imaging the salivary glands, Dentomaxillofac Radiol 20:3-10, 1991.

Roebker JJ, Hall LC and Lukin RR: Fractured submandibular gland: CT findings, J Comput Assist Tomogr 15:1068-1069, 1991.

Traxler M et al: Magnetic resonance in lesions of the parotid gland, Int J Oral Maxillofac Surg 20:170-174, 1991.

1992 Aasen S and Kolbenstvedt A: CT appearances of normal and obstructed submandibular duct, Acta Radiol 33:414-419, 1992.

Buckenham TM, Page JE and Jeddy T: Technical report: interventional sialography: balloon dilatation of a Stensen's duct stricture using digital subtraction sialography, Clin Radiol 45:34, 1992.

Califano L, Zupi A and Giardino C: Accuracy in the diagnosis of parotid tumours, J Craniomaxillofac Surg 20:354-359, 1992.

Chisin R et al: Contribution of nuclear medicine to the diagnosis and management of extracranial head and neck diseases (excluding thyroid and parathyroid), Isr J Med Sci 28:254-261, 1992.

Gibbs SJ: Comparative imaging of the jaws, Curr Opin Dent 2:55-63, 1992.

Ilgit ET et al: Digital subtraction sialography: technique, advantages and results in 107 cases, Eur J Radiol 15:244-247, 1992.

Pellegrini V, Harris I and Lipton M: Can we reduce the number of routine films required for contrast sialography? Clin Radiol 45:254-255, 1992.

Takashima S et al: Sjogren syndrome: comparison of sialography and ultrasonography, JCU 20:99-109, 1992.

Walker GD: Sialography using a paediatric intravenous cannula, Br J Radiol 65:1130, 1992.

Weber AL: Imaging of the salivary glands, Curr Opin Radiol 4:117-122, 1992.

Yasumoto M et al: Computed tomography and ultrasonography in submandibular tumours, Clin Radiol 46:114-120, 1992.

1993   Ino C et al: Approach to the diagnosis of sialadenosis using sialography, Acta Otolaryngol Suppl Stockh 500:121-125, 1993.

Markusse HM et al: Digital subtraction sialography of the parotid glands in primary Sjogren's syndrome, J Rheumatol 20:279-283, 1993.

CRANIUM
General

For bibliographic citations before 1964, please see the fifth edition of this atlas. For citations from 1964 through 1974, see the sixth or seventh edition.

1975   Haller JO and Slovis TL: Importance of horizontal beam for lateral view of skull in pediatric radiography, Radiol Technol 47:150-152, 1975.

Potter GD and Gold RP: Radiographic analysis of the skull, Med Radiogr Photogr 51:2-15, 1975.

1976   Lanksch W and Kazner E, editors: Cranial computerized tomography, New York, 1976, Springer-Verlag.

Tator CH and Rowed DW: Fluoroscopy of foramen ovale as an aid to thermocoagulation of the Gasserian ganglion, J Neurosurg 44:254-257, 1976.

1977   Davis KR et al: Computed tomography in head trauma, Semin Roentgenol 12:53-62, 1977.

Jergens ME, Morgan MT and McElroy CE: Selective use of radiography of the skull and cervical spine, West J Med 127:1-4, 1977.

1978   Bradac GB et al: CT of the base of the skull, Neuroradiology 17:1-5, 1978.

Moody DM et al: Emergency plain film radiology of the nontraumatized patient with altered consciousness, Radiol Clin North Am 16:49-64, 1978.

Osborn AG, Brinton WR and Smith WH: Radiology of the jugular tubercles, AJR 131:1037-1040, 1978.

Tomsick TA, Chambers AA and Lukin RR: Skull fractures, Semin Roentgenol 13:27-36, 1978.

1979   DeSmet AA, Fryback DG and Thornbury JR: A second look at the utility of radiographic skull examination for trauma, AJR 132:95-97, 1979.

Masters SJ: Evaluation of head trauma: efficacy of skull films, AJR 135:539-547, 1980.

Palmer A and Munro L: The principles of tomographic positioning with particular reference to skull tomography, Radiography 45(531):51-60, 1979.

1980   Bruce DA and Schut L: The value of CAT scanning following pediatric head injury, Clin Pediatr (Phila) 19:719-725, 1980.

Cummins RO: Clinicians' reasons for overuse of skull radiographs, AJR 135:549-552, 1980.

Cummins RO et al: High-yield referral criteria for posttraumatic skull roentgenography: response of physicians and accuracy of criteria, JAMA 244:673-676, 1980.

de Campo J and Petty PG: How useful is the skull x-ray examination in trauma? Med J Aust 2:553-555, 1980.

de Lacey G et al: Mild head injuries: a source of excessive radiography? (Analysis of a series and review of the literature), Clin Radiol 31:457-462, 1980.

Eckerdal O and Nelvig P: Reproducible positioning of the skull at tomography, Acta Radiol [Diagn] (Stockh) 21:557-559, 1980.

Fischer HW: Occurrence of seizure during cranial computed tomography, Radiology 137:563-564, 1980.

Freed HA: Skull x-ray criteria endorsed by the Food and Drug Administration: some flaws and proposed modifications, Neurosurgery 7:636-638, 1980.

Ghoshhajra K: CT in trauma of the base of the skull and its complications, CT 4:271-276, 1980.

Jennatt B: Skull x-rays after recent head injury, Clin Radiol 31:463-469, 1980.

Kaiser M, Veiga-Pires JA and Silvestre ME: The value of three-dimensional CT scanning in head pathology, ROEFO 132:406-410, 1980.

Lee RT: The superimposition of lateral skull radiographs by subtraction: a new method, Br J Orthod 7:121-124, 1980.

Masters SJ: Evaluation of head trauma: efficacy of skull films, AJR 135:539-547, 1980.

Rao KC: The role and limitation of CT in craniocerebral trauma, CT 4:253-260, 1980.

Shindler E and Reck R: Value and limits of computer-assisted tomography, Head Neck Surg 2:287-292, 1980.

A study of the utilization of skull radiography in nine accident-and-emergency units in the UK: a national study by the Royal College of Radiologists, Lancet 2:1234-1236, 1980.

Tsai FY et al: Computed tomography in child abuse head trauma, CT 4:277-286, 1980.

van Hassel-Strijbosch M and van de Werf K: Value of reconstruction modes in CT scanning of the head, Radiography 46:209-212, 1980.

1981   Balasubramaniam S et al: Efficacy of skull radiography, Am J Surg 142:366-369, 1981.

Burrows EH: Clinical relevance of radiological abnormalities of the craniovertebral junction, Br J Radiol 54:195-202, 1981.

Cordon IW: Skull roentgenography for patients with head trauma: the use of high-yield criteria, Can Med Assoc J 124:584-589, 1981.

Costs and benefits of skull radiography for head injury: a national study by the Royal College of Radiologists, Lancet 2:791-795, 1981.

Kaiser MC et al: CT for trauma to the base of the skull and spine in children, Neuroradiology 22:27-31, 1981.

Olmsted WW: Some skeletogenic lesions with common calvarial manifestations, Radiol Clin North Am 19:703-713, 1981.

Robson TW et al: Fungal infections of the base of the skull: two case reports, J Laryngol Otol 95:109-114, 1981.

Sandor T et al: Automated calvaria analysis from computerized axial tomographic scans, Comput Biomed Res 14:119-124, 1981.

Young IR et al: Magnetic resonance properties of hydrogen: imaging the posterior fossa, AJR 137:895-901, 1981.

1982   Bessen HA and Rothstein RJ: Futility of skull radiography for nontraumatic conditions, Ann Emerg Med 11:605-609, 1982.

Carmel PW and Mawad M: CT scanning of the posterior fossa, Clin Neurosurg 29:51-102, 1982.

Ferry BC: Skull roentgenograms in pediatric head trauma: a vanishing necessity? Pediatrics 69:237-238, 1982.

Healy JF and Crudale AS: Computed tomographic evaluation of depressed skull fractures and associated intracranial injury, Comput Radiol 6:323-330, 1982.

LaMasters DL et al: Multiplanar metrizamide-enhanced CT imaging of the foramen magnum, AJNR 3:485-494, 1982.

Shaffer MA and Doris PE: Increasing the diagnostic yield of portable skull films, Ann Emerg Med 11:303-306, 1982.

Tunturi T et al: Head injuries and skull radiography: clinical factors predicting a fracture, Injury 13:478-483, 1982.

1983   Bligh AS et al: Patient selection for skull radiography in uncomplicated head injury, Lancet 1:115-118, 1983.

Cooper PR and Ho V: Role of emergency skull x-ray films in the evaluation of the head-injured patient: a retrospective study, Neurosurgery 13:136-140, 1983.

Cooper PW and Kassel EE: CT of the cranium in head injury, J Can Assoc Radiol 34:167-177, 1983.

DeLuca SA and Rhea JT: Skull fractures, Am Fam Physician 28:125-126, 1983.

Gibson TC: Skull x-rays in minor head injury: a review of their use and interpretation by casualty officers, Scott Med J 28:132-137, 1983.

Iko BO and Teal JS: Computed tomography of the calvarium: a prospective study, Comput Radiol 7:323-324, 1983.

North S and Pollak EW: Skull roentgenography in the evaluation of head injury, South Med J 76:468-470, 1983.

Tress BM: The need for skull radiography in patients presenting for CT, Radiology 146:87-89, 1983.

1984 De la Cruz A: Polytomographic evaluation of the clivus and petrous apices: a new view, Laryngoscope 94:153-164, 1984.

Marglin SI and Phillips LA: Radiologic assessment of head trauma, Nurse Pract 9:64-65, 68, 1984.

Pastakia B and Herdt JR: Radiolucent "zones" in parietal bones seen on computed tomography: a normal anatomic variant, J Comput Assist Tomogr 8:108-109, 1984.

Whelan MA et al: CT of the base of the skull, Radiol Clin North Am 22:177-217, 1984.

1986 Harding G and Tischler R: Dual-energy Compton scatter tomography, Phys Med Biol 31:477-489, 1986.

Lufkin R and Hanafee W: Magnetic resonance imaging of the nasopharynx and skull base, Acta Radiol Suppl (Stockh) 369:325-326, 1986.

Virapongse C et al: Three-dimensional computed tomographic reformation of the spine, Neurosurgery 18:53-58, 1986.

1987 Honda H et al: Optimal positioning for CT examinations of the skull base: experimental and clinical studies, Eur J Radiol 7:225-228, 1987.

Kimber PM: Isocentric neuroradiography, Radiography 53:201-210, 1987.

Teatini G et al: Computed tomography of the ethmoid labyrinth and adjacent structures, Ann Otol Rhinol Laryngol 96:239-250, 1987.

1988 Lufkin R et al: Magnetic resonance imaging of the craniocervical junction, Comput Med Imaging Graph 12:281-292, 1988.

Valvassori GE and Guzman M: Magnetic resonance imaging of the posterior cranial fossa, Ann Otol Rhinol Laryngol 97:594-598, 1988.

1989 Deck MD: Computed tomography and magnetic resonance imaging of the skull and brain, Clin Imaging 13:95-113, 1989.

Fezoulidis I et al: Diagnostic imaging of the occipito-cervical junction in patients with rheumatoid arthritis: plain films, computed tomography, magnetic resonance imaging, Eur J Radiol 9:5-11, 1989.

Masala W et al: Multiplanar reconstructions in the study of ethmoid anatomy, Neuroradiology 31:151-155, 1989.

1990 de Lacey G et al: Testing a policy for skull radiography (and admission) following mild head injury, Br J Radiol 63:14-18, 1990.

Kimura F et al: MR imaging of the normal and abnormal clivus, AJR 155:1285-1291, 1990.

Kinnunen J et al: Improved visualization of posterior fossa with clivoaxial CT scanning plane, Roentgenblatter 43:539-542, 1990.

Kirsch DL et al: MRI of the skull, Magn Reson Imaging 8:217-222, 1990.

Laine FJ, Nadel L and Braun IF: CT and MR imaging of the central skull base. I. Techniques, embryologic development, and anatomy, Radiographics 10:591-602, 1990.

Laine FJ, Nadel L and Braun IF: CT and MR imaging of the central skull base. II. Pathologic spectrum, Radiographics 10:797-821, 1990.

Lewis S: The radiographic demonstration of the pterygopalatine fossa and canal, Radiogr Today 56:21-22, 1990.

Medearis AL and Platt LD: Ultrasound imaging of the cranium and spine, Clin Perinatol 17:597-609, 1990.

Saab MH, Dietrich RB and Lufkin RB: MR imaging of the calvarium: pictorial essay, Surg Radiol Anat 12:215-218, 1990.

Unger JM, Gentry LR and Grossman JE: Sphenoid fractures: prevalence, sites, and significance, Radiology 175:175-180, 1990.

1991 Bonnier L et al: Three-dimensional reconstruction in routine computerized tomography of the skull and spine: experience based on 161 cases, J Neuroradiol 18:250-266, 1991.

Goncalves-Ferreira A: Stereotactic anatomy of the posterior cranial fossa: a study of the transcerebellar approach to the brainstem, Acta Neurochir 113:149-165, 1991.

Grevers G et al: Three-dimensional magnetic resonance imaging in skull base lesions, Am J Otolaryngol 12:139-145, 1991.

Hackney DB: Skull radiography in the evaluation of acute head trauma: a survey of current practice, Radiology 181:711-714, 1991.

Kaplan SB, Kemp SS and Oh KS: Radiographic manifestations of congenital anomalies of the skull, Radiol Clin North Am 29:195-218, 1991.

Leonardi M et al: Curved CT reformatted images of head scans, J Comput Assist Tomogr 15:1074-1076, 1991.

Levy JM and Hupke R: Composite addition technique: a new method in CT scanning of the posterior fossa, AJNR 12:686-688, 1991.

Lloyd GA and Barker PB: Subtraction magnetic resonance for tumours of the skull base and sinuses: a new imaging technique, J Laryngol Otol 105:628-631, 1991.

Merenich WM et al: The foramen ovale: MR and CT correlation, Clin Imaging 15:20-30, 1991.

Rosenorn J et al: Is a skull X-ray necessary after milder head trauma? Br J Neurosurg 5:135-139, 1991.

Rozeik C et al: Cranial CT artifacts and gantry angulation, J Comput Assist Tomogr 15:381-386, 1991.

1992 Berlis A, Putz R and Schumacher M: Direct and CT measurements of canals and foramina of the skull base, Br J Radiol 65:653-661, 1992.

Chowdhury V et al: Cranial sonography in preterm infants, Indian Pediatr 29:411-415, 1992.

Ros SP and Cetta F: Are skull radiographs useful in the evaluation of asymptomatic infants following minor head injury? Pediatr Emerg Care 8:328-330, 1992.

1993 Okudera H, Takemae T and Kobayashi S: Intraoperative computed tomographic scanning during transsphenoidal surgery: technical note, Neurosurgery 32:1041-1043, 1993.

Ray CE et al: Applications of three-dimensional CT imaging in head and neck pathology, Radiol Clin North Am 31:181-194, 1993.

Tiede U et al: A computerized three-dimensional atlas of the human skull and brain, AJNR 14:551-559, 1993.

Sella turcica

For bibliographic citations before 1964, please see the fifth edition of this atlas. For citations from 1964 through 1974, see the sixth or seventh edition.

1976 Dublin AB and Poirier VC: Fracture of the sella turcica, AJR 127:969-972, 1976.

1977 Leeds NE and Naidich TP: Computerized tomography in the diagnosis of sellar and parasellar lesions, Semin Roentgenol 12:121-135, 1977.

Teal JS: Radiology of the adult sella turcica, Bull Los Angeles Neurol Soc 42:111-174, 1977.

1979 Bruneton JN et al: Normal variants of the sella turcica, Radiology 131:99-104, 1979.

1980 Davis JR et al: Metrizamide sagittal tomography: adjunct to CT cisternography of the sellar region, AJR 134:1205-1208, 1980.

Hoffman JC Jr and Tindall GT: Diagnosis of empty sella syndrome using Amipaque cisternography combined with computerized tomography, J Neurosurg 52:99-102, 1980.

Penley MW and Pribram HF: Diagnosis of empty sella with small amounts of air at computed tomography, Surg Neurol 14:296-301, 1980.

Sage MR, Chan ES and Reilly PL: The clinical and radiological features of the empty sella syndrome, Clin Radiol 31:513-519, 1980.

Tindall GT and Hoffman JC Jr: Evaluation of the abnormal sella turcica, Arch Intern Med 140:1078-1083, 1980.

1981 Dietemann JL et al: Anatomy and radiology of the sellar spine, Neuroradiology 21:5-7, 1981.

Earnest F IV, McCullough EC and Frank DA: Fact or artifact: an analysis of artifact in high-resolution computed tomographic scanning of the sella, Radiology 140:109-113, 1981.

Ghoshhajra, K: High-resolution metrizamide CT cisternography in sellar and suprasellar abnormalities, J Neurosurg 54:232-239, 1981.

Goodrich I and Lee KJ: The differential diagnosis of sellar and parasellar diseases: clinical and radiographic features, Otolaryngol Clin North Am 14:355-378, 1981.

Kuuliala I, Katevuo K and Ketonen L: Metrizamide cisternography with hypocycloid and computed tomography in sellar and suprasellar lesions, Clin Radiol 32:403-407, 1981.

Miller JH: Radiological evaluation of sellar lesions, CRC Crit Rev Diagn Imaging 16:311-347, 1981.

Turski PA, Newton TH and Horten BH: Sellar contour: anatomic-polytomographic correlation, AJR 137:213-216, 1981.

1982 Chambers EF et al: Regions of low density in the contrast-enhanced pituitary gland: normal and pathologic processes, Radiology 144:109-113, 1982.

Cohen WA, Pinto RS and Kricheff II: The value of dynamic scanning, Radiol Clin North Am 20:23-35, 1982.

Dutton JJ et al: Evaluation of the suprasellar cistern by computed tomography, Ophthalmology (Rochester) 89:1220-1225, 1982.

LaMasters DL, Boggan JE and Wilson CB: Computerized tomography of a sellar spine: case report, J Neurosurg 57:407-409, 1982.

Smaltino F et al: CT in the diagnosis of sellar and parasellar lesions, J Neurosurg Sci 26:159-164, 1982.

Taylor S: High resolution computed tomography of the sella, Radiol Clin North Am 20:207-236, 1982.

1983 Banna M et al: Anatomico-radiological study of the borderline sella, Br J Radiol 56:1-5, 1983.

Chilton LA, Dorst JP and Garn SM: The volume of the sella turcica in children: new standards, AJR 140:797-801, 1983.

Dietemann JL et al: Computed tomography of the sellar spine, Neuroradiology 24:173-174, 1983.

Grossman RI and Lynch RM: Neuroimaging in neuroophthalmology, Neurol Clin 1:831-857, 1983.

Price MJ, Corbett JJ and Thompson HS: Diagnosis of the empty sella with intrathecal metrizamide computed tomography, Surv Ophthalmol 28:42-44, 1983.

Roppolo HM et al: Normal pituitary gland. I. Macroscopic anatomy-CT correlation, AJNR 4:927-935, 1983.

1984 De la Cruz A: Polytomographic evaluation of the clivus and petrous apices: a new view, Laryngoscope 94:153-164, 1984.

1987 Daniels DL and Haughton VM: Magnetic resonance imaging of the sella and temporal bone, Magn Reson Annu 1-47, 1987.

1989 Chakeres DW, Curtin A and Ford G: Magnetic resonance imaging of pituitary and parasellar abnormalities, Radiol Clin North Am 27:265-281, 1989.

Scotti G et al: New imaging techniques in endocrinology: magnetic resonance of the pituitary gland and sella turcica, Acta Pediatr Scand Suppl 356:5-14, 1989.

Zachariades N: Fracture of the sella turcica, Oral Surg Oral Med Oral Pathol 67:228, 1989.

1990 Baldwin JE and Freer CE: Pituitary computed tomography: is contrast enhancement necessary? Clin Radiol 42:20-23, 1990.

1991 Ambrosetto P et al: CT and MR of the sellar spine, Neuroradiology 33:465, 1991.

Guy RL et al: A comparison of CT and MRI in the assessment of the pituitary and parasellar region, Clin Radiol 43:156-161, 1991.

Johnsen DE et al: MR imaging of the sellar and juxtasellar regions, Radiographics 11:727-758, 1991.

ORBIT AND OPTIC CANAL
General

For bibliographic citations before 1964, please see the fifth edition of this atlas. For citations from 1964 through 1974, see the sixth or seventh edition.

1975 Lloyd GA: Radiology of the orbit, Philadelphia, 1975, WB Saunders Co.

Yeh HC and Butt WP: A modified Towne's view for radiography of the orbit and maxillary antrum, Radiology 116:724-728, 1975.

1976 Lame EL and Redick TJ: A new radiographic technique for fractures of the orbit and maxilla, AJR 127:473-480, 1976.

Lloyd GA: The impact of CT scanning and ultrasonography on orbital diagnosis, Clin Radiol 28:583-593, 1977.

1977 Strother CM, Sackett JF and Appen RE: Anatomic considerations for computed tomography of the optic chiasm, Arch Neurol 34:713-714, 1977.

Van Damme W, Kosmann P and Wackenheim C: A standardized method for computed tomography of the orbits, Neuroradiology 13:139-140, 1977.

1978 Haverling M and Johanson H: Computed sagittal tomography of the orbit, AJR 131:346-347, 1978.

1980 Alper MG: Computed tomography in planning and evaluating orbital surgery, Ophthalmology (Rochester) 87:418-431, 1980.

Grove AS, Jr: Orbital trauma and computed tomography, Ophthalmology (Rochester) 87:403-411, 1980.

Leo JS, Halpern J and Sackler JP: Computed tomography in the evaluation of orbital infections, Comput Tomogr 4:133-138, 1980.

Trokel SL and Hilal SK: Submillimeter resolution CT scanning of orbital diseases, Ophthalmology (Rochester) 87:412-417, 1980.

Unsold R, Norman D and Berninger W: Multiplanar evaluation of the optic canal from axial transverse CT sections, J Comput Assist Tomogr 4:418, 1980.

Wende S, Kazner E and Grumme T: The diagnostic value of computed tomography in orbital diseases: a cooperative study of 520 cases, Neurosurg Rev 3:43-49, 1980.

1981 Alker GJ et al: Computed tomography of the orbit, CRC Crit Rev Diagn Imaging 15:27-93, 1981.

Fernbach SK and Naidich TP: CT diagnosis of orbital inflammation in children, Neuroradiology 22:7-13, 1981.

Macpherson P: Improvements in technique developed over a series of 500 orbital venograms–cavernous sinograms, Clin Radiol 32:107-111, 1981.

Moos KF, Le May M and Ord RA: Investigation and management of orbital trauma, Int J Oral Surg 10(Suppl 1):229-234, 1981.

Nicolle DA, Ethier R and Peters TM: Clinical application of multiplanar computerized tomography of the orbit, Can J Ophthalmol 16:124-131, 1981.

Ord RA et al: Computerized tomography and B-scan ultrasonography in the diagnosis of fractures of the medial orbital wall, Plast Reconstr Surg 67:281-288, 1981.

Weinstein MA et al: Visualization of the arteries, veins, and nerves of the orbit by sector computed tomography, Radiology 138:83-87, 1981.

Zilkha A: Computed tomography of blow-out fracture of the medial orbital wall, AJR 137:963-965, 1981.

1982 Beck TJ, Rosenbaum AE and Miller NR: Orbital computed tomography: technical aspects, Int Ophthalmol Clin 22:7-43, 1982.

Forbes G: Computed tomography of the orbit, Radiol Clin North Am 20:37-49, 1982.

Forbes GS, Earnest F IV and Waller RR: Computed tomography of orbital tumors, including late-generation scanning techniques, Radiology 142:387-394, 1982.

Hammerschlag SB et al: Another look at blow-out fractures of the orbit, AJR 139:133-137, 1982.

Hammerschlag SB et al: Blow-out fractures of the orbit: a comparison of computed tomography and conventional radiography with anatomical correlation, Radiology 143:487-492, 1982.

Healy JF: Computed tomography of orbital trauma, CT 6:1-10, 1982.

Laurin S and Johansen CC: Oblique lateral projection of the orbital floor, Acta Radiol [Diagn] (Stockh) 23:423-432, 1982.

Unsold R: Computed tomographic anatomy of the orbit, Int Ophthalmol Clin 22:45-80, 1982.

Weber AL, Dallow RD and Hammerschlag SB: Evaluation of orbital and eye lesions by radiographic examination, ultrasound, and computerized tomography, CRC Crit Rev Diagn Imaging 17:277-321, 1982.

1983 Coker NJ, Brooks BS and El Gammal T: Computed tomography of orbital medial wall fractures, Head Neck Surg 5:383-389, 1983.

Fryczkowski AW et al: Experimental intravenous digital subtraction angiography (DSA) of orbital and choroidal circulation: preliminary study, Invest Radiol 18:512-516, 1983.

Grossniklaus H, Makley T and Johnson J: Computed axial tomography in ophthalmology, Ann Ophthalmol 15:904-906, 1983.

Laurin S and Johansen CC: A new method for demonstration of blow-out fractures, Ann Radiol (Paris) 26:231-234, 1983.

Marsh JL and Gado M: The longitudinal orbital CT projection: a versatile image for orbital assessment, Plast Reconstr Surg 71:308-317, 1983.

Xeroradiography for ophthalmic applications, Radiography 49:176, 1983.

Yamamoto Y, Sakurai M and Asari S: Towne (half-axial) and semisagittal computed tomography in the evaluation of blow-out fractures of the orbit, J Comput Assist Tomogr 7:306-309, 1983.

1984 Berges O, Vignaud J and Aubin ML: Comparison of sonography and computed tomography in the study of orbital space-occupying lesions, AJNR 5:247-251, 1984.

Han JS et al: Magnetic resonance imaging of the orbit: a preliminary experience, Radiology 150:755-759, 1984.

1985 Keene J and Doris PE: A simple radiographic diagnosis of occult blow-out fractures, Ann Emerg Med 14:335-338, 1985.

1986 Citrin CM: High resolution orbital computed tomography, J Comput Assist Tomogr 10:810-816, 1986.

Leib ML: Computed tomography of the orbit, Int Ophthalmol Clin 26:103-121, 1986.

1987 Levine RA: Orbital ultrasonography, Radiol Clin North Am 25:447-469, 1987.

Lindahl S: Computed tomography of intraorbital foreign bodies, Acta Radiol 28:235-240, 1987.

Weiss RA et al: Advanced diagnostic imaging techniques in ophthalmology, Adv Ophthalmic Plast Reconstr Surg 6:207-263, 1987.

Zonneveld FW et al: Normal direct multiplanar CT anatomy of the orbit with correlative anatomic cryosections, Radiol Clin North Am 25:381-407, 1987.

1988 Berardo N, Leban SG and Williams FA: A comparison of radiographic treatment methods for evaluation of the orbit, J Oral Maxillofac Surg 46:844-849, 1988.

MacManus D and Bartlett P: Magnetic resonance imaging (MRI) of the orbit, Radiogr Today 54:40-41, 1988.

1989 Antonyshyn O, Gruss JS and Kassel EE: Blow-in fractures of the orbit, Plast Reconstr Surg 84:10-20, 1989.

Atlas SW: Magnetic resonance imaging of the orbit: current status, Magn Reson Q 5:39-96, 1989.

Dortzbach RK, Kronish JW and Gentry LR: Magnetic resonance imaging of the orbit. I. Physical principles, Ophthalmic Plast Reconstr Surg 5:151-159, 1989.

Etherington RJ and Hourihan MD: Localisation of intraocular and intraorbital foreign bodies using computed tomography, Clin Radiol 40:610-614, 1989.

1990 Daly BD et al: Thin section computed tomography in the evaluation of naso-ethmoidal trauma, Clin Radiol 41:272-275, 1990.

DeMarco JK and Dillon WP: Orbital magnetic resonance imaging, Curr Opin Radiol 2:112-117, 1990.

Dorfman RE and Spickler EM: Current status of magnetic resonance imaging of the orbit, Top Magn Reson Imaging 2:17-26, 1990.

Moseley I: Diagnostic value of 'optic foramen views': experience from an eye hospital, Br J Ophthalmol 74:235-237, 1990.

1991 Hopper KD, Sherman JL and Boal DK: Abnormalities of the orbit and its contents in children: CT and MR imaging findings, AJR 156:1219-1224, 1991.

Kincaid W and Dutton GN: Optic foraminal radiography—a redundant investigation? Br J Ophthalmol 75:665-666, 1991.

Lieb WE et al: Color Doppler imaging of the eye and orbit: technique and normal vascular anatomy, Arch Ophthalmol 109:527-531, 1991.

Zentner J, Hassler W and Petersen D: A wooden foreign body penetrating the superior orbital fissure, Neurochirurgia 34:188-190, 1991.

1992 Hopper KD et al: CT and MR imaging of the pediatric orbit, Radiographics 12:485-503, 1992.

Otto PM et al: Screening test for detection of metallic foreign objects in the orbit before magnetic resonance imaging, Invest Radiol 27:308-311, 1992.

Roberts CF and Leehey PJ: Intraorbital wood foreign body mimicking air at CT, Radiology 185:507-508, 1992.

Specht CS et al: Orbitocranial wooden foreign body diagnosed by magnetic resonance imaging: dry wood can be isodense with air and orbital fat by computed tomography, Surv Ophthalmol 36:341-344, 1992.

1993 Fox LA: Images in clinical medicine: three-dimensional CT diagnosis of maxillofacial trauma, N Engl J Med 329:102, 1993.

Temporal bone

For bibliographic citations before 1964, please see the fifth edition of this atlas. For citations from 1964 through 1974, see the sixth or seventh edition.

1975 Coin CG and Scanlan RL: Technique for internal auditory cisternography, Acta Radiol [Suppl] 347:53-57, 1975.

Gado MH and Arenberg IK: Radiological visualization of the vestibular aqueduct, Radiology 117:621-626, 1975.

Johnson DH and Hunter DR: Temporal bone radiography: a screening survey approach, South Med J 68:1385-1387, 1975.

1976 Schatz CJ and Vignaud J: The inclined lateral projection: a new view in temporal bone tomography, Radiology 118:355-361, 1976.

1978 Jensen GL: An improved method for examining the mastoid process in the posterior tangential projection, Radiol Technol 49:631-633, 1978.

1980 Bentson JR et al: Combined gas cisternography and edge-enhanced computed tomography of the internal auditory canal, Radiology 136:777-779, 1980.

Hanafee WN et al: Edge enhancement computed tomography scanning in inflammatory lesions of the middle ear, Radiology 136:771-775, 1980.

Lloyd GA: High resolution computerized tomography of the petrous bone, J R Soc Med 73:699-700, 1980.

Naidich TP: Air CT canalography for the evaluation of the internal auditory canals, Laryngoscope 90:526-530, 1980.

Shaffer KA and Haughton VM: Thin section computed tomography of the temporal bone, Laryngoscope 90:1099-1105, 1980.

Shaffer KA, Haughton VM and Wilson CR: High resolution computed tomography of the temporal bone, Radiology 134:409-414, 1980.

Shaffer KA, Volz DJ and Haughton VM: Manipulation of CT data for temporal-bone imaging, Radiology 137:825-829, 1980.

1981 Gilmor RL, Yune HY and Holden RW: Computed tomography of the temporal bone, CRC Crit Rev Diagn Imaging 15:1-25, 1981.

Kinney SE et al: Sector computerized tomography of temporal bone and base of skull, Otolaryngol Head Neck Surg 89:453-456, 1981.

Littleton JT et al: Temporal bone: comparison of pluridirectional tomography and high resolution computed tomography, AJR 137:835-845, 1981.

Tatezawa T: Temporal bone radiography using the orthopantomograph, AJR 137:589-594, 1981.

Thomsen J et al: Tomography of the internal acoustic meatus: a critical evaluation of the radiological appearance in normals and in patients with acoustic neuromas, J Laryngol Otol 95:1191-1204, 1981.

1982 Clement PA and De Smedt E: High-resolution computerized tomographic scans of the normal and abnormal ear, Am J Otolaryngol 3:286-294, 1982.

Dixon HS: Otolaryngologic plain film radiography, with an emphasis on the temporal bone—how to do it. I. Am J Otol 3:318-338, 1982.

Lufkin R et al: Comparison of computed tomography and pluridirectional tomography of the temporal bone, Radiology 143:715-718, 1982.

Olson JE, Dorwart RH and Brant WE: Use of high resolution thin section CT scanning of the petrous bone in temporal bone anomalies, Laryngoscope 92:1274-1278, 1982.

Russell EJ et al: Transverse axial plane anatomy of the temporal bone employing high spatial resolution computed tomography, Neuroradiology 22:185-191, 1982.

Shaffer KA et al: Temporal bone anatomy: comparison of computed tomography and complex motion tomography, Head Neck Surg 4:296-300, 1982.

Valvassori GE, Mafee MF and Dobben GD: Computerized tomography of the temporal bone, Laryngoscope 92:562-565, 1982.

Viraponse C et al: Computed tomographic anatomy of the temporal bone, AJR 139:739-749, 1982.

Virapongse C et al: The role of high resolution computed tomography in evaluating disease of the middle ear, J Comput Assist Tomogr 6:711-720, 1982.

Wright JW Jr, Wright JW III and Hicks G: Polytomography and congenital anomalies of the ear, Ann Otol Rhinol Laryngol 91:480-484, 1982.

1983 Chakeres DW and Spiegel PK: A systematic technique for comprehensive evaluation of the temporal bone by computed tomography, Radiology 146:97-106, 1983.

Jazrawy H et al: Computed tomography of the temporal bone, J Otolaryngol 12:37-44, 1983.

Lamothe A et al: High resolution CT scan of the temporal bone, J Otolaryngol 12:119-124, 1983.

Lindeman P and Haglund M: Size of the mastoid air cell system obtained with two types of x-ray equipment, Acta Otolaryngol (Stockh) 95:101-104, 1983.

Swartz JD: High-resolution computed tomography of the middle ear and mastoid, Radiology 148:449-454, 1983.

Valavanis A, Kubik S and Schubiger O: High-resolution CT of the normal and abnormal fallopian canal, AJNR 4:748-751, 1983.

Virapongse C et al: High-resolution computed tomography of the temporal bone: its role in the evaluation of middle ear disease, Am J Otolaryngol 4:107-112, 1983.

Virapongse C et al: Temporal bone disease: a comparison between high resolution tomography and pluridirectional tomography, Radiology 147:743-748, 1983.

Zonneveld FW: The value of non-reconstructive multiplanar CT for the evaluation of the petrous bone, Neuroradiology 25:1-10, 1983.

1984 Archer A: Panoramic zonography of the middle and inner ear, Radiography 50:107-109, 1984.

Chakeres DW and Kapila A: Computed tomography of the temporal bone, Med Radiogr Photogr 60:1-32, 1984.

Curtin HD: CT of acoustic neuroma and other tumors of the ear, Radiol Clin North Am 22:77-105, 1984.

De la Cruz A: Polytomographic evaluation of the clivus and petrous apices: a new view, Laryngoscope 94:153-164, 1984.

Johnson DW et al: Temporal bone trauma: high-resolution computed tomographic evaluation, Radiology 151:411-415, 1984.

Lewis S: Cephalic index and how it may be of relevance in radiography of the petrous bone, Radiography 50:180-184, 1984.

1985 Manzione JV, Rumbaugh CL and Katzberg RW: Direct sagittal computed tomography of the temporal bone, J Comput Assist Tomogr 9:417-419, 1985.

Zonneveld FW: The technique of direct multiplanar high resolution CT of the temporal bone, Neurosurg Rev 8:5-13, 1985.

1987 Cooper MH, Archer CR and Kveton JF: Correlation of high-resolution computed tomography and gross anatomic sections of the temporal bone. I. The facial nerve, Am J Otol 8:375-384, 1987.

Daniels DL and Haughton VM: Magnetic resonance imaging of the sella and temporal bone, Magn Reson Annu 1-47, 1987.

Kobayashi H and Zusho H: Measurements of internal auditory meatus by polytomography, Br J Radiol 60:209-214, 1987.

O'Donoghue GM: Imaging the temporal bone, Clin Otolaryngol 12:157-160, 1987.

Phelps PD: Computerized imaging of the ear, Clin Otolaryngol 12:401-404, 1987.

Savic D, Jasovic A and Djeric D: The value of computerized tomography (CT) in the evaluation of the anatomic structure of the attic, J Laryngol Otol 101:1118-1124, 1987.

Todd NW et al: Mastoid size determined with lateral radiographs and computerized tomography, Acta Otolaryngol (Stockh) 103:226-231, 1987.

1988 Archer CR, Cooper MH and Kveton JF: Correlation of high-resolution computed tomography and gross anatomic sections of the temporal bone. II. Vestibular apparatus, Am J Otol 9:276-281, 1988.

Daniels DL et al: The effect of patient positioning on MR imaging of the internal auditory canal, Neuroradiology 30:395-398, 1988.

Hasso AN and Ledington JA: Imaging modalities for the study of the temporal bone, Otolaryngol Clin North Am 21:219-244, 1988.

Jackler RK: CT and MRI of the ear and temporal bone: current state of the art and future prospects, Am J Otol 9:232-239, 1988.

Mafee MF et al: Direct sagittal CT in the evaluation of temporal bone disease, AJR 150:1403-1410, 1988.

1989 Brogan M and Chakeres DW: Computed tomography and magnetic resonance imaging of the normal anatomy of the temporal bone, Semin Ultrasound CT MR 10:178-194, 1989.

Dolan KD: Temporal bone fractures, Semin Ultrasound CT MR 10:262-279, 1989.

Eelkema EA and Curtin HD: Congenital anomalies of the temporal bone, Semin Ultrasound CT MR 10:195-212, 1989.

Esfahani F and Dolan KD: Air CT cisternography in the diagnosis of vascular loop causing vestibular nerve dysfunction, AJNR 10:1045-1049, 1989.

Holliday RA and Reede DL: MRI of mastoid and middle ear disease, Radiol Clin North Am 27:283-299, 1989.

Lee BC et al: CT evaluation of the temporal bone ossicles by using oblique reformations: a technical note, AJNR 10:431-433, 1989.

Louryan SM et al: Comprehensive and interpretative radiology of middle ear malformations, Acta Otorhinolaryngol Belg 43:569-577, 1989.

Meyerhoff WL et al: Magnetic resonance imaging in the diagnosis of temporal bone and skull base lesions, Am J Otol 10:131-137, 1989.

Millen SJ, Daniels DL and Meyer GA: Gadolinium-enhanced magnetic resonance imaging in temporal bone lesions, Laryngoscope 99:257-260, 1989.

Pyhtinen J, Laitinen J and Jokinen K: Plain radiography and tomography of the internal auditory canal for the diagnosis of acoustic neuroma, Roentgenblatter 42:339-342, 1989.

Smith IM et al: CT air meatography: review of side effects in 60 patients, J Laryngol Otol 103:173-174, 1989.

Swartz JD: Current imaging approach to the temporal bone, Radiology 171:309-317, 1989.

1990 Ali QM: Radiography of the auditory ossicles: a review, East Afr Med J 67:794-800, 1990.

Alvord LS: Uses of ultrasound in audiology, J Am Acad Audiol 1:227-235, 1990.

Goligher JE and Lloyd GA: Fractures of the petrous temporal bone, J Laryngol Otol 104:438-439, 1990.

Howard JD, Elster AD and May JS: Temporal bone: three-dimensional CT. I. Normal anatomy, techniques, and limitations, Radiology 177:421-425, 1990.

Howard JD, Elster AD and May JS: Temporal bone: three-dimensional CT. II. Pathologic alterations, Radiology 177:427-430, 1990.

Hughes K: A simplified anatomical approach to thin section, high resolution CT of the ear and facial nerve, Radiogr Today 56:18-23, 1990.

Isono M et al: High resolution computed tomography of auditory ossicles, Acta Radiol 31:27-31, 1990.

Litt AW et al: Role of slice thickness in MR imaging of the internal auditory canal, J Comput Assist Tomogr 14:717-720, 1990.

Swartz JD: The petrous bone, Curr Opin Radiol 2:83-92, 1990.

Swartz JD: The temporal bone: imaging considerations, CRC Crit Rev Diagn Imaging 30:341-417, 1990.

Swartz JD and Harnsberger HR: The temporal bone: magnetic resonance imaging, Top Magn Reson Imaging 2:1-16, 1990.

1991 Bryan RN: MR of the temporal bone, AJNR 12:17-18, 1991.

Cripps D: The use of macro-radiography in the initial examination of the petrous temporal region, Radiogr Today 57:17-22, 1991.

Jabour BA: Imaging of the temporal bone, Curr Opin Radiol 3:57-60, 1991.

Monsour PA and Mendoza AR: Visualization of the maxillary sinus and styloid processes using rotational panoramic radiography, Austr Dent J 36:5-10, 1991.

1992 Hayran M, Onerci M and Ozturk C: Evaluation of the temporal bone by anatomic sections and computed tomography, Surg Radiol Anat 14:169-173, 1992.

Torizuka T et al: High-resolution CT of the temporal bone: a modified baseline, Radiology 184:109-111, 1992.

Weber AL: Magnetic resonance imaging and computed tomography of the internal auditory canal and cerebellopontine angle, Isr J Med Sci 28:173-182, 1992.

Zanella FE: Imaging of the temporal bone, Curr Opin Radiol 4:103-111, 1992.

1993 Ali QM, Ulrich C and Becker H: Three-dimensional CT of the middle ear and adjacent structures, Neuroradiology 35:238-241, 1993.

Jugular foramen

For bibliographic citations before 1964, please see the fifth edition of this atlas. For citations from 1964 through 1974, see the sixth or seventh edition.

1978 Sutton JS: The normal jugular spur, jugular foramen, and jugular bulb as visualized on skull and temporal bone radiographs, Radiology 128:109-117, 1978.

1984 Daniels DL, Williams AL and Haughton VM: Jugular foramen: anatomic and computed tomographic study, AJR 142:153-158, 1984.

Lo WW and Solti-Bohman LG: High-resolution CT of the jugular foramen: anatomy and vascular variants and anomalies, Radiology 150:743-747, 1984.

1989 Matsushima T et al: Magnetic resonance imaging of jugular foramen neurinomas, Acta Neurochir 96:83-87, 1989.

HYPOGLOSSAL CANAL
General

For bibliographic citations before 1964, please see the fifth edition of this atlas. For citations from 1964 through 1974, see the sixth or seventh edition.

1978 Tanzer A: Roentgen diagnosis of hypoglossal nerve canal (English abstract), Radiologe 18:42-48, 1978.

1980 Fujiwara S, Hachisuga S and Numaguchi Y: Intracranial hypoglossal neurinoma: report of a case, Neuroradiology 20:87-90, 1980.

1982 Berger MS, Edwards MS and Bingham WG: Hypoglossal neurilemmoma: case report and review of the literature, Neurosurgery 10:617-620, 1982.

1987 Honda H et al: Optimal positioning for CT examinations of the skull base: experimental and clinical studies, Eur J Radiol 7:225-228, 1987.

Facial bones

For bibliographic citations before 1964, please see the fifth edition of this atlas. For citations from 1964 through 1974, see the sixth or seventh edition.

1975 Yeh HC and Butt WP: A modified Towne's view for radiography of the orbit and maxillary antrum, Radiology 116:724-728, 1975.

1976 Lame EL and Redick TJ: A new radiographic technique for fractures of the orbit and maxilla, AJR 127:473-480, 1976.

1978 Dolan KD and Jacoby CG: Facial fractures, Semin Roentgenol 13:37-51, 1978.

Marshall KA, Sadowsky NL and Sigman D: Xeroradiography in the diagnosis of facial fractures, Plast Reconstr Surg 62:207-211, 1978.

1979 Osborn AG: Radiology of the pterygoid plates and pterygopalatine fossa, AJR 132:389-394, 1979.

1980 Jacoby CG and Dolan KD: Fragment analysis in maxillofacial injuries: the tripod fracture, J Trauma 20:292-296, 1980.

1981 Charlton OP et al: Panoramic zonography of fractures of the facial skeleton, AJR 137:109-112, 1981.

Fitz CR: Radiological evaluation of craniofacial anomalies, Scand J Plast Reconstr Surg 15:199-204, 1981.

Fitz CR: Radiology of the asymmetrical face, Scand J Plast Reconstr Surg 15:205-210, 1981.

Fujii N and Yamashiro M: Computed tomography for the diagnosis of facial fractures, J Oral Surg 39:735-741, 1981.

Mafee MF and Valvassori GE: Radiology of the craniofacial anomalies, Otolaryngol Clin North Am 14:939-988, 1981.

Rowe LD, Miller E and Brandt-Zawadzki MN: Computed tomography in maxillofacial trauma, Laryngoscope 91:745-757, 1981.

1982 Brandt-Zawadzki MN et al: High resolution CT with image reformation in maxillofacial pathology, AJR 138:477-483, 1982.

Frame JW and Wake MJ: Evaluation of maxillofacial injuries by use of computerized tomography, J Oral Maxillofac Surg 40:482-486, 1982.

Horowitz I, Abrahami E and Mintz SS: Demonstration of condylar fractures of the mandible by computed tomography, Oral Surg 54:263-268, 1982.

Moilanen A: Errors in the primary x-ray diagnosis of maxillofacial fractures, ROEFO 137:129-135, 1982.

Moilanen A: Skull radiology in patients with facial trauma, Int J Oral Surg 11:89-95, 1982.

Neumann PR and Zilkha A: Use of the CAT scan for diagnosis in the complicated facial fracture patient, Plast Reconstr Surg 70:683-693, 1982.

Noyek AM et al: Sophisticated CT in complex maxillofacial trauma, Laryngoscope 92:1-17, 1982.

Rowe LD and Brandt-Zawadzki MN: Spatial analysis of midfacial fractures with multidirectional and computed tomography: clinicopathologic correlates in 44 cases, Otolaryngol Head Neck Surg 90:651-660, 1982.

Zilkha A: Computed tomography in facial trauma, Radiology 144:545-548, 1982.

1983 Cooper PW, Kassel EE and Gruss JS: High-resolution CT scanning of facial trauma, AJNR 4:495-498, 1983.

Daffner RH, Apple JS and Gehweiler JA: Lateral view of facial fractures: new observations, AJR 141:587-591, 1983.

Daffner RH et al: Computed tomography in the evaluation of severe facial trauma, Comput Radiol 7:91-102, 1983.

Gentry LR et al: High-resolution CT analysis of facial struts in trauma. I. Normal anatomy, AJR 140:523-532, 1983.

Gentry LR et al: High-resolution CT analysis of facial struts in trauma. II. Osseous and soft-tissue complications, AJR 140:533-541, 1983.

Hemmy DC, David DJ and Herman GT: Three-dimensional reconstruction of craniofacial deformity using computed tomography, Neurosurgery 13:534-541, 1983.

Hryshko FG and Deeb ZL: Computed tomography in acute head injuries, CT 7:331-344, 1983.

Kassel EE, Noyek AM and Cooper PW: CT in facial trauma, J Otolaryngol 12:2-15, 1983.

Moilanen A: Midfacial fractures in supine panoramic zonography, Roentgenblatter 36:184-187, 1983.

Noyek AM et al: Contemporary radiologic evaluation in maxillofacial trauma, Otolaryngol Clin North Am 16:473-508, 1983.

Paukku P et al: Comparison of the visibility of the anatomical structures of the facial skeleton in panoramic zonography and linear tomography, Eur J Radiol 3:177-179, 1983.

1984 Johnson DH Jr: CT of maxillofacial trauma, Radiol Clin North Am 22:131-144, 1984.

Kreipke DL et al: Computed tomography and thin-section tomography in facial trauma, AJR 142:1041-1045, 1984.

Moilanen A: Midfacial fractures in dental panoramic radiography, Oral Surg 57:106-110, 1984.

Sataloff RT et al: Computed tomography of the face and paranasal sinuses. I. Normal anatomy, Head Neck 7:110-122, 1984.

Vannier MW, Marsh JL and Warren JO: Three-dimensional CT reconstruction images for craniofacial surgical planning and evaluation, Radiology 150:179-184, 1984.

1987 Flaxman NA and Kattan KR: Metallic objects seen in radiographs of the maxilla and mandible, Am Fam Physician 35:197-203, 1987.

Hart CW and Gillespie JE: Three-dimensional cranio-facial reformations, Radiography 53:173-175, 1987.

Hemmy DC: Three-dimensional imaging in craniofacial disorders: a brief review, Aust N Z J Surg 57:101-104, 1987.

Luffingham JK: Stereoradiography of the anterior maxilla, Eur J Orthod 9:193-199, 1987.

Moilanen A: The role of primary head CT-scans in facial fractures, Int J Oral Maxillofac Surg 16:572-576, 1987.

1988 Frank DA, Kern EB and Kispert DB: Measurement of large or irregular-shaped septal perforations, Radiol Technol 59:409-412, 1988.

Partinen M: Obstructive sleep apnea and cephalometric roentgenograms: the role of anatomic upper airway abnormalities in the definition of abnormal breathing during sleep, Chest 93:1199-1205, 1988.

Rubesin SE et al: Contrast examination of the soft palate with cross sectional correlation, Radiographics 8:641-665, 1988.

1990 Carter LC, Dennison M and Carter JM: Panoramic zonography of the midface: a clinician's guide to vertical magnification, Todays FDA 2:1C-3C, 1990.

Daly BD et al: Thin section computed tomography in the evaluation of naso-ethmoidal trauma, Clin Radiol 41:272-275, 1990.

Henze E et al: The orthopan tomoscintigram—a new application of emission computed tomography for facial bone scanning, Eur J Nucl Med 16:97-101, 1990.

Hyde JS et al: Facial surface coil for MR imaging, Radiology 174:276-279, 1990.

Russell JL et al: Computed tomography in the diagnosis of maxillofacial trauma, Br J Oral Maxillofac Surg 28:287-291, 1990.

1991 Eppley BL and Sadove AM: Computerized digital enhancement in craniofacial cephalometric radiography, J Oral Maxillofac Surg 49:1038-1043, 1991.

Haug RH et al: Cervical spine fractures and maxillofacial trauma, J Oral Maxillofac Surg 49:725-729, 1991.

Ponsford A and Clements R: A modified view of the facial bones in the seriously injured, Radiogr Today 57:10-12, 1991.

1992 Gilda JE and Maillie HD: Dosimetry of absorbed radiation in radiographic cephalometry, Oral Surg Oral Med Oral Pathol 73:638-643, 1992.

Zinreich SJ: 3-D reconstruction for evaluation of facial trauma, AJNR 13:893-895, 1992.

1993 DelBalso AM and Hall RE: Advances in maxillofacial imaging, Curr Probl Diagn Radiol 22:91-142, 1993.

Fox LA: Images in clinical medicine: three-dimensional CT diagnosis of maxillofacial trauma, N Engl J Med 329:102, 1993.

Yanagisawa K et al: DentaScan imaging of the mandible and maxilla, Head Neck 15:1-7, 1993.

Nasal bones

For bibliographic citations before 1964, please see the fifth edition of this atlas. For citations from 1964 through 1974, see the sixth or seventh edition.

1977 de Lacey GJ et al: The radiology of nasal injuries: problems of interpretation and clinical relevance, Br J Radiol 50:412-414, 1977.

1981 Facer GW: A blow to the nose: common injury requiring skillful management, Postgrad Med 70:83, 92, 1981.

1982 Nash P: Diagnosis and treatment of fractures of the nose, Aust Fam Physician 11:663, 665, 670, 1982.

1983 Kassel EE, Cooper PW and Kassel RN: CT of the nasal cavity, J Otolaryngol 12:16-36, 1983.

Zygomatic bone (zygoma)

For bibliographic citations before 1964, please see the fifth edition of this atlas. For citations from 1964 through 1974, see the sixth or seventh edition.

1980 Jacoby CG and Dolan KD: Fragment analysis in maxillofacial injuries: the tripod fracture, J Trauma 20:292-296, 1980.

1981 Ryan WJ and Jones CA: A radiodiagnostic technique to show the zygomatic process, Radiography 47:165-168, 1981.

1982 Hughes LK: Simplified radiography of the zygomatic arches (the rat's head view), Radiol Technol 53:513-516, 1982.

1987 Tyndall DA and Matteson SR: The zygomatic air cell defect (ZACD) on panoramic radiographs, Oral Surg Oral Med Oral Pathol 64:373-376, 1987.

1990 Akizuki H, Yoshida H and Michi K: Ultrasonographic evaluation during reduction of zygomatic arch fractures, J Craniomaxillofac Surg 18:263-266, 1990.

Mandible

For bibliographic citations before 1964, please see the fifth edition of this atlas. For citations from 1964 through 1974, see the sixth or seventh edition.

1976 Gerlock AJ: The flared mandible sign of the flail mandible, Radiology 117:299-300, 1976.

1977 Trapnell DH: The "magnification sign" of triple mandibular fracture, Br J Radiol 50:97-100, 1977.

1979 Sweeney RJ: One more look at the mandibular condyle, Radiol Technol 51:321-327, 1979.

1980 Johnston CC and Doris PE: Clinical trial of pantomography for the evaluation of mandibular trauma, Ann Emerg Med 9:415-418, 1980.

Reiskin AB and Valachovic RW: Radiologic considerations in evaluation of radiolucent lesions of the mandible, J Am Dent Assoc 101:771-776, 1980.

Stalker WH, Cutright DE and Goodwin DW: Tomography of the alveolar process, Oral Surg 49:184-186, 1980.

1981 Higashi T et al: Experimental use of CT scan for definition of dento-maxillomandibular anatomy, J Oral Surg 39:568-571, 1981.

1982 Bertolami CN and Kaban LB: Chin trauma: a clue to associated mandibular and cervical spine injury, Oral Surg 53:122-126, 1982.

Chomenko AG: Structure of the TMJ as viewed on the pantomograph, J Prosthet Dent 48:332-335, 1982.

Moilanen A: Primary radiographic diagnosis of fractures in the mandible, Int J Oral Surg 11:299-303, 1982.

Moilanen A: Skull radiology in patients with facial trauma, Int J Oral Surg 11:89-95, 1982.

Osborn AG, Hanafee WH and Mancuso AA: Normal and pathologic CT anatomy of the mandible, AJR 139:555-559, 1982.

Shinozima M et al: Tomorex (curved rotational tomography apparatus) in experimental and clinical practice, Oral Surg 53:94-110, 1982.

1983 Grondahl HG and Grondahl K: Subtraction radiography for the diagnosis of periodontal bone lesions, Oral Surg Oral Med Oral Pathol 55:208-213, 1983.

Hausmann E et al: Techniques for assessing alveolar bone mass changes in periodontal disease, J Clin Periodontol 10:455-464, 1983.

1984 Moilanen A: Midfacial fractures in dental panoramic radiography, Oral Surg 57(1):106-110, 1984.

1985 Mori S et al: Enlargement radiography with special reference to lateral oblique radiography of the mandible, Dentomaxillofac Radiol 14:59-63, 1985.

1986 Hadeed GJ, Pipko DJ and Zullo TJ: A method for determining anterior mandibular height using a radiographic paralleling measuring system, J Oral Maxillofac Surg 44:188-192, 1986.

Patel JR and Manson Hing LR: The horizontal plane in patient positioning for panoramic radiography, Oral Surg Oral Med Oral Pathol 62:350-353, 1986.

Ponce AZ et al: Adaptation of the Panorex II for use with rare earth screen-film, Oral Surg Oral Med Oral Pathol 61:645-648, 1986.

Ponce AZ et al: Kodak T-Mat G film in rotational panoramic radiography, Oral Surg Oral Med Oral Pathol 61:649-652, 1986.

Schiff T et al: Common positioning and technical errors in panoramic radiography, J Am Dent Assoc 113:422-426, 1986.

1987 Chilvarquer I et al: Intercondylar dimension as a positioning factor for panoramic images, Oral Surg Oral Med Oral Pathol 64:768-773, 1987.

Fernandes RJ et al: A cephalometric tomographic technique to visualize the buccolingual and vertical dimensions of the mandible, J Prosthet Dent 58:466-470, 1987.

Flaxman NA and Kattan KR: Metallic objects seen in radiographs of the maxilla and mandible, Am Fam Physician 35:197-203, 1987.

Markus AF, Poswillo DE and Semple J: The reverse panoral radiograph, Br Dent J 162:145-148, 1987.

Ordman J et al: Head holder for panoramic dental radiography, Angle Orthod 57:322-331, 1987.

Reijnen AL and Sanderink GC: The variation in appearance of the hard palate and the nasal floor, Oral Surg Oral Med Oral Pathol 63:115-119, 1987.

Taylor VE: Improving your radiography. II. Panoramic technique [i], Dent Update 14:341-343, 345-350, 1987.

Taylor VE: Improving your radiography. III. Panoramic technique [ii], Dent Update 14:429-435, 1987.

Tyndall DA and Bedsole SM: Exposure reduction and image quality for pantomographic radiography, Radiol Technol 59:51-53, 1987.

Tyndall DA and Matteson SR: The zygomatic air cell defect (ZACD) on panoramic radiographs, Oral Surg Oral Med Oral Pathol 64:373-376, 1987.

1988 Chilvarquer I et al: A new technique for imaging the temporomandibular joint with a panoramic x-ray machine. I. Description of the technique, Oral Surg Oral Med Oral Pathol 65:626-631, 1988.

Chilvarquer I et al: A new technique for imaging the temporomandibular joint with a panoramic x-ray machine. II. Positioning with the use of patient data, Oral Surg Oral Med Oral Pathol 65:632-636, 1988.

Rosenquist B et al: Accuracy of the oblique lateral transcranial projection, lateral condyle displacement, J Oral Maxillofac Surg 46:862-867, 1988.

Underhill TE et al: Radiobiologic risk estimation from dental radiology. I. Absorbed doses to critical organs, Oral Surg Oral Med Oral Pathol 66:111-120, 1988.

1989 Christianson R et al: MRI of the mandible, Surg Radiol Anat 11:163-169, 1989.

1990 Kapa SF and Platin E: Exposure reduction in panoramic radiography, Radiol Technol 62:130-133, 1990.

1991 Tal H and Moses O: A comparison of panoramic radiography with computed tomography in the planning of implant surgery, Dentomaxillofac Radiol 20:40-42, 1991.

1992 Gibbs SJ: Comparative imaging of the jaws, Curr Opin Dent 2:55-63, 1992.

1993 Yanagisawa K et al: DentaScan imaging of the mandible and maxilla, Head Neck 15:1-7, 1993.

Temporomandibular joint

For bibliographic citations before 1964, please see the fifth edition of this atlas. For citations from 1964 through 1974, see the sixth or seventh edition.

1976 Stanson AW and Baker HL: Routine tomography of the temporomandibular joint, Radiol Clin North Am 14:105-127, 1976.

1978 Collins VA: Transpharyngeal radiography of the temporomandibular joint, Radiography 44(527):259-260, 1978.

Lynch TP and Chase DC: Arthrography in the evaluation of the temporomandibular joint, Radiology 126:667-672, 1978.

1979 Katzberg RW et al: Arthrotomography of the temporomandibular joint: new technique and preliminary observations, AJR 132:949, 1979.

Murphy WA et al: Magnification radiography of the temporomandibular joint: technical considerations, Radiology 133:524-527, 1979.

1980 Beckwith PJ, Monfort DR and Williams BH: Accurate depth of cut in temporomandibular joint laminagraphs, Angle Orthod 50:16-22, 1980.

Blaschke DD, Solberg WK and Sanders B: Arthrography of the temporomandibular joint: review of current status, J Am Dent Assoc 100:388-395, 1980.

Bussard DA et al: Technique and use of "corrected-axis" tomograms of the mandibular condyles, Oral Surg 49:394-397, 1980.

Helms CA et al: Arthrotomographic diagnosis of meniscus perforations in the temporomandibular joint, Br J Radiol 53:283-285, 1980.

Katzberg RW et al: Arthrotomography of the temporomandibular joint, AJR 134:995-1003, 1980.

Rasmussen OC: Semiopaque arthrography of the temporomandibular joint, Scand J Dent Res 88:521-534, 1980.

Westesson PL, Omnell KA and Rohlin M: Double-contrast tomography of the temporomandibular joint: a new technique based on autopsy specimen examinations, Acta Radiol [Diagn] (Stockh) 21:777-784, 1980.

1981 Barrs DM et al: Arthrotomography of the temporomandibular joint, Arch Otolaryngol 107:337-339, 1981.

Duffy MT and Taupmann RE: Temporomandibular joint arthrography in the diagnosis of internal derangements of the temporomandibular joint, J Okla State Med Assoc 74:161-168, 1981.

Dunn MJ et al: Polycycloidal corrected tomography of the temporomandibular joint, Oral Surg 51:375-384, 1981.

Katzberg RW et al: New observations with routine and CT-assisted arthrography in suspected internal derangements of the temporomandibular joint, Oral Surg 51:569-574, 1981.

Kinnie BH: Laminagraphic x-ray procedures in the diagnosis and treatment of the TMJ syndrome, Dent Radiogr Photogr 54:65-79, 1981.

Larheim TA: Radiographic appearance of the normal temporomandibular joint in newborns and small children, Acta Radiol [Diagn] (Stockh) 22:593-599, 1981.

Larheim TA: Temporomandibular joint space in children without joint disease, Acta Radiol [Diagn] (Stockh) 22:85-88, 1981.

Mongini F: The importance of radiography in the diagnosis of TMJ dysfunctions: a comparative evaluation of transcranial radiographs and serial tomography, J Prosthet Dent 45:186-198, 1981.

Murphy WA: Arthrography of the temporomandibular joint, Radiol Clin North Am 19:365-378, 1981.

1982 Chomenko AG: Structure of the TMJ as viewed on the pantomograph, J Prosthet Dent 48:332-335, 1982.

Helms CA et al: Computed tomography of the meniscus of the temporomandibular joint: preliminary observations, Radiology 145:719-722, 1982.

Rosenberg HM and Silha RE: TMJ radiography with emphasis on tomography, Dent Radiogr Photogr 55:1-24, 1982.

1983 Bell KA and Walters PJ: Videofluoroscopy during arthrography of the temporomandibular joint, Radiology 147:879, 1983.

Berrett A: Radiology of the temporomandibular joint, Dent Clin North Am 27:527-540, 1983.

Campbell RL and Alexander JM: Temporomandibular joint arthrography: negative pressure, nontomographic techniques, Oral Surg 55:121-126, 1983.

Doyle T: Arthrography of the temporomandibular joint: a simple technique, Clin Radiol 34:147-151, 1983.

Doyle T and Hase M: The use of arthrography in management of temporomandibular joint problems, Aust Dent J 28:9-12, 1983.

Goldman SM and Taylor R: Radiographic examination of the abnormal temporomandibular joint, J Prosthet Dent 49:711-714, 1983.

Gusching AC: Frontal tomography of articulating temporomandibular joint surfaces, Angle Orthod 53:234-239, 1983.

Helms CA et al: Computed tomography of the temporomandibular joint meniscus, J Oral Maxillofac Surg 41:512-517, 1983.

Manzione JV et al: Direct sagittal computed tomography of the temporomandibular joint, AJR 140:165-167, 1983.

Nance EP Jr: Temporomandibular joint arthrography, J Craniomandibular Pract 1:35-50, 1983.

Preti G, Fava C and Pera P: Accuracy and repeatability of a new procedure for temporomandibular joint laminagraphy, J Prosthet Dent 49:715-725, 1983.

Updegrave WJ: Radiography of the temporomandibular joints individualized and simplified, Compend Contin Educ Dent 4:23-29, 1983.

van Sickels JE, Bianco HJ Jr and Pifer RG: Transcranial radiographs in the evaluation of craniomandibular (TMJ) disorders, J Prosthet Dent 49:244-249, 1983.

Westesson PL: Double-contrast arthrotomography of the temporomandibular joint: introduction of an arthrographic technique for visualization of the disc and articular surfaces, J Oral Maxillofac Surg 41:163-172, 1983.

1984 Bramwit DN: Direct sagittal (lateral) computer tomography of the temporomandibular joints, J Bergen Cty Dent Soc 50:11-13, 1984.

Bussard DA, Yune HY and Whitehead D: Comparison of corrected-axis and straight lateral TMJ tomograms, J Clin Orthod 18:894-898, 1984.

Doyle T: A simplified method for temporomandibular joint arthrography, Australas Radiol 28:12-15, 1984.

Katzberg RW: Preliminary evaluation of Hexabrix for temporomandibular joint arthrography, Invest Radiol 19:S387-S388, 1984.

Manzione JV, Katzberg RW and Brodsky GL: Internal derangements of the temporomandibular joint: diagnosis by direct sagittal computed tomography, Radiology 150:111-115, 1984.

Roberts D et al: Radiologic techniques used to evaluate the temporomandibular joint, Anesth Prog 31:197-206, 1984.

Roberts D et al: Three-dimensional imaging and display of the temporomandibular joint, Oral Surg Oral Med Oral Pathol 58:461-474, 1984.

Sartoris DJ, Neumann CH and Riley RW: The temporomandibular joint: true sagittal computed tomography with meniscus visualization, Radiology 150:250-254, 1984.

Thompson JR et al: Dislocation of the temporomandibular joint disk demonstrated by CT, AJNR 5:115-116, 1984.

Thompson JR et al: Temporomandibular joints: high-resolution computed tomographic evaluation, Radiology 150:105-110, 1984.

Tucker TN: Head position for transcranial temporomandibular joint radiographs, J Prosthet Dent 52:426-431, 1984.

1985 Burke RH: Cinefluorography of the temporomandibular joint, Cranio 3:396-397, 1985.

Conover GL: Direct sagittal CT scanning of the temporomandibular joint, CDS Rev 78:28-31, 1985.

Kaplan P et al: Temporomandibular joint arthrography of normal subjects: prevalence of pain with ionic versus nonionic contrast agents, Radiology 156:825-826, 1985.

Katzberg RW et al: Temporomandibular joint arthrography: comparison of morbidity with ionic and low osmolality contrast media, Radiology 155:245-246, 1985.

Kofler TJ and Howard JA: Temporomandibular joint arthrography, Curr Probl Diagn Radiol 14:1-54, 1985.

Pettigrew J et al: Identification of an anteriorly displaced meniscus in vitro by means of three-dimensional image reconstructions, Oral Surg Oral Med Oral Pathol 59:535-542, 1985.

Simon DC et al: Direct sagittal CT of the temporomandibular joint, Radiology 157:545, 1985.

1986 Bardach M and Beltran J: Radiologic evaluation of the temporomandibular joint, Radiol Technol 57:252-256, 1986.

Christiansen EL et al: Correlative thin section temporomandibular joint anatomy and computed tomography, Radiographics 6:703-723, 1986.

Gillespy T III and Helms CA: Oblique head position in temporomandibular joint arthrography, Radiology 158:541-543, 1986.

Helms CA III et al: Cine-CT of the temporomandibular joint, Cranio 4:246-250, 1986.

Kursunoglu S et al: Three-dimensional computed tomographic analysis of the normal temporomandibular joint, J Oral Maxillofac Surg 44:257-259, 1986.

Rosenberg HM and Graczyk RJ: Temporomandibular articulation tomography: a corrected anteroposterior and lateral cephalometric technique, Oral Surg Oral Med Oral Pathol 62:198-204, 1986.

Willetts PG: Arthrography of the temporomandibular joint, Radiography 52:229-231, 1986.

1987 Chilvarquer I et al: Intercondylar dimension as a positioning factor for panoramic images, Oral Surg Oral Med Oral Pathol 64:768-773, 1987.

Christiansen EL et al: Computed tomography of condylar and articular disk positions within the temporomandibular joint, Oral Surg Oral Med Oral Pathol 64:757-767, 1987.

Harms SE and Wilk RM: Magnetic resonance imaging of the temporomandibular joint, Radiographics 7:521-542, 1987.

Heffez L et al: Accuracy of temporomandibular joint space measurements using corrected hypocycloidal tomography, J Oral Maxillofac Surg 45:137-142, 1987.

Heffez L, Mafee MF and Langer B: Use of a new head holder for obtaining direct sagittal CT images of the TMJ, J Oral Maxillofac Surg 45:822-824, 1987.

Jacobs JM and Manaster BJ: Digital subtraction arthrography of the temporomandibular joint, AJR 148:344-346, 1987.

Keller DC et al: Quantitative radionuclide scanning of the temporomandibular joint. An initial study, Cranio 5:152-156, 1987.

O'Ryan FS and Croall DV: Enhancement of the TMJ region in lateral cephalograms, J Clin Orthod 21:60-62, 1987.

Redlund Johnell I: Radiographic measurements of severe temporomandibular joint destruction at cervical radiography, Scand J Rheumatol 16:355-359, 1987.

Schellhas KP et al: Temporomandibular joint imaging: practical application of available technology, Arch Otolaryngol Head Neck Surg 113:744-748, 1987.

Southard TE, Harris EF and Walter RG: Image enhancement of the mandibular condyle through digital subtraction, Oral Surg Oral Med Oral Pathol 64:645-647, 1987.

Westesson PL and Bronstein SL: Temporomandibular joint: comparison of single- and double-contrast, Radiology 164:65-70, 1987.

1988 Chilvarquer I et al: A new technique for imaging the temporomandibular joint with a panoramic x-ray machine. I. Description of the technique, Oral Surg Oral Med Oral Pathol 65:626-631, 1988.

Chilvarquer I et al: A new technique for imaging the temporomandibular joint with a panoramic x-ray machine. II. Positioning with the use of patient data, Oral Surg Oral Med Oral Pathol 65:632-636, 1988.

Cohen HV et al: Diagnostic imaging of the temporomandibular joint, Clin Prevent Dent 10:25-28, 1988.

Fava C and Preti G: Lateral transcranial radiography of temporomandibular joints. II. Image formation studied with computerized tomography, J Prosthet Dent 59:218-227, 1988.

Harms SE: Temporomandibular joint imaging, Magn Reson Annu 271-297, 1988.

Heffez L, Mafee MF and Langer B: Double-contrast arthrography of the temporomandibular joint, Oral Surg Oral Med Oral Pathol 65:511-514, 1988.

Jumean F, Hatjigiorgis CG and Neff PA: Comparative study of two radiographic techniques to actual dissections of the temporomandibular joint, Cranio 6:141-147, 1988.

Leary JM, Johnson WT and Harvey BV: An evaluation of temporomandibular joint radiographs, J Prosthet Dent 60:94-97, 1988.

Lott CW, Wilson DJ and Juniper RP: Temporomandibular joint arthrography: dynamic study by videorecording, Clin Radiol 39:73-76, 1988.

Ludlow JB: Vertical tomography of the temporomandibular joint with the use of a dental chair and intraoral x-ray unit, Oral Surg Oral Med Oral Pathol 65:358-365, 1988.

Mafee MF et al: Temporomandibular joint: role of direct sagittal CT air-contrast, Otolaryngol Clin North Am 21:575-588, 1988.

Preti G and Fava C: Lateral transcranial radiography of temporomandibular joints. I. Validity in skulls and patients, J Prosthet Dent 59:85-93, 1988.

Rosenquist B et al: Accuracy of the oblique lateral transcranial projection, lateral condyle displacement, J Oral Maxillofac Surg 46:862-867, 1988.

Schellhas KP and Wilkes CH: Temporomandibular joint arthrography: analysis of procedure-related discomfort in abnormal joints, Cranio 6:308-311, 1988.

Walter E et al: CT and MR imaging of the temporomandibular joint, Radiographics 8:327-348, 1988.

1989 Bledsoe WS: The transcranial radiograph: the diagnostic difference between 'corrected' vs 'uncorrected' films, Funct Orthod 6:14-26, 1989.

Fulmer JM and Harms SE: The temporomandibular joint, Top Magn Reson Imaging 1:75-84, 1989.

Hasso AN, Christiansen EL and Alder ME: The temporomandibular joint, Radiol Clin North Am 27:301-314, 1989.

Kaplan PA, Lieberman RP and Chu WK: Comparison of omnipaque with hypaque in temporomandibular arthrography, AJR 153:1225-1227, 1989.

1990 Duvoisin B, Klaus E and Schnyder P: Coronal radiographs and videofluoroscopy improve the diagnostic quality of temporomandibular joint arthrography, AJR 155:105-107, 1990.

Ebner KA et al: Axial temporomandibular joint morphology: a correlative study of radiographic and gross anatomic findings, Oral Surg Oral Med Oral Pathol 69:247-252, 1990.

Helms CA and Kaplan P: Diagnostic imaging of the temporomandibular joint: recommendations for use of the various techniques, AJR 154:319-322, 1990.

Lynn J: TMJ tomography, a standard of the future: a review of the A-P projection of the mandibular condyle, Funct Orthod 7:32-40, 1990.

Pollei SR and Schellhas KP: Magnetic resonance imaging of the temporomandibular joint, Semin Ultrasound CT MR 11:346-361, 1990.

van der Kuijl B et al: Temporomandibular joint computed tomography: development of a direct sagittal technique, J Prosthet Dent 64:709-715, 1990.

van der Kuijl B et al: Temporomandibular joint direct sagittal computed tomography: evaluation of image-processing modalities, J Prosthet Dent 64:589-595, 1990.

1991 Betz BW and Wiener MD: Air in the temporomandibular joint fossa: CT sign of temporal bone fracture, Radiology 180:463-466, 1991.

Dixon DC: Diagnostic imaging of the temporomandibular joint, Dent Clin North Am 35:53-74, 1991.

Knoernschild KL, Aquilino SA and Ruprecht A: Transcranial radiography and linear tomography: a comparative study, J Prosthet Dent 66:239-250, 1991.

Ludlow JB et al: Digitally subtracted linear tomograms: three techniques for measuring condylar displacement, Oral Surg Oral Med Oral Pathol 72:614-620, 1991.

Thorburn DN et al: Exposure factors and screen-film combinations in temporomandibular joint radiography, Dentomaxillofac Radiol 20:87-92, 1991.

1992 Engelke W et al: An experimental study of new diagnostic methods for the examination of osseous lesions in the temporomandibular joint, Oral Surg Oral Med Oral Pathol 73:348-359, 1992.

Keesler JT et al: A transcranial radiographic examination of the temporal portion of the temporomandibular joint, J Oral Rehabil 19:71-84, 1992.

Lieberman JM et al: MR imaging of the juvenile temporomandibular joint: preliminary report, Radiology 182:531-534, 1992.

1993 Brady AP et al: A technique for magnetic resonance imaging of the temporomandibular joint, Clin Radiol 47:127-133, 1993.

Brooks SL and Westesson PL: Temporomandibular joint: value of coronal MR images, Radiology 188:317-321, 1993.

TEETH

For bibliographic citations before 1964, please see the fifth edition of this atlas. For citations from 1964 through 1974, see the sixth or seventh edition.

1975 Maw J: Profile radiography, Br J Orthod 2:119-120, 1975.

1976 Biggerstaff RH and Phillips JR: A quantitative comparison of paralleling long-cone and bisection of angle periapical radiography, Oral Surg 62:673-677, 1976.

Weinstein S and Colanche D: Special radiological methods, Oral Sci Rev 8:63-87, 1976.

1977 Horton PS, Sippy FH and Higa LH: panoramic radiography—an adjunct, Oral Surg 43:473-477, 1977.

Snyder MB et al: The advantages of xeroradiography for panoramic examination of jaws and teeth, J Periodontol 48:467-472, 1977.

1979 Jensen TW: The free focus concept in dental and maxillofacial radiography: the present status of the miniaturized dental x-ray machines, Oral Surg 47:282-293, 1979.

1980 Benkel HD et al: Comparison of endodontic measurement controls using a paralleling technique with a grid and a conventional measurement, Oral Surg 49:157-161, 1980.

Nakasima A et al: Radiologic exposure conditions and resultant skin doses in application of xeroradiography to the orthodontic diagnosis, Am J Orthod 78:646-656, 1980.

Westesson PL and Carlsson LE: Anatomy of mandibular third molars: a comparison between radiographic appearance and clinical observations, Oral Surg 49:90-94, 1980.

1981 Bhakdinaronk A and Manson-Hing LR: Effect of radiographic technique upon prediction of tooth length in intraoral radiography, Oral Surg 51:100-107, 1981.

Spyropoulos ND, Patsakas AJ and Angelopoulos AP: findings from radiographs of the jaws of edentulous patients, Oral Surg 52:455-459, 1981.

1982 Chomenko AG: Structure of the TMJ as viewed on the pantomograph, J Prosthet Dent 48:332-335, 1982.

Matteson SR: Pantomographic radiology. I. Theory of pantomographic imaging, normal radiographic anatomy, and developmental abnormality interpretation, Dent Radiogr Photogr 55:45-59, 1982.

Stoneman DW: Radiology of trauma to the teeth and jaws, Dent Clin North Am 26:591-611, 1982.

1984 Archer A: Panoramic zonography of the middle and inner ear, Radiography 50:107-109, 1984.

Buenviaje TM and Rapp R: Dental anomalies in children: a clinical and radiographic survey, ASDC J Dent Child 51:42-46, 1984.

Clow IM: A radiographic survey of third molar development: a comparison, Br J Orthod 11:9-15, 1984.

Coupland MA: Localisation of misplaced maxillary canines: orthopantomograph and PA: skull views compared, Br J Orthod 11:27-32, 1984.

1985 Borglin K et al: Radiation dosimetry in tomography of the teeth and jaws using a multi-film cassette, Acta Radiol [Diagn] 26:739-743, 1985.

1986 Mittal RK, Givila CP and Mathur RM: A study of orthopantomography in conservative dentistry, J Indian Dent Assoc 58:107-110, 1986.

Patel JR and Manson Hing LR: The horizontal plane in patient positioning for panoramic radiography, Oral Surg Oral Med Oral Pathol 62:350-353, 1986.

Ponce AZ et al: Adaptation of the Panorex II for use with rare earth screen-film, Oral Surg Oral Med Oral Pathol 61:645-648, 1986.

Ponce AZ et al: Kodak T-Mat G film in rotational panoramic radiography, Oral Surg Oral Med Oral Pathol 61:649-652, 1986.

Schiff T et al: Common positioning and technical errors in panoramic radiography, J Am Dent Assoc 113:422-426, 1986.

1987 Chilvarquer I et al: Intercondylar dimension as a positioning factor for panoramic images, Oral Surg Oral Med Oral Pathol 64:768-773, 1987.

Jeffcoat MK et al: Extraoral control of geometry for digital subtraction radiography, J Periodont Res 22:396-402, 1987.

Markus AF, Poswillo DE and Semple J: The reverse panoral radiograph, Br Dent J 162:145-148, 1987.

Ordman J et al: Head holder for panoramic dental radiography, Angle Orthod 57:322-331, 1987.

Reijnen AL and Sanderink GC: The variation in appearance of the hard palate and the nasal floor, Oral Surg Oral Med Oral Pathol 63:115-119, 1987.

Taylor VE: Improving your radiography. II. Panoramic technique [i], Dent Update 14:341-343, 345-350, 1987.

Taylor VE: Improving your radiography. III. Panoramic technique [ii], Dent Update 14:429-435, 1987.

Tyndall DA and Bedsole SM: Exposure reduction and image quality for pantomographic radiography, Radiol Technol 59:51-53, 1987.

Tyndall DA and Matteson SR: The zygomatic air cell defect (ZACD) on panoramic radiographs, Oral Surg Oral Med Oral Pathol 64:373-376, 1987.

1988 Chilvarquer I et al: A new technique for imaging the temporomandibular joint with a panoramic x-ray machine. I. Description of the technique, Oral Surg Oral Med Oral Pathol 65:626-631, 1988.

Chilvarquer I et al: A new technique for imaging the temporomandibular joint with a panoramic x-ray machine. II. Positioning with the use of patient data, Oral Surg Oral Med Oral Pathol 65:632-636, 1988.

Underhill TE et al: Radiobiologic risk estimation from dental radiology. I. Absorbed doses to critical organs, Oral Surg Oral Med Oral Pathol 66:111-120, 1988.

1989 DeConinck AT: The benefit of radiographs in endodontics, J Macomb Dent Soc 26:28-29, 31, 1989.

Kelly WH: Radiographic asepsis in endodontic practice, Gen Dent 37:302-303, 1989.

1990 Kapa SF and Platin E: Exposure reduction in panoramic radiography, Radiol Technol 62:130-133, 1990.

Zanella FE: Dental radiology, Curr Opin Radiol 2:140-144, 1990.

1991 Velders XL, van Aken J and van der Stelt PF: Absorbed dose to organs in the head and neck from bitewing radiography, Dentomaxillofac Radiol 20:161-165, 1991.

1992 Lew KK: The prediction of eruption-sequence from panoramic radiographs, ASDC J Dent Child 59:346-349, 1992.

AUDITORY (EUSTACHIAN) TUBE

For bibliographic citations before 1964, please see the fifth edition of this atlas. For citations from 1964 through 1974, see the sixth or seventh edition.

1977 Khoo FY et al: Radiology of the eustachian fossa, Clin Radiol 28:151-160, 1977.

1980 Pinckney LE and Currarino G: Reflux of barium into the middle ear during upper gastrointestinal series, Radiology 135:653-654, 1980.

1985 Khan NA: Technique and clinical importance of eustachian tube radiography, Am J Otol 6:222-224, 1985.

1987 Naito Y et al: Magnetic resonance imaging of the eustachian tube: a correlative anatomical study, Arch Otolaryngol Head Neck Surg 113:1281-1284, 1987.

1989 Conticello S et al: Computed tomography in the study of the eustachian tube, Arch Otorhinolaryngol 246:259-261, 1989.

1992 Paludetti G et al: Functional study of the eustachian tube with sequential scintigraphy, ORL 54:76-79, 1992.

EYES
General

For bibliographic citations before 1964, please see the fifth edition of this atlas. For citations from 1964 through 1974, see the sixth or seventh edition.

1979 Belkin M: A retention modification for the limbal ring method of foreign body localization, Am J Ophthalmol 88:124-125, 1979.

1983 Sevel D et al: Value of computed tomography for the diagnosis of a ruptured eye, J Comput Assist Tomogr 7:870-875, 1983.

1989 Etherington RJ and Hourihan MD: Localisation of intraocular and intraorbital foreign bodies using computed tomography, Clin Radiol 40:610-614, 1989.

1990 King SJ and Haigh SF: Technical report: digital subtraction dacryocystography, Clin Radiol 42:351-353, 1990.

Siddle KJ and Sim L: Radiation dose to the lens of the eye during computerised tomography examinations of the orbit, the pituitary fossa and the brain on a General Electric 9800 Quick CT scanner, Australas Radiol 34:326-330, 1990.

Siddle KJ, Sim LH and Case CC: Radiation doses to the lens of the eye during computerised tomography of the orbit: a comparison of four modern computerised tomography units, Australas Radiol 34:323-325, 1990.

1991 Bray LC and Griffiths PG: The value of plain radiography in suspected intraocular foreign body, Eye 5:751-754, 1991.

Moseley IF: The plain radiograph in ophthalmology: a wasteful and potentially dangerous anachronism, J R Soc Med 84:76-80, 1991.

Zentner J, Hassler W and Petersen D: A wooden foreign body penetrating the superior orbital fissure, Neurochirurgia 34:188-190, 1991.

1992 Otto PM et al: Screening test for detection of metallic foreign objects in the orbit before magnetic resonance imaging, Invest Radiol 27:308-311, 1992.

Specht CS et al: Orbitocranial wooden foreign body diagnosed by magnetic resonance imaging: dry wood can be isodense with air and orbital fat by computed tomography, Surv Ophthalmol 36:341-344, 1992.

1993 Massoud TF, Whittet HB and Anslow P: CT-dacryocystography for nasolacrimal duct obstruction following paranasal sinus surgery, Br J Radiol 66:223-227, 1993.

Lacrimal drainage system

For bibliographic citations before 1964, please see the fifth edition of this atlas. For citations from 1964 through 1974, see the sixth or seventh edition.

1975 Gerlock AJ: A simple radiographic technic for visualization of the lacrimal foramen, South Med J 68:118-120, 1975.

Hurwitz JJ, Welham AN and Lloyd GA: The role of intubation macrodacryocystography in management of problems of the lacrimal system, Can J Ophthalmol 10:361-366, 1975.

1976 Fisch AE and Sondheimer FK: Evaluation of the nasolacrimal canal in the basal projection, Radiology 118:230-231, 1976.

Veirs ER: Lacrimal disorders: diagnosis and treatment, Saint Louis, 1976, Mosby.

1977 Johansen JG and Udnaes I: Dacryocystography with Amipaque (metrizamide), Acta Ophthalmol 55:683-687, 1977.

1979 Montanara A, Catalino P and Gualdi M: Improved radiological technique for evaluating the lacrimal pathways with special emphasis on functional disorders, Acta Ophthalmol 57:547-563, 1979.

1981 Sekaran C and Janosik J: Lacrimal drainage system. I. Macrodacryocystography, Radiography 47:125-137, 1981.

1983 Balchunas WR, Quencer RM and Byrne SF: Lacrimal gland and fossa masses: evaluation by computed tomography and A-mode echography, Radiology 149:751-758, 1983.

Montanara A, Mannino G and Contestabile MT: Macrodacryocystography and echography in diagnosis of disorders of the lacrimal pathways, Surv Ophthalmol 28:33-41, 1983.

1985 Heyman S, Katowitz JA and Smoger B: Dacryoscintigraphy in children, Ophthalmic Surg 16:703-709, 1985.

Russell EJ et al: CT of the inferomedial orbit and the lacrimal drainage apparatus: normal and pathologic anatomy, AJR 145:1147-1154, 1985.

1987 Millman AL, Liebeskind A and Putterman AM: Dacryocystography: the technique and its role in the practice of ophthalmology, Radiol Clin North Am 25:781-786, 1987.

1988 Lewis S: A lateral oblique radiographic projection for use in dacrocystography, Radiogr Today 54:37-38, 1988.

1989 Jackson A et al: Reduction of ocular lens dosage in dacryocystography, Clin Radiol 40:615-618, 1989.

Munk PL et al: Dacryocystography: comparison of water-soluble and oil-based contrast agents, Radiology 173:827-830, 1989.

1990 King SJ and Haigh SF: Technical report: digital subtraction dacryocystography, Clin Radiol 42:351-353, 1990.

Montecalvo RM et al: Evaluation of the lacrimal apparatus with digital subtraction macrodacryocystography, Radiographics 10:483-490, 1990.

1991 Ashenhurst M et al: Combined computed tomography and dacryocystography for complex lacrimal problems, Can J Ophthalmol 26:27-31, 1991.

1993 Goldberg RA, Heinz GW and Chiu L: Gadolinium magnetic resonance imaging dacryocystography, Am J Ophthalmol 115:738-741, 1993.

Massoud TF, Whittet HB and Anslow P: CT-dacryocystography for nasolacrimal duct obstruction following paranasal sinus surgery, Br J Radiol 66:223-227, 1993.

EXTERNAL EAR

For bibliographic citations before 1964, please see the fifth edition of this atlas. For citations from 1964 through 1974, see the sixth or seventh edition.

1981 Wright JW, Jr: Polytomography and congenital external and middle ear anomalies, Laryngoscope 91:1806-1811, 1981.

1982 Wright JW Jr, Wright JW III and Hicks G: Polytomography and congenital anomalies of the ear, Ann Otol Rhinol Laryngol 91:480-484, 1982.

1983 Virapongse C et al: High resolution computed tomography of the osseous external auditory canal. 2. Pathology, J Comput Assist Tomogr 7:493-497, 1983.

1984 Chakeres DW: CT of ear structures: a tailored approach, Radiol Clin North Am 22:3-14, 1984.

Curtin HD: CT of acoustic neuroma and other tumors of the ear, Radiol Clin North Am 22:77-105, 1984.

1985 Fileni A et al: Tomography in the preoperative evaluation of ear malformations, J Laryngol Otol 99:433-438, 1985.

1989 Vanneste F et al: High resolution CT findings in diseases of the external auditory canal: a review of 31 cases, J Belge Radiol 72:199-205, 1989.

PARANASAL SINUSES

For bibliographic citations before 1964, please see the fifth edition of this atlas. For citations from 1964 through 1974, see the sixth or seventh edition.

1975 Yeh HC and Butt WP: A modified Towne's view for radiography of the orbit and maxillary antrum, Radiology 116:724-728, 1975.

Yune HY, Holden RW and Smith JA: Normal variations and lesions of the sphenoid sinus, AJR 124:129-138, 1975.

1976 Ohba T and Katayama H: Comparison of panoramic radiography and Water's projection in the diagnosis of maxillary sinus disease, Oral Surg 42:534-538, 1976.

1977 Crooks HE and Ardran GM: An air-gap technique for nasal sinus radiography, Radiography 43:195-202, 1977.

Yanagisawa E, Gaudet PT and Eibling DE: Zygomatic arch simulating air-fluid level in the sphenoid sinus, Ear Nose Throat J 56:487-492, 1977.

1980 Shapiro R and Schorr S: A consideration of the systemic factors that influence frontal sinus pneumatization, Invest Radiol 15:191-202, 1980.

Sperber GH: Applied anatomy of the maxillary sinus, Can Dent Assoc J 46:381-386, 1980.

1981 Nehen AM et al: Computed tomography and hypocycloid tomography in lesions of the nose, paranasal sinuses, and nasopharynx, Acta Radiol [Diagn] (Stockh) 22:285-287, 1981.

Potter GD: Sinus anatomy and pathology, Bull NY Acad Med 57:591-594, 1981.

1982 Bilaniuk LT and Zimmerman RA: Computed tomography in evaluation of the paranasal sinuses, Radiol Clin North Am 20:51-66, 1982.

Dolan KD: Paranasal sinus radiology. Ia. introduction and the frontal sinuses, Head Neck Surg 4:301-311, 1982.

Dolan KD: Paranasal sinus radiology. IIIa. Sphenoidal sinus, Head Neck Surg 5:164-176, 1982.

Jannert M et al: Ultrasonic examination of the paranasal sinuses, Acta Otolaryngol [Suppl] (Stockh) 389:1-52, 1982.

Kondo M et al: Computed tomography of malignant tumors of the nasal cavity and paranasal sinuses, Cancer 50:226-231, 1982.

Laasonen EM, Servo A and Sumuvuori H: Sphenoid sinus fluid level in skull-base fractures, Eur J Radiol 2:5-7, 1982.

Noyek AM and Kassel EE: Computed tomography in frontal sinus fractures, Arch Otolaryngol 108:378-379, 1982.

Rieder-Grosswasser I, Godel V and Lazar M: Computed tomography in ethmoid cell trauma, Comput Radiol 6:171-179, 1982.

Schneider G, Sager WD and Lepuschutz H: Multidirectional tomography and high resolution CT in lesions of the paranasal sinuses and the pharyngeal cavity, Acta Radiol [Diagn] (Stockh) 23:63-69, 1982.

Som PM: The role of CT in the diagnosis of carcinoma of the paranasal sinuses and nasopharynx, J Otolaryngol 11:340-348, 1982.

1983 Carter BL, Bankoff MS and fisk JD: Computed tomographic detection of sinusitis responsible for intracranial and extracranial infections, Radiology 147:739-742, 1983.

Eddleston B and Johnson RJ: A comparison of conventional radiographic imaging and computed tomography in malignant disease of the paranasal sinuses and the postnasal space, Clin Radiol 34:161-172, 1983.

Kondo M et al: Value of computed tomography for radiation therapy of tumors of the nasal cavity and paranasal sinuses, Acta Radiol [Oncol] 22:3-7, 1983.

1984 Gibson W Jr: Sphenoid sinus revisited, Laryngoscope 94:185-191, 1984.

Hasso AN: CT of tumors and tumor-like conditions of the paranasal sinuses, Radiol Clin North Am 22:119-130, 1984.

Kuijpers D, Blickman JG and Camps JA: The five degree rule: optimization of the paranasal sinus examination of children, Radiology 152:814, 1984.

Moilanen A: Panoramic zonography in the diagnosis of the maxillary sinus disease, Int J Oral Surg 13:432-436, 1984.

Sataloff RT et al: Computed tomography of the face and paranasal sinuses. I. Normal anatomy, Head Neck 7:110-122, 1984.

Schatz CJ and Becker TS: Normal CT anatomy of the paranasal sinuses, Radiol Clin North Am 22:107-118, 1984.

1985 Chakeres DW: Computed tomography of the ethmoid sinuses, Otolaryngol Clin North Am 18:29-42, 1985.

Dolan KD: The ethmoid sinus: plain film and tomographic radiology, Otolaryngol Clin North Am 18:15-28, 1985.

Kalender WA, Rettinger G and Suess C: Measurement of paranasal sinus ventilation by xenon-enhanced dynamic computed tomography, J Comput Assist Tomogr 9:524-529, 1985.

1986 Kuhn JP: Imaging of the paranasal sinuses: current status, J Allerg Clin Immunol 77:6-8, 1986.

Singh AP et al: Computerized axial tomography of the nose, paranasal sinuses, nasopharynx and pterygoid regions, J Laryngol Otol 100:907-914, 1986.

1987 Jensen C and von Sydow C: Radiography and ultrasonography in paranasal sinusitis, Acta Radiol 28:31-34, 1987.

Teatini G et al: Computed tomography of the ethmoid labyrinth and adjacent structures, Ann Otol Rhinol Laryngol 96:239-250, 1987.

1988 Carter BL and Runge VS: Imaging modalities for the study of the paranasal sinuses and nasopharynx, Otolaryngol Clin North Am 21:395-420, 1988.

Kopp W, Stammberger H and Fotter R: Special radiologic imaging of paranasal sinuses: a prerequisite for functional endoscopic sinus surgery, Eur J Radiol 8:153-156, 1988.

1989 Lloyd GA: Diagnostic imaging of the nose and paranasal sinuses, J Laryngol Otol 103:453-460, 1989.

Masala W et al: Multiplanar reconstructions in the study of ethmoid anatomy, Neuroradiology 31:151-155, 1989.

Shapiro MD and Som PM: MRI of the paranasal sinuses and nasal cavity, Radiol Clin North Am 27:447-475, 1989.

1990 Beahm E et al: MR of the paranasal sinuses, Surg Radiol Anat 12:203-208, 1990.

Hayward MW et al: Radiography of the paranasal sinuses—one or three views? Clin Radiol 41:163-164, 1990.

Philippou M et al: Cross-sectional anatomy of the nose and paranasal sinuses: a correlative study of computer tomographic images and cryosections, Rhinology 28:221-230, 1990.

Veillon F, Bintner M and Bourjat P: The paranasal sinuses, Curr Opin Radiol 2:100-104, 1990.

Weissman JL, Tabor EK and Curtin HD: Magnetic resonance imaging of the paranasal sinuses, Top Magn Reson Imaging 2:27-38, 1990.

White PS et al: Computerized tomography mini-series: an alternative to standard paranasal sinus radiographs, Aust N Z J Surg 60:25-29, 1990.

Zinreich SJ: Paranasal sinus imaging, Otolaryngol Head Neck Surg 103:863-868, 1990.

1991 Bolger WE, Butzin CA and Parsons DS: Paranasal sinus bony anatomic variations and mucosal abnormalities: CT analysis for endoscopic sinus surgery, Laryngoscope 101:56-64, 1991.

Lloyd GA and Barker PB: Subtraction magnetic resonance for tumours of the skull base and sinuses: a new imaging technique, J Laryngol Otol 105:628-631, 1991.

MacLeod B: Paranasal sinus radiography, Emerg Med Clin North Am 9:743-755, 1991.

Monsour PA and Mendoza AR: Visualization of the maxillary sinus and styloid processes using rotational panoramic radiography, Aust Dent J 36:5-10, 1991.

1992 Lazar RH, Younis RT and Parvey LS: Comparison of plain radiographs, coronal CT, and intraoperative findings in children with chronic sinusitis, Otolaryngol Head Neck Surg 107:29-34, 1992.

Riechelmann H and Mann W: Ultrasonography of paranasal sinus lesions, Rhinology Suppl 14:136-140, 1992.

1993 Earwaker J: Anatomic variants in sinonasal CT, Radiographics 13:381-415, 1993.

MAMMOGRAPHY

For bibliographic citations before 1964, please see the fifth edition of this atlas. For citations from 1964 through 1974, see the sixth or seventh edition.

1975 Egan RL: Mammography, xeroradiography, and thermography, Clin Obstet Gynecol 18:197-209, 1975.

Lawrence W Jr and Horsley JS: The use of xeromammography in early detection of breast cancer, Va Med Mon 102:313-321, 1975.

1976 Egan RL: Mammography and radiation dose, J Med Assoc Ga 65:328-329, 1976.

Hermel MB and Murdock MG: Microdose mammography, Cancer 38:1947-1951, 1976.

Puretz DH: Mammography, history, current events, and recommendations, N Y State J Med 76:1985-1991, 1976.

1977   Baum G: Ultrasound mammography, Radiology 122:199-205, 1977.

Chang CH et al: Computed tomography of the breast: a preliminary report, Radiology 124:827-829, 1977.

Kalisher L and Schaffer D: Indications and guidelines for mammographic examinations, Am J Surg 133:326-330, 1977.

Lester RG: Risk vs. benefit in mammography, Radiology 124:1-6, 1977.

Matallana RH: Negative technique in xeroradiography of the breast, Cancer 39:112-122, 1977.

Wilson P: Some application problems and solutions in xeromammography, Radiol Technol 48:389-403, 1977.

1978   Arnold BA, Webster EW and Kalisher L: Evaluation of mammographic screen-film systems, Radiology 129:179-185, 1978.

Lundgren B: Malignant features of breast tumors at radiography, Acta Radiol 19:623-633, 1978.

Moskowitz M: Mammography in medical practice: a rational approach, JAMA 240:1898-1899, 1978.

Quimet-Oliva D, Hebert G and Ladouceur J: Radiographic characteristics of male breast cancer, Radiology 129:37-40, 1978.

1979   Askins BS et al: Autoradiographic enhancement of mammograms: investigation of a new dose reduction technique, Radiology 130:103-107, 1979.

Bassett LW and Axelrod S: A modification of the craniocaudal view in mammography, Radiology 132:222-224, 1979.

Bigongiari L et al: Dependent compression mammography: a new look at an old idea, J Kans Med Soc 80:336-340, 1979.

Greens RA et al: Efficacy of the lateral view mammogram in the detection of breast malignancy, Radiology 130:793-794, 1979.

Palmer DS: Needle localization of nonpalpable breast lesions, Clin Radiol 30:291-293, 1979.

Sickles EA: Microfocal spot magnification mammography using xeroradiographic and screen recording systems, Radiology 131:599-607, 1979.

Sickles EA and Genant HK: Controlled single-blind clinical evaluation of low-dose mammographic screen-film systems, Radiology 130:347-351, 1979.

1980   Bassett LW, Pagani JJ and Gold RH: Pitfalls in mammography: demonstrating deep lesions, Radiology 136:641-645, 1980.

Chang CH et al: Computed tomography in detection and diagnosis of breast cancer, Cancer 46:939-946, 1980.

Fatouros PP, Rao GU and Kao CC: Xeromammographic image quality, Med Phys 7:331-340, 1980.

Hassani SN, Bard RL and Flynn GS, Jr: High-resolution breast ultrasonography, Diagn Gynecol Obstet 2:303-312, 1980.

Moores BM, Ramsden JA and Asbury DL: An atmospheric pressure ionography system suitable for mammography, Phys Med Biol 25:893-902, 1980.

Pagani JJ et al: Efficacy of combined film-screen/xeromammography: preliminary report, AJR 135:141-146, 1980.

Sickles EA: Further experience with microfocal spot magnification mammography in the assessment of clustered breast microcalcifications, Radiology 137:9-14, 1980.

Weshler Z and Sulkes A: Contrast mammography and the diagnosis of male breast cysts, Clin Radiol 31:341-343, 1980.

Wyatt CC: Xero and film mammography: two images with one exposure, Radiol Technol 51:621-625, 1980.

1981   Blomerus JM: Office mammography: report of 2,621 examinations, Appl Radiol 10:39-42, 1981.

Bragg DG: Tumor imaging in diagnostic radiology, Cancer 47:1159-1163, 1981.

Broadbent RV and Reid MH: Mammography—misunderstood and underutilized, Postgrad Med 70:93-97, 100-101, 1981.

Cole-Beuglet C et al: Ultrasound mammography: a comparison with radiographic mammography, Radiology 139:693-698, 1981.

Dodd GD: Radiation detection and diagnosis of breast cancer, Cancer 47:1766-1769, 1981.

Doust BD, Milbrath JR and Doust VL: CT scanning of the breast using a conventional CT scanner, CT 5:296-302, 1981.

Friedrich M: The XERG-mammography system: a solution to the dose-quality problem? Eur J Radiol 1:143-151, 1981.

Goldberg IM et al: Contact plate thermography: a new technique for diagnosis of breast masses, Arch Surg 116:271-273, 1981.

Jennings RJ et al: Optimal x-ray spectra for screen-film mammography, Med Phys 8:629-639, 1981.

Loughry CW et al: Breast cancer detection utilizing biostereometric analysis, Cancer Detect Prev 4:589-594, 1981.

Meyer JE and Munzenrider JE: Computed tomographic demonstration of internal mammary lymph-node metastasis in patients with locally recurrent breast carcinoma, Radiology 139:661-663, 1981.

Ouimet-Oliva D et al: Effect of danazol on the radiographic density of breast parenchyma, J Can Assoc Radiol 32:159-161, 1981.

Schmarsow R, Wessels G and Bielke G: A new applicator for ultrasound mammography, Rev Interam Radiol 6:59-60, 1981.

Shrivastava PN: Radiation dose in mammography: an energy-balance approach, Radiology 140:483-490, 1981.

Tabar L et al: The diagnostic and therapeutic value of breast cyst puncture and pneumocystography, Radiology 141:659-663, 1981.

1982   Alberti GP and Troiso A: Secreting breast: the role of galactography, Eur J Gynaecol Oncol 3:96-100, 1982.

Barnes GT and Chakraborty DP: Radiographic mottle and patient exposure in mammography, Radiology 145:815-821, 1982.

Beaman SA and Lillicrap SC: Optimum x-ray spectra for mammography, Phys Med Biol 27:1209-1220, 1982.

Breyer B, Cepulic E and Zunter F: Ultrasonic mammography without specialized equipment: comparison with clinical examination and x-rays, Ultrasound Med Biol 8:377-379, 1982.

Chang CH et al: Computed tomographic mammography using a conventional body scanner, AJR 138:553-558, 1982.

Cole-Beuglet D et al: Ultrasound mammography for male breast enlargement, J Ultrasound Med 1:301-305, 1982.

Homer MJ: Mammographic detection of breast cancer, Clin Obstet Gynecol 25:393-400, 1982.

Karila KT: Performance of automatic exposure controls in mammography, Med Phys 9:898-903, 1982.

Karila KT: Performance of x-ray generators and unnecessary dose in mammography, Radiology 144:395-401, 1982.

Lundgren B and Helleberg A: Single oblique-view mammography for periodic screening for breast cancer in women, JNCI 68:351-355, 1982.

Ross RJ et al: Nuclear magnetic resonance imaging and evaluation of human breast tissue: preliminary clinical trials, Radiology 143:195-205, 1982.

Schuy S: Medical ultrasonic imaging, Med Prog Technol 9:161-164, 1982.

Sterns EE et al: Thermography in breast diagnosis, Cancer 50:323-325, 1982.

1983   Bassett LW and Gold RH: Breast radiography using the oblique projection, Radiology 149:585-587, 1983.

Beaman S, Lillicrap SC and Price JL: Tungsten anode tubes with K-edge filters for mammography, Br J Radiol 56:721-727, 1983.

Egan RL, McSweeney MB and Sprawls P: Grids in mammography, Radiology 146:359-362, 1983.

Fritz SL, Chang CH and Livingston WH: Scatter/primary ratios for x-ray spectra modified to enhance iodine contrast in screen-film mammography, Med Phys 10:866-870, 1983.

Jewell WR, Thomas JH and Chang CH: Computed tomographic mammography directed biopsy of the breast, Surg Gynecol Obstet 157:75-76, 1983.

Kapdi CC and Parekh NJ: The male breast, Radiol Clin North Am 21:137-148, 1983.

McSweeney MB, Sprawls P and Egan RL: Enhanced image mammography, AJR 140:9-14, 1983.

Muller JW, van Waes PF and Koehler PR: Computed tomography of breast lesions: comparison with x-ray mammography, J Comput Assist Tomogr 7:650-654, 1983.

Muntz EP et al: On the significance of very small angle scattered radiation to radiographic imaging at low energies, Med Phys 10:819-823, 1983.

Novak D: Indications for and comparative diagnostic value of combined ultrasound and X-ray mammography, Eur J Radiol 3:299-302, 1983.

Symposium on mammography, Radiol Clin North Am 21:1-194, 1983.

Tabar L, Dean PB and Pentek Z: Galactography: the diagnostic procedure of choice for nipple discharge, Radiology 149:31-38, 1983.

1984 Bloomberg TJ, Chivers RC and Price JL: Real-time ultrasonic characteristics of the breast, Clin Radiol 35:21-27, 1984.

Dodd GD: Mammography: state of the art, Cancer 53:652-657, 1984.

El-Yousef SJ et al: Magnetic resonance imaging of the breast. Work in progress, Radiology 150:761-766, 1984.

Feig SA: Radiation risk from mammography: is it clinically significant? AJR 143:469-475, 1984.

Hatton PD, Harford FJ Jr and Sheppard JR: Xeromammographic screening: is it helping? South Med J 77:857-859, 1984.

Kopans DB: "Early" breast cancer detection using techniques other than mammography, AJR 143:465-468, 1984.

Kopans DB, Meyer JE and Sadowsky N: Breast imaging, N Engl J Med 310:960-967, 1984.

McLelland R: Mammography 1984: challenge to radiology, AJR 143:1-4, 1984.

McSweeney MB, Sprawls P and Egan RL: Enhanced-image mammography, Recent Results Cancer Res 90:79-89, 1984.

Muir BB et al: Oblique-view mammography: adequacy for screening. Work in progress, Radiology 151:39-41, 1984.

Rasmussen OS and Seerup A: Preoperative radiographically guided wire marking of nonpalpable breast lesions, Acta Radiol [Diagn] 25:13-16, 1984.

Schreiman JS et al: Ultrasound transmission computed tomography of the breast, Radiology 150:523-530, 1984.

Sickles EA: Mammographic features of "early" breast cancer, AJR 143:461-464, 1984.

Stanton L et al: Dosage evaluation in mammography, Radiology 150:577-584, 1984.

1985 Chan HP et al: Ultra-high–strip-density radiographic grids: a new antiscatter technique for mammography, Radiology 154:807-815, 1985.

Dershaw DD et al: Mammography using an ultrahigh-strip-density, stationary, focused grid, Radiology 156:541-544, 1985.

Kirkpatrick AE and Law J: The usefulness of a moving grid in mammography, Br J Radiol 58:257-258, 1985.

Kowalczyk N: Patients' perceptions of a mammographic examination, Radiol Technol 56(4):212-216, 1985.

Niklason LT, Barnes GT and Rubin E: Mammography phototimer technique chart, Radiology 157:539-540, 1985.

1986 Baker SR: Screening mammography—potential problems on the horizon, Invest Radiol 21:891-892, 1986.

Cuttino JT Jr, Yankaskas BC and Hoskins EO: Screen-film mammography versus xeromammography in the detection of breast cancer, Br J Radiol 59:1159-1162, 1986.

Dershaw DD: Male mammography, AJR 146:127-131, 1986.

Dershaw DD and Malik S: Stationary and moving mammography grids: comparative radiation dose, AJR 147:491-492, 1986.

Fritz SL et al: A digital radiographic imaging system for mammography, Invest Radiol 21:581-583, 1986.

Gisvold JJ et al: Comparison of mammography and transillumination light scanning in the detection of breast lesions, AJR 147:191-194, 1986.

Homer MJ and Pile-Spellman ER: Needle localization of occult breast lesions with a curved-end retractable wire: technique and pitfalls, Radiology 161:547-548, 1986.

Jackson VP et al: Mammography and ultrasonography for breast cancer detection, Indiana Med 79:749-752, 1986.

Massa T, Pino G and Boccardo F: Correlation between mammographic and thermographic patterns: use of thermography as a possible pre-screening procedure in patients at risk for breast cancer, Eur J Gynaecol Oncol 7:39-44, 1986.

Nielsen B and Fagerberg G: Image quality in mammography with special reference to anti-scatter grids and the magnification technique, Acta Radiol [Diagn] 27:467-479, 1986.

Sickles EA and Weber WN: High-contrast mammography with a moving grid: assessment of clinical utility, AJR 146:1137-1139, 1986.

Sickles EA et al: Baseline screening mammography: one vs two views per breast, AJR 147:1149-1153, 1986.

Smathers RL et al: Mammographic microcalcifications: detection with xerography, screen-film, and digitized film display, Radiology 159:673-677, 1986.

Walker QJ and Langlands AO: The misuse of mammography in the management of breast cancer, Med J Aust 145:185-187, 1986.

Wallberg H et al: The value of diaphanography as an adjunct to mammography in breast diagnostics, Acta Chir Scand Suppl 530:83-87, 1986.

Williams SM et al: Mammography in women under age 30: is there clinical benefit? Radiology 161:49-51, 1986.

1987 Asaga T et al: Breast imaging: dual-energy projection radiography with digital radiography, Radiology 164:869-870, 1987.

Bassett LW et al: Automated and hand-held breast US: effect on patient management, Radiology 165:103-108, 1987.

Bassett LW et al: Breast cancer detection: one versus two views, Radiology 165:95-97, 1987.

Bassett LW et al: Survey of mammography practices, AJR 149:1149-1152, 1987.

Breast imaging, Radiol Clin North Am 25:897-1048, 1987.

Chan HP et al: Image feature analysis and computer-sided diagnosis in digital radiography. I. Automated detection of microcalcifications in mammography, Med Phys 14:538-548, 1987.

Chang CH: Computed tomographic mammography in the diagnosis of breast diseases, Yonsei Med J 28:243-248, 1987.

Feig SA: Mammography equipment: principles, features, selection, Radiol Clin North Am 25:897-911, 1987.

Galkin BM et al: Imaging capabilities and dose considerations of different mammographic units, Recent Results Cancer Res 105:25-30, 1987.

Haus AG: Recent advances in screen-film mammography, Radiol Clin North Am 25:913-928, 1987.

Haus AG: Recent trends in screen-film mammography: technical factors and radiation dose, Recent Results Cancer Res 105:37-51, 1987.

Homer MJ: Preoperative needle localization of lesions in the lower half of the breast: needle entry from below, AJR 149:43-45, 1987.

Kimme-Smith C, Bassett LW and Gold RH: Evaluation of radiation dose, focal spot, and automatic exposure of newer film-screen mammography units, AJR 149:913-917, 1987.

Kimme-Smith C et al: Mammographic dual-screen-dual-emulsion-film combination: visibility of simulated microcalcifications and effect on image contrast, Radiology 165:313-318, 1987.

Kirkpatrick AE and Law J: A comparative study of films and screens for mammography, Br J Radiol 60:73-78, 1987.

Logan WW and Janus J: Use of special mammographic views to maximize radiographic information, Radiol Clin North Am 25:953-959, 1987.

Melville RP and Burch W: Modern mammography, Aust Fam Physician 16:1478, 1987.

Monsees B, Destouet JM and Totty WG: Light scanning versus mammography in breast cancer detection, Radiology 163:463-465, 1987.

Nielsen B: Image quality in mammography: physical and technical limitations, Recent Results Cancer Res 105:1-14, 1987.

Nishikawa RM et al: Scanned-projection digital mammography, Med Phys 14:717-727, 1987.

Pennes DR and Homer MJ: Disappearing breast masses caused by compression during mammography, Radiology 165:327-328, 1987.

Pope TL Jr, Fechner RE and Brenbridge AN: Carcinosarcoma of the breast: radiologic, ultrasonographic, and pathologic correlation, Can Assoc Radiol J 38:50-51, 1987.

Rebner M et al: Two-view specimen radiography in surgical biopsy of nonpalpable breast masses, AJR 149:283-285, 1987.

Sickles EA: Comparison of mammographic screen-film systems, Recent Results Cancer Res 105:52-57, 1987.

Sickles EA: The role of magnification technique in modern mammography, Recent Results Cancer Res 105:19-24, 1987.

Stanton L et al: Screen-film mammographic technique for breast cancer screening, Radiology 163:471-479, 1987.

Wolfe JN: History and recent developments in xeroradiography of the breast, Radiol Clin North Am 25:929-937, 1987.

Wolfe JN et al: Xeroradiography of the breast: overview of 21,057 consecutive cases, Radiology 165:305-311, 1987.

1988 Bassett LW and Gold RH: The evolution of mammography, AJR 150:493-498, 1988.

Ciatto S et al: The role of galactography in the detection of breast cancer, Tumori 74:177-181, 1988.

Dhawan AP and Le Royer E: Mammographic feature enhancement by computerized image processing, Comput Methods Programs Biomed 27:23-35, 1988.

Dodd GD: Is screening mammography routinely indicated for women between 40 and 50 years of age? An affirmative view, J Fam Pract 27:313-316, 1988.

Eklund GW et al: Improved imaging of the augmented breast, AJR 151:469-473, 1988.

Feig SA: The importance of supplementary mammographic views to diagnostic accuracy, AJR 151:40-41, 1988.

Guyer PB: Direct-contact B-scan sonomammography—an aid to X-ray mammography, Ultrasound Med Biol 14 (Suppl 1): 49-52, 1988.

Hendee WR and Kellie SE: Mammographic screening in women 40-49 years old, AJR 151:683-684, 1988.

Homer MJ: Localization of nonpalpable breast lesions with the curved-end, retractable wire: leaving the needle in vivo, AJR 151:919-920, 1988.

Jackson VP, Lex AM and Smith DJ: Patient discomfort during screen-film mammography, Radiology 168:421-423, 1988.

Karila KT: Manual or automatic exposure controller imaging in mammography, Radiogr Today 54:35-40, 1988.

LaFrance R, Gelskey DE and Barnes GT: A circuit modification that improves mammographic phototimer performance, Radiology 166:773-776, 1988.

Oestmann JW et al: Comparison of two screen-film combinations in contact and magnification mammography: detectability of microcalcifications, Radiology 168:657-659, 1988.

Prado KL et al: Breast radiation dose in film/screen mammography, Health Phys 55:81-83, 1988.

Sickles EA: Practical solutions to common mammographic problems: tailoring the examination, AJR 151:31-39, 1988.

Stomper PC et al: Is mammography painful? A multicenter patient survey, Arch Intern Med 148:521-524, 1988.

Turner DA et al: Carcinoma of the breast: detection with MR imaging versus xeromammography, Radiology 168:49-58, 1988.

1989 Berna JD, Guirao J and Garcia V: A coaxial technique for performing galactography, AJR 153:273-274, 1989.

Chakraborty DP and Barnes GT: An energy sensitive cassette for dual-energy mammography, Med Phys 16:7-13, 1989.

Champ CS et al: A Perspex grid for localization of non-palpable mammographic lesions, Histopathology 14:311-315, 1989.

Chen HH et al: Needle localization of non-palpable breast lesions with a portable, Radiology 170:687-690, 1989.

Cooper RA: Mammography, Clin Obstet Gynecol 32:768-785, 1989.

Dodd GD: Quality assurance in mammography, Cancer 64:2707-2709, 1989.

Gilula LA, Destouet JM and Monsees B: Nipple simulating a breast mass on a mammogram, Radiology 170:272, 1989.

Kimme-Smith C et al: Digital mammography: a comparison of two digitization methods, Invest Radiol 24:869-875, 1989.

Kimme-Smith C et al: Film-screen mammography x-ray tube anodes: molybdenum versus tungsten, Med Phys 16:279-283, 1989.

Kimme-Smith C et al: Mammographic film-processor temperature, development time, and chemistry: effect on dose, contrast, and noise, AJR 152:35-40, 1989.

Lam KL and Chan HP: Exposure equalization technique in mammography, Invest Radiol 24:154-157, 1989.

Law J and Kirkpatrick AE: films, screens and cassettes for mammography, Br J Radiol 62:163-167, 1989.

Linden SS and Sullivan DC: Breast skin calcifications: localization with a stereotactic device, Radiology 171:570-571, 1989.

Martin JE: A demonstration comparing film mammography with the new high sensitivity xeromammography, Radiographics 9:153-168, 1989.

Parks S: A practical guide to mammography training, Radiogr Today 55:31, 1989.

Reid AW, McKellar NJ and Sutherland GR: Breast ductography—its role in the diagnosis of breast disease, Scott Med J 34:497-499, 1989.

Rickard MT: The quality mammographic image: a review of its components, Australas Radiol 33:328-334, 1989.

Tabar L and Haus AG: Processing of mammographic films: technical and clinical considerations, Radiology 173:65-69, 1989.

Vilaro MM et al: Hand-held and automated sonomammography: clinical role relative to X-ray mammography, J Ultrasound Med 8:95-100, 1989.

1990 Alveryd A et al: Lightscanning versus mammography for the detection of breast cancer in screening and clinical practice: a Swedish multicenter study, Cancer 65:1671-1677, 1990.

Brower TD: Positioning techniques for the augmented breast, Radiol Technol 61:209-211, 1990.

Gold RH, Bassett LW and Widoff BE: Highlights from the history of mammography, Radiographics 10:1111-1131, 1990.

Haiart DC and Kirkpatrick AE: Mammographic screening for breast cancer: recall rates using two views compared with the oblique view alone, Br J Clin Pract 44:213-215, 1990.

Haus AG: Technologic improvements in screen-film mammography, Radiology 174:628-637, 1990.

Hendrick RE: Standardization of image quality and radiation dose in mammography, Radiology 174:648-654, 1990.

Hubbard LB: AAPM tutorial: mammography as a radiographic system, Radiographics 10:103-113, 1990.

Kimme-Smith C: Mammographic image receptors and image processing, Curr Opin Radiol 2:719-725, 1990.

Law J: Recent films and screens for mammography, Br J Radiol 63:966-967, 1990.

Law J and Kirkpatrick AE: Further comparisons of films, screens and cassettes for mammography, Br J Radiol 63:128-131, 1990.

Lofgren M, Andersson I and Lindholm K: Stereotactic, x-ray guided, fine needle aspiration biopsy of nonpalpable breast lesions: comparison with the coordinate grid localization technique, Recent Results Cancer Res 119:100-104, 1990.

McLelland R and Pisano ED: Issues in mammography, Cancer 66:1341-1344, 1990.

Nickoloff EL et al: Mammographic resolution: influence of focal spot intensity distribution and geometry, Med Phys 17:436-447, 1990.

Rothenberg LN: AAPM tutorial: patient dose in mammography, Radiographics 10:739-746, 1990.

Sickles EA: One versus two views per breast for screening mammography, Recent Results Cancer Res 119:81-87, 1990.

Skubic SE et al: Value of increasing film processing time to reduce radiation dose during mammography, AJR 155:1189-1193, 1990.

Villafana T: Generators, x-ray tubes, and exposure geometry in mammography, Radiographics 10:539-554, 1990.

Yaffe MJ: AAPM tutorial: physics of mammography: image recording process, Radiographics 10:341-363, 1990.

1991 Boone JM: Color mammography: image generation and receiver operating characteristic evaluation, Invest Radiol 26:521-527, 1991.

Cranley K: Measuring the filtration of mammographic X-ray tubes with molybdenum targets, Br J Radiol 64:842-845, 1991.

Datoc PD et al: Mammographic follow-up of nonpalpable low-suspicion breast abnormalities: one versus two views, Radiology 180:387-391, 1991.

Frederick EE et al: Accurate automatic exposure controller for mammography: design and performance, Radiology 178:393-396, 1991.

Friedrich MA: Mammographic equipment, technique, and quality control, Curr Opin Radiol 3:571-578, 1991.

Gaw VP et al: A program to improve mammography skills of practicing radiologic technologists, QRB 17:48-53, 1991.

Grumbach Y and Nguyen HT: Mammography in younger women, Curr Opin Radiol 3:602-610, 1991.

Hachiya J et al: MR imaging of the breast with Gd-DTPA enhancement: comparison with mammography and ultrasonography: the abnormal mammogram—what to do, Radiat Med 20:1431-1435, 1991.

Jarlman O, Samuelsson L and Braw M: Digital luminescence mammography: early clinical experience, Acta Radiol 32:110-113, 1991.

Law J: Patient dose and risk in mammography, Br J Radiol 64:360-365, 1991.

McLelland R et al: The American College of Radiology Mammography Accreditation Program, AJR 157:473-479, 1991.

Nielsen BB et al: Pain and discomfort associated with film-screen mammography, J Natl Cancer Inst 83:1754-1756, 1991.

Reitherman RW: No one is immune from breast cancer, Radiol Technol 63:41-42, 1991.

Young VL et al: Effect of breast implants on mammography, South Med J 84:707-714, 1991.

1992 Bates BF and Gaskin H: A modified technique for breast compression during needle localization, AJR 159:1189-1190, 1992.

Blinov NN, Kozlovsky EB and Leonov BI: Optimization of X-ray mammography conditions, Med Prog Technol 18:69-72, 1992.

Cardenosa G and Eklund GW: Effects of a defective filter on magnification image quality in mammography, Radiology 182:894-895, 1992.

Clark R, Nemec L and Love N: Breast imaging: a practical look at its capabilities and its limitations, Postgrad Med 92:117-122, 127-134, 1992.

Eklund GW and Cardenosa G: The art of mammographic positioning, Radiol Clin North Am 30:21-53, 1992.

Fajardo LL, Jackson VP and Hunter TB: Interventional procedures in diseases of the breast: needle biopsy, pneumocystography, and galactography, AJR 158:1231-1238, 1992.

Faulk RM and Sickles EA: Efficacy of spot compression-magnification and tangential views in mammographic evaluation of palpable breast masses, Radiology 185:87-90, 1992.

Gold RH: The evolution of mammography, Radiol Clin North Am 30:1-19, 1992.

Heggie JC: The selection of kV in mammography, Australas Phys Eng Sci Med 15:214-216, 1992.

Heywang-Kobrunner SH: Nonmammographic breast imaging techniques, Curr Opin Radiol 4:146-154, 1992.

Horton JA, Romans MC and Cruess DF: Mammography attitudes and usage study, Women Health 2:180-186, 1992.

Husien AM: Stereotactic localization mammography: interpreting the check film, Clin Radiol 45:387-389, 1992.

Kimme-Smith C: New and future developments in screen-film mammography equipment and techniques, Radiol Clin North Am 30:55-66, 1992.

Kimme-Smith C et al: Effect of poor control of film processors on mammographic image quality, Radiographics 12:1137-1146, 1992.

Kimme-Smith C et al: Mammography screen-film selection: individual facility testing technique, Med Phys 19:1195-1199, 1992.

Kuhn H and Knupfer W: Imaging characteristics of different mammographic screens, Med Phys 19:449-457, 1992.

Lagendik JJ and Hofman P: A standardized multifield irradiation technique for breast tumours using asymmetrical collimators and beam angulation, Br J Radiol 65:56-62, 1992.

Leaney BJ and Martin M: Breast pain associated with mammographic compression, Australas Radiol 36:120-123, 1992.

Moskovic E, Parsons C and Baum M: Chest radiography in the management of breast cancer, Br J Radiol 65:30-32, 1992.

Nielsen B: Technical aspects of mammography, Curr Opin Radiol 4:118-122, 1992.

Nielsen BB et al: Mobile mammography: the technologist's role, Radiol Technol 63:316-323, 1992.

Panayiotakis G et al: An anatomical filter for exposure equalization in mammography, Eur J Radiol 15:15-17, 1992.

Pastore G: Digital radiography in mammography, Rays 17:539-546, 1992.

Peart O: Stereostatic localization pinpoints breast lesions, Radiol Technol 63:234-238, 1992.

Pollack AH: Localization of breast lesions identified on one mammographic view: the skin-pinch technique, Radiology 185:278-280, 1992.

Reitherman RW: The forces behind accreditation, Radiol Technol 63:203-204, 1992.

Reitherman RW: Will mammographers be ready? Radiol Technol 63:336-338, 1992.

Rutter DR et al: Discomfort and pain during mammography: description, prediction, and prevention, BMJ 305:443-445, 1992.

Schueler BA, Gray JE and Gisvold JJ: A comparison of mammography screen-film combinations, Radiology 184:629-634, 1992.

Shtern F: Digital mammography and related technologies: a perspective from the National Cancer Institute, Radiology 183:629-630, 1992.

van Dijck JA et al: One-view versus two-view mammography in baseline screening for breast cancer: a review, Br J Radiol 65:971-976, 1992.

Zinninger MD: Mammography quality assurance, J Am Med Wom Assoc 47:155-157, 164, 1992.

1993 Albertyn LE: Radiology and the breast, Aust Fam Physician 22:27-34, 1993.

Bassett LW, Jessop NW and Wilcox PA: Mammography film-labeling practices, Radiology 187:773-775, 1993.

Bassett LW et al: Mammographic positioning: evaluation from the view box, Radiology 188:803-806, 1993.

Beral V: Mammographic screening, Lancet 341:1509-1510, 1993.

Cowen AR, Brettle DS and Workman A: Technical note: compensation for field non-uniformity on a mammographic X-ray unit, Br J Radiol 66:150-154, 1993.

D'Orsi CJ et al: A complication involving a braided hook-wire localization device, Radiology 187:580-581, 1993.

Dershaw DD et al: Use of digital mammography in needle localization procedures, AJR 161:559-562, 1993.

Hendrick RE: Mammography quality assurance: current issues, Cancer 72:1466-1474, 1993.

Hussman K et al: MR mammographic localization. Work in progress, Radiology 189:915-917, 1993.

Jackson VP et al: Imaging of the radiographically dense breast, Radiology 188:297-301, 1993.

Karssemeijer N, Frieling JT and Hendriks JH: Spatial resolution in digital mammography, Invest Radiol 28:413-419, 1993.

Kimme-Smith C and Chatziioannou A: Mammography focal spot measurement with a star pattern: techniques to avoid inaccuracies, Med Phys 20:93-97, 1993.

Kotre CJ, Robson KJ and Faulkner K: Technical note: assessment of X-ray field alignment in mammography, Br J Radiol 66:155-157, 1993.

Kuni CC: Mammography in the 1990s: a plea for objective doctors and informed patients, Am J Prevent Med 9:185-190, 1993.

Law J: The influence of focal spot size on image resolution and test phantom scores in mammography, Br J Radiol 66:441-446, 1993.

Law J: Measurement of focal spot size in mammography X-ray tubes, Br J Radiol 66:44-50, 1993.

Liddell MJ: Mass mammographic screening—the other side of the argument, Aust Fam Physician 22:1168-1175, 1993.

Nielsen B, Miaskowski C and Dibble SL: Pain with mammography: fact or fiction? Oncol Nurs Forum 20:639-642, 1993.

Patient education for screening mammography: the unmet need, R I Med J 76:366-367, 1993.

Persliden J et al: Comparison of image quality and mean absorbed dose to the breast for two mammographic films, Acta Radiol 34:351-355, 1993.

Reitherman RW: Health care reform and mammography, Radiol Technol 64:311-312, 1993.

Reitherman RW: Your patient deserves no less than the best, Radiol Technol 64:251-252, 1993.

Reynolds HE, Jackson VP and Musick BS: A survey of interventional mammography practices, Radiology 187:71-73, 1993.

Robinson JD et al: Improved mammography with a reduced radiation dose, Radiology 188:868-871, 1993.

Simeoni RJ and Thiele DL: Scatter radiation in mammography, Australas Phys Eng Sci Med 16:33-36, 1993.

Yin FF et al: Comparison of bilateral-subtraction and single-image processing techniques in the computerized detection of mammographic masses, Invest Radiol 28:473-481, 1993.

Young VL et al: The relative radiolucencies of breast implant filler materials, Plast Reconstr Surg 91:1066-1072, 1993.

BRAIN AND SPINAL CORD
General

For stereotactic bibliographic citations, see Volume 3 bibliography of this atlas.

1985   Altman N et al: Evaluation of the infant spine by direct sagittal computed tomography, AJNR 6:65-69, 1985.

Grundy D, Russell J and Swain A: ABC of spinal cord injury: radiological investigations, BMJ 291:1702-1705, 1985.

1986   Beltramello A et al: Iopamidol 150: a low iodine content non-ionic water-soluble contrast medium for CT myelocisternography, Acta Radiol Suppl 369:542-544, 1986.

Benson DF: Neuroimaging and dementia, Neurol Clin 4:341-353, 1986.

Bradley WG Jr: Magnetic resonance imaging in the central nervous system: comparison with computed tomography, Magn Reson Ann 81-122, 1986.

Panzer RJ, Kido DK and Hindmarsh T: A methodologic assessment of studies comparing magnetic resonance imaging and computed tomography of the brain, Acta Radiol Suppl 369:269-274, 1986.

Ruggiero R, Piscitelli G and Ambrosio A: Iopamidol for intrathecal use in pediatric neuroradiology, Acta Radiol Suppl 369:532-536, 1986.

Spiegel SM et al: Increased density of tentorium and falx: a false positive CT sign of subarachnoid hemorrhage, Can Assoc Radiol J 37:243-247, 1986.

Tadmor R et al: Magnetic resonance imaging of the thoracical spinal cord and spine with surface coils, Acta Radiol Suppl 369:475-480, 1986.

Takahashi M, Bussaka H and Miyawaki M: Stereoscopic DSA of the central nervous system, Neuroradiology 28:105-108, 1986.

Virapongse C et al: Three-dimensional computed tomographic reformation of the spine, skull, and brain from axial images, Neurosurg 18:53-58, 1986.

Zimmerman RA et al: Magnetic resonance imaging of the pediatric spinal cord and canal, Acta Radiol Suppl 369:649-650, 1986.

1987   Banks G, Vries JK and McLinden S: Radiologic automated diagnosis (RAD), Comput Methods Programs Biomed 25:157-167, 1987.

Hopper JL et al: Analysis of dynamic computed tomography scan brain images, Invest Radiol 22:651-657, 1987.

Kawahara H et al: Normal development of the spinal cord in neonates and infants seen on ultrasonography, Neuroradiology 29:50-52, 1987.

Moseley I: Interpreting the skull X-ray, Br J Hosp Med 37:340-348, 1987.

Valenti RM: Lumbar myelography: contrast agents used in the past, present, and future, Radiol Technol 58:493-496, 1987.

1988   Alexander MP and Warren RL: Localization of callosal auditory pathways: a CT case study, Neurology 38:802-804, 1988.

Czervionke LF et al: The MR appearance of gray and white matter in the cervical spinal cord, AJNR 9:557-562, 1988.

Duthoy MJ and Lund G: MR imaging of the spine in children, Eur J Radiol 8:188-195, 1988.

Ishida Y, Suzuki K and Ohmori K: Dynamics of the spinal cord: an analysis of functional myelography by CT scan, Neuroradiology 30:538-544, 1988.

Nakstad PH and Kjartansson O: Accidental spinal cord injection of contrast material during cervical myelography with lateral C1-C2 puncture, AJNR 9:410, 1988.

Slappendel R et al: Spread of radiopaque dye in the thoracic epidural space, Anaesthesia 43:939-942, 1988.

Tawn DJ, Snow M and Jeans WD: Computed tomography of the internal auditory canals, Bristol Med Chir J 103:13-15, 1988.

van der Knaap MS and Valk J: Classification of congenital abnormalities of the CNS, AJNR 9:315-326, 1988.

1989   Carvlin MJ et al: High-resolution MR of the spinal cord in humans and rats, AJNR 10:13-17, 1989.

Curtin AJ et al: MR imaging artifacts of the axial internal anatomy of the cervical spinal cord, AJR 152:835-842, 1989.

Esfahani F and Dolan KD: Air CT cisternography in the diagnosis of vascular loop causing vestibular nerve dysfunction, AJNR 10:1045-1049, 1989.

Finch IJ, Sun Y and Shatsky SA: Technique for cranial CT scanning of excessively obese patients, AJNR 10:434, 1989.

Fredericks BJ et al: Diseases of the spinal canal in children: diagnosis with noncontrast CT scans, AJNR 10:1233-1238, 1989.

Ho PS et al: MR appearance of gray and white matter at the cervicomedullary region, AJNR 10:1051-1055, 1989.

Jensen PR, Owre A and Ahlgren P: Reaction to contrast media in contrast-enhanced CT of the brain: a comparative investigation of non-ionic ultravist and ionic urografinmeglumin, Eur J Radiol 9:144-146, 1989.

Kanpolat Y et al: CT-guided percutaneous cordotomy, Acta Neurochir Suppl 46:67-68, 1989.

Lemansky E: Contrast agents used for myelography: an historical perspective, Radiol Technol 60:489-496, 1989.

Miller GM, Forbes GS and Onofrio BM: Magnetic resonance imaging of the spine, Mayo Clin Proc 64:986-1004, 1989.

Raghavan N et al: MR imaging in the tethered spinal cord syndrome, AJR 152:843-852, 1989.

Tien R et al: A simple method for spinal localization in MR imaging, AJNR 10:1232, 1989.

Tiver K: Treatment of CNS tumours with conventional radiotherapy: the importance of dose & volume factors in tumour control & CNS radiation tolerance, Australas Radiol 33:15-22, 1989.

1990   Belanger JG et al: Adult myelography with iohexol, Can Assoc Radiol J 41:191-194, 1990.

Croft MJ: Stereotactic radiosurgery of arteriovenous malformations, Radiol Technol 61:375-379, 1990.

Glasier CM et al: Screening spinal ultrasound in newborns with neural tube defects, J Ultrasound Med 9:339-343, 1990.

Kuhn MJ and Baker MR: Optimization of low-osmolality contrast media for cranial CT: a dose comparison of two contrast agents, AJNR 11:847-849, 1990.

Nagata K et al: Clinical value of magnetic resonance imaging for cervical myelopathy, Spine 15:1088-1096, 1990.

Simon JH: Technologic advances in computed tomography and magnetic resonance imaging in the central nervous system, Curr Opin Radiol 2:518-525, 1990.

Sze G: New applications of MR contrast agents in neuroradiology, Neuroradiology 32:421-438, 1990.

Wall EJ et al: Cauda equina anatomy. I. Intrathecal nerve root organization, Spine 15:1244-1247, 1990.

1991   Bernard MS, Hourihan MD and Adams H: Computed tomography of the brain: does contrast enhancement really help? Clin Radiol 44:161-164, 1991.

Giles LG: Review of tethered cord syndrome with a radiological and anatomical study: case report, Surg Radiol Anat 13:339-343, 1991.

Mountz JM and Wilson MW: Brain structure localization in positron emission tomography: comparison of magnetic resonance imaging and a stereotactic method, Comput Med Imaging Graph 15:17-22, 1991.

Prager JM and Mikulis DJ: The radiology of headache, Med Clin North Am 75:525-544, 1991.

Spiegelmann R and Friedman WA: Rapid determination of thalamic CT-stereotactic coordinates: a method, Acta Neurochir 110:77-81, 1991.

Wardle S and Carty H: CT scanning in meningitis, Eur J Radiol 12:113-119, 1991.

1992 Anson JA and Spetzler RF: Interventional neuroradiology for spinal pathology, Clin Neurosurg 39:388-417, 1992.

Berk M: Indications for computed tomographic brain scanning in psychiatric inpatients, S Afr Med J 82:338-340, 1992.

Castillo M and Dominguez R: Imaging of common congenital anomalies of the brain and spine, Clin Imaging 16:73-88, 1992.

Cormack J et al: Evaluating the clinical efficacy of diagnostic imaging procedures, Eur J Radiol 16:1-9, 1992.

Dietemann JL et al: CT, myelography and CT-myelography in the evaluation of common cervicobrachial neuralgia, J Neuroradiol 19:167-176, 1992.

Engel PA and Gelber J: Does computed tomographic brain imaging have a place in the diagnosis of dementia? Arch Intern Med 152:1437-1440, 1992.

Larsson EM: Magnetic resonance imaging of the cervical and thoracic spine and the spinal cord: a study using a 0.3 T vertical magnetic field, Acta Radiol Suppl (Stockh) 378:71-92, 1992.

Martin DS et al: Current imaging concepts of thoracic intervertebral disks, CRC Crit Rev Diagn Imaging 33:109-181, 1992.

Patil A et al: The value of intraoperative scans during CT-guided stereotactic procedures, Neuroradiology 34:453-456, 1992.

Sze G: MR imaging of the spinal cord: current status and future advances, AJR 159:149-159, 1992.

VanDyke CW et al: 3D MR myelography, J Comput Assist Tomogr 16:497-500, 1992.

Wilson TA and Branch CL Jr: Thoracic disk herniation, Aust Fam Physician 45:2162-2168, 1992.

Yone K et al: Preoperative and postoperative magnetic resonance image evaluations of the spinal cord in cervical myelopathy, Spine 17:388-392, 1992.

Zisch RJ, Hollenbach HP and Artmann W: Lumbar myelography with three-dimensional MR imaging, JMR 2:731-734, 1992.

1993 Baleriaux D, Matos C and De Greef D: Gadodiamide injection as a contrast medium for MRI of the central nervous system: a comparison with gadolinium-DOTA, Neuroradiology 35:490-494, 1993.

Cantrell P et al: The value of baseline CT head scans in the assessment of shunt complications in hydrocephalus, Pediatr Radiol 23:485-486, 1993.

Fulbright R, Ross JS and Sze G: Application of contrast agents in MR imaging of the spine, JMR 3:219-232, 1993.

Garcia FF et al: Diagnostic imaging of childhood spinal infection, Orthop Rev 22:321-327, 1993.

Ghaziuddin M et al: Utility of the head computerized tomography scan in child and adolescent psychiatry, J Am Acad Child Adolesc Psychiatry 32:123-126, 1993.

Hamano K et al: A comparative study of linear measurement of the brain and three-dimensional measurement of brain volume using CT scans, Pediatr Radiol 23:165-168, 1993.

Jackson A et al: CT appearances of haematomas in the corpus callosum in patients with subarachnoid haemorrhage, Neuroradiology 35:420-423, 1993.

Tso EL et al: Cranial computed tomography in the emergency department evaluation of HIV-infected patients with neurologic complaints, Ann Emerg Med 22:1169-1176, 1993.

1994 Glantz MJ et al: The radiographic diagnosis and treatment of paraneoplastic central nervous system disease, Cancer 73:168-175, 1994.

Myelography

For bibliographic citations before 1964, please see volume 3 of the fifth edition of this atlas. For citations from 1964 through 1974, see volume 3 of the sixth or seventh edition.

1975 Coin CG and Scanlan RL: Technique for internal auditory cisternography, Acta Radiol [Suppl] 347:53-57, 1975.

Novy S and Jensen KM: filling defects and nonfilling of the internal auditory canal in posterior fossa myelography, AJR 124:265-270, 1975.

Peterson HO: The hazards of myelography, Radiology 115:237-239, 1975.

Skalpe IO and Amundsen P: Lumbar radiculography with metrizamide, a nonionic water-soluble contrast medium, Radiology 115:91-95, 1975.

1977 Boyd WR and Gardiner GA Jr: Metrizamide myelography, AJR 129:481-484, 1977.

Mosely J: The oil myelogram after operation for lumbar disc lesions, Clin Radiol 28:267-276, 1977.

Scher A and Vambeck V: An approach to the radiological evaluation of the cervicodorsal junction following injury, Clin Radiol 28:243-246, 1977.

1978 Deeb ZL et al: Reduced morbidity in gas myelography, Neuroradiology 16:352-353, 1978.

Eldevik OP, Nakken KO and Haughton VM: The effect of dehydration on side effects of metrizamide myelography, Radiology 129:715-716, 1978.

Kieffer SA et al: Contrast agents for myelography: clinical and radiological evaluation of Amipaque and Pantopaque, Radiology 129:695-705, 1978.

McClendon LK: Flying lateral technique for thoracic myelography, Radiol Technol 50:9-16, 1978.

McCormick CC: Radiology in low back pain and sciatica: an analysis of the relative efficacy of spinal venography, discography, and epidurography in patients with a negative or equivocal myelogram, Clin Radiol 29:393-406, 1978.

1979 Gelmers HJ: Adverse side effects of metrizamide in myelography, Neuroradiology 18:119-123, 1979.

Pilling JR: Water-soluble radiculography in the erect posture: a clinicoradiological study, Clin Radiol 30:665-670, 1979.

Rice JF and Bathia AL: Lateral C1-2 puncture for myelography: posterior approach, Radiology 132:760-762, 1979.

Schmidt RC: Cervical double contrast myelocisternography by the lateral approach, Neuroradiology 17:183-184, 1979.

1980 El Gammal T: Cervical myelography and posterior fossa examinations with Amipaque using magnification and subtraction, Radiology 136:219-222, 1980.

Taylor AJ, Haughton VM and Doust BD: CT imaging of the thoracic spinal cord without intrathecal contrast media, J Comput Assist Tomogr 4:223-224, 1980.

1981 Ahn HS et al: Lumbar myelography with metrizamide: supplemental techniques, AJR 136:547-551, 1981.

Amundsen P: Cervical myelography with Amipaque: seven years experience, Radiologe 21:282-287, 1981.

Khan A et al: Total myelography with metrizamide through the lumbar route, AJR 136:771-776, 1981.

Sykes RH et al: Incidence of adverse effects following metrizamide myelography in nonambulatory and ambulatory patients, Radiology 138:625-627, 1981.

1982 Chrzanowski R: The contrast media used for myelography, Eur Neurol 21:194-197, 1982.

Drayer B et al: Clinical trial of iopamidol for lumbar myelography, AJNR 3:59-64, 1982.

Hatten HP Jr: Routine cervical myelography with overhead oblique projections and Pantopaque, Spine 7:512-514, 1982.

Katevuo K and Kuuliala I: Lateral C1-C2 puncture: a technique to reduce adverse reactions in metrizamide sellar cisternography, Neuroradiology 24:43-44, 1982.

Lotz PR: Intracranial delivery of metrizamide from the lumbar subarachnoid space: prone versus supine positioning, J Comput Assist Tomogr 6:920-922, 1982.

Valk J: Lateral cervical, C1-C2, puncture in cervical myelography, Eur Neurol 21:175-180, 1982.

1983 Alenghat JP, Kim HS and Duda EE: Cervical and lumbar metrizamide myelography: split-dose technique, Radiology 149:852-853, 1983.

Bannon KR et al: Comparison of radiographic quality and adverse reactions in myelography with iopamidol and metrizamide, AJNR 4:312-313, 1983.

Bockenheimer SA and Hillesheimer W: Clinical experience with iopamidol for myelography, AJNR 4:314-316, 1983.

Capek V et al: Computed air myelography of the lumbosacral spine, AJNR 4:609-610, 1983.

Ericson K, Hindmarsh T and Hannerz J: Experience with iohexol in lumbar myelography, Acta Radiol 24:503-505, 1983.

Orrison WW, Eldevik OP and Sackett JF: Lateral C1-2 puncture for cervical myelography. III. Historical, anatomic, and technical considerations, Radiology 146: 401-408, 1983.

Orrison WW, Sackett JF and Amundsen P: Lateral C1-2 puncture for cervical myelography. II. Recognition of improper injection of contrast material, Radiology 146:395-400, 1983.

Osborne D: Improved head support for prone myelographic and CT examinations, AJR 141:1025-1026, 1983.

Parks RE and Dublin AB: Residual myelographic contrast material seen on the chest radiograph, Radiology 148:617-620, 1983.

Skutta T et al: Clinical trial of lotrol for lumbar myelography, AJNR 4:302-303, 1983.

Tan WS et al: Computed air myelography of the lumbosacral spine, AJNR 4:609-610, 1983.

Teasdale E and Macpherson P: Incidence of side effects following direct puncture cervical myelography: bed rest versus normal mobility, Neuroradiology 25:85-86, 1983.

Virapongse C, Bhimani SM and Vliem C: Cervical metrizamide myelography via a C1-2 puncture for patients in a seated position, Radiology 149:854, 1983.

1984   Barmeir E et al: Prone computed tomography metrizamide myelography: a technique for improved diagnosis of lumbar disc herniation, Clin Radiol 35:479-481, 1984.

Daniels DL et al: Cervical radiculopathy: computed tomography and myelography compared, Radiology 151:109-113, 1984.

Gabrielsen TO et al: Iohexol versus metrizamide for lumbar myelography: double-blind trial, AJR 142:1047-1049, 1984.

Shapiro R: Myelography, Chicago, 1984, Mosby.

Teasdale E and Macpherson P: Guidelines for cervical myelography: lumbar versus cervical puncture, Br J Radiol 57:789-793, 1984.

1985   Doyle T, Tress B and Gillot R: Combined discography and metrizamide myelography in evaluation of confusing low back pain, Australas Radiol 29:217-222, 1985.

Laasonen EM: Iohexol and metrizamide in lumbar myelography: comparison of side effects, Acta Radiol [Diagn] (Stockh) 26:761-765, 1985.

Macpherson P and Teasdale E: Routine bed rest is unnecessary after cervical myelography, Neuroradiology 27:214-216, 1985.

Nakstad P et al: Functional cervical myelography with iohexol, Neuroradiology 27: 220-225, 1985.

Petras AF, Westmoreland LH and Sobel DF: Simplified cervical metrizamide myelography: decubitus approach, Spine 10:860-862, 1985.

1986   Acikgoz B et al: Unusual neurological complications of lumbar myelography with dimeglumine iocarmate (Dimer X), Paraplegia 24:379-382, 1986.

Beltramello A et al: Iopamidol 150: a low iodine content non-ionic water-soluble contrast medium for CT myelocisternography, Acta Radiol Suppl (Stockh) 369:542-544, 1986.

Burt TB et al: Dural infolding during C1-2 myelography, Radiology 158:546-547, 1986.

Coolens D et al: Cervical myelography and the lateral approach on a conventional examination table, J Belge Radiol 69:163-165, 1986.

Crane R and Margolis MT: Use of sitting position to relieve myelographic obstruction, AJNR 7:502-503, 1986.

Dombrowski ET et al: Efficacy and morbidity of water soluble and oil-based myelography: study compares both methods in 314 patients, Orthop Rev 15:24-29, 1986.

Green J et al: Comparison of neurothermography and contrast myelography, Orthopedics 9:1699-1704, 1986.

Hoe JW, Ng AM and Tan LK: A comparison of iohexol and iopamidol for lumbar myelography, Clin Radiol 37:505-507, 1986.

Kendall B: Iohexol in paediatric myelography: an open non-comparative trial, Neuroradiology 28:65-68, 1986.

Lamb J et al: A prospective comparison of iotrolan, iohexol and iopamidol for lumbar myelography, Acta Radiol Suppl (Stockh) 369:524-527, 1986.

Lilleas F, Bach-Gansmo T and Weber H: Lumbar myelography with Omnipaque (iohexol), Neuroradiology 28:344-346, 1986.

Numaguchi Y et al: Myelography with metrizamide: effect of contrast removal on side effects, AJNR 7:498-501, 1986.

Peeters F: Myelography using iohexol (Omnipaque), Diagn Imaging 55:348-351, 1986.

Ramsey RG and Rabin DN: Removal of water-soluble contrast media after cervical myelography using cervical injection, AJNR 7:141, 1986.

Reicher MA et al: The push-up view: a superior cross-table lateral projection for cervical myelography, AJNR 7:899-900, 1986.

Wang AM and Zamani AA: Intradural herniation of thoracic disc: CT metrizamide myelography, Comput Radiol 10:115-118, 1986.

Wang H et al: Low dose cervical CT myelography: how acceptable are adverse effects at this juncture? Acta Radiol Suppl (Stockh) 369:539-541, 1986.

1987   Hodges SD and Berasi CC: Complications of myelography after partial metrizamide withdrawal, Spine 12:53-55, 1987.

Ilkko E, Leinonen K and Lahde S: Comparison of the radiation doses in lumbar CT and myelography, Eur J Radiol 7:119-120, 1987.

Jinkins JR: Large volume full columnar lumbar myelography, Neuroradiology 29:371-373, 1987.

Kuuliala IK and Goransson HJ: Adverse reactions after iohexol lumbar myelography: influence of postprocedural positioning, AJR 149:389-390, 1987.

Raininko R and Sonninen P: Dorsal CSF space at CI-II level: technique of cervical myelography, Neuroradiology 29:73-75, 1987.

Sand T et al: Side effects after diagnostic lumbar puncture and lumbar iohexol myelography, Neuroradiology 29:385-388, 1987.

Simon JH et al: High-dose iohexol myelography, Radiology 163:455-458, 1987.

Valenti RM: Lumber myelography: contrast agents used in the past, present, and future, Radiol Technol 58:493-496, 1987.

Wright CJ: Epidurography, Radiography 53:131-132, 1987.

1988   de Baas PD et al: Cervical myelography: run-up technique, Ann Radiol 31:393-401, 1988.

Diament MJ, Bird CR and Stanley P: Outpatient performance of invasive radiologic procedures in pediatric patients, Radiology 166:401-403, 1988.

Karnaze MG et al: Comparison of MR and CT myelography in imaging the cervical and thoracic spine, AJR 150:397-403, 1988.

Maly P, Bach-Gansmo T and Elmqvist D: Risk of seizures after myelography: comparison of iohexol and metrizamide, AJNR 9:879-883, 1988.

Minken TJ and Ahlgren P: Cross-table cervical myelography: a technique to improve visualization, AJNR 9:874, 1988.

Provinciali L et al: Lumbar myelography with iopamidol: a methodological approach to the investigation of side effects, Neuroradiology 30:528-533, 1988.

Schick RM et al: CT guided lateral C1-C2 puncture, J Comput Assist Tomogr 12:715-716, 1988.

Skalpe IO and Nakstad P: Myelography with iohexol (Omnipaque): a clinical report with special reference to the adverse effects, Neuroradiology 30:169-174, 1988.

Takahashi T et al: Localization of dural fistulas using metrizamide digital subtraction fluoroscopic cisternography, J Neurosurg 68:721-725, 1988.

Weisz GM, Lamond TS and Kitchener PN: Spinal imaging: will MRI replace myelography? Spine 13:65-68, 1988.

1989 Bien S et al: Iotrolan, a nonionic dimeric contrast medium in myelography, Fortschr Geb Rontgenstr 128:158-160, 1989.

Fagerlund MK and Thelander UE: Comparison of myelography and computed tomography in establishing lumbar disc herniation, Acta Radiol 30:241-246, 1989.

Fredericks BJ et al: Diseases of the spinal canal in children: diagnosis with noncontrast CT scans, AJNR 10:1233-1238, 1989.

Jackson RP et al: The neuroradiographic diagnosis of lumbar herniated nucleus pulposus. I. A comparison of computed tomography (CT), myelography, CT-myelography, discography, and CT-discography, Spine 14:1356-1361, 1989.

Jackson RP et al: The neuroradiographic diagnosis of lumbar herniated nucleus pulposus. II. A comparison of computed tomography (CT), myelography, CT-myelography, and magnetic resonance imaging, Spine 14:1362-1367, 1989.

Lemansky E: Contrast agents used for myelography: an historical perspective, Radiol Technol 60:489-496, 1989.

Sand T: Which factors affect reported headache incidences after lumbar myelography? A statistical analysis of publications in the literature, Neuroradiology 31:55-59, 1989.

Vezina JL, Fontaine S and Laperriere J: Outpatient myelography with fine-needle technique: an appraisal, AJNR 10:615-617, 1989.

1990 Altschuler EM and Segal R: Generalized seizures following myelography with iohexol (Omnipaque), J Spinal Disord 3:59-61, 1990.

Berlanger JG et al: Adult myelography with iohexol, Can Assoc Radiol J 41:191-194, 1990.

Hashimoto K et al: Magnetic resonance imaging of lumbar disc herniation: comparison with myelography, Spine 15:1166-1169, 1990.

Hilz MJ et al: Fatal complications after myelography with meglumine diatrizoate, Neuroradiology 32:70-73, 1990.

Katoh Y et al: Complications of lateral C1-2 puncture myelography, Spine 15:1085-1087, 1990.

Kelly TJ: Post-myelogram CT and the incidence of headache, Radiol Technol 62:32-34, 1990.

Robertson HJ and Smith RD: Cervical myelography: survey of modes of practice and major complications, Radiology 174:79-83, 1990.

Sand T et al: Side effects after lumbar iohexol myelography: relation to radiological diagnosis, sex and age, Neuroradiology 31:523-528, 1990.

1991 Breidahl WH, Low V and Khangure MS: Imaging the cervical spine: a comparison of MR with myelography and CT myelography, Australas Radiol 35:306-314, 1991.

Dalen K et al: Seizure activity after iohexol myelography, Spine 16:384, 1991.

Foote S: Myelography—an assessment of communication with a view to improving patient care and standardising information, Radiogr Today 57:20-24, 1991.

Halpin SF, Guest PJ and Byrne JV: Theory and practice: how much contrast for myelography? Neuroradiology 33:411-413, 1991.

Larsen JL and Olsen KO: Radiographic anatomy of the distal dural sac: a myelographic investigation of dimensions and termination, Acta Radiol 32:214-219, 1991.

Lee T et al: Post-myelogram headache—physiological or psychological? Neuroradiology 33:155-158, 1991.

Tamura T: A simple technique for cervical myelography, Spine 16:1267-1268, 1991.

Vestergaard A et al: Central nervous system reactions to cervical myelography, Acta Radiol 32:411-414, 1991.

Wang H et al: Iohexol cervical myelography in adult outpatients, Spine 16:1356-1358, 1991.

Wilkinson AG and Sellar RJ: The influence of needle size and other factors on the incidence of adverse effects caused by myelography, Clin Radiol 44:338-341, 1991.

1992 Bell GR and Ross JS: Diagnosis of nerve root compression: myelography, computed tomography, and MRI, Orthop Clin North Am 23:405-419, 1992.

Curnes JT: Modification of the standard myelography tray for universal precautions: technical note, Neurosurgery 31:158-159, 1992.

Dietemann JL et al: CT, myelography and CT-myelography in the evaluation of common cervicobrachial neuralgia, J Neuroradiol 19:167-176, 1992.

Dube LJ, Blair IG and Geoffroy G: Paediatric myelography with iohexol, Pediatr Radiol 22:290-292, 1992.

Martin DS et al: Current imaging concepts of thoracic intervertebral disks, CRC Crit Rev Diagn Imaging 33:109-181, 1992.

McGann GM et al: The influence of needle size on post-myelography headache: a controlled trial, Br J Radiol 65:1102-1104, 1992.

Perneczky G et al: Diagnosis of cervical disc disease: MRI versus cervical myelography, Acta Neurochir 116:44-48, 1992.

Rosati G, Leto di Priolo S and Tirone P: Serious or fatal complications after inadvertent administration of ionic water-soluble contrast media in myelography, Eur J Radiol 15:95-100, 1992.

Wilson TA and Branch CL Jr: Thoracic disk herniation, Aust Fam Physician 45:2162-2168, 1992.

1993 Esposito DP and Millner MR: Use of lumbar run-up technique for cervical myelography, South Med J 86:875-879, 1993.

Harrison PB: The contribution of needle size and other factors to headache following myelography, Neuroradiology 35:487-489, 1993.

Hecht ST and Greenspan A: Digital subtraction lumbar diskography: technical note, J Spinal Disord 6:68-70, 1993.

Holtas S: Radiology of the degenerative lumbar spine, Acta Orthop Scand Suppl 251:16-18, 1993.

Kido DK, Wippold FJ and Wood RC Jr: The role of nonionic myelography in the diagnosis of lumbar disc herniation, Invest Radiol 28 Suppl 5:S62-66, 1993.

Milants WP et al: Epidural and subdural contrast in myelography and CT myelography, Eur J Radiol 16:147-150, 1993.

Provinciali L et al: Electrophysiological and cognitive effects of lumbar myelography with iopamidol: comparison with diagnostic lumbar puncture, Neuroradiology 35:483-486, 1993.

Thornbury JR et al: Disk-caused nerve compression in patients with acute low-back pain: diagnosis with MR, CT myelography, and plain CT, Radiology 186:731-738, 1993.

DISKOGRAPHY
General

For bibliographic citations before 1964, please see volume 3 of the fifth edition of this atlas. For citations from 1964 through 1974, see volume 3 of the sixth or seventh edition.

1975 Collins HR: An evaluation of cervical and lumbar discography, Clin Orthop 107:133-138, 1975.

Jacobs GB, Pillone PR and Mazzola R: Lumbar discography in the diagnosis of herniated disks, Int Surg 60:6-9, 1975.

1978 McCormick CC: Radiology in low back pain and sciatica: an analysis of the relative efficacy of spinal venography, discography, and epidurography in patients with a negative or equivocal myelogram, Clin Radiol 29:393-406, 1978.

1981 Mosley GT: Technical considerations of epidural venography, Radiol Technol 52:371-374, 1981.

1982 Landherr EJ and Smigiel MR, Jr: New concepts in diagnosis and treatment of back ailments in the elderly, Surg Clin North Am 62:291-295, 1982.

Raininko R and Torma T: Contrast enhancement around a prolapsed disk, Neuroradiology 24:49-51, 1982.

1983 Hartjes H et al: Cervical disk syndromes: value of metrizamide myelography and diskography, AJNR 4:644-645, 1983.

Quinnell RC and Stockdale: Flexion and extension radiograph of the lumbar spine: a comparison with lumbar discography, Clin Radiol 34:405-411, 1983.

1985 Doyle T, Tress B and Gillot R: Combined discography and metrizamide myelography in evaluation of confusing low back pain, Australas Radiol 29:217-222, 1985.

1986 Bosacco SJ: Lumbar discography: redefining its role with intradiscal therapy, Orthopedics 9:399-401, 1986.

Gibson MJ et al: Magnetic resonance imaging and discography in the diagnosis of disc degeneration: a comparative study of 50 discs, J Bone Joint Surg Br 68:369-373, 1986.

Gillstrom P, Ericsson K and Hindmarsh T: A comparison of computed tomography and myelography in the diagnosis of lumbar disc herniation, Arch Orthop Trauma Surg 106:12-14, 1986.

1987 Bhoopat W et al: Lumbar disc herniation: a prospective comparison of computed tomography and myelography, J Med Assoc Thai 70:9-13, 1987.

Carroll G: Discography of the lumbar spine and chemonucleolysis of the intervertebral discs, Radiography 53:225-228, 1987.

Fraser RD, Osti OL and Vernon-Roberts B: Discitis after discography, J Bone Joint Surg [Br] 69:26-35, 1987.

Kornberg M: Computed tomography of the lumbar spine following discography: clinical application in selective cases, Spine 12:823-825, 1987.

Matsui H et al: Significance of tangential views in lumbar discography, Clinical Orthop 165-171, 1987.

Videman T, Malmivaara A and Mooney V: The value of the axial view in assessing discograms: an experimental study with cadavers, Spine 12:299-304, 1987.

1988 Buirski G and Watt I: Dynamic CT discography: an evaluation of a new technique, Australas Radiol 32:197-202, 1988.

Guyer RD et al: Discitis after discography, Spine 13:1352-1354, 1988.

McFadden JW: The stress lumbar discogram, Spine 13:931-933, 1988.

1989 Jackson RP et al: The neuroradiographic diagnosis of lumbar herniated nucleus pulposus. I. A comparison of computed tomography (CT), myelography, CT-myelography, discography, and CT-discography, Spine 14:1356-1361, 1989.

Jackson RP et al: The neuroradiographic diagnosis of lumbar herniated nucleus pulposus. II. A comparison of computed tomography (CT), myelography, CT-myelography, and magnetic resonance imaging, Spine 14:1362-1367, 1989.

Johnson RG: Does discography injure normal discs? An analysis of repeat discograms, Spine 14:424-426, 1989.

Kornberg M: Discography and magnetic resonance imaging in the diagnosis of lumbar disc disruption, Spine 14:1368-1372, 1989.

Nachemson A: Lumbar discography—where are we today? Spine 14:555-557, 1989.

1990 Bernard TN Jr: Lumbar discography followed by computed tomography: refining the diagnosis of low-back pain, Spine 15:690-707, 1990.

Collins CD et al: The role of discography in lumbar disc disease: a comparative study of magnetic resonance imaging and discography, Clin Radiol 42:252-257, 1990.

Linson MA and Crowe CH: Comparison of magnetic resonance imaging and lumbar discography in the diagnosis of disc degeneration, Clinical Orthop 160-163, 1990.

Sachs BL et al: Techniques for lumbar discography and computed tomography/discography in clinical practice, Orthopaedic Review 19:775-778, 1990.

1991 el-Khoury GY and Renfrew DL: Percutaneous procedures for the diagnosis and treatment of lower back pain: diskography, facet-joint injection, and epidural injection, AJR 157:685-691, 1991.

Simmons JW et al: Awake discography: a comparison study with magnetic resonance imaging, Spine 16:S216-S221, 1991.

Soini J et al: Disc degeneration and angular movement of the lumbar spine: comparative study using plain and flexion-extension radiography and discography, J Spinal Disord 4:183-187, 1991.

Tervonen O, Lahde S and Vanharanta H: Ultrasound diagnosis of lumbar disc degeneration: comparison with computed tomography/discography, Spine 16:951-954, 1991.

Tournade A et al: Contribution of discography to the diagnosis and treatment of lumbar disc herniation, J Neuroradiol 18:1-11, 1991.

1992 Birney TJ et al: Comparison of MRI and discography in the diagnosis of lumbar degenerative disc disease, J Spinal Disord 5:417-423, 1992.

Castro WH et al: Restriction of indication for automated percutaneous lumbar discectomy based on computed tomographic discography, Spine 17:1239-1243, 1992.

Greenspan A et al: Is there a role for diskography in the era of magnetic resonance imaging? Prospective correlation and quantitative analysis of computed tomography-diskography, magnetic resonance imaging, and surgical findings, J Spinal Disord 5:26-31, 1992.

Horton WC and Daftari TK: Which disc as visualized by magnetic resonance imaging is actually a source of pain? A correlation between magnetic resonance imaging and discography, Spine 17:S164-S171, 1992.

Maezawa S and Muro T: Pain provocation at lumbar discography as analyzed by computed tomography/discography, Spine 17:1309-1315, 1992.

Tehranzadeh J: Current status of discography, West J Med 156:300, 1992.

1993 Bogduk N and Aprill C: On the nature of neck pain, discography and cervical zygapophysial joint blocks, Pain 54:213-217, 1993.

Connor PM and Darden BV: Cervical discography complications and clinical efficacy, Spine 18:2035-2038, 1993.

Shinomiya K et al: evaluation of cervical diskography in pain origin and provocation, J Spinal Disord 6:422-426, 1993.

Cerebral pneumography

For bibliographic citations before 1964, please see the fifth edition of this atlas. For citations from 1964 through 1974, see the sixth or seventh edition.

1978 Swalingam S et al: Computer assisted ventriculography, J Comput Assist Tomogr 2:162-164, 1978.

1979 Quencer RM et al: Lateral decubitus pneumoencephalography: angiography for localizing atrial and para-atrial vascular lesions, AJR 132:617-622, 1979.

1980 Bentson JR et al: Combined gas cisternography and edge-enhanced computed tomography of the internal auditory canal, Radiology 136:777-779, 1980.

Kricheff II et al: Air-CT cisternography and canalography for small acoustic neuromas, AJNR 1:57-63, 1980.

Savolaine ER and Gerber AM: Need for complementary use of air ventriculography and computerized tomographic scanning in infected hydrocephalus, Neurosurgery 6:96-98, 1980.

1982 Anderson R et al: CT air-contrast scanning of the internal auditory canal, Ann Otol Rhinol Laryngol 91:501-505, 1982.

1983 Robertson HJ, Hatten HP Jr and Keating JW: False-positive CT gas cisternogram, AJNR 4:474-477, 1983.

Ruggiero G and Manfredini M: Focused encephalography, AJNR 4:767-769, 1983.

1984 Johnson DW: Air cisternography of the cerebellopontine angle using high-resolution computed tomography, Radiology 151:401-403, 1984.

Solti-Bohman LG et al: Gas-CT cisternography for detection of small acoustic nerve tumors, Radiology 150:403-407, 1984.

1985 Bassi P et al: High resolution O2 computed meatocisternography in the differential diagnosis of internal auditory canal pathology, Neuroradiology 27:26-31, 1985.

Johnson DW, Voorhees RL and Wong ML: Virtues and vagaries of high-resolution CT air cisternography in the diagnosis of acoustic neuromas, Otolaryngol Head Neck Surg 93:156-160, 1985.

1987 Greenberger R, Khangure MS and Chakera TM: The morbidity of CT air meatography: a follow-up of 84 patients, Clin Radiol 38:535-536, 1987.

1989 Esfahani F and Dolan KD: Air CT cisternography in the diagnosis of vascular loop causing vestibular nerve dysfunction, AJNR 10:1045-1049, 1989.

Hillel AD and Schwartz AN: Trumpet maneuver for visual and CT examination of the pyriform sinus and retrocricoid area, Head Neck 11:231-236, 1989.

1992 Maurer HJ and Pulst W: The first description and introduction into clinical use of air encephalography, Neuroradiology 34:168-169, 1992.

1993 Hariz MI, Bergenheim AT and Fodstad H: Air-ventriculography provokes an anterior displacement of the third ventricle during functional stereotactic procedures, Acta Neurochir 123:147-152, 1993.

CIRCULATORY SYSTEM
Anatomy

For bibliographic citations before 1964 please see volume 3 of the fifth edition of this atlas. For citations from 1964 through 1974, see volume 3 of the sixth or seventh edition.

1979 Moncada R et al: Normal vascular anatomy of the abdomen on computed tomography, Radiol Clin North Am 17:25-37, 1979.

1988 Holmes RL: Computer-assisted quantitation of coronary artery stenosis, Radiol Technol 60:37-41, 1988.

1989 Felson B: Aortic arch anomalies: a few facts and a lot of speculation, Semin Roentgenol 24:69-74, 1989.

1990 Teefey SA et al: Differentiating pelvic veins and enlarged lymph nodes: optimal CT techniques, Radiology 175:683-685, 1990.

1992 Bogaert J et al: Pictorial essay: right aortic arch, J Belge Radiol 75:406-409, 1992.

Carpenter JP et al: Magnetic resonance angiography of peripheral runoff vessels, J Vasc Surg 16:807-813, 1992.

Harms SE and Flamig DP: Magnetic resonance angiography: application to the peripheral circulation, Invest Radiol 27 (Suppl 2):S80-S83, 1992.

Schiebler ML et al: Magnetic resonance angiography of the pelvis and lower extremities. Work in progress, Invest Radiol 27 (Suppl 2):S90-S96, 1992.

Cerebral angiography

For bibliographic citations before 1964, please see the fifth edition of this atlas. For citations from 1964 through 1974, see the sixth or seventh edition.

1976 Long JM: Routine magnification cerebral angiography: a practical system designed for community hospital application, South Med J 69:911-913, 1976.

Takahashi M et al: Serial cerebral angiography in stereoscopic magnification, AJR 126:1211-1218, 1976.

1977 Doi K, Rossmann K and Duda EE: Application of longitudinal magnification effect to magnification stereoscopic angiography: a new method for cerebral angiography, Radiology 124:395-401, 1977.

Larson EB et al: Impact of computed tomography on utilization of cerebral angiograms, AJR 129:1-3, 1977.

1979 Quencer RM, Rosomoff HL and Green BA: Lateral decubitus pneumoencephalography-angiography for localizing atrial and para-atrial vascular lesions, AJR 132:617-622, 1979.

1980 Christenson PC et al: Intravenous angiography using digital video subtraction: intravenous cervicocerebrovascular angiography, AJR 135:1145-1152, 1980.

Cochran RM: Determining cerebral death with radiologic diagnostic procedures, Radiol Technol 51:777-790, 1980.

Jensen HP et al: Computerized tomography in vascular malformations of the brain, Neurosurg Rev 3:119-127, 1980.

Lantz BM et al: Angiographic determination of cerebral blood flow, Acta Radiol [Diagn] 21:147-153, 1980.

Numaguchi Y et al: Prolonged injection angiography for diagnosing intracranial neoplasms, Radiology 136:387-393, 1980.

Rubin JM et al: Clinical applications of combined cerebral angiograms and brain CT scans, AJNR 1:83-87, 1980.

Savolaine ER, Gerber AM and Nowak SF: Pitfalls in the angiographic diagnosis of serious head injury, J Neurosurg 53:53-57, 1980.

Takahashi M and Ozawa Y: Routine biplane cerebral angiography with stereoscopic magnification, Radiology 136:113-117, 1980.

1981 Turnipseed WD, Sackett JF, Strother CM: Computerized arteriography of the cerebrovascular system: its use with intravenous administration of contrast material, Arch Surg 116:470-473, 1981.

1982 Ahlgren P: Iohexol compared to urografin meglumine in cerebral angiography: a randomized, double-blind cross-over study, Neuroradiology 23:195-198, 1982.

Amundsen P et al: Cerebral angiography with iohexol: a multicentre clinical trial, Acta Radiol [Diagn] 23:529-534, 1982.

Forbes GS et al: Digital angiography: introducing digital techniques to clinical cerebral angiography practice, Mayo Clin Proc 57:683-693, 1982.

Ingstrup HM and Hauge P: Clinical testing of iohexol, Conray meglumine and Amipaque in cerebral angiography, Neuroradiology 23:75-79, 1982.

Molyneux AJ and Sheldon PW: A randomized blind trial of iopamidol and meglumine calcium metrizoate (Triosil 280, Isopaque Cerebral) in cerebral angiography, Br J Radiol 55:117-119, 1982.

Molyneux AJ, Sheldon PW and Yates DA: A comparative trial of sodium meglumine ioxaglate (Hexabrix) and iopamidol (Niopam) for cerebral angiography, Br J Radiol 55:881-884, 1982.

Nakstad P et al: Cerebral angiography with the non-ionic water-soluble contrast medium iohexol and meglumine-Cametrizoate: a randomized double-blind parallel study in man, Neuroradiology 23:199-202, 1982.

Turnipseed WD et al: A comparison of standard cerebral arteriography with noninvasive Doppler imaging and intravenous angiography, Arch Surg 117:419-421, 1982.

Yamamoto Y et al: Minimum dose contrast bolus in computed angiotomography of the brain, J Comput Assist Tomogr 6:575-585, 1982.

Yamamoto Y et al: Normal anatomy of cerebral vessels by computed angiotomography in the coronal, Towne, and semi-sagittal planes, J Comput Assist Tomogr 6:1049-1057, 1982.

1983 Amundsen P et al: Randomized double-blind cross-over study of iohexol and Amipaque in cerebral angiography, AJNR 4:342-343, 1983.

Brant-Zawadzki M et al: Digital subtraction cerebral angiography by intraarterial injection: comparison with conventional angiography, AJR 140:347-353, 1983.

Bryan RN et al: Neuroangiography with iohexol, AJNR 4:344-346, 1983.

Doi K and Duda EE: Detectability of depth information by use of magnification stereoscopic technique in cerebral angiography, Radiology 146:91-95, 1983.

Hahn FJ: "Squirt-pull" technique for left carotid catheterization, AJNR 4:1129, 1983.

Hindmarsh T et al: Comparative double-blind investigation of meglumine metrizoate, metrizamide, and iohexol in carotid angiography, AJNR 4:347-349, 1983.

Holtas S, Cronqvist S and Renaa T: Cerebral angiography with iohexol: a comparison with metrizamide in man, Neuroradiology 24:201-204, 1983.

Ingstrup HM and Laulund S: Clinical testing of Omnipaque and Amipaque in external carotid and vertebral angiography: randomized double-blind cross-over study, AJNR 4:1097-1099, 1983.

Nakstad P, Sortland O and Aaserud O: Iohexol compared to meglumine-Cametrizoate in common carotid angiography: a randomized double-blind cross-over study in man, Neuroradiology 25:33-36, 1983.

Skalpe IO and Anke IM: Complications in cerebral angiography: a comparison between the non-ionic contrast medium iohexol and meglumine metrizoate (Isopaque Cerebral), Neuroradiology 25:157-160, 1983.

Thron A and Voigt K: Rotational cerebral angiography: procedure and value, AJNR 4:289-291, 1983.

Yamaki T, Yoshino E and Higuchi T: Extravasation of contrast medium during both computed tomography and cerebral angiography, Surg Neurol 19:247-250, 1983.

1984 Chakeres DW and Wiatrowski W: Cerebral angiography: a device to reduce exposure to the eye lens, Radiology 152:534-535, 1984.

Earnest F IV et al: Complications of cerebral angiography: prospective assessment of risk, AJR 142:247-253, 1984.

Glover JL et al: Duplex ultrasonography, digital subtraction angiography, and conventional angiography in assessing carotid atherosclerosis, Arch Surg 119:664-669, 1984.

Higa T et al: A femocerebral catheter for middle-aged patients of relatively small stature, Neuroradiology 26:55-56, 1984.

Maravilla KR et al: Digital tomosynthesis: technique modifications and clinical applications for neurovascular anatomy, Radiology 152:719-724, 1984.

O'Connor MK et al: Digital fluoroscopy with a conventional fluoroscopic room and a nuclear medicine computer system, Br J Radiol 57:553-560, 1984.

Schonfeld SM et al: Iopamidol and Conray 60: comparison in superselective angiography, Radiology 152:809-811, 1984.

Takahashi M, Bussaka H and Nakagawa N: Evaluation of the cerebral vasculature by intraarterial DSA—with emphasis on in vivo resolution, Neuroradiology 26:253-259, 1984.

Tsai FY et al: Arterial digital subtraction angiography with particulate intravascular embolization and angioplasty, Surg Neurol 22:204-212, 1984.

Valk J, Crezee F and Olislagers-de Slegte RGM: Comparison of iohexol 300 mg I/ml and Hexabrix 320 mg I/ml in central angiography: a double-blind trial, Neuroradiology 26:217-221, 1984.

Zubkov YN, Nikiforov BM and Shustin VA: Balloon catheter technique for dilatation of constricted cerebral arteries after aneurysmal SAH, Acta Neurochir 70:65-79, 1984.

1985 Karoll MP et al: Air gap technique for digital subtraction angiography of the extra-cranial carotid arteries, Invest Radiol 20:742-745, 1985.

1986 Andreula CF: Contrast media tolerability in cerebral angiography, Radiol Med 72:30-31, 1986.

Dion J et al: Clinical events following neuroangiography: a prospective study, Acta Radiol Suppl (Stockh) 369:29-33, 1986.

Foley KT, Cahan LD and Hieshima GB: Intraoperative angiography using a portable digital subtraction unit, J Neurosurg 64:816-818, 1986.

Fukui K, Sadamoto K and Sakaki S: Development of the new cerebral angio-CT technique and magnetic resonance angio-imaging, Acta Radiol Suppl 369:67-68, 1986.

Hicks ME et al: Cerebrovascular disease: evaluation with transbrachial intraarterial digital subtraction angiography using a 4-F catheter, Radiology 161:545-546, 1986.

Hinck VC: Single catheter for aortic arch and selective cerebral angiography, AJNR 7:159-160, 1986.

Lovrencic M, Jakovac I and Klanfar Z: Iohexol versus meglumine-Ca-metrizoate in cerebral angiography: a randomized double-blind cross-over study, Acta Radiol Suppl 369:521-523, 1986.

Mueller DL et al: The application of i.v. digital subtraction angiography to cranial disease in children, AJNR 7:669-674, 1986.

Nakstad P et al: Intra-arterial digital subtraction angiography of the carotid arteries: special reference to contrast media, Neuroradiology 28:195-198, 1986.

Plunkett MB, Gray JE and Kispert DB: Radiation exposure from conventional and digital subtraction angiography of cerebral vessels, AJNR 7:665-668, 1986.

Ruggiero G et al: fifty-five thousand cerebral angiographies, Acta Radiol Suppl (Stockh) 369:285-288, 1986.

Takahashi M, Miyawaki M and Bussaka H: Development of a new universal neuroangiographic unit, Neuroradiology 28:351-354, 1986.

1987 Barry R and Nel CJ: Comparison of duplex Doppler scanning with contrast angiography in carotid artery disease, S Afr Med J 72:851-852, 1987.

Butler P et al: Intravenous digital subtraction angiography in intracranial aneurysms, Br J Radiol 60:323-326, 1987.

de Lange EE: Radiographic position of the trigeminal nerve in the skull for angiographic determination of arterial-nerve relationship in trigeminal neuralgia: results of a radiologic-anatomic study, Surg Radiol Anat 9:193-200, 1987.

Delcour C et al: Comparison of iohexol and ioxaglate for intravenous digital subtraction angiography of the neck and head, Invest Radiol 22:811-813, 1987.

Doyon D et al: Comparative trial of Hexabrix (320 mg iodine/ml), iohexol (300 mg iodine/ml) and iopamiron (300 mg iodine/ml) in cerebral and spinal angiography: a preliminary report, Br J Radiol 60:671-675, 1987.

Edvinsson L, Golman K and Jansen I: Site of action of contrast media on cerebral vessels, Cephalalgia 7:83-85, 1987.

Hieshima GB et al: Intraoperative digital subtraction neuroangiography: a diagnostic and therapeutic tool, AJNR 8:759-767, 1987.

Kim KS and Weinberg PE: A simple method to form an open loop with the sidewinder catheter for cerebral angiography, Neuroradiology 29:76-77, 1987.

Kleefield J et al: Biplane stereoscopic magnification cerebral angiography, Radiology 165:576-577, 1987.

Stillman MJ et al: Cerebral infarction: shortcomings of angiography in the evaluation of intracranial cerebrovascular disease in 25 cases, Medicine 66:297-308, 1987.

Vandermeulen D et al: Angiographic localizer ring for the BRW stereotactic system, Acta Neurochir Suppl 39:15-17, 1987.

1988 Bakke SJ, Nakstad PH and Aakhus T: Intravenous digital subtraction angiography of the precerebral and cerebral arteries in patients with TIA: a comparison with conventional angiography, Eur J Radiol 8:140-144, 1988.

Bishop S: Cerebral angiography using the femoral catheterisation technique, Radiography 54:52-60, 1988.

Moringlane JR, Lippitz B and Ostertag CB: Cerebral angiography under stereotactic conditions: technical note, Acta Neurochir 91:147-150, 1988.

Pelz DM et al: A comparison of iopamidol and iohexol in cerebral angiography, AJNR 9:1163-1166, 1988.

Skalpe IO: Complications in cerebral angiography with iohexol (Omnipaque) and meglumine metrizoate (Isopaque cerebral), Neuroradiology 30:69-72, 1988.

Touho H et al: Transbrachial artery approach for selective cerebral angiography in outpatients, AJNR 9:334-336, 1988.

1989 Betramello A et al: Interventional angiography in neuropediatrics, Childs Nerv Syst 5:87-93, 1989.

Bredenberg CE et al: Operative angiography by intraarterial digital subtraction angiography: a new technique for quality control of carotid endarterectomy, J Vasc Surg 9:530-534, 1989.

Cerebral arteriography: a report for health professionals by the Executive Committee of the Stroke Council, American Heart Association, Circulation 79:474, 1989.

Mewissen MW, Zavitz WR and Lipchik EO: Brachiocephalic vessels in the elderly: technique for catheterization, Radiology 170:887, 1989.

Nakstad PH: The reaction of cerebral arteries to non-ionic contrast media during cerebral angiography, Neuroradiology 31:247-249, 1989.

Phillips MH et al: Heavy charged-particle stereotactic radiosurgery: cerebral angiography and CT in the treatment of intracranial vascular malformations, Int J Radiat Oncol Biol Phys 17:419-426, 1989.

Ross JS et al: Magnetic resonance angiography of the extracranial carotid arteries and intracranial vessels: a review, Neurology 39:1369-1376, 1989.

Schumacher M, Kutluk K and Ott D: Digital rotational radiography in neuroradiology, AJNR 10:644-649, 1989.

Stevens JM et al: Relative safety of intravenous digital subtraction angiography over other methods of carotid angiography and impact on clinical management of cerebrovascular disease, Br J Radiol 62:813-816, 1989.

Zanette EM et al: Comparison of cerebral angiography and transcranial Doppler sonography in acute stroke, Stroke 20:899-903, 1989.

Zeitler E et al: The value of angiography in cerebrovascular disease, Thor Cardiovasc Surg 37:259-263, 1989.

1990 Colosimo C, Moschini M and Rollo M: Angiography of the intracranial vessels, Rays 15:243-267, 1990.

Kirsch WM and Zhu YH: Intraoperative digital subtraction angiography for neurosurgery, West J Med 153:547-548, 1990.

1991 Link KM et al: Clinical utility of three-dimensional magnetic resonance angiographic imaging, Clin Neurosurg 37:275-288, 1991.

McElveen JT Jr et al: Magnetic resonance angiography: technique and skull-base applications, Am J Otol 12:323-328, 1991.

Mitsumori M, Hayakawa K and Abe M: ECG changes during cerebral angiography: a comparison of low osmolality contrast media, Eur J Radiol 13:55-58, 1991.

Ottomo M et al: Rotatostereoradiography: a new radiodiagnostic method—development of a new three-dimensional radiodiagnostic device and evaluation in neurosurgical clinics, Neurol Med Chir 31:69-76, 1991.

1992 Feygelman VM, Huda W and Peters KR: Effective dose equivalents to patients undergoing cerebral angiography, AJNR 13:845-849, 1992.

Guo WY et al: Stereotaxic angiography in gamma knife radiosurgery of intracranial arteriovenous malformations, AJNR 13:1107-1114, 1992.

Harbaugh RE et al: Three-dimensional computerized tomography angiography in the diagnosis of cerebrovascular disease, J Neurosurg 76:408-414, 1992.

Mattle HP and Edelman RR: Cerebral magnetic resonance angiography, Neurol Res 14:118-121, 1992.

Riles TS et al: Comparison of magnetic resonance angiography, conventional angiography, and duplex scanning, Stroke 23:341-346, 1992.

Wolpert SM and Caplan LR: Current role of cerebral angiography in the diagnosis of cerebrovascular diseases, AJR 159:191-197, 1992.

1993 Blatter DD et al: Cervical carotid MR angiography with multiple overlapping thin-slap acquisition: comparison with conventional angiography, AJR 161:1269-1277, 1993.

Buijs PC et al: Carotid bifurcation imaging: magnetic resonance angiography compared to conventional angiography and Doppler ultrasound, Eur J Vasc Surg 7:245-251, 1993.

Durgun B et al: Evaluation by angiography of the lateral dominance of the drainage of the dural venous sinuses, Surg Radiol Anat 15:125-130, 1993.

MacDonald RL, Wallace MC and Kestle JR: Role of angiography following aneurysm surgery, J Neurosurg 79:826-832, 1993.

Markus H et al: Microscopic air embolism during cerebral angiography and strategies for its avoidance, Lancet 341:784-787, 1993.

Nemzek WR and Hecht ST: Radiopaque markers facilitate intraoperative angiography: technical note, Surg Neurol 40:81-82, 1993.

VISCERAL AND PERIPHERAL ANGIOGRAPHY

For bibliographic citations before 1964, please see volume 3 of the fifth edition of this atlas. For citations from 1964 through 1974, see volume 3 of the sixth or seventh edition.

1975 Guistra PE et al: Outpatient arteriography at a small community hospital, Radiology 116:581-583, 1975.

Sheedy FP II, Fulton RE and Atwell DT: Angiographic evaluation of patients with chronic gastrointestinal bleeding, AJR 123:338-347, 1975.

Staple TM: Vascular radiological procedures in orthopedic surgery, Clin Orthop 107:48-61, 1975.

Wendth AJ Jr: Peripheral arteriography: an overview of its origins and present status, CRC Crit Rev Radiol Nucl Med 6:369-401, 1975.

1976 Athanasoulis CA et al: Angiography: its contribution to the emergency management of gastrointestinal hemorrhage, Radiol Clin North Am 14:265-280, 1976.

Erikson V: Technique of coronary angiography, Acta Radiol 17:781-785, 1976.

Janicki P and Alfidi RJ: Selective visceral angiography in the diagnosis and treatment of gastroduodenal hemorrhage, Surg Clin North Am 56:1365-1373, 1976.

Mojab K and Ghosh BC: Thyroid angiography, Am J Surg 132:620-622, 1976.

1977 Eisenberg RL and Mani RL: Pressure dressings and postangiographic care of the femoral puncture site, Radiology 122:677-678, 1977.

Fitzgerald DE and Carr J: Peripheral arterial disease: assessment by arteriography and alternative noninvasive measurements, AJR 128:385-388, 1977.

Leslie J et al: A new simple power injector, AJR 128:381-384, 1977.

Tegtmeyer CJ: A simplified technique for selective and superselective abdominal angiography, J Can Assoc Radiol 28:224-226, 1977.

1978 Frasson F et al: Angiography versus computerized tomography, Ann Radiol 21:387-392, 1978.

Holgate RC et al: Angiography in otolaryngology: anatomy, methodology, complications, and contraindications, Otolaryngol Clin North Am 11:457-475, 1978.

Oleaga JA et al: Renal venography: new applications in pathologic conditions, Urology 12:609-613, 1978.

Rees R et al: Angiography in extremity trauma: a prospective study, Am J Surg 44:661-663, 1978.

1979 Boyle RN: Arteriography in the small hospital, Surg Clin North Am 59:495-500, 1979.

Cohen DB: Transcatheter therapy in angiography: indications, techniques, and illustrations, Radiol Technol 51:29-35, 1979.

Lang EK: Current and future applications of angiography in the abdomen, Radiol Clin North Am 17:55-76, 1979.

1980 Boijsen E and Gothlin J: Abdominal angiography after intra-arterial injection of vasopressin, Acta Radiol 21:523-533, 1980.

Fitzer PM: Contrast venography: a "golden oldie," Va Med (Mon) 107:210-214, 1980.

Herman RJ et al: Descending venography: a method of evaluating lower extremity venous valvular function, Radiology 137:63-69, 1980.

1981 Chuang VP: Basic rule of catheter selection for visceral angiography, AJR 136:423-433, 1981.

Elliott LP: Significance of caudal left anterior oblique view in analyzing the left main coronary artery and its major branches, Radiology 139:39-43, 1981.

Hessel SJ et al: Complications of angiography, Radiology 138:273-281, 1981.

LeVeen RF et al: Pressure-infusion venography of the leg with remote control fluoroscopy, Radiology 138:730-731, 1981.

Mosely GT: Technical considerations of epidural venography, Radiol Technol 52:371-374, 1981.

Nathan MH: Pressure infusion venography, Radiology 138:731-732, 1981.

Suzuki S and Mine H: Roll-film changer for whole-limb angiography: a trial production and its clinical application, Cardiovasc Intervent Radiol 4:66-70, 1981.

Turnipseed WD et al: Computerized intravenous arteriography: a technique for visualizing the peripheral vascular system, Surgery 89:118-123, 1981.

1982 Abaskaron M: Catheter modification to improve the performance of aorto-ileofemoral examinations, Radiology 144:420, 1982.

Gordon DH et al: Descending varicose venography of the lower extremities: an alternative method to evaluate the deep venous system, Radiology 145:832-834, 1982.

Kaseff LG: Positional variations of the common carotid artery bifurcation, Radiology 145:377-378, 1982.

Lantz BM et al: Vasodilator response in the lower extremity induced by contrast medium, Acta Radiol [Diagn] 23:185-191, 1982.

Laskey WK et al: A safe and rapid technique for retrograde catheterization of the left ventricle in aortic stenosis, Cathet Cardiovasc Diagn 8:429-435, 1982.

Slack JD, Slack LA and Orr C: Recurrent severe reaction to iodinated contrast media during cardiac catheterization, Heart Lung 11:348-352, 1982.

1983 Egsgaard H, Hrup A and Praestholm J: A controlled clinical trial of iohexol and diatrizoate in aortofemoral angiography, Eur J Radiol 3:14-17, 1983.

Elliott LP, Bargeron LM Jr and Green CE: Angled angiography: general approach and findings, Cardiol Clin 1:361-385, 1983.

Foley WD et al: Digital subtraction angiography of the portal venous system, AJR 140:497-499, 1983.

Hagen B: Iohexol and iopromide—two new non-ionic water-soluble radiographic contrast media: randomized, intraindividual double-blind study versus ioxaglate in peripheral angiography, Fortschr Geb Rontgenstr Nuklearmed Erganzungsband 118:107-114, 1983.

Harrington DP et al: Compound angulation for the angiographic evaluation of renal artery, Radiology 146:829-831, 1983.

Higgins CB and Buonocore E: Digital subtraction angiography: techniques and applications for evaluating cardiac anatomy and function, Cardiol Clin 1:413-425, 1983.

Kolbenstvedt A: Iohexol in lower extremity, renal, and visceral angiography: survey and present state, Acta Radiol 366:153-157, 1983.

Mardini MK and Rao PS: Left ventricular and aortic catheterization and angiography via a patent ductus arteriosus: a new technique, Cathet Cardiovasc Diagn 9:89-95, 1983.

Saibil EA, Maggisano R and Witchell SJ: Angiography in the diagnosis and treatment of trauma, J Can Assoc Radiol 34:218-227, 1983.

Seigel RS and Williams AG: Efficacy of prone positioning for intravenous digital angiography of the abdomen, Radiology 148:295, 1983.

Seldin DW et al: Left ventricular volume determined from scintigraphy and digital angiography by a semiautomated geometric method, Radiology 149:809-813, 1983.

Skjennald A, Heldaas J and Hiseth A: Comparison of iohexol and meglumine-Na-Cametrizoate in visceral angiography, Acta Radiol 366:158-163, 1983.

Widrich WC et al: Iopamidol and meglumine diatrizoate: comparison of effects on patient discomfort during aortofemoral arteriography, Radiology 148:61-64, 1983.

1984 Brandt PW: Axially angled angiocardiography, Cardiovasc Intervent Radiol 7:166-169, 1984.

Cragg AH et al: Rotational kymography: technique for automated analysis of cine left ventriculograms, Radiology 150:260-262, 1984.

Hillman BJ: Digital imaging of the kidney, Radiol Clin North Am 22:341-364, 1984.

Kinnunen J et al: A double curve catheter for the left axillary artery approach to aortofemoral, selective renal, and visceral angiography, Eur J Radiol 4:229-231, 1984.

Nelson JA and Kruger RA: Digital angiography, Radiologe 24:149-154, 1984.

Schatz SL et al: A subtraction technique in conventional angiography, Radiology 151:531, 1984.

Soto B, Coghlan CH and Bargeron LM: Present status of axially angled angiocardiography, Cardiovasc Intervent Radiol 7:156-165, 1984.

Vetrovec GW and Strash AM: Modification of cradle angiographic tables to more easily obtain axial coronary views, Cathet Cardiovasc Diagn 10:607-611, 1984.

1985 Block RW et al: A device for positioning the breast during angiography, Radiology 155:824, 1985.

Detrano R et al: Cardiac digital subtraction angiography: peripheral versus central intravenous dye injections, Cardiovasc Intervent Radiol 8:55-58, 1985.

Fisher M et al: Arteriography of the carotid bifurcation: oblique projections, Neurology 35:1201-1204, 1985.

Guthaner DF, Wexler L and Bradley B: Digital subtraction angiography of coronary grafts: optimization of technique, AJR 145:1185-1190, 1985.

Karoll MP et al: Air gap technique for digital subtraction angiography of the extra-cranial carotid arteries, Invest Radiol 20:742-745, 1985.

McCorkell SJ et al: Indications for angiography in extremity trauma, AJR 145:1245-1247, 1985.

Mendelson EB et al: Evaluation of the prone position in digital subtraction angiography, Cardiovasc Intervent Radiol 8:72-75, 1985.

Passariello R: Angio-CT techniques, Eur J Radiol 5:193-198, 1985.

Saddekni S et al: Contrast administration and techniques of digital subtraction angiography performance, Radiol Clin North Am 23:275-291, 1985.

Smith DC and Simmons CR: The quick aortic turn: a rapid method for reformation of the sidewinder catheter, Radiology 155:247-248, 1985.

Wilson P: Equipment for digital angiography, Radiography 51:193-196, 1985.

1986 Afshani E and Berger PE: Gastrointestinal tract angiography in infants and children, J Pediatr Gastroenterol Nutr 5:173-186, 1986.

Amiel MJ: Contrast media in angiography: state of the art and future prospects, Radiol Med 72:2-8, 1986.

Anonymous: Vascular imaging: angiography and the new modalities, Radiol Clin North Am 24:337-525, 1986.

Bowles JN, Thomas ML and Treweeke PS: A comparative trial of the diagnostic quality of and tolerance for two low concentration low osmolality contrast media for phlebography, Eur J Radiol 6:301-302, 1986.

Chakravarty M: Utilization of angiography in trauma, Radiol Clin North Am 24:383-396, 1986.

Cittadini G et al: Side effects from angiographic contrast media: subjective, objective, instrumental and laboratorial, Radiol Med 72:14-19, 1986.

Cohen MI and Vogelzang RL: A comparison of techniques for improved visualization of the arteries of the distal lower extremity, AJR 147:1021-1024, 1986.

Cope C: Minipuncture angiography, Radiol Clin North Am 24:359-367, 1986.

Cruz C et al: Contrast media for angiography: effect on renal function, Radiology 158:109-112, 1986.

Favilla I, Barry WR and Turner IJ: Video and digital fluorescein angiography, Aust N Z J Ophthalmol 14:229-234, 1986.

Feldman L: Digital vascular imaging of the great vessels and heart, Cardiovasc Clin 17:357-384, 1986.

Gerard P and Lefkovitz Z: The optical push device: an aid to the angiographer, Cardiovasc Intervent Radiol 9:111-112, 1986.

Gersten K et al: Crossed-leg technique for digital subtraction angiography, AJR 146:843-844, 1986.

Glanz S and Gordon DH: Utility of foot venography as part of the routine lower-extremity venogram: a prospective study, Cardiovasc Intervent Radiol 9:15-16, 1986.

Gmelin E, Weiss HD and Buchmann F: Cardiac gating in intravenous DSA, Eur J Radiol 6:24-29, 1986.

Godwin JD and Chen JT: Thoracic venous anatomy, AJR 147:674-684, 1986.

Gomes AS, Lois JF and McCoy RD: Angiographic treatment of gastrointestinal hemorrhage: comparison of vasopressin infusion and embolization, AJR 146:1031-1037, 1986.

Gonzalez CF et al: Extracranial vascular angiography, Radiol Clin North Am 24:419-451, 1986.

Grainger RG: The optimal concentration of contrast medium for aortography and femoral arteriography: a comparison of Hexabrix 320 and Hexabrix 250, Clin Radiol 37:281-284, 1986.

Gray A, Dugdale LM and Roberts A: Erect angiography and the thoracic outlet syndrome, Australas Radiol 30:307-309, 1986.

Grime JS et al: A method of radionuclide angiography and comparison with contrast aortography in the assessment of aorto-iliac disease, Nucl Med Commun 7:45-52, 1986.

Kendall B: Spinal angiography with iohexol, Neuroradiology 28:72-73, 1986.

Kimme-Smith C et al: Diagnostic effects of edge sharpening filtration and magnification, Med Phys 13:850-856, 1986.

Kinnison ML et al: Upper-extremity venography using digital subtraction angiography, Cardiovasc Intervent Radiol 9:106-108, 1986.

Kistner RL et al: A method of performing descending venography, J Vasc Surg 4:464-468, 1986.

Lesak F and Andresen J: The value of angiography in gastrointestinal and urological bleeding, Diagn Imaging 55:126-131, 1986.

Mills CS and Van Aman ME: Modified technique for percutaneous transfemoral pulmonary angiography, Cardiovasc Intervent Radiol 9:52-53, 1986.

Ovitt TW and Newell JD II: Digital subtraction angiography: technology, equipment, and techniques, Med Instrum 20:199-205, 1986.

Petty W et al: Arterial digital angiography in the evaluation of potential renal donors, Invest Radiol 21:122-124, 1986.

Reuter SR: Some legal aspects of angiography and interventative radiology, Leg Med 124-133, 1986.

Rossi P et al: Present and future prospects for angiographic techniques, Radiol Med 72: 51-53, 1986.

Simunic S et al: Vessel imaging, Radiol Med 72:39-43, 1986.

Smith TP et al: Lower-extremity venography: value of femoral-vein compression, AJR 147:1025-1026, 1986.

Sussman SK et al: Digital indirect portography, AJR 147:39-43, 1986.

Takahashi M et al: Biplane digital subtraction angiography, Comput Radiol 10:221-225, 1986.

1987 Akins EW et al: Preoperative evaluation of the thoracic aorta using MRI and angiography, Ann Thor Surg 44:499-507, 1987.

Andrews JC, Williams DM and Cho KJ: Digital subtraction venography of the upper extremity, Clin Radiol 38:423-424, 1987.

Bettmann MA et al: Contrast venography of the leg: diagnostic efficacy, tolerance, and complication rates with ionic and nonionic contrast media, Radiology 165:113-116, 1987.

Boesmi B et al: Digital angiography in children, Rays 12:47-52, 1987.

Brazzini A et al: Safe splenoportography, Radiology 162:607-609, 1987.

Compton SC: Bit conversion of technical factors in vascular procedures, Radiol Technol 58:413-416, 1987.

Dean PB and Sickles EA: Breast lesions examined by digital angiography, Invest Radiol 22:698-699, 1987.

Dixon PM and Fletcher EW: Peripheral angiography in a standard fluoroscopy room, Br J Radiol 60:923-924, 1987.

Dorros G and Lewin RF: Angiography of the internal mammary artery via the contralateral brachial artery, Cathet Cardiovasc Diagn 13:138-140, 1987.

Dumoulin CL, Souza SP and Hart HR: Rapid scan magnetic resonance angiography, Magn Reson Med 5:238-245, 1987.

Harrington DP and Kandarpa K: Quantification in peripheral angiography, Cardiovasc Intervent Radiol 10:400-408, 1987.

Interventional radiology in the thorax, J Thorac Imaging 2:1-80, 1987.

Lieberman RP and Kaplan PA: Superficial peroneal nerve block for leg venography, Radiology 165:578-579, 1987.

Mauro MA and Jaques PF: New technique for left adrenal vein catheterization, Cardiovasc Intervent Radiol 10:86-88, 1987.

Miller DL and Wall RT: Fentanyl and diazepam for analgesia and sedation during radiologic procedures, Radiology 162: 195-198, 1987.

Miller K: Advantages of a low-osmolality ionic contrast medium in intra-arterial applications, Radiol Technol 59:43-48, 1987.

Nilsson P et al: Addition of local anesthetics to contrast media. I. Effects on patient discomfort and hemodynamics in aorto-femoral angiography, Acta Radiol 28:209-214, 1987.

Orofino L et al: Digital angiography and hemodialysis vascular access, Nephron 46:394, 1987.

Pillari G et al: Lower extremity swelling: computerized tomography following negative venography, Cardiovasc Intervent Radiol 10:261-263, 1987.

Pruneau D et al: A practical approach to direct magnification radiography, Radiol Technol 59:121-127, 1987.

Puyau FA et al: Dynamic corpus cavernosography: effect of papaverine injection, Radiology 164:179-182, 1987.

Reiss H: Role of spongiosography in study of penile veins, Urology 29:146-149, 1987.

Robertson HJ: Blood clot formation in angiographic syringes containing nonionic contrast media, Radiology 162:621-622, 1987.

Smith TP et al: Improved vessel dilator for percutaneous catheterization, Radiology 163:271-272, 1987.

Stiris MG and Laerum F: Iohexol and ioxaglate in peripheral angiography, Acta Radiol 28:767-770, 1987.

Tempkin DL and Ladika JE: New catheter design and placement technique for pulmonary arteriography, Radiology 163: 275-276, 1987.

Thomas ML and Hicks P: Limb muscle compression: an alternative technique for intravenous digital subtraction angiography, Br J Radiol 60:123-125, 1987.

Trigaux JP: Angiography in thyroid and parathyroid pathology, Acta Otorhinolaryngol Belg 41:669-676, 1987.

Vlahos L et al: Comparative study between iohexol and iopromide for aortofemoral arteriography, Radiologe 27:581-582, 1987.

Witte G et al: The use of the Fourier transform in cardiac digital angiography, Cardiovasc Intervent Radiol 10:59-64, 1987.

Zagoria RJ, D'Souza VJ and Baker AL: Recommended precautions when using low-osmolality or nonionic contrast agents with vasodilators, Invest Radiol 22:513-514, 1987.

1988 Bettmann MA: Noninvasive and venographic diagnosis of deep vein thrombosis, Cardiovasc Intervent Radiol 11 (Suppl): S 15-S20, 1988.

Bonomo L et al: Identification and minimization of risk factors in angiography, Rays 13:81-86, 1988.

Bookstein JJ: Penile angiography: the last angiographic frontier, AJR 150:47-54, 1988.

Bookstein JJ and Lurie AL: Selective penile venography: anatomical and hemodynamic observations, J Urol 140:55-60, 1988.

Bowman LK: Peak filling rate normalized to mitral stroke volume: a new Doppler angiographic technique, J Am Coll Cardiol 12:937-943, 1988.

Britton CA and Wholey MH: Radiation exposure of personnel during digital subtraction angiography, Cardiovasc Intervent Radiol 11:108-110, 1988.

Cardella JF et al: Lower-extremity venous thrombosis: comparison of venography, impedance plethysmography, and intravenous manometry, Radiology 168:109-112, 1988.

Colapinto RF and Harty PW: Femoral artery compression device for outpatient angiography, Radiology 166:890-891, 1988.

Delcour C et al: Technical advances in penile arteriography, AJR 150:803-804, 1988.

Diament MJ, Bird CR and Stanley P: Outpatient performance of invasive radiologic procedures in pediatric patients, Radiology 166:401-403, 1988.

Dondelinger RF and Kurdziel JC: Computed tomographic arteriography (CTA) of the liver, Bull Soc Sci Med Grand Duche Luxemb 125:27-34, 1988.

Dumay AC et al: Three-dimensional reconstruction of myocardial contrast perfusion techniques, Int J Card Imaging 3:141-152, 1988.

Dumoulin CL et al: Time-resolved magnetic resonance angiography, Magn Reson Med 6:275-286, 1988.

Essinger A et al: Conventional renal angiography versus renal digital subtraction angiography (DSA) in the study of renovascular hypertension, Ann Radiol 31:104-106, 1988.

Forbes G et al: Complications of spinal cord arteriography: prospective assessment of risk for diagnostic procedures, Radiology 169:479-484, 1988.

Foster CJ, Butler P and Freer CE: Digital subtraction angiography of the left ventricle, Br J Radiol 61:1009-1013, 1988.

Frahm J: Rapid line scan NMR angiography, Magn Reson Med 7:79-87, 1988.

Gmelin E and Rinast E: Translumbar catheter angiography with a needle-sheath system, Radiology 166:888-889, 1988.

Grollman JH Jr and Marcus R: Transbrachial arteriography: techniques and complications, Cardiovasc Intervent Radiol 11:32-35, 1988.

Johnson RL et al: Silicone rubber catheter venography using standard angiographic techniques, Cardiovasc Intervent Radiol 11:45-49, 1988.

Kido DK et al: The role of catheters and guidewires in the production of angiographic thromboembolic complications, Invest Radiol 23:359-365, 1988.

Kozak BE and Rosch J: Curved guide wire for percutaneous pulmonary angiography, Radiology 167:864-865, 1988.

Kumpe DA, Zwerdlinger S and Griffin DJ: Blue digit syndrome: treatment with percutaneous transluminal angioplasty, Radiology 166:37-44, 1988.

Lea-Thomas M, Tanqueray AB and Burnand KG: Visualization of the plantar arch by aortography: technique and value, Br J Radiol 61:469-472, 1988.

Lechner G et al: The relationship between the common femoral artery, the inguinal crease, and the inguinal ligament: a guide to accurate angiographic puncture, Cardiovasc Intervent Radiol 11:165-169, 1988.

McClennan GL and Scalapino MC: Pulmonary artery catheterization: a modified technique, Radiology 169:264-265, 1988.

Murphy G, Campbell DR and Fraser DB: Pain in peripheral arteriography: an assessment of conventional versus ionic and non-ionic low-osmolality contrast agents, Can Assoc Radiol J 39:103-106, 1988.

Naidich JB et al: Contrast venography: reassessment of its role, Radiology 168:97-100, 1988.

Nakhjavan FK: Use of angioplasty guidewire for technically difficult angiography, Cathet Cardiovasc Diagn 14:213, 1988.

Olsen WL, Jeffrey RB Jr and Tolentino CS: Closed system for arterial puncture in patients at risk for AIDS, Radiology 166:551-552, 1988.

Piao ZE et al: Hemodynamic effects of contrast media during coronary angiography: a comparison of three nonionic agents to Hypaque-76, Cathet Cardiovasc Diagn 14:53-58, 1988.

Raby N et al: Assessment of portal vein patency: comparison of arterial portography and ultrasound scanning, Clin Radiol 39:381-385, 1988.

Robertson HJ: Nonionic contrast media in radiology: procedural considerations, Invest Radiol 23:S374-S377, 1988.

Rosen MP, Walker TG and Greenfield AJ: Arteriography and radiology of impotence, Urol Radiol 10:136-143, 1988.

Schnell N et al: Requirements on resolution of digital imaging equipment in the cardiac catheterization laboratory, Int J Card Imaging 3:111-116, 1988.

Spies JB, Rosen RJ and Lebowitz AS: Antibiotic prophylaxis in vascular and interventional radiology: a rational approach, Radiology 166:381-387, 1988.

Takayasu K et al: Plastic-coated guide wire for hepatic arteriography, Radiography 166:545-546, 1988.

Takeda T: Intraarterial digital subtraction angiography with carbon dioxide, Cardiovasc Intervent Radiol 11:101-107, 1988.

Thijssen HO et al: Comparison of brachiocephalic angiography and IVDSA in the same group of patients, Neuroradiology 30:91-97, 1988.

Tsai FY et al: Aberrant placement of a Kimray-Greenfield filter in the right atrium: percutaneous retrieval, Radiology 167:423-424, 1988.

Vogel RA: Left ventricular imaging by digital subtraction angiography, Int J Card Imaging 3:29-38, 1988.

Wondrow MA et al: Technical consideration for a new x-ray video progressive scanning, Cathet Cardiovasc Diagn 14:126-134, 1988.

1989   Anand R: Fluorescein angiography. I. Technique and normal study, J Ophthalmic Nurs Technol 8:48-52, 1989.

Bettmann MA: Clinical experience with ioversol for angiography, Invest Radiol 24:61-66, 1989.

Cossman DV et al: Comparison of contrast arteriography to arterial mapping with color-flow duplex imaging in the lower extremities, J Vasc Surg 10:522-528, 1989.

Dawson P and Dunn G: Intraarterial digital subtraction venography (i.a.-DSV) of abdominal vessels, Acta Radiol 30:109-111, 1989.

Dedrick CG: Adrenal arteriography and venography, Urol Clin North Am 16:515-526, 1989.

Dion JE et al: Progressive Suppleness Pursil catheter: a new tool for superselective angiography and embolization, AJNR 10:1068-1070, 1989.

Duptat G Jr, Merette G and Roy P: Phentolamine for enhanced visualization of distal arteries in lower extremity arteriography, Can Assoc Radiol J 40:32-33, 1989.

Fellmeth B, Bookstein JJ and Lurie A: Ultralong, reverse-curve angiographic catheter, Radiology 172:872-873, 1989.

Fink U et al: Subtracted versus nonsubtracted digital imaging in peripheral angiography, Eur J Radiol 9:236-240, 1989.

Gavant ML: Digital subtraction angiography of the foot in atherosclerotic occlusive disease, South Med J 82:328-334, 1989.

Gomes AS et al: Acute renal dysfunction in high-risk patients after angiography: comparison of ionic and nonionic contrast media, Radiology 170:65-68, 1989.

Goyal AK et al: Can sonography replace splenoportovenography in evaluation of patients with portal hypertension? Indian J Gastroenterol 8:157-159, 1989.

Grassi CJ et al: Ioversol: double-blind study of a new low osmolar contrast agent for peripheral and visceral arteriography, Invest Radiol 24:133-137, 1989.

Hansen EC et al: New high-flow "cloud" catheter for safer delivery of contrast material, Radiology 173:461-464, 1989.

Hawkins IF Jr and Akins EW: Miniaturization of catheter systems for angiography, Radiology 172:1015-1021, 1989.

Huff JA, Kasemeyer B and Lutjen G: Bilateral femoral angiography: a step-by-step approach, Radiol Technol 61:35-39, 1989.

Hwang MH et al: The potential risk of thrombosis during coronary angiography using nonionic contrast media, Cathet Cardiovasc Diagn 16:209-213, 1989.

Ireland MA et al: Safety and convenience of a mechanical injector pump for coronary angiography, Cathet Cardiovasc Diagn 16:199-201, 1989.

Joyce PF et al: Comparison of Hexabrix 320 and Hexabrix 250 in aortoperipheral arteriography: towards cheaper low osmolar contrast media? Cardiovasc Intervent Radiol 12:161-163, 1989.

Langer M et al: Renal and hepatic tolerance of nonionic and ionic contrast media in intravenous digital subtraction angiography, Fortschr Geb Rontgenstr 128:95-100, 1989.

Lee KR et al: Digital venography of the lower extremity, AJR 153:413-417, 1989.

Mewissen MW, Zavitz WR and Lipchik EO: Brachiocephalic vessels in the elderly: technique for catheterization, Radiology 170:887, 1989.

Miller DL: Heparin in angiography: current patterns of use, Radiology 172:1007-1011, 1989.

Okuda K, Takayasu K and Iwamoto S: Angiography in the diagnosis of liver disease, Semin Liver Dis 9:50-62, 1989.

Parker LA Jr, Delany D and Friday JM: Oblique projections in aortography following blunt thoracic trauma, Can Assoc Radiol J 40:172-173, 1989.

Pinto RS, Robbins E and Seidenwurm D: Thrombogenicity of Teflon versus copolymer-coated guidewires: evaluation with scanning electron microscopy, AJNR 10:407-410, 1989.

Pond GD et al: Intraoperative arteriography: comparison of conventional screen-film with photostimulable imaging plate radiographs, Radiology 170:367-370, 1989.

Rosengarten PL, Tuxen DV and Weeks AM: Whole lung pulmonary angiography in the intensive care unit with two portable chest x-rays, Crit Care Med 17:274-278, 1989.

Sharma S et al: The influence of buscopan on adverse reactions to intravascular contrast media, Br J Radiol 62:1056-1058, 1989.

Tamura S et al: New projection for portography, Radiology 173:279-281, 1989.

Taylor CR: Assessment of portal vein patency: pitfalls and problems in diagnostic comparative studies, Hepatology 10:117-118, 1989.

Thomas ML and Tung KT: The value of the lateral projection in preoperative assessment of abdominal aortic aneurysms by IV-DSA, VASA 18:13-17, 1989.

Tomac B and Hebrang A: New catheter technique for transcubital intraarterial DSA of the aortic arch and the supraaortic vessels, Neuroradiology 31:80-84, 1989.

Wilson AJ et al: Ascending lower limb phlebography: comparison of ioversol and iothalamate meglumine, Can Assoc Radiol J 40:142-144, 1989.

Yashiro N et al: Development of multipurpose catheter for visceral arteriography, Radiat Med 7:278-281, 1989.

Zierler RE: Doppler techniques for lower extremity arterial diagnosis, Herz 14:126-133, 1989.

1990   Angiography and interventional radiology, Curr Opin Radiol 2:319-331, 1990.

Bergqvist D and Bergentz SE: Diagnosis of deep vein thrombosis, World J Surg 14:679-687, 1990.

Carella A, Resta M and D'Aprile P: Contrast materials with low iodine concentration and intra-arterial digital subtraction angiography, J Neuroradiol 17:201-211, 1990.

Cascade PN and Kastan DJ: Monitoring and evaluating the quality and appropriateness of angiographic/interventional radiologic procedures, Radiology 174:926-928, 1990.

Dake MD: Peripheral angiography, angioplasty, atherectomy, laser techniques, thrombolysis, and stents, Curr Opin Radiol 2:239-249, 1990.

de Valois JC et al: Contrast venography: from gold standard to 'golden backup' in clinically suspected deep vein thrombosis, Eur J Radiol 11:131-137, 1990.

Del Campo C: Intraoperative angiography: a simplified technique, Can J Surg 33:259-260, 1990.

Druy EM: Renal tract intervention and genitourinary angiography, Curr Opin Radiol 2:266-273, 1990.

Fahlman M, Samuelsson L and Svedman P: An angiographic technique for three-dimensional determination of arterial supply patterns in cadaver soft tissue, Plast Reconstr Surg 86:785-792, 1990.

Falappa PG, Macis G and Cotroneo AR: Diagnostic and interventional angiography of hepatocellular carcinoma, Rays 15:381-398, 1990.

Glickstein MF, McLean GK and Sussman SK: Optimizing heparin utilization in angiographic flush solutions, Angiology 41:825-828, 1990.

Interventional radiography of the liver. I. Cardiovasc Intervent Radiol 13:133-207, 1990.

Klein JS: Pulmonary angiography, Curr Opin Radiol 2:284-290, 1990.

Kohler TR et al: Can duplex scanning replace arteriography for lower extremity arterial disease? Ann Vasc Surg 4:280-287, 1990.

Krieger RA et al: CO2 power-assisted hand-held syringe: better visualization during diagnostic and interventional angiography, Cathet Cardiovasc Diagn 19:123-128, 1990.

Lensing AW et al: Lower extremity venography with iohexol: results and complications, Radiology 177:503-505, 1990.

Lunderquist A: Angiography in lesions of the small bowel, Radiologe 30:286-289, 1990.

Maroney TP: Venography and venous intervention, Curr Opin Radiol 2:279-283, 1990.

McConnell EA: Assessing groin pain after an arteriogram, Nursing 20:86-88, 1990.

Mori H et al: Embolization of a thoracic aortic aneurysm: the straddling coil technique: technical note, Cardiovasc Intervent Radiol 13:50-52, 1990.

Patel YD: Technical development: a modified pigtail catheter for transbrachial aortography, Clin Radiol 41:128-129, 1990.

Prevost DB: Diagnostic arteriography and percutaneous transluminal angioplasty of the lower extremities, J Vasc Nurs 8:6-12, 1990.

Routh WD and Keller FS: Abdominal angiography and embolization, Curr Opin Radiol 2:291-299, 1990.

Sanders C: Current role of conventional and digital aortography in the diagnosis of aortic disease, J Thorac Imaging 5:48-59, 1990.

Smith TP et al: Techniques for lower-limb angiography: a comparative study, Radiology 174:951-955, 1990.

Stevenson AJ, Moss JG and Kirkpatrick AE: Comparison of temperature profiles (DeVeTherm) and conventional venography in suspected lower limb thrombosis, Clin Radiol 42:37-39, 1990.

Thomas ML: Techniques of phlebography: a review, Eur J Radiol 11:125-130, 1990.

Trerotola SO, Kuhlman JE and fishman EK: Bleeding complications of femoral catheterization: CT evaluation, Radiology 174:37-40, 1990.

Wilms G et al: Outpatient angiography, J Belge Radiol 73:125-128, 1990.

1991 Aston NO, Thomas ML and Burnand KG: A modified technique of pre-operative aortography to demonstrate the complete arterial tree of the lower limb, J Cardiovasc Surg 32:360-365, 1991.

Bales J and Greening N: A practical approach to dose reduction for imaging staff, Radiogr Today 57:15-17, 1991.

Bhargava R and Millward SF: Contrast venography in patients with very edematous feet: use of transdermal illumination to aid in vein puncture, Radiology 179:583, 1991.

Cragg AH et al: Hematoma formation after diagnostic angiography: effect of catheter size, J Vasc Interv Radiol 2:231-233, 1991.

Cragg AH et al: Radomized double-blind trial of midazolam/placebo and midazolam/fentanyl for sedation and analgesia in lower-extremity angiography, AJR 157:173-176, 1991.

Darcy MD: Lower-extremity arteriography: current approach and techniques, Radiology 178:615-621, 1991.

Dawson P and Strickland NH: Thromboembolic phenomena in clinical angiography: role of materials and technique, J Vasc Interv Radiol 2:125-132, 1991.

Dawson P: Embolic problems in angiography, Semin Hemat 28:31-37, 1991.

Frood LR et al: Use of angiographic needles with or without stylets: pathologic assessment of vessel walls after puncture, J Vasc Interv Radiol 2:269-272, 1991.

Goldberg MA et al: Importance of daily rounds by the radiologist after interventional procedures of the abdomen and chest, Radiology 180:767-770, 1991.

Grabowski EF, Kaplan KL and Halpern EF: Anticoagulant effects of nonionic versus ionic contrast media in angiography syringes, Invest Radiol 26:417-421, 1991.

Jaffe RB: Radiographic manifestations of congenital anomalies of the aortic arch, Radiol Clin North Am 29:319-334, 1991.

Johns CM and Sumkin JH: US-guided venipuncture for venography in the edematous leg, Radiology 180:573, 1991.

Johnston JM et al: Open-floored concave compensating filter for angiography, Radiology 178:578-579, 1991.

Kim D et al: Renal artery imaging: a prospective comparison of intra-arterial digital subtraction angiography with conventional angiography, Angiology 42:345-357, 1991.

Naisby GP et al: Transfemoral digital subtraction aortography: are diluted high osmolar contrast media acceptable? Acta Radiol 32:137-140, 1991.

Pincus D et al: Comparison of nonsubtracted digital angiography and conventional screen-film angiography for the evaluation of patients with peripheral vascular disease, J Vasc Interv Radiol 2:359-364, 1991.

Richardson P et al: Value of CT in determining the need for angiography when findings of mediastinal hemorrhage on chest radiographs are equivocal, AJR 156:273-279, 1991.

Siegel EL, Cook LT and Parsa MB: Conventional screen/film vs reduced exposure photostimulable phosphor plate imaging in lower extremity venography: an ROC analysis, AJR 156:1095-1099, 1991.

Tomac B and Hebrang A: Selective catheterization and digital subtraction angiography of supraaortic arteries via the transcubital approach: a technical note, AJNR 12:843-844, 1991.

Vogelzang RL: Arteriography of the hand and wrist, Hand Clin 7:63-86, 1991.

Watkinson AF and Hartnell GG: Complications of direct brachial artery puncture for arteriography: a comparison of techniques, Clin Radiol 44:189-191, 1991.

Westhoff-Bleck M, Bleck JS and Jost S: The adverse effects of angiographic radiocontrast media, Drug Saf 6:28-36, 1991.

Yedlicka JW Jr et al: Nonselective and semiselective catheters for renal artery evaluation: experimental study, J Vasc Interv Radiol 2:273-276, 1991.

Zemel G et al: Compact contrast material bolus with a new 5-F angiographic catheter, J Vasc Interv Radiol 2:279-280, 1991.

1992 Albrechtsson U et al: Iodixanol—a new nonionic dimer—in aortofemoral angiography, Acta Radiol 33:611-613, 1992.

Alcorn JM et al: Beam-shaping device for long-film angiography, Radiographics 12:323-328, 1992.

Blinov NN et al: New equipment for stereophlebography, Med Prog Technol 18:111-114, 1992.

Bounameaux H et al: Venography of the lower limbs: pitfalls of the diagnostic standard: the ETTT Trial Investigators, Invest Radiol 27:1009-1011, 1992.

Coldwell DM: Visceral angiography and embolization, Curr Opin Radiol 4:97-101, 1992.

Falappa PG et al: Digital imaging: digital angiography, Rays 17:393-415, 1992.

Kandarpa K et al: Prospective double-blinded comparison of MR imaging and aortography in the preoperative evaluation of abdominal aortic aneurysms, J Vasc Interv Radiol 3:83-89, 1992.

Kudo S et al: Digital subtraction angiography for leg venography, Radiat Med 10:1-5, 1992.

Manotti C et al: Variation in hemostatic parameters after intra-arterial and intravenous administration of iodinated contrast media, Invest Radiol 27:1025-1030, 1992.

Maubon A et al: Trans-uterine venography: normal anatomy and pathologic appearances, Surg Radiol Anat 14:259-263, 1992.

Murray KK and Hawkins IF Jr: angiography of the lower extremity in atherosclerotic vascular disease: current techniques, Surg Clin North Am 72:767-789, 1992.

Mussurakis S: Combined superficial peroneal and saphenous nerve block for ascending venography, Eur J Radiol 14:56-59, 1992.

Nakamura H et al: Pancreatic angiography using balloon catheter occlusion and a vasoconstrictor, Radiat Med 10:48-49, 1992.

Pais SO: Diagnostic and therapeutic angiography in the trauma patient, Semin Roentgenol 27:211-232, 1992.

Rieser R, Beinborn W and Ney N: A double-blind comparative study on the contrast quality, tolerance and safety of ioversol 300 versus iohexol 300 in central venous angiography (C.V. DSA), Ann Radiol 35:311-314, 1992.

Segall GM et al: Functional imaging of peripheral vascular disease: a comparison between exercise whole-body thallium perfusion imaging and contrast arteriography, J Nucl Med 33:1797-1800, 1992.

Smith DC et al: Effects of angiographic needle size and subsequent catheter insertion on arterial walls: an in vitro experiment in human cadavers, Invest Radiol 27:763-767, 1992.

Spijkerboer AM: Peripheral angiography and angioplasty, Curr Opin Radiol 4:81-87, 1992.

Sugai Y et al: Digital angiography using hand-operated table movement for vascular disease of the pelvis and lower extremities, Radiat Med 10:82-86, 1992.

Tamura S et al: Right anterior caudocranial oblique projection for portal venography: its indications and advantages, Eur J Radiol 15:215-219, 1992.

Treiman GS et al: Examination of the patient with a knee dislocation: the case for selective arteriography, Arch Surg 127:1056-1062, 1992.

van Tussenbroek FM et al: Transbrachial approach for aortic and selective supraaortic vessel catheterization using a safe and easy technique to reform the Simmons II catheter tip, Eur J Radiol 15:59-64, 1992.

Waugh JR and Sacharias N: Arteriographic complications in the DSA era, Radiology 182:243-246, 1992.

1993   AbuRahma AF et al: Complications of arteriography in a recent series of 707 cases: factors affecting outcome, Ann Vasc Surg 7:122-129, 1993.

Carpenter JP et al: Magnetic resonance venography for the detection of deep venous thrombosis: comparison with contrast venography and duplex Doppler ultrasonography, J Vasc Surg 18:734-741, 1993.

Chan TY et al: Position of skin puncture in translumbar aortography, Acta Radiol 34:631-632, 1993.

Eschelman DJ and Sullivan KL: Exchange of an occluded nephroureteral stent by using a snare, Radiology 186:894-895, 1993.

Gillespie DL et al: Role of arteriography for blunt or penetrating injuries in proximity to major vascular structures: an evolution in management, Ann Vasc Surg 7:145-149, 1993.

Graeter T et al: Three-dimensional vascular imaging—an additional diagnostic tool, Thorac Cardiovasc Surg 41:183-185, 1993.

Holder LE, Merine DS and Yang A: Nuclear medicine, contrast angiography, and magnetic resonance imaging for evaluating vascular problems in the hand, Hand Clin 9:85-113, 1993.

Jurriaans E and Wells IP: Bolus chasing: a new technique in peripheral angiography, Clin Radiol 48:182-185, 1993.

McBride KD, Gaines PA and Beard JD: Pneumatic phlebography: a possible new technique for the assessment of recurrent varicose veins, Eur J Radiol 17:101-105, 1993.

Minakuchi K et al: Intra-arterial digital subtraction portography with a blood-isotonic, non-ionic, dimeric contrast medium, Radiat Med 11:43-48, 1993.

Mistretta CA: Relative characteristics of MR angiography and competing vascular imaging modalities, J Magn Reson Imaging 3:685-698, 1993.

Montefusco von Kleist CM et al: Comparison of duplex ultrasonography and ascending contrast venography in the diagnosis of venous thrombosis, Angiology 44:169-175, 1993.

Nikonoff T et al: Effects of femoral arteriography and low osmolar contrast agents on renal function, Acta Radiol 34:88-91, 1993.

Pallan TM et al: Incompatibility of Isovue 370 and papaverine in peripheral arteriography, Radiology 187:257-259, 1993.

Quigley MJ, Sniderman KW and Yeung EY: Translumbar aortography: experience with a steerable pigtail catheter, Can Assoc Radiol J 44:29-34, 1993.

Raininko R and Soder H: Clot formation in angiographic catheters—an in vitro comparative study: effects of heparin and protein coating of the catheter, Acta Radiol 34:78-82, 1993.

Santilli SM et al: Comparison of preoperative standard angiography with preoperative balloon occlusion femoral angiography of the lower extremity, J Invest Surg 6:83-95, 1993.

Schwartz MR et al: Refining the indications for arteriography in penetrating extremity trauma: a prospective analysis, J Vasc Surg 17:116-122, 1993.

Singh K et al: Iodixanol in abdominal digital subtraction angiography: a randomized, double-blind, parallel trial with iodixanol and iohexol, Acta Radiol 34:242-245, 1993.

Standards of Practice Committee of the Society of Cardiovascular and Interventional Radiology: Standard for diagnostic arteriography in adults, J Vasc Interv Radiol 4:385-395, 1993.

Steele HR and Temperton DH: Technical note: patient doses received during digital subtraction angiography, Br J Radiol 66:452-456, 1993.

Weintraub WS et al: Long-term clinical follow-up in patients with angiographic restudy after successful angioplasty, Circulation 87:831-840, 1993.

INTERVENTIONAL RADIOGRAPHY

For bibliographic citations before 1964, please see volume 3 of the fifth edition of this atlas. For citations from 1964 through 1974, see volume 3 of the sixth or seventh edition.

1980   Abele JE: Balloon catheters and transluminal dilatation: technical considerations, AJR 135:901-906, 1980.

Athanasoulis CA: Percutaneous transluminal angioplasty: general principles, AJR 135:893-900, 1980.

Jander HP and Russinovich NA: Transcatheter gelfoam embolization in abdominal, retroperitoneal, and pelvic hemorrhage, Radiology 136:337-344, 1980.

Weber J and Novak D: Occlusion arteriography: diagnostic and therapeutic applicability of balloon catheters to arterial disease of the lower extremities, AJR 142:23-25, 1980.

1981   Ring EJ and McLean GK: Interventional radiology, Boston, 1981, Little, Brown & Co.

Vlietstra RE et al: Percutaneous transluminal coronary angioplasty: initial Mayo clinic experience, Mayo Clin Proc 56:287-293, 1981.

1982   Miller K and Pruneau D: Transcatheter therapy in the angiographic suite, Radiol Technol 53:469-476, 1982.

Sclafani SJ et al: Interventional radiology in trauma victims: analysis of 51 consecutive patients, J Trauma 22:353-360, 1982.

1983   Comazzi JL et al: Percutaneous transluminal angioplasty of a large septal artery, Cathet Cardiovasc Diagn 9:181-186, 1983.

Health and Public Policy Committee, American College of Physicians: Percutaneous transluminal angioplasty, Ann Intern Med 99:864-869, 1983.

Lock JE et al: Balloon dilatation angioplasty of hypoplastic and stenotic pulmonary arteries, Circulation 67:962-967, 1983.

Rogers PA: Percutaneous needle aspiration biopsy of pulmonary lesions, Radiol Technol 55:527-531, 1983.

Rose JS: Invasive radiology: risks and patient care, Chicago, 1983, Mosby.

1984 Fellows KE, Jr: Therapeutic catheter procedures in congenital heart disease: current status and future prospects, Cardiovasc Intervent Radiol 7:170-177, 1984.

Katzen BT: Percutaneous transluminal angioplasty for arterial disease of the lower extremities, AJR 142:23-25, 1984.

McAuley BJ, Oesterle S and Simpson JB: Advances in guidewire technology, Am J Cardiol 53:94C-96C, 1984.

Nichols DM et al: The safe intercostal approach? Pleural complications in abdominal interventional radiology, AJR 142:1013-1018, 1984.

O'Neill DM: Percutaneous transluminal angioplasty: development, technique, and application, Radiol Technol 55:10-16, 1984.

1986 Boretos JW et al: Jet-directed catheter for interventional radiology, Ann Biomed Eng 14:323-338, 1986.

Ingram C and Burkhalter: Percutaneous nephrostolithotomy, Radiol Technol 58:11-15, 1986.

Quinn SF et al: Interventional radiology in the spleen, Radiology 161:289-291, 1986.

Reuter SR: Some legal aspects of angiography and interventative radiology, Leg Med 124-133, 1986.

Rosch J et al: Interventional angiography in the diagnosis of acute lower gastrointestinal bleeding, Eur J Radiol 6:136-141, 1986.

Singh H and Ruttley MS: Intracoronary thrombolytic treatment: another hazard, Br Heart J 56:182-184, 1986.

1987 Burke DR et al: Percutaneous transluminal angioplasty of subclavian arteries, Radiology 164:699-704, 1987.

Dreesen RG and Becker GJ: Effects of streptokinase in thrombolytic therapy: a radiology research project, Radiol Technol 58:211-214, 1987.

Fisher RG and Ben-Menachem Y: Interventional radiology in appendicular skeletal trauma, Radiol Clin North Am 25:1203-1209, 1987.

Interventional radiology in the thorax, J Thorac Imaging 2:1-80, 1987.

Weiner RI and Maranhao V: A modified hand injector for percutaneous transluminal coronary angioplasty, Cathet Cardiovasc Diagn 13:145-147, 1987.

Wilms G et al: Percutaneous transluminal angioplasty of the subclavian artery: early and late results, Cardiovasc Intervent Radiol 10:123-128, 1987.

1988 Ben-Menachem Y: Pelvic fractures: diagnostic and therapeutic angiography, Instr Course Lect 37:139-141, 1988.

Collins JD, Graves WA and Shaver ML: The importance of the "sloping rib" in interventional radiology procedures of the chest, J Natl Med Assoc 80:1293-1296, 1988.

Gibson RN: Interventional radiology in the biliary tract, Br J Hosp Med 40:374-378, 1988.

Kumpe DA, Zwerdlinger S and Griffin DJ: Blue digit syndrome: treatment with percutaneous transluminal angioplasty, Radiology 166:37-44, 1988.

Murphy FB and Bernardino ME: Interventional computed tomography, Curr Probl Diagn Radiol 17:121-154, 1988.

Spies JB, Rosen RJ and Lebowitz AS: Antibiotic prophylaxis in vascular and interventional radiology: a rational approach, Radiology 166:381-387, 1988.

Tsai FY et al: Aberrant placement of a Kimray-Greenfield filter in the right atrium: percutaneous retrieval, Radiology 167:423-424, 1988.

1989 Adam A: Percutaneous techniques in the liver and biliary system: recent advances, Br J Hosp Med 42:102-110, 1989.

Angelini P: Use of mechanical injectors during percutaneous transluminal coronary angioplasty (PTCA), Cathet Cardiovasc Diagn 16:193-194, 1989.

Betramello A et al: Interventional angiography in neuropediatrics, Childs Nerv Syst 5:87-93, 1989.

Dunnick NR et al: Interventional uroradiology, Invest Radiol 24:831-841, 1989.

Hall-Craggs MA: Interventional abdominal ultrasound: recent advances, Br J Hosp Med 42:176-182, 1989.

Hruby W: Interventional uroradiology, Curr Opin Radiol 1:290-292, 1989.

Kozarek RA et al: Endoscopic placement of pancreatic stents and drains in the management of pancreatitis, Ann Surg 209:261-266, 1989.

Rickards D and Jones SN: Percutaneous interventional uroradiology, Br J Radiol 62:573-581, 1989.

Teplick SK: Diagnostic and therapeutic interventional gall bladder procedures, AJR 152:913-916, 1989.

vanSonnenberg E et al: Interventional radiology in the gallbladder, Radiographics 9:39-49, 1989.

1990 Angiography and interventional radiology, Curr Opin Radiol 2:319-331, 1990.

Burhenne HJ: The history of interventional radiology of the biliary tract, Radiol Clin North Am 28:1139-1144, 1990.

Cascade PN and Kastan DJ: Monitoring and evaluating the quality and appropriateness of angiographic/interventional radiologic procedures, Radiology 174:926-928, 1990.

Cwikiel W, Ivancev K and Lunderquist A: Interventional radiology of the biliary tract: metallic stents, Radiol Clin North Am 28:1203-1210, 1990.

Dake MD: Peripheral angiography, angioplasty, atherectomy, laser techniques, thrombolysis, and stents, Curr Opin Radiol 2:239-249, 1990.

Dalman RL, Taylor LM Jr and Proter JM: Will interventional angiology replace vascular surgery? Acta Chir Scand Suppl 555:25-35, 1990.

Druy EM: Renal tract intervention and genitourinary angiography, Curr Opin Radiol 2:266-273, 1990.

Eskridge JM: Advances in interventional radiology, Curr Opin Radiol 2:62-67, 1990.

Fache JS: Interventional radiology of the biliary tract: transcholecystic intervention, Radiol Clin North Am 28:1157-1169, 1990.

Falappa PG, Macis G and Cotroneo AR: Diagnostic and interventional angiography of hepatocellular carcinoma, Rays 15:381-398, 1990.

Frink NC, Paolella LP and Dorfman GS: Angioplasty sites: assessment with the dual-access technique, Radiology 174:264, 1990.

Hopper KD and Yakes WF: The posterior intercostal approach for percutaneous renal procedures: risk of puncturing the lung, spleen, and liver as determined by CT, AJR 154:115-117, 1990.

Interventional radiology of the liver. I. Cardiovasc Intervent Radiol 13:133-207, 1990.

Krieger RA et al: CO2 power-assisted hand-held syringe: better visualization during diagnostic and interventional angiography, Cathet Cardiovasc Diagn 19:123-128, 1990.

Matalon TA and Silver B: US guidance of interventional procedures, Radiology 174:43-47, 1990.

Mori H et al: Embolization of a thoracic aortic aneurysm: the straddling coil technique: technical note, Cardiovasc Intervent Radiol 13:50-52, 1990.

Prevost DB: Diagnostic arteriography and percutaneous transluminal angioplasty of the lower extremities, J Vasc Nurs 8:6-12, 1990.

Rafert JA et al: Balloon expandable intraluminal vascular stent, Radiol Technol 62:114-119, 1990.

Richter GM et al: The transjugular intrahepatic portosystemic stent-shunt (TIPSS): results of a pilot study, Cardiovasc Intervent Radiol 13:200-207, 1990.

Selby JB, Tegtmeyer CJ and Bittner GM: Experience with new retrieval forceps for foreign body removal in the vascular, urinary, and biliary systems, Radiology 176:535-538, 1990.

Selby JB Jr and Tegtmeyer CJ: New balloon-through-balloon angioplasty technique for the treatment of segmental lesions, Radiology 177:276-277, 1990.

van Sonnenberg E, D'Agostino H and Casola G: Interventional gallbladder procedures, Radiol Clin North Am 28:1185-1190, 1990.

Wholey MH: Controversies in peripheral vascular intervention, Radiology 174:929-931, 1990.

Yee AC and Ho CS: Percutaneous transhepatic biliary drainage: a review, CRC Crit Rev Diagn Imaging 30:247-279, 1990.

1991   Angiography and interventional radiology, Curr Opin Radiol 3:289-306, 1991.

Burke DR: Biliary and other gastrointestinal interventions, Curr Opin Radiol 3:151-159, 1991.

Dawson P and Strickland NH: Thromboembolic phenomena in clinical angiography: role of materials and technique, J Vasc Interv Radiol 2:125-132, 1991.

Fleck E, Maier-Rudolf W and Oswald H: Coronary angiography and interventional cardiology, Curr Opin Radiol 3:550-560, 1991.

Goldberg MA et al: Importance of daily rounds by the radiologist after interventional procedures of the abdomen and chest, Radiology 180:767-770, 1991.

Kagetsu NJ, Berenstein A and Choi IS: Interventional radiology of the extracranial head and neck, Cardiovasc Intervent Radiol 14:325-333, 1991.

Kelly IM and Dick R: Technical report: interventional sialography: dormia basket removal of Wharton's duct calculus, Clin Radiol 43:205-206, 1991.

LaBerge JM, Ring EJ and Gordon RL: Percutaneous intrahepatic portosystemic shunt created via a femoral vein approach, Radiology 181:679-681, 1991.

Long BW, Rafert JA and Cory D: Percutaneous feeding tube method for use in children, Radiol Technol 62:274-278, 1991.

McLellan GL: A new percutaneous access set for interventional procedures, AJR 156:397-399, 1991.

Patel A and Cholankeril J: Case of the migrating embolic filter, Hosp Pract [Off] 26:129-132, 1991.

Reed JG, Rubin SA and Schnadig VJ: Interventional procedures used for diagnosing and treating lung cancer, J Thorac Imaging 7:48-56, 1991.

Takahashi M et al: Development of a ceiling-suspended angiographic unit for interventional neuroradiology, Neuroradiology 33:507-509, 1991.

Towbin RB: Pediatric interventional radiology, Curr Opin Radiol 3:931-935, 1991.

Wimmer B and Wenz W: CT-guided interventions: present and future aspects, Acta Radiol Suppl 377:46-49, 1991.

Zemel G et al: Percutaneous transjugular portosystemic shunt, JAMA 266:390-393, 1991.

1992   Abramson AF and Mitty HA: Update on interventional treatment of urinary obstruction, Urol Radiol 14:234-236, 1992.

Akiyama H, Itoh M and Tazuma S: Gallbladder and biliary interventional radiology, Curr Opin Radiol 4:116-124, 1992.

Anson JA and Spetzler RF: Interventional neuroradiology for spinal pathology, Clin Neurosurg 39:388-417, 1992.

Bennett JD et al: Deep pelvic abscesses: transrectal drainage with radiologic guidance, Radiology 185:825-828, 1992.

Bounameaux H et al: Venography of the lower limbs: pitfalls of the diagnostic standard: the ETTT Trial Investigators, Invest Radiol 27:1009-1011, 1992.

Chalmers N et al: Transjugular intrahepatic portosystemic stent shunt (TIPSS): early clinical experience, Clin Radiol 46:166-169, 1992.

Chopra PS, Kandarpa K and Harrington DP: Quality assurance in cardiovascular and interventional radiology, CRC Crit Rev Diagn Imaging 33:183-200, 1992.

Fajardo LL, Jackson VP and Hunter TB: Interventional procedures in diseases of the breast: needle biopsy, pneumocystography, and galactography, AJR 158:1231-1238, 1992.

Gunther RW: Percutaneous interventions in the thorax: seventh annual Charles Dotter Memorial Lecture, J Vasc Interv Radiol 3:379-390, 1992.

Harman JT et al: Localization of the portal vein for transjugular catheterization: percutaneous placement of a metallic marker with real-time US guidance, J Vasc Interv Radiol 3:545-547, 1992.

Haskal ZJ et al: Role of parallel transjugular intrahepatic portosystemic shunts in patients with persistent portal hypertension, Radiology 185:813-817, 1992.

Interventional radiology, Curr Opin Radiol 4:151-163, 1992.

Klein JS: Thoracic intervention, Curr Opin Radiol 4:94-103, 1992.

Klein JS, Schultz S: Interventional chest radiology, Curr Probl Diagn Radiol 21:219-277, 1992.

LaBerge JM et al: Nonoperative treatment of enteric fistulas: results in 53 patients, J Vasc Interv Radiol 3:353-357, 1992.

Lees WR: Interventional radiology of the gallbladder, Baillieres Clin Gastroenterol 6:383-401, 1992.

Mahler F, Do DD and Triller J: Interventional angiology, Eur J Med 1:295-301, 1992.

Marx MV and Williams D: Percutaneous transjugular portosystemic shunt: commentary on the technical aspects of this new procedure, Hepatology 15:557-558, 1992.

McKay RH et al: Contrast injection around mandril wire of an Accustick system using an extension tubing: technical note, Cardiovasc Intervent Radiol 15:254-255, 1992.

Montgomery TA: TIPSS: use of metallic stents offers non-surgical alternative, Radiol Technol 64:38-45, 1992.

Nakamura H et al: Pancreatic angiography using balloon catheter occlusion and a vasoconstrictor, Radiat Med 10:48-49, 1992.

Noeldge G et al: Morphologic and clinical results of the transjugular intrahepatic portosystemic stent-shunt (TIPSS), Cardiovasc Intervent Radiol 15:342-348, 1992.

Pais SO: Diagnostic and therapeutic angiography in the trauma patient, Semin Roentgenol 27:211-232, 1992.

Richter GM et al: Transjugular intrahepatic portosystemic stent shunt, Baillieres Clin Gastroenterol 6:403-419, 1992.

Rossle M and Haag K: Interventional treatment of portal hypertension, Dig Dis 10 (Suppl) 1:94-102, 1992.

Sanders C: Transthoracic needle aspiration, Clin Chest Med 13:11-16, 1992.

Selby JB Jr: Interventional radiology of trauma, Radiol Clin North Am 30:427-439, 1992.

Spijkerboer AM: Peripheral angiography and angioplasty, Curr Opin Radiol 4:81-87, 1992.

Stanley P: Advances in pediatric interventional radiology, Curr Opin Radiol 4:73-78, 1992.

Thomas S: A new development in radiology: TIPS, Nurs Stand 7:25-28, 1992.

Thomsen HS and Dorph S: Interventional uroradiology today, Ann Med 24:167-169, 1992.

Tomaru T et al: Laser recanalization of thrombosed arteries using thermal and/or modified optical probes: angiographic and angioscopic study, Angiology 43:412-420, 1992.

vanSonnenberg E et al: Interventional radiology in the chest, Chest 102:608-612, 1992.

Vehmas T and Tikkanen H: Measuring radiation exposure during percutaneous drainages: can shoulder dosemeters be used to estimate finger doses? Br J Radiol 65:1007-1010, 1992.

Waller BF et al: Anatomy, histology, and pathology of coronary arteries: a review relevant to new interventional and imaging techniques. II. Clin Cardiol 15:535-540, 1992.

Waller BF et al: Anatomy, histology, and pathology of coronary arteries: a review relevant to new interventional and imaging techniques. III. Clin Cardiol 15:607-615, 1992.

Wenz F et al: US-guided paraumbilical vein puncture: an adjunct to transjugular intrahepatic portosystemic shunt (TIPS) placement, J Vasc Interv Radiol 3:549-551, 1992.

Zemel G et al: Technical advances in transjugular intrahepatic portosystemic shunts, Radiographics 12:615-622, 1992.

1993   Adams L and Soulen MC: TIPS: a new alternative for the variceal bleeder, Am J Crit Care 2:196-201, 1993.

Barnwell SL: Interventional neuroradiology, West J Med 158:162-170, 1993.

Becker GJ: Suggested standard terms for interventional procedures [editorial], J Vasc Interv Radiol 4:616, 1993.

Brown KT et al: Infrapopliteal angioplasty: long-term follow-up, J Vasc Interv Radiol 4:139-144, 1993.

Buckenham TM et al: Infrapopliteal angioplasty for limb salvage, Eur J Vasc Surg 7:21-25, 1993.

Cardella JF, Fox PS and Lawler JB: Interventional radiologic placement of peripherally inserted central catheters, J Vasc Interv Radiol 4:653-660, 1993.

Conn HO: Transjugular intrahepatic portal-systemic shunts: the state of the art, Hepatology 17:148-158, 1993.

Donald JJ, Fache JS and Burhenne HJ: Percutaneous transluminal biopsy of the biliary tract, Can Assoc Radiol J 44:185-188, 1993.

Eschelman DJ and Sullivan KL: Exchange of an occluded nephroureteral stent by using a snare, Radiology 186:894-895, 1993.

Gordon RL et al: Recanalization of occluded intrahepatic portosystemic shunts: use of the Colapinto needle, J Vasc Interv Radiol 4:441-443, 1993.

Haskal ZJ, Pentecost MJ and Rubin RA: Hepatic arterial injury after transjugular intrahepatic portosystemic shunt placement: report of two cases, Radiology 188:85-88, 1993.

Hieshima GB: Future directions of neurointerventional radiology, Invest Radiol 28 (Suppl 3):S150, 1993.

Hunink MG et al: Risks and benefits of femoropopliteal percutaneous balloon angioplasty, J Vasc Surg 17:183-192, 1993.

Insall RL, Loose HW and Chamberlain J: Long-term results of double-balloon percutaneous transluminal angioplasty of the aorta and iliac arteries, Eur J Vasc Surg 7:31-36, 1993.

Kaye RD, Grifka RG and Towbin R: Intervention in the thorax in children, Radiol Clin North Am 31:693-712, 1993.

Korogi Y and Takahashi M: A double-guide-wire technique in renal angioplasty: a modified approach, Acta Radiol 34:196-197, 1993.

Koutrouvelis PG et al: A three-dimensional stereotactic device for computed tomography-guided invasive diagnostic and therapeutic procedures, Invest Radiol 28:845-847, 1993.

Krige JE and Beningfield SJ: Surgery and interventional radiology for benign bile duct strictures, HPB Surgery 7:94-97, 1993.

LaBerge JM et al: Creation of transjugular intrahepatic portosystemic shunts with the wallstent endoprosthesis: results in 100 patients, Radiology 187:413-420, 1993.

LaPlante JS et al: Migration of the Simon nitinol vena cava filter to the chest, AJR 160:385-386, 1993.

Martin M et al: Transjugular intrahepatic portosystemic shunt in the management of variceal bleeding: indications and clinical results, Surgery 114:719-726, 1993.

Mauro MA and Jaques PF: Radiologic placement of long-term central venous catheters: a review, J Vasc Interv Radiol 4:127-137, 1993.

May J et al: Isolated limb perfusion with urokinase for acute ischemia, J Vasc Surg 17:408-413, 1993.

Maynar M et al: Transjugular intrahepatic portosystemic shunt: early experience with a flexible trocar/catheter system, AJR 161:301-306, 1993.

Murphy TP, Dorfman GS and Becker J: Use of preprocedural tests by interventional radiologists, Radiology 186:213-220, 1993.

Pallan TM et al: Incompatibility of Isovue 370 and papaverine in peripheral arteriography, Radiology 187:257-259, 1993.

Patel YD: Vascular interventions in the abdomen: current status, Ann Acad Med Singapore 22:768-775, 1993.

Rosch J et al: Coaxial catheter-needle system for transjugular portal vein entrance, J Vasc Interv Radiol 4:145-147, 1993.

Rozenblit G and Del Guercio LR: Combined transmesenteric and transjugular approach for intrahepatic portosystemic shunt placement, J Vasc Interv Radiol 4:661-666, 1993.

Santilli SM et al: Comparison of preoperative standard angiography with preoperative balloon occlusion femoral angiography of the lower extremity, J Invest Surg 6:83-95, 1993.

Selby JB Jr et al: Balloon angioplasty above the aortic arch: immediate and long-term results, AJR 160:631-635, 1993.

Teitelbaum GP et al: Portal venous branch targeting with a platinum-tipped wire to facilitate transjugular intrahepatic portosystemic shunt (TIPS) procedures, Cardiovasc Intervent Radiol 16:198-200, 1993.

Tytle TL, Loeffler C and Thompson WM: Transjugular intrahepatic portosystemic shunt (TIPS): a promising nonsurgical treatment for bleeding gastroesophageal varices, J Okla State Med Assoc 86:220-224, 1993.

van der Heijden FH et al: Value of Duplex scanning in the selection of patients for percutaneous transluminal angioplasty, Eur J Vasc Surg 7:71-76, 1993.

Weintraub WS et al: Long-term clinical follow-up in patients with angiographic restudy after successful angioplasty, Circulation 87:831-840, 1993.

Yankelevitz DF, Henschke CI and Davis SD: Percutaneous CT biopsy of chest lesions: an in vitro analysis of the effect of partial volume averaging on needle positioning, AJR 161:273-278, 1993.

1994 Rossle M et al: The transjugular intrahepatic portosystemic stent-shunt procedure for variceal bleeding, N Engl J Med 330:165-171, 1994.

Sadler MA and Shapiro RS: Images in clinical medicine: transjugular intrahepatic portosystemic shunt, N Engl J Med 330:182, 1994.

SUBTRACTION TECHNIQUE

For bibliographic citations before 1964, please see volume 3 of the fifth edition of this atlas. For citations from 1964 through 1974, see volume 3 of the sixth or seventh edition.

1977 Mikkelsen WJ et al: Subtraction technique in intravenous aortography, Radiology 123:231-232, 1977.

Mojab K, Garcia L and Talge G: A new subtraction technique using duplicating film as a final print, AJR 129:528-530, 1977.

Ort MG: Subtraction radiography techniques and limitations, Radiology 124:65-72, 1977.

1980 El Gammal T: Cervical myelography and posterior fossa examinations with Amipaque using magnification and subtraction, Radiology 136:219-222, 1980.

1981 Brody WR: Hybrid subtraction for improved arteriography, Radiology 141:828-831, 1981.

1983 Foley WD et al: Digital subtraction angiography of the portal venous system, AJR 140:497-499, 1983.

Grondahl HG and Grondahl K: Subtraction radiography for the diagnosis of periodontal bone lesions, Oral Surg 55:208-213, 1983.

McSweeney MB, Sprawls P and Egan RL: Enhanced image mammography, AJR 140:9-14, 1983.

Thron A and Voigt K: Rotational cerebral angiography: procedure and value, AJNR 4:289-291, 1983.

1984 Fallone BG and Podgorsak EB: Image subtraction by solid state electroradiography, Phys Med Biol 29:703-709, 1984.

Fallone BG and Podgorsak EB: Radiographic image subtraction in gas ionography, Med Phys 11:47-49, 1984.

McSweeney MB, Sprawls P and Egan RL: Enhanced-image mammography, Recent Results Cancer Res 90:79-89, 1984.

Schatz SL et al: A subtraction technique in conventional angiography, Radiology 151:531, 1984.

1985 Lightfoote JB, Friedenberg RM and Smolin MF: Digital subtraction ductography, AJR 144:635-638, 1985.

1986 Blakeman BM, Littooy FN and Baker WH: Intra-arterial digital subtraction angiography as a method to study peripheral vascular disease, J Vasc Surg 4:168-173, 1986.

Butler P: Intravenous digital subtraction angiography, Br J Hosp Med 35:30-36, 1986.

Dardik H et al: Primary and adjunctive intra-arterial digital subtraction arteriography of the lower extremities, J Vasc Surg 3:599-604, 1986.

de Jong TE, Appelman PT and Lampmann LE: Subtraction pitfalls in venous DSA of the renal arteries, ROFO 145:21-25, 1986.

Feldman L: Digital vascular imaging of the great vessels and heart, Cardiovasc Clin 17:357-384, 1986.

Feltrin G: Evaluation of the influence of contrast media viscosity on DSA: suggestions for an ideal angiographic contrast, Radiol Med 72:54-57, 1986.

Foley KT, Cahan LD and Hieshima GB: Intraoperative angiography using a portable digital subtraction unit: technical note, J Neurosurg 64:816-818, 1986.

Gordon TA et al: The use of intravenous digital subtraction angiography in the evaluation of tetralogy of Fallot, Am Heart J 112:89-96, 1986.

Hicks ME et al: Cerebrovascular disease: evaluation with transbrachial intraarterial digital subtraction angiography using a 4-F catheter, Radiology 161:545-546, 1986.

Hoogland PH and Tans JT: The role of digital subtraction angiography in neuroradiology: an evaluation of intravenous and intraarterial digital subtraction angiography, Acta Radiol Suppl (Stockh) 369:4-7, 1986.

Karle A et al: Intravenous digital subtraction angiography with iohexol (Omnipaque) and sodium meglumin diatrizoate (Urografin), Diagn Imaging 55:352-359, 1986.

Kinnison ML et al: Upper-extremity venography using digital subtraction angiography, Cardiovasc Intervent Radiol 9:106-108, 1986.

Mistretta CA and Crummy AB: Basic concepts of digital angiography, Progr Cardiovasc Dis 28:245-255, 1986.

Nelson JA: Newer subtraction and filtration techniques, Med Instrum 20:192-198, 1986.

Ohara K et al: Investigation of basic imaging properties in digital radiography: detection of simulated low-contrast objects in digital subtraction angiographic images, Med Phys 13:304-311, 1986.

Passariello R et al: Digital subtraction angiography in cerebral and peripheral vascular diseases, Monogr Atheroscl 14:101-106, 1986.

Petty W et al: Arterial digital angiography in the evaluation of potential renal donors, Invest Radiol 21:122-124, 1986.

Plunkett MB, Gray JE and Kispert DB: Radiation exposure from conventional and digital subtraction angiography of cerebral vessels, AJNR 7:665-668, 1986.

Rossi P, Pavone P and Castrucci M: Intraarterial digital subtraction angiography (DSA) for total body vascular imaging, Ann Radiol 29:112-114, 1986.

Scholz FJ: Digital subtraction angiography, Med Clin North Am 70:1253-1265, 1986.

Sinonetti G et al: Intra-arterial digital subtraction angiography, Radiol Med 72:67-69, 1986.

Sniderman KW, Morse SS and Strauss EB: Comparison of intra-arterial digital subtraction angiography and conventional filming in peripheral vascular disease, Can Assoc Radiol J 37:76-82, 1986.

Struyven JJ et al: Digital subtraction angiography (DSA) of the heart and coronary arteries, Ann Radiol 29:107-111, 1986.

Takahashi M et al: Automatic reregistration for correction of localized misregistration artifacts in digital subtraction angiography of the head and neck, Acta Radiol Suppl (Stockh) 369:281-284, 1986.

Takahashi M et al: Evaluation of high resolution digital subtraction angiography in neuroradiology, Acta Radiol Suppl (Stockh) 369:278-280, 1986.

Tonkin IL et al: Pediatric digital subtraction angiography: intraarterial and intracardiac applications, Pediatr Radiol 16:126-130, 1986.

1987 Andrews JC, Williams DM and Cho KJ: Digital subtraction venography of the upper extremity, Clin Radiol 38:423-424, 1987.

Butler P: Digital subtraction angiography (DSA): a neurosurgical perspective, Br J Neurosurg 1:323-333, 1987.

Butler P et al: Intravenous digital subtraction angiography in intracranial aneurysms, Br J Radiol 60:323-326, 1987.

Doris I et al: Intravenous digital subtraction angiography by peripheral injection, Can Assoc Radiol J 38:7-10, 1987.

Gritter KJ, Laidlaw WW and Peterson NT: Complications of outpatient transbrachial intraarterial digital subtraction angiography. Work in progress, Radiology 162:125-127, 1987.

Hemingway AP: Digital subtraction angiography in gastrointestinal disease, Ann Radiol 30:156-157, 1987.

Hieshima GB et al: Intraoperative digital subtraction neuroangiography: a diagnostic and therapeutic tool, AJNR 8:759-767, 1987.

Hunt AH: Digital subtraction angiography: patient preparation and care, J Neurosci Nurs 19:222-225, 1987.

Jacobs JM and Manaster BJ: Digital subtraction arthrography of the temporomandibular joint, AJR 148:344-346, 1987.

Levin AR: Digital subtraction angiography, Pediatr Ann 16:563-569, 1987.

Pincus D et al: Use of digital subtraction angiography for evaluation of vascular access for hemodialysis, Cardiovasc Intervent Radiol 10:210-214, 1987.

Southard TE, Harris EF and Walter RG: Image enhancement of the mandibular condyle through digital subtraction, Oral Surg Oral Med Oral Pathol 64:645-647, 1987.

Thomas ML and Hicks P: Limb muscle compression: an alternative technique for intravenous digital subtraction angiography, Br J Radiol 60:123-125, 1987.

Wattie WJ: Digital subtraction angiography, N Z Med J 100:238-239, 1987.

1988 Bakke SJ, Nakstad PH and Aakhus T: Intravenous digital subtraction angiography of the precerebral and cerebral arteries in patients with TIA: a comparison with conventional angiography, Eur J Radiol 8:140-144, 1988.

Beyer D, Gross-Fengels W and Neufang KF: Digital subtraction angiography: the intravenous approach, Int J Card Imaging 3:13-20, 1988.

Britton CA and Wholey MH: Radiation exposure of personnel during digital subtraction angiography, Cardiovasc Intervent Radiol 11:108-110, 1988.

Dawson P: Digital angiography—myth and reality, Australas Radiol 32:18-20, 1988.

Dawson P: Digital subtraction angiography—a critical analysis, Clin Radiol 39:474-477, 1988.

Essinger A et al: Conventional renal angiography versus renal digital subtraction angiography (DSA) in the study of renovascular hypertension, Ann Radiol 31:104-106, 1988.

Gattoni F et al: Digital subtraction angiography of the kidney, Br J Urol 62:214-218, 1988.

Ishigaki T, Sakuma S and Ikeda M: One-shot dual-energy subtraction chest imaging with computed radiography: clinical evaluation of film images, Radiology 168:67-72, 1988.

Motson RW et al: Digital subtraction cholangiography: a new technique for visualising the common bile duct during cholecystectomy, Ann R Coll Surg Engl 70:135-138, 1988.

Perri G et al: Digital subtraction radiography in voiding cystourethrography, Eur J Radiol 8:175-178, 1988.

Pittman CC et al: Digital subtraction wrist arthrography: use of double contrast technique as a supplement to single contrast arthrography, Skeletal Radiol 17:119-122, 1988.

Skau T, Bolin T and Karner G: Digital subtraction angiography versus standard contrast arteriography in evaluation of peripheral vascular disease, Int Angiol 7:42-45, 1988.

Svetkey LP et al: Comparison of intravenous digital subtraction angiography and conventional arteriography in defining renal anatomy, Transplantation 45:56-58, 1988.

Takahashi T et al: Localization of dural fistulas using metrizamide digital subtraction fluoroscopic cisternography, J Neurosurg 68:721-725, 1988.

Takeda T et al: Intraarterial digital subtraction angiography with carbon dioxide: superior detectability of arteriovenous shunting, Cardiovasc Intervent Radiol 11:101-107, 1988.

Thijssen HO et al: Comparison of brachiocephalic angiography and IVDSA in the same group of patients, Neuroradiology 30:91-97, 1988.

Thijssen HO et al: Improvement of IVDSA of the brachiocephalic arteries using a non-ionic contrast medium, Neuroradiology 30:211-213, 1988.

1989 Barber CJ: Central venous catheter placement for intravenous digital subtraction angiography: an assessment of technical problems and success rate, Br J Radiol 62:599-602, 1989.

Barth KH et al: Quantitative digital subtraction arteriography with a calibration catheter, Cardiovasc Intervent Radiol 12:281-285, 1989.

Bredenberg CE et al: Operative angiography by intraarterial digital subtraction angiography: a new technique for quality control of carotid endarterectomy, J Vasc Surg 9:530-534, 1989.

Fink U et al: Subtracted versus non-subtracted digital imaging in peripheral angiography, Eur J Radiol 9:236-240, 1989.

Gavant ML: Digital subtraction angiography of the foot in atherosclerotic occlusive disease, South Med J 82:328-334, 1989.

Howard CA et al: Intra-arterial digital subtraction angiography in the evaluation of peripheral vascular trauma, Ann Surg 210:108-111, 1989.

King JN et al: Arteriography with portable DSA equipment, Radiology 172:1023-1025, 1989.

Langer M et al: Renal and hepatic tolerance of nonionic and ionic contrast media in intravenous digital subtraction angiography, Fortschr Geb Rontgenstr 128:95-100, 1989.

Menanteau BP et al: Imaging of the digital arteries: digital subtraction angiography versus conventional arteriography, Can Assoc Radiol J 40:34-37, 1989.

Miekos E et al: Usefulness of digital subtraction angiography for diagnosis of renal tumours, Int Urol Nephrol 21:353-358, 1989.

Parker PM et al: Intravenous digital subtraction angiography: its use in evaluating vascular injuries in children, J Pediatr Surg 24:423-427, 1989.

Rees CR et al: Nonselective digital subtraction angiography: compact contrast material bolus for improved image quality, Invest Radiol 24:277-281, 1989.

Sharma S et al: The influence of buscopan on adverse reactions to intravascular contrast media, Br J Radiol 62:1056-1058, 1989.

Stevens JM et al: Relative safety of intravenous digital subtraction angiography over other methods of carotid angiography and impact on clinical management of cerebrovascular disease, Br J Radiol 62:813-816, 1989.

Stiel GM et al: Digital flashing tomosynthesis (DFTS)—a technique for three-dimensional coronary angiography, Int J Card Imaging 5:53-61, 1989.

Thomas ML and Tung KT: The value of the lateral projection in preoperative assessment of abdominal aortic aneurysms by IV-DSA, VASA 18:13-17, 1989.

Tomac B and Hebrang A: New catheter technique for transcubital intraarterial DSA of the aortic arch and the supraaortic vessels, Neuroradiology 31:80-84, 1989.

Turner WH and Murie JA: Intravenous digital subtraction angiography for extracranial carotid artery disease, Br J Surg 76:1247-1250, 1989.

Vowden P et al: A comparison of three imaging techniques in the assessment of an abdominal aortic aneurysm, J Cardiovasc Surg 30:891-896, 1989.

1990 Belsole RJ et al: Digital subtraction arthrography of the wrist, J Bone Joint Surg [Am] 72:846-851, 1990.

Carella A, Resta M and D'Aprile P: Contrast materials with low iodine concentration and intra-arterial digital subtraction angiography, J Neuroradiol 17:201-211, 1990.

Grzyska U, Freitag J and Zeumer H: Selective cerebral intraarterial DSA: complication rate and control of risk factors, Neuroradiology 32:296-299, 1990.

Jeans WD: The development and use of digital subtraction angiography, Br J Radiol 63:161-168, 1990.

King SJ and Haigh SF: Technical report: digital subtraction dacryocystography, Clin Radiol 42:351-353, 1990.

Kirsch WM and Zhu YH: Intraoperative digital subtraction angiography for neurosurgery, West J Med 153:547-548, 1990.

Kolar J et al: Digital subtraction angiography in musculoskeletal tumors and other conditions, Arch Orthop Trauma Surg 109:89-93, 1990.

Olcott EW: Magnetic resonance angiography, angiographic contrast media, and digital angiography, Curr Opin Radiol 2:252-258, 1990.

Peters TM et al: Integration of stereoscopic DSA with three-dimensional image reconstruction for stereotactic planning, Stereotact Funct Neurosurg 55:471-476, 1990.

Sanders C: Current role of conventional and digital aortography in the diagnosis of aortic disease, J Thorac Imaging 5:48-59, 1990.

Takahashi K et al: Hepatic neoplasms: detection with hepatoportal subtraction angiography—a new technique of DSA, Radiology 177:243-248, 1990.

Weaver FA, Pentecost MJ and Yellin AE: Carbon dioxide digital subtraction arteriography: a pilot study, Ann Vasc Surg 4:437-441, 1990.

Yong OY et al: Clinical application of DSA and evaluation of its methods: analysis of 160 cases and review of literature, Radiat Med 8:71-78, 1990.

1991 Ameli FM et al: Intravenous digital subtraction arteriography in the evaluation of vascular grafts, Ann Vasc Surg 5:223-228, 1991.

Baxter GM et al: Comparison of colour Doppler ultrasound with venography in the diagnosis of axillary and subclavian vein thrombosis, Br J Radiol 64:777-781, 1991.

Bjork L: Arterial phlebography of the leg, Acta Radiol 32:141-142, 1991.

Fink U et al: Peripheral DSA with automated stepping, Eur J Radiol 13:50-54, 1991.

Harries S et al: An evaluation of intravenous digital subtraction angiography in assessing lower limb ischaemia, Eur J Vasc Surg 5:205-207, 1991.

Kido DK et al: Evaluation of the carotid artery bifurcation: comparison of magnetic resonance angiography and digital subtraction arch aortography, Neuroradiology 33:48-51, 1991.

Kim D et al: Renal artery imaging: a prospective comparison of intra-arterial digital subtraction angiography with conventional angiography, Angiology 42:345-357, 1991.

Meguro K et al: Portable digital subtraction angiography in the operating room and intensive care unit, Neurol Med Chir 31:768-772, 1991.

Naisby GP et al: Transfemoral digital subtraction aortography: are diluted high osmolar contrast media acceptable? Acta Radiol 32:137-140, 1991.

Said R and Hamzeh Y: Digital subtraction venography in the diagnosis of renal vein thrombosis, Am J Nephrol 11:305-308, 1991.

Sharma S and Rajani M: Invasive imaging of abdominal aortic occlusions: intravenous versus intra-arterial route, Int Angiol 10:54-58, 1991.

Sheikh KH et al: Comparison of intravascular ultrasound, external ultrasound and digital angiography for evaluation of peripheral artery dimensions and morphology, Am J Cardiol 67:817-822, 1991.

Tomac B and Hebrang A: Selective catheterization and digital subtraction angiography of supraaortic arteries via the transcubital approach: a technical note, AJNR 12:843-844, 1991.

Walker CW et al: Arthrography of painful hips following arthroplasty: digital versus plain film subtraction, Skeletal Radiol 20:403-407, 1991.

Weaver FA et al: Clinical applications of carbon dioxide/digital subtraction arteriography, J Vasc Surg 13:266-272, 1991.

1992 Dacoronias D et al: Iomeprol vs iopamidol in intraarterial peripheral digital subtraction angiography, Angiology 43:734-740, 1992.

Falappa PG et al: Digital imaging: digital angiography, Rays 17:393-415, 1992.

Ilgit ET et al: Digital subtraction sialography: technique, advantages and results in 107 cases, Eur J Radiol 15:244-247, 1992.

Kudo S et al: Digital subtraction angiography for leg venography, Radiat Med 10:1-5, 1992.

Lanzieri CF et al: Use of the delayed mask for improved demonstration of aneurysms on intraarterial DSA, AJNR 13:1589-1593, 1992.

Perri G et al: Digital subtraction radiography in pediatric cystourethrography, Child Nephrol Urol 12:40-42, 1992.

Rieser R, Beinborn W and Ney N: A double-blind comparative study on the contrast quality, tolerance and safety of ioversol 300 versus iohexol 300 in central venous angiography (C.V. DSA), Ann Radiol 35:311-314, 1992.

Simmons MJ et al: Double blind comparison of Iomeprol 350 and Iopamidol 340 in intravenous digital subtraction angiography for peripheral vascular disease, Clin Radiol 45:338-339, 1992.

Smith TP et al: Comparison of the efficacy of digital subtraction and film-screen angiography of the lower limb: prospective study in 50 patients, AJR 158:431-436, 1992.

Waugh JR and Sacharias N: Arteriographic complications in the DSA era, Radiology 182:243-246, 1992.

1993 Coste E et al: Frameless method of stereotaxic localization with DSA, Radiology 189:829-834, 1993.

Hecht ST and Greenspan A: Digital subtraction lumbar diskography: technical note, J Spinal Disord 6:68-70, 1993.

Ito W et al: Improvement of detection in computed radiography by new single-exposure dual-energy subtraction, J Digit Imaging 6:42-47, 1993.

Kinno Y et al: Gadopentetate dimeglumine as an alternative contrast material for use in angiography, AJR 160:1293-1294, 1993.

Langer R et al: Femoral head perfusion in patients with femoral neck fracture and femoral head necrosis, J Belge Radiol 76:145-149, 1993.

Minakuchi K et al: Intra-arterial digital subtraction portography with a blood-isotonic, non-ionic, dimeric contrast medium, Radiat Med 11:43-48, 1993.

Singh K et al: Iodixanol in abdominal digital subtraction angiography: a randomized, double-blind, parallel trial with iodixanol and iohexol, Acta Radiol 34:242-245, 1993.

Steele HR and Temperton DH: Technical note: patient doses received during digital subtraction angiography, Br J Radiol 66:452-456, 1993.

LYMPHOGRAPHY

For bibliographic citations before 1964, please see volume 3 of the fifth edition of this atlas. For citations from 1964 through 1974, see volume 3 of the sixth or seventh edition.

1975 Göthlin J et al: Retrograde angiography of the human thoracic duct, AJR 124:472-476, 1975.

Grant W: Lymphography: technique, indications, and principles of interpretation, S Afr Med J 49:1341-1346, 1975.

Laurin S: Cavography and lymphangiography in Hodgkin's disease, Acta Radiol 16:98-106, 1975.

1976 Beeckman P et al: Critical evaluation of different x-ray methods in exploration of mediastinal lymphadenopathy, J Belge Radiol 59:459-465, 1976.

1977 Blank N and Castellino RA: Mediastinal lymphadenopathy, Semin Roentgenol 12:215-223, 1977.

Gandhi MG: Testicular lymphography: a clinical study, J Urol 117:174, 1977.

Kinmonth JB: Lymphography 1977: a review of some technical points, Lymphology 10:102-106, 1977.

1978 Farah RN and Cerny JC: Lymphangiography in staging patients with carcinoma of the bladder, J Urol 119:40-41, 1978.

Nuttall J et al: Lymphography in tumours of the urogenital tract, J R Soc Med 71:41-43, 1978.

Rubin BE: Extravasation of Ethiodol into deep tissues of the foot: a complication of lymphangiography, AJR 131:342-343, 1978.

1979 Knochel JQ, Koehler PR and Miller FJ: Need for chest radiographs during and after lymphography, AJR 132:981-982, 1979.

Raghavaiah NV and Jordan WP Jr: Prostatic lymphography, J Urol 121:178-181, 1979.

1980 Carr D and Davidson JK: Magnification lymphography, Clin Radiol 31:535-539, 1980.

Castaneda-Zuniga WR et al: Routine magnification lymphangiography with a swinging slot x-ray machine, Radiology 137:231-234, 1980.

Lee JK et al: Limitations of the postlymphangiogram plain abdominal radiograph as an indicator of recurrent lymphoma: comparison to computed tomography, Radiology 134:155-158, 1980.

McIvor J: Changes in lymph node size induced by lymphography, Clin Radiol 31:541-544, 1980.

Ritsema GH: Ether-thinned ethiodol in lymphangiography: a prospective comparative study, Diagn Imaging 49:316-319, 1980.

Siefert HM et al: Iotasul, a water-soluble contrast agent for direct and indirect lymphography: results of preclinical investigations, Lymphology 13:150-157, 1980.

1981 Bollinger A et al: Fluorescence microlymphography, Circulation 64:1195-1200, 1981.

Hoekstra WJ and Schroeder FH: The role of lymphangiography in the staging of prostatic cancer, Prostate 2:433-440, 1981.

1982 Hirsch JI et al: Use of Isosulfan Blue for identification of lymphatic vessels: experimental and clinical evaluation, AJR 139:1061-1064, 1982.

Magnusson A et al: Computed tomography, ultrasound and lymphography in the diagnosis of malignant lymphoma, Acta Radiol [Diagn] 23:29-35, 1982.

1983 Eichner E, Danese C and Katz G: Vulvar lymphatics as demonstrated by vital dyes and lymphangiography, Int Surg 68:175-177, 1983.

Kinsman P: Lymphangiography—the last decade. I. Anatomy, uses, procedure, Radiography 49:203-209, 1983.

Magnusson A: Size of normal retroperitoneal lymph nodes, Acta Radiol 24:315-318, 1983.

Strijk SP, Debruyne FM and Herman CJ: Lymphography in the management of urologic tumors: radiological-pathological correlation, Radiology 146:39-45, 1983.

Zoretic SN et al: filling of the obturator nodes in pedal lymphangiography: fact or fiction, J Urol 129:533-535, 1983.

1984 Castellino RA et al: Computed tomography, lymphography, and staging laparotomy: correlations in initial staging of Hodgkin disease, AJR 143:37-41, 1984.

Staton R: Lymphography, Radiol Technol 55:233-238, 1984.

1985 Clouse ME et al: Lymphangiography, ultrasonography, and computed tomography in Hodgkin's disease and non-Hodgkin's lymphoma, J Comput Tomogr 9:1-8, 1985.

Dixon AK: The current practice of lymphography: a survey in the age of computed tomography, Clin Radiol 36:287-290, 1985.

Groote AD et al: Radiographic imaging of lymph nodes in lymph node dissection specimens, Lab Invest 52:326-329, 1985.

Kono M et al: Mediastinal lymphography using non-ionic, water-soluble contrast medium, Lymphology 18:132-135, 1985.

Lien HH and Lund G: Computed tomography of mediastinal lymph nodes. Anatomic review based on contrast enhanced nodes following foot lymphography, Acta Radiol [Diagn] 26:641-647, 1985.

Miller DL et al: The upright film in lymphangiographic detection of lymphangiomatosis, AJR 145:847-848, 1985.

Taaning E et al: Comparison of 99Tcm lymphoscintigraphy and lymphangiography in patients with malignant lymphomas, Acta Radiol [Diagn] 26:79-83, 1985.

1986 Barigozzi P et al: Lymphography in pelvic oncology: some recent developments, Rays 11:93-97, 1986.

Wells RG, Ruskin JA and Sty JR: Lymphoscintigraphy: lower extremity lymphangioma, Clin Nucl Med 11:523, 1986.

1987 Lanning P and Lanning M: Lymphography and its prognostic value in childhood leukemia, Rontgenblatter 40:118-120, 1987.

Pera A, Capek M and Shirkhoda A: Lymphangiography and CT in the follow-up of patients with lymphoma, Radiology 164:631-633, 1987.

1988 Bruna J and Dvorakova V: Oil contrast lymphography and respiratory function, Lymphology 21:178-180, 1988.

Cooper SG, Maitem AN and Richman AH: Fluorescein labeling of lymphatic vessels for lymphangiography, Radiology 167:559-560, 1988.

Lanning P et al: The value of lymphography in childhood solid tumours, Rontgenblatter 41:46-49, 1988.

Ngan H, Fok M and Wong J: The role of lymphography in chylothorax following thoracic surgery, Br J Radiol 61:1032-1036, 1988.

1989 Barber CJ: Serious adverse reaction to patent blue violet at lymphography, Clin Radiol 40:631, 1989.

Harzmann R, Hirnle P and Geppert M: Retroperitoneal lymph nodal visualization using 30% Guajazulen blue (chromolymphography), Lymphology 22:147-149, 1989.

Weissleder H and Weissleder R: Interstitial lymphangiography: initial clinical experience with a dimeric nonionic contrast agent, Radiology 170:371-374, 1989.

Weissleder R and Thrall JH: The lymphatic system: diagnostic imaging studies, Radiology 172:315-317, 1989.

1990 Kramer EL: Lymphoscintigraphy: radiopharmaceutical selection and methods, Int J Rad Appl Instrum [B] 17:57-63, 1990.

Teefey SA et al: Differentiating pelvic veins and enlarged lymph nodes: optimal CT techniques, Radiology 175:683-685, 1990.

Weinstein JN: Antibody lymphoscintigraphy, Cancer Treat Res 51:365-385, 1990.

1991 Moskovic E et al: Lymphography—current role in oncology, Br J Radiol 64:422-427, 1991.

1992 Case TC et al: Magnetic resonance imaging in human lymphedema: comparison with lymphangioscintigraphy, Magn Reson Imaging 10:549-558, 1992.

North LB et al: Current use of lymphography for staging lymphomas and genital tumors, AJR 158:725-728, 1992.

1993 Cambria RA et al: Noninvasive evaluation of the lymphatic system with lymphoscintigraphy: a prospective, semiquantitative analysis in 386 extremities, J Vasc Surg 18:773-782, 1993.

Hanna SL et al: MR imaging of infradiaphragmatic lymphadenopathy in children and adolescents with Hodgkin disease: comparison with lymphography and CT, JMR 3:461-470, 1993.

Murray JG and Breatnach E: The American Thoracic Society lymph node map: a CT demonstration, Eur J Radiol 17:61-68, 1993.

North LB et al: Lymphography for staging lymphomas: is it still a useful procedure? AJR 161:867-869, 1993.

Peh WC and Ngan H: Lymphography—still useful in the diagnosis of lymphangiomatosis, Br J Radiol 66:28-31, 1993.

Pendlebury SC: Role of bipedal lymphangiogram in radiation treatment planning for cervix cancer, Int J Radiat Oncol Biol Phys 27:959-962, 1993.

Sombeck MD et al: Correlation of lymphangiography, computed tomography, and laparotomy in the staging of Hodgkin's disease, Int J Radiat Oncol Biol Phys 25:425-429, 1993.

West JH, Seymour JC and Drane WE: Combined transmission-emission imaging in lymphoscintigraphy, Clin Nucl Med 18:762-764, 1993.

SECTIONAL ANATOMY

For bibliographic citations before 1964, please see volume 3 of the fifth edition of this atlas. For citations from 1964 through 1974, see volume 3 of the sixth or seventh edition.

1985 Goldberg RP and Austin RM: Computed tomography of axillary and supraclavicular adenopathy, Clin Radiol 36:593-596, 1985.

Heger L and Wulff K: Computed tomography of the calcaneus: normal anatomy, AJR 145:123-129, 1985.

Zirinsky K et al: The portacaval space: CT with MR correlation, Radiology 156:453-460, 1985.

1986 Christiansen EL et al: Correlative thin section temporomandibular joint anatomy and computed tomography, Radiographics 6:703-723, 1986.

Dillon WP: Magnetic resonance imaging of head and neck tumors, Cardiovasc Intervent Radiol 8:275-282, 1986.

Rholl KS et al: Oblique magnetic resonance imaging of the cardiovascular system, Radiographics 6:177-188, 1986.

Schilling JF and Wechsler RJ: Computed tomographic anatomy of the buttock, Skeletal Radiol 15:613-618, 1986.

Unger JM: Computed tomography of the parapharyngeal space, CRC Crit Rev Diagn Imaging 26:265-290, 1986.

1987 Cooper MH, Archer CR and Kveton JF: Correlation of high-resolution computed tomography and gross anatomic sections of the temporal bone. I. The facial nerve, Am J Otol 8:375-384, 1987.

Daniels DL et al: Computed tomography and magnetic resonance imaging of the orbital apex, Radiol Clin North Am 25:803-817, 1987.

Olszewski J: Sectional anatomy of the human temporal bone, Folia Morphol 46:235-239, 1987.

Sartoris DJ and Resnick D: Pictorial review: cross-sectional imaging of the foot and ankle, Foot Ankle 8:59-80, 1987.

1988 Baker EJ et al: The cross sectional anatomy of ventricular septal defects: a reappraisal, Br Heart J 59:339-351, 1988.

Karssemeijer N, van Erning LJ and Eijkman EG: Recognition of organs in CT-image sequences: a model guided approach, Comput Biomed Res 21:434-448, 1988.

Rubesin SE et al: Contrast examination of the soft palate with cross sectional correlation, Radiographics 8:641-665, 1988.

Sartoris DJ and Resnick D: Cross-sectional imaging of the foot: test of anatomical knowledge, J Foot Surg 27:374-383, 1988.

Zlatkin MB et al: Cross-sectional imaging of the capsular mechanism of the glenohumeral joint, AJR 150:151-158, 1988.

1989 Collins JD et al: Anatomy of the abdomen, back, and pelvis as displayed by magnetic resonance imaging. I. J Natl Med Assoc 81:680-684, 1989.

Collins JD et al: Anatomy of the abdomen, back and pelvis as displayed by magnetic resonance imaging. II. J Natl Med Assoc 81:809-813, 1989.

Collins JD et al: Anatomy of the abdomen, back, and pelvis as displayed by magnetic resonance imaging. III. J Natl Med Assoc 81:857-861, 1989.

Johnson ND et al: MR imaging anatomy of the infant hip, AJR 153:127-133, 1989.

Lipton RJ, McCaffrey TV and Cahill DR: Sectional anatomy of the larynx: implications for the transcutaneous approach to endolaryngeal structures, Ann Otol Rhinol Laryngol 98:141-144, 1989.

Rapp JH et al: "Angiography" by magnetic resonance imaging: detailed vascular anatomy without ionizing radiation or contrast media, Surgery 105:662-667, 1989.

Wechsler RJ and Steiner RM: Cross-sectional imaging of the chest wall, J Thorac Imaging 4:29-40, 1989.

1990 Bhalla M et al: Counting ribs on chest CT, J Comput Assist Tomogr 14:590-594, 1990.

Ebner KA et al: Axial temporomandibular joint morphology: a correlative study of radiographic and gross anatomic findings, Oral Surg Oral Med Oral Pathol 69:247-252, 1990.

Kimura F et al: MR imaging of the normal and abnormal clivus, AJR 155:1285-1291, 1990.

Laine FJ, Nadel L and Braun IF: CT and MR imaging of the central skull base. I. Techniques, embryologic development, and anatomy, Radiographics 10:591-602, 1990.

Logan BM, Liles RP and Bolton I: A photographic technique for teaching topographical anatomy from whole body transverse sections, J Audiov Media Med 13:45-48, 1990.

Philippou M et al: Cross-sectional anatomy of the nose and paranasal sinuses: a correlative study of computer tomographic images and cryosections, Rhinology 28:221-230, 1990.

Prescher A and Adam G: Cross-sectional anatomy of the knee, Surg Radiol Anat 12:19-29, 1990.

Saab MH, Dietrich RB and Lufkin RB: MR imaging of the calvarium: pictorial essay, Surg Radiol Anat 12:215-218, 1990.

Wall EJ et al: Cauda equina anatomy. I. Intrathecal nerve root organization, Spine 15:1244-1247, 1990.

1991 Chevallier JM et al: The thoracic esophagus: sectional anatomy and radiosurgical applications, Surg Radiol Anat 13:313-321, 1991.

Conway WF et al: Cross-sectional imaging of the patellofemoral joint and surrounding structures, Radiographics 11:195-217, 1991.

Freeny PC: Angio-CT: diagnosis and detection of complications of acute pancreatitis, Hepatogastroenterology 38:109-115, 1991.

Goncalves-Ferreira A: Stereotactic anatomy of the posterior cranial fossa: a study of the transcerebellar approach to the brainstem, Acta Neurochir 113:149-165, 1991.

Spring BI and Schiebler ML: Normal anatomy of the thoracic inlet as seen on transaxial MR images, AJR 157:707-710, 1991.

1992   Cooper DE et al: Anatomy, histology, and vascularity of the glenoid labrum: an anatomical study, J Bone Joint Surg Am 74:46-52, 1992.

Hayran M, Onerci M and Ozturk C: Evaluation of the temporal bone by anatomic sections and computed tomography, Surg Radiol Anat 14:169-173, 1992.

Sartoris DJ: Diagnostic imaging insight: cross-sectional imaging of the foot (computed tomography-magnetic resonance), J Foot Surg 31:190-202, 1992.

1993   Murray JG and Breatnach E: The American Thoracic Society lymph node map: a CT demonstration, Eur J Radiol 17:61-68, 1993.

Tiede U et al: A computerized three-dimensional atlas of the human skull and brain, AJNR 14:551-559, 1993.

Bibliography

INDEX

Index

Index

Index

Index

Index

Index

Index

Index

Research applications of ionizing radiation, **1:**22-23
Resistive magnet
    defined, **3:**203
    in magnetic resonance imaging, **3:**185
Resnick method for lungs, **1:**467
Resolution, **3:**247
    in computed tomography, **3:**130, **3:**143, **3:**144
    defined, **3:**207, **3:**320
    focal spot size and, **3:**316
    positron emission tomography and, **3:**277, **3:**290
    spatial, **3:**130, **3:**143
        defined, **3:**152
Resonance, **3:**183
    defined, **3:**203
Resonant frequency, **3:**210, **3:**247
Respirations; *see also* Breathing
    gravid patient and, **2:**204
Respiratory excursion, **1:**404
Respiratory system, **1:**436-439; *see also* Lung
    nuclear medicine and, **3:**267
Response time, defined, **3:**126
Rete testis, **2:**197
Retention catheters, **2:**122
Retention tips, rectal, **2:**122
Retina, **2:**288
Retinoblastoma, **3:**300
Retrieval, defined, **3:**152
Retrograde cystography, **2:**157, **2:**183
    contrast injection method for, **2:**183
    contrast media for, **2:**182
Retrograde urography, **2:**158, **2:**179-182
    contrast media for, **2:**160-161
Retroperitoneum, ultrasound of, **3:**227-231
Reverberation, **3:**247
Reverberation artifact, **3:**212
Reverse Caldwell position for skull tomography, **3:**68
Reverse Waters method for facial bones, **2:**308, **2:**309
Rhese method
    for ethmoidal, frontal, and sphenoidal sinuses, **2:**392, **2:**393
    for optic foramen, **2:**272-275
Rheumatoid arthritis, thermography in, **3:**82
RIA; *see* Radioimmunoassay
Rib, **1:**420-431
    anatomy of, **1:**402
    axillary portion of, **1:**428-429
    false, **1:**403
    floating, **1:**403
    posterior, **1:**426-427
    projection for
        AP, **1:**426-427
        AP oblique, **1:**428-429
        PA, **1:**424-425
        PA oblique, **1:**430-431
        in RAO or LAO positions, **1:**460-461
        in RPO or LPO positions, **1:**428-429
    respiration in radiography of, **1:**422, **1:**423
    true, **1:**403
    upper anterior, **1:**424-425
Rib tubercle articular facet; *see* Costal facet
Richards method for localization of eye foreign body, **2:**293
Right anterior oblique position, **1:**53
Right colic flexure, **2:**61; *see also* Intestine, large
Right lateral decubitus position, **1:**55

Right posterior oblique position, **1:**54
Rigler method for pneumothorax, **1:**476
Rima glottidis, **2:**14; *see also* Neck
Rima vestibuli, **2:**14
Ring biliary drainage catheter, **2:**568
Risk versus benefit
    defined, **2:**492
    in mammography, **2:**458-459
RMI; *see* Radiation Measurements Incorporated
Road mapping in digital subtraction angiography, **3:**177
Robinson, Meares, and Goree method for sphenoidal sinus effusion, **2:**240
Roentgen, **1:**24
    defined, **3:**304
ROI; *see* Region of interest
Rolleston and Reay technique for hydronephrosis, **2:**174
ROM; *see* Read only memory
Roseno and Jepkins introduction of intravenous pyelography, **2:**160
Rotation, **1:**57
Rotational tomography, **2:**368-369
Rotator cuff, sectional anatomy of, **2:**602
Round window; *see* Fenestra cochlea
Rowntree first use of contrast media in urinary tract, **2:**160
Rubin, Gray, and Green method for shoulder, **1:**142, **1:**143
Rugae; *see* Gastric folds
Runström method for otitis media, **2:**406

S

Saccule; *see* Sacculus
Sacculus, **2:**229; *see also* Ear
Sacral cornu; *see* Sacral horns
Sacral horns, **1:**323; *see also* Sacrum and coccyx
Sacral promontory, **1:**275
Sacral vertebral canal
    axial projection for, **1:**390-391
    Nölke method for, **1:**390-391
Sacroiliac joint, **1:**274, **1:**323, **1:**378-383
    Brower and Kransdorf method for, **1:**378-379
    Chamberlain method for, **1:**384-385
    Meese method for, **1:**378-379
    Nölke method for, **1:**390-391
    projection for
        AP axial, **1:**378-379
        AP oblique, **1:**380-381
        axial, **1:**390-391
        PA oblique, **1:**382-383
        in RAO or LAO positions, **1:**382-383
        in RPO or LPO positions, **1:**380-381
    sectional anatomy of, **2:**614
Sacroiliac motion, Chamberlain method for, **1:**384-385
Sacrum, sectional anatomy of, **2:**618
Sacrum and coccyx, **1:**275, **1:**386-389
    anatomy of, **1:**312, **1:**322-323
    female, **1:**322
    male, **1:**322
    projection for
        AP and PA axial, **1:**386-387
        lateral, **1:**388-389
Saddle joint, **1:**47
Sagittal image plane, **3:**213
    of neonatal skull, **3:**238
Sagittal sinuses, sectional anatomy of, **2:**599
Sagittal suture, **2:**216

Salivary glands, **2:**1-10
    anatomy of, **2:**3
    calculi of, **2:**4
    diverticulae of, **2:**4
    fistulae of, **2:**4
    function of, nuclear medicine studies of, **3:**268
    Iglauer method for, **2:**8
    parotid, **2:**5-9
    sectional anatomy of, **2:**596, **2:**599, **2:**600
    sialography and, **2:**4
    strictures of, **2:**4
    sublingual, **2:**10
    submandibular, **2:**8-9
Salter-Harris fracture, **3:**33
Sampling in positron emission tomography, **3:**286
Sandbags in pediatric immobilization, **3:**14
Sansregret modification of Chaussé method for temporal bone, **2:**418-419
Santorini's duct, **2:**35
Scan
    defined, **3:**152, **3:**247
    myocardial perfusion, **3:**258
Scan converter, **3:**211, **3:**247
Scan diameters, **3:**144
    defined, **3:**152
Scanner
    components of, **3:**135-139
    generations of, **3:**131-132
    positron emission, **3:**284-285; *see also* Positron emission tomography
    rectilinear, **3:**255, **3:**273
Scanning
    dynamic, in computed tomography, **3:**145, **3:**152
    whole-body, **3:**284, **3:**288
Scaphoid, **1:**180, **1:**181; *see also* Wrist
    anatomy of, **1:**60
    PA axial projection for, **1:**91-92
    Stecher method for, **1:**91-92
Scapula, **1:**164-173
    anatomy of, **1:**122-123
    Lilienfeld method of, **1:**168-169
    Lorenz and Lilienfeld methods for, **1:**168-169
    Marzujian method for, **1:**166, **1:**167
    McLaughlin method for, **1:**166
    projection for
        AP, **1:**164, **1:**165
        AP axial, **1:**172, **1:**173
        AP oblique, **1:**170, **1:**171
        lateral, **1:**166, **1:**167
        PA oblique, **1:**166-169
Scapular notch, **1:**123; *see also* Scapula
Scapular spine, **1:**174-177
    Laquerrière-Pierquin method for, **1:**174-175
Scapular Y projection, **1:**142, **1:**143
Scapulohumeral articulation, **1:**125; *see also* Shoulder
Scatter, **3:**247
    defined, **3:**304
    of ultrasound wave, **3:**209
Scatter radiation, **1:**24
Schencker infusion nephrotomography and nephrourography, **2:**175
Schilling's test, nuclear medicine and, **3:**269
School-age child
    approach to, **3:**6
    limb radiography in, **3:**31
    upright chest radiography of, **3:**16, **3:**17
Schüller method
    for cranial base, **2:**253-254, **2:**255

Index

Index